HANDBOOK OF SOCIAL WORK WITH GROUPS

Handbook of Social Work with Groups

Edited by

CHARLES D. GARVIN
LORRAINE M. GUTIÉRREZ
MAEDA J. GALINSKY

THE GUILFORD PRESS
New York   London

© 2004 The Guilford Press
A Division of Guilford Publications, Inc.
72 Spring Street, New York, NY 10012
www.guilford.com

Printed in the United States of America

This book is printed on acid-free paper.

Last digit is print number: 9   8   7   6   5   4   3   2   1

Library of Congress Cataloging-in-Publication Data

Handbook of social work with groups / edited by Charles D. Garvin, Lorraine
M. Gutiérrez, Maeda J. Galinsky.
   p. cm.
  Includes bibliographical references and indexes.
  ISBN 1-59385-004-2 (hardcover : alk. paper)
  1. Social group work. I. Garvin, Charles D. II. Gutiérrez, Lorraine M.
(Lorraine Margot) III. Galinsky, Maeda J.
  HV45.H26 2004
  361.4—dc22
                                        2003027525

About the Editors

Charles D. Garvin, PhD, is Professor Emeritus at the School of Social Work of the University of Michigan. He is the author or coauthor of such books as *Contemporary Group Work, Interpersonal Practice in Social Work, Social Work in Contemporary Society,* and *Generalist Practice: A Task-Centered Approach*, and is coeditor of *The Handbook of Social Work Direct Practice* and *Integrating Knowledge and Practice: The Case of Social Work and Social Science*, among other works. He has also written journal articles and book chapters about many social work topics, especially group work. Dr. Garvin taught group work courses at the master's and doctoral levels for almost 40 years at the University of Michigan. He is the past chair and a current board member of the International Association for the Advancement of Social Work with Groups. His current research focuses on the use of group work in two areas: to reduce tensions among ethnic groups, and to enhance the functioning of people suffering from severe mental illness.

Lorraine M. Gutiérrez, PhD, is Professor at the School of Social Work and the Department of Psychology at the University of Michigan, where she also directs the Edward Ginsberg Center for Community Service and Learning. Her teaching and research focus on multicultural and community organization practice. Dr. Gutiérrez has been involved in social work practice and research in multiethnic communities in New York, Chicago, San Francisco, Detroit, and Seattle. Her current projects include identifying methods for multicultural community-based research and practice, defining multicultural education for social work practice, and identifying effective methods for learning about social justice. She has published over 30 articles, chapters, and books on topics such as empowerment, group work, multicultural practice, and women of color.

Maeda J. Galinsky, PhD, is Kenan Distinguished Professor at the University of North Carolina at Chapel Hill, where she has taught social work group practice at the School of Social Work for about 40 years. She has published widely in the area of group work theory, practice, and research, including articles on support groups, open-ended groups, and evaluations of innovative interventions. Her recent publications focus on technology-based groups, the use of the risk and resilience framework as a foundation for social work practice, and the design and development of a structured intervention geared to the prevention and reduction of aggressive behavior in children. Dr. Galinsky is co-principal investigator of the Making Choices Project, a program aimed at the prevention of violence in elementary school children. She has been on the editorial boards of *Social Work with Groups, Small Group Research, American Journal of Orthopsychiatry*, and *Social Work Research*, and is currently a board member of the International Association for the Advancement of Social Work with Groups.

Contributors

Julie S. Abramson, PhD, School of Social Welfare, State University of New York—The University at Albany, Albany, New York

Robin G. Arndt, BSW, School of Social Work, University of Wisconsin, Madison, Wisconsin

David Bargal, PhD, Paul Baerwald School of Social Work, The Hebrew University, Jerusalem, Israel

Margot Breton, MSW, Faculty of Social Work, University of Toronto, Toronto, Ontario, Canada

Laura R. Bronstein, PhD, Division of Social Work, School of Education and Human Development, State University of New York—Binghamton University, Binghamton, New York

Aaron M. Brower, PhD, School of Social Work and Department of Integrated Liberal Studies, University of Wisconsin, Madison, Wisconsin

Gale Burford, PhD, MSW, Department of Social Work, University of Vermont, Burlington, Vermont

Jillian Dean Campana, MA, Department of Drama/Dance, University of Montana, Missoula, Montana

Ruth Campbell, MSW, University of Michigan Geriatrics Center, Ann Arbor, Michigan

E. Summerson Carr, MA, MSW, School of Social Work and Department of Anthropology, University of Michigan, Ann Arbor, Michigan

Michael Chovanec, PhD, School of Social Work, University of St. Thomas, St. Paul, Minnesota

Doreen Elliott, PhD, Graduate School of Social Work, University of Texas at Arlington, Arlington, Texas

Paul H. Ephross, PhD, School of Social Work, University of Maryland, Baltimore, Maryland

Janet L. Finn, PhD, Department of Social Work, University of Montana, Missoula, Montana

Maurice S. Fisher, PhD, LCSW, Insight Physicians, Richmond, Virginia

Maeda J. Galinsky, PhD, School of Social Work, University of North Carolina, Chapel Hill, North Carolina

Larry M. Gant, PhD, School of Social Work, University of Michigan, Ann Arbor, Michigan

Charles D. Garvin, PhD, School of Social Work, University of Michigan, Ann Arbor, Michigan

Zvi D. Gellis, PhD, School of Social Welfare, State University of New York— The University at Albany, Albany, New York

George S. Getzel, DSW, emeritus, School of Social Work, City University of New York— Hunter College, New York, New York

Alex Gitterman, EdD, School of Social Work, University of Connecticut, West Hartford, Connecticut

Lorraine M. Gutiérrez, PhD, School of Social Work and Department of Psychology, University of Michigan, Ann Arbor, Michigan

Barbara A. Israel, DPH, Health Behavior and Health Education, School of Public Health, University of Michigan, Ann Arbor, Michigan

Maxine Jacobson, PhD, Department of Social Work, University of Montana, Missoula, Montana

Lani V. Jones, PhD, LICSW, School of Social Welfare, State University of New York— The University at Albany, Albany, New York

Annemarie Ketterhagen, BA, English and Secondary Education, University of Wisconsin, Madison, Wisconsin

Linda Farris Kurtz, DPA, ACSW, School of Social Work, Eastern Michigan University, Ypsilanti, Michigan

Paula Lantz, PhD, Health Management and Policy, School of Public Health, University of Michigan, Ann Arbor, Michigan

Randy Magen, PhD, School of Social Work, University of Alaska, Anchorage, Alaska

Andrew Malekoff, MSW, North Shore Child and Family Guidance Center, Roslyn Heights, New York

Nazneen S. Mayadas, DSW, ACSW, LMSW-ACP, Graduate School of Social Work, University of Texas at Arlington, Arlington, Texas

Andrea Meier, PhD, School of Social Work, University of North Carolina, Chapel Hill, North Carolina

James K. Nash, PhD, MSW, Graduate School of Social Work, Portland State University, Portland, Oregon

Helen Northen, PhD, MSW, emeritus, School of Social Work, University of Southern California, Los Angeles, California

Joan Pennell, PhD, Social Work Program, North Carolina State University, Raleigh, North Carolina

Barbara Rittner, PhD, LCSW, School of Social Work, State University of New York— The University at Buffalo, Buffalo, New York

Roger Roffman, DSW, School of Social Work, University of Washington, Seattle, Washington

Ron Rooney, PhD, School of Social Work, University of Minnesota, Minneapolis, Minnesota

Sheldon D. Rose, PhD, School of Social Work, University of Wisconsin, Madison, Wisconsin

Amy J. Schulz, PhD, Health Behavior and Health Education, School of Public Health, University of Michigan, Ann Arbor, Michigan

Rebecca Smith, PhD, Department of Social Work, Northeastern State University, Tahlequah, Oklahoma

Susie E. Snyder, LCSW, Graduate School of Social Work, Portland State University, Portland, Oregon

Lee H. Staples, PhD, MSW, School of Social Work, Boston University, Boston, Massachusetts

Ronald W. Toseland, PhD, School of Social Welfare, State University of New York— The University at Albany, Albany, New York

John E. Tropman, PhD, School of Social Work, University of Michigan, Ann Arbor, Michigan

Thomas V. Vassil, PhD, School of Social Work, University of Maryland, Baltimore, Maryland

Contents

Introduction

CHARLES D. GARVIN
LORRAINE M. GUTIÉRREZ
MAEDA J. GALINSKY

A BROAD VIEW

In this book we portray what we see as the critical dimensions of social work with groups, and we take a broad view of this domain of social work. We see it as encompassing any and all of the types of groups in which social workers participate as part of their professional activities, either as members or facilitators. This view of group work consequently incorporates groups that individuals join to enhance their functioning, enrich their lives, ameliorate problems experienced by organizations and communities, produce social change, and promote social justice.

There are currently no books that fully portray this range of group work. This is undoubtedly due to the space constraints imposed on texts, as well as to the limitations of books with a single author or only a few authors. A handbook such as this one, with multiple authors, is required to fill this void. Such a handbook should be a valuable resource to scholars and practitioners who seek knowledge about any and all aspects of group work, including the knowledge base, the nature of existing models, the practice of group work in different contexts, and the ways in which knowledge of group work can be extended through research.

We do not believe that a single model of practice can encompass this range, and, therefore, we have commissioned chapters that explicate different models of practice. Chapters that discuss various practice settings also draw on a wide array of practice models.

There has been a good deal of debate as to what constitutes social work with groups and how this practice differs from the way other professionals, such as those in counseling and clinical psychology, perform this service. We believe that there is considerable similarity in the ways different human service professions do group work. We do not wish to define each profession's practice but only to assert what we regard as being social work with groups. We are also mindful of a long tradition of referring to social work with groups as *social group work*, and some writers have referred to contemporary practice that stems from this tradition as *mainstream practice* (Papell & Rothman, 1980). We believe, however, that social workers, because of the many ways in which they are asked to provide group services, have had to develop many different group modalities.

Our position is that social work practice with groups first and foremost conforms to the ethical guidelines of the profession, and this principle is expanded on in great detail in Chapter 5, inasmuch as there are issues that are unique to ethical practice with groups. There are additional boundaries to social work practice with groups. One is that this practice places a strong emphasis on the importance of the quality of interactions among the members. These interactions should be characterized by mutual respect and the recognition of the value of each individual to the group. Whenever appropriate to the purpose of the group, this quality includes the principle of *mutual aid*, which sees members as helping one another. This principle draws on a vision of a democratic society in which individuals come to understand their interdependence.

Professional social workers who work with groups consequently seek to carry these ideas out in the groups they facilitate or in which they participate as members. Some groups, such as task groups, may not draw on the mutual aid concept so much when members are committed to accomplishing some purpose external to the group. In any case, however, group workers must be mindful of group processes, especially those that pertain to the quality of relationships among members, as well as of how groups evolve over time.

Group work takes place in all the types of settings in which social workers work. This is a result of the fact that humans are interdependent beings and can benefit from working with others in groups to attain their goals.[1] At times, however, they may choose not to do so. Others with whom they are compatible may not be available; a person may fear the consequences of others knowing about some aspect of his or her life that creates extreme vulnerability; or the person's behavior may be such that at a given time working in a group may place other group members in some jeopardy. Whether some problem situations best lend themselves to a search for solutions in a group is a matter not yet fully resolved (Toseland & Siporin, 1986).

In planning this book, we sought to cover the following area: (1) the knowledge base for practice; (2) the variations in group work that are related to the cultures found in various parts of the world; (3) the value and philosophical premises of group work; (4) the major models of practice; (5) the ways practice differs when the purposes for creating groups varies and when it is conducted in different types of practice settings; (6) the varied use of groups employed to further organizational or community purposes; (7) the issues faced by researchers and evaluators related to group work; and (8) the ways in which technological advances can be employed by groups.

Consequently, we have organized the book into several parts related to these areas. Part I presents the intellectual contexts of group work in the social sciences, as well as in the realm of values, including the all-important value placed on empowerment. We have included two chapters on the social science base. Chapter 1 focuses on content from group dynamics; Chapter 2 takes a systems and environmental context perspective. Chapter 3 provides a global perspective on group work and indicates that social work with groups is a major activity in every society in the world, albeit there are differences in how group work is perceived because of the various cultures and social and political conditions present in societies.

Part II presents two of the major models driving contemporary practice theory. One, referred to as the "mutual aid" model, focuses on the processes that occur among group members. The other, referred to as a "cognitive-behavioral model," focuses on the way that member behaviors and thoughts are altered by individual and group processes so as to attain desired outcomes. There are other models of practice, and these are referred to in chapters in this book devoted to various settings and purposes. The two models presented at this point, however, seemed to us to represent clearly different approaches to group work that require practitioners to think about their work in substantially different ways.

Part III discusses three types of groups that may be found in many settings but that require different sets of practice principles. These are support and self-help groups, psychoeducational groups, and groups for the prevention of individual problems.

Part IV describes the specifics of group work practice in some of the major social welfare service areas. These include group work focused on physical and mental health, on involuntary clients, on children and families, on child welfare, on substance abuse, on older adults, and on the reduction of intergroup conflicts.

Part V presents groups formed to support organizational and community-oriented goals. These include community collaboration, popular education, social action, relief of poverty, improvement in team functioning, empowerment of consumers, and accomplishment of tasks.

Part VI presents chapters on group work research and evaluation methods. Included in this section are chapters on measurement and design. Part VII is devoted to the emerging importance of the use of technology in group work.

CHAPTER STRUCTURE

We believe that effective group work requires the practitioner to draw on many sources of knowledge about how humans interact in groups. These sources include psychology and sociology—particularly the overlap of these disciplines, namely, social psychology. In addition, however, economists, political scientists, and anthropologists have contributed to our understanding of the context and meaning of groups. Other professions, such as nursing, psychiatry, and public health, also work with groups and add to our conceptualization (or comprehension) of ways of helping in groups. The authors in this book, therefore, were asked to selectively draw on all these sources of knowledge.

We also believe that evidence of effectiveness of group work practices is vital to improving group work. Thus progress in group work or, for that matter, in any form of professional practice is rooted both in the wisdom of its practitioners as they reflect on their professional actions and in the careful collection of data about the impact of the practice on members and their environments. These data can be in the form of either qualitative or quantitative information or both. Consequently, we asked all the authors in this handbook to attend to these areas of research as they relate to their foci.

This emphasis is closely related to a development in many professions referred to as "evidence-based practice." This approach affirms the idea that the practitioner should examine studies of the effectiveness of a particular intervention when utilizing it. A number of social work scholars have examined the utility of this type of practice, and we hope this book will extend the application of such practice to group work (Fraser, 2003; Gambrill, 1999, 2003).

Since the pioneering work of writers such as Grace Coyle, Gertrude Wilson, Gladys Ryland, Hy Weiner, and Alan Klein, group workers have been concerned with helping group members become more effective in challenging oppressive environments. The modern-day term related to this is *empowerment*, and we have asked the contributors to attend to this issue and have also devoted a full chapter to this subject.

Last, and perhaps of the greatest importance, we emphasized to the authors that all practice must take into account human differences related to culture, race, ethnicity, gender, and physical and mental abilities, as well as other sources of human variation, and how these are used to privilege some and oppress others, and have also asked them to discuss how these issues affect their domains. We chose this way of dealing with this set of issues rather than commissioning separate chapters on diversity that would, of necessity, be too general. We believe that this issue is so central to good group work practice that it should be attended to in all of the chapters, with the greater degree of specificity that can be attained in this way.

In summary, we asked the authors to prepare chapters based on the most advanced ideas and research about the topic. We also asked them to incorporate a vision of the developments they anticipate will occur with respect to theoretical issues, as well as in the social sciences and other fields of knowledge, in the years ahead. We emphasized that the issues of diversity and social justice were very important to this book. We then supplied the following general outline for them to follow, although we recognized that the chapters would vary based on the nature of their content:

1. Overview of the chapter
2. Description of the purpose of group work in the context of the chapter
3. Interventions
4. Empirical evidence and theoretical base
5. Examples
6. Future directions

FUTURE CHALLENGES TO GROUP WORK

We planned in this volume not only to report what is already known but also to stimulate the future development of the theory and practice of social work with groups. One of the most important ways in which this must happen is through the development of practice theory and practice research, and we believe that these are inextricable.

Practice Theory

The recent focus on evidence-based practice in social work discussed previously—practice grounded in the best available research evidence and integrated with practitioner wisdom and consumer preferences—illustrates one promising approach to greater specificity. Our practice theory in social group work has tended to be broad; we have applied a number of principles to a wide variety of situations. We have drawn from social science theory, as already stated, about group norms, group goals, group development, and other aspects of group dynamics, and we have utilized group work concepts such as group composition, mutual aid, and programming. We have also considered system levels and the interactions among them such as group–agency–environmental interactions. Although this approach has served us well up to a point, we now recognize the need to create specific practice theory and precise practice principles. In this process, we can use the rapidly increasing number of descriptive accounts of group work with specific populations and the slowly growing body of empirical literature from studies of process and outcomes.

An important aspect of our ability to meet this challenge is the increasing recognition and acceptance among group workers of the need for theoretical specificity and more precise practice principles—the recognition that there is not one all-purpose theory to which every group worker must adhere, no one overarching or "mainstream" model of practice. Group problem solving in a task group is not the same as individual psychological or behavioral change in a therapeutic group. Group work with an open-ended group is not the same as group work with a closed group. Group work on the computer is not the same as group work face-to-face. And community empowerment and social action groups are not the same, for example, as support groups in a hospital setting. We are more frequently asking such questions as: What works with different populations? What interventions should be used to achieve different purposes—whether, for example, to provide support, to complete organizational tasks, or to enable interpersonal change? What kinds of more standardized practice principles can we develop for a particular problem or task? How do we modify or develop new practice principles for different group formats, such as open-ended groups or groups with a set agenda? How does the context affect the delivery of group services?

Writers on group work are beginning to give more explicit directions to group workers. They are also developing practice manuals that are based on social science and on practice theory and research. These manuals give social group workers an overview of the latest information on the topic of the manual, delineate goals and objectives for each of a series of topical sessions, suggest content and activities to help achieve the objectives, and supply evaluation tools. As many authors in this book point out, however, these resources must not be used rigidly but in ways that recognize how members of one group differ from those of another and how members set in motion processes that must be respected. In other words, any structured approach to practice must be used with full recognition of the importance of worker sensitivity to the wishes and inputs of members of every group.

As we work to improve our practice theory and to strive for increased specificity, we again encounter a series of issues and their associated tasks. Topics here include the degree of flexibility of the group work practice principles, the necessity to keep practice guidelines up to date, and the call for culturally competent practice.

The first issue concerns the degree of flexibility promoted in the use of practice guidelines. Specificity is a desirable quality and practitioners need to be sufficiently directed by accumulated knowledge; prescriptiveness can be a virtue. We may aim for the kinds of practice guidelines that represent statements to help practitioner and patient decisions about appropriate interventions in specific situations. In view of the lack of data, and because it is always imperative that group workers understand the distinctive qualities of each group, practitioners will have to continue to make choices and exercise judgment, to assess unique individual and group factors, and to build on their own experience. Furthermore, evidence-based practice requires that client choice is a primary consideration for action.

Because of the complexity of human behavior and the many ways in which practice situations vary, we may not ever be able to create precise directives that fit most narrowly defined practice situations. Thus there is an art to the application of practice guidelines. In essence, as we work to create clear directives for practice that can serve as a guide to group workers, we also need to be aware of the flexibility required for their usage in the real world of meeting client and group goals.

Group workers must engage in critical thinking. They must have a broad theoretical perspective, be aware of specific practice principles already developed from research evidence, thoughtfully consider the uniqueness of a particular practice situation, take into account their own practice experience with similar situations, and incorporate client wishes for intervention. Furthermore, in novel situations, such as technology-based practice, group workers need to be able to determine whether practice principles apply or need to be modified to fit the particular individual and group conditions that they face.

A major challenge to group work in the coming years will be to make appropriate use of technology, and we have included a full chapter on this subject. Group work has been a practice modality that helps people draw from each other's strengths through face-to-face interactions. We now have the opportunity to broaden the scope of that helping interaction with the aid of advances in technology. We have all seen our world change and reshape itself with new and improved forms of technology. We can foresee the enormous promise of technology as it becomes an integral part of group work practice.

A second important issue for the development of practice theory is the need to keep our practice guidelines current. Ideally, a book such as this will be revised every few years. Each time that we construct practice principles, we must use the knowledge then available. We have to continually update our practice theory with new findings from research in the social sciences, in social work, and in related practice disciplines—as, for example, findings on the nature of computer group interactions from social work and clinical psychology. Evidence-based practice is built on this foundation of current knowledge.

We have tried to show throughout this introductory statement that we need a body of empirically tested knowledge to develop practice principles. We do not have sufficient empirical research on group work to support a strong foundation for evidence-based practice. Clearly, we need to conduct more and better research. We are getting increased support from funding sources, including governmental agencies, and recently a number of centers and institutes have been established at schools of social work.

A third critical issue involves the impetus to cultural competence, the attention of group work to racial and ethnic diversity in practice theory. The recent census data have underscored the diversity in our current society. We are beginning to focus more on this area of cultural competence through workshops and academic courses. Although group workers have always had the mission to be inclusive and respectful of all racial and ethnic groups and to promote intercultural understanding, we need to articulate more clearly concepts that apply to diversity. We need to be more specific in addressing cultural factors that affect particular racial and ethnic populations. For example, familism and cultural assimilation are two concepts currently in use to examine diverse populations. In group work, we also need to consider the complexities of heterogeneous racial and ethnic composition as people meet together. Practice principles for cultural competence must be built on an empirical foundation as we gather data from and about diverse ethnic and racial groups. Practice wisdom is critical given that people's identities are not determined by any one attribute, such as gender or ethnicity, but are an amalgam of many different attributes, including age, physical ability, and social class. Evidence about one group must be put into perspective by the group worker with each new group. Thus the ways people seek to give and take help in groups are complex and not easily understood.

Practice Research

We must begin to create a strong empirical foundation for group work practice. We must, consequently, increase our productivity and our ability to conduct research relevant to the practice of group work. Four issues on which we must simultaneously work are: (1) the training of researchers, (2) the development of appropriate research methodology, (3) the nurturing of a research–practice partnership, and (4) the translation of research findings into practice language. The scope of this research agenda calls for a broad range of approaches, including qualitative and quantitative methods, ethnography, experimental research, and action research.

We need to build a cadre of trained researchers who are interested in studying group work processes and outcomes. Although our capacity is growing, still, at the current time, our abilities are limited. We need to increase the number of persons interested in doing research on social group work practice, and we need to foster an interest in intervention research, so that our findings are more directly applicable to the practice world. We need to create a climate in which an interest in testing and refining practice principles is valued and rewarded.

The second task in the empirical area relates to research methodology—design and measurement issues—and several chapters in this handbook relate to these issues. We need to promote research designs that capture real-life practice situations and that also give us an accurate assessment of effectiveness. We need to go beyond practitioner descriptions and free-flowing subjective evaluations to well-developed ethnographies and well-formulated evaluations. We need to listen to those who are sophisticated about intervention research and to carry out more systematically conducted pilot studies. We then need to conduct studies in which we rigorously test our interventions in several sites, but few enough so that intervention and data collection can be carefully monitored. We need to train researchers in both quantitative and qualitative methods of data collection, researchers who can decide which method or combination of methods to use to answer the research question at hand. We need to use comparison and wait-list groups when we cannot randomly assign participants to a control group condition, and we must devise and be open to new variations in research designs.

Measurement tools to study both group processes and outcomes are also of methodological importance. We do not have enough validated measures that adequately capture the processes that occur in our group interventions, processes such as cohesion and supportive interactions. We also need to develop more valid and reliable measures of individual and group outcomes. Although the currently published measures may fit or approximate outcomes that are related to our goals of service, these measures often do not pinpoint the specifically stated goals of our interventions.

A third issue for empirical research in social group work is that of the extent and types of collaboration between practitioners and researchers. Practice research must be relevant to practitioners. The best way to begin to make this happen is to use methods from action research to involve practitioners in all phases of the research process. They need to be involved in the choice of research questions, in the selection of research sites and of research methodology, in the conduct of the interventions, in the evaluation of process and outcome, and in the interpretation of findings for practice. In essence, we need to draw on group workers' knowledge, skill, and experience. Practitioners, too, have the responsibility for creating a hospitable climate for intervention research by participating in the research, following the agreed-upon plan, cooperating in the collection of data, engaging in interpretation of data, and, of course, using the findings in their group work practice.

Finally, researchers need to be able to translate the findings of their research into the language of the world of practice. Involving practitioners, they need to be able to interpret the findings, translate them into practice principles, and disseminate these principles. Researchers often complain that practitioners do not pay attention to research and that they do not read the literature. It is essential that we articulate the implications for practice of our research findings and publish and teach practice principles in a usable form.

Although the traditional focus of intervention research has been in clinical settings, these suggestions are equally applicable to groups in organizations and communities. The use of groups for purposes of community action and organizational functioning is significant. The chapters on work with organizations and communities provide some examples of how multiple case studies, ethnography, and other qualitative methods can be used to study and understand these forms of group work. An important challenge for our field is to continue to develop research-based group methods for work on the organizational and community levels.

The reverse is also true—that researchers may not adequately appreciate what has been termed "practice wisdom." This represents information that practitioners convey to each other about what they have done and "what works." Through these means, a set of group work practice principles have evolved out of practice, and we have a great deal of respect for these principles.

To summarize, the areas of challenge we have addressed and to which we hope this volume contributes are (1) the challenge of using technology for group work practice, (2) the challenge of creating more specific group work practice theory, and (3) the challenge of increasing the empirical base of group work practice.

We believe that those of us in practice and those of us in research can work together to meet these challenges. We can flourish in an environment that supports both the group work practitioner and the social work researcher, that respects the worlds of practice and of academia, that encourages interchange, and that values what each person has to bring to the common pursuit of effective group work practice. We need a perspective of mutual esteem and cooperation. We must draw on the legacy of luminaries, such as the authors of the chapters in this book. With a spirited devotion to practice and to research, we believe that group work can meet the challenges we face in building a practice theory anchored in research and open to new and exciting possibilities for expanding services.

NOTE

1. We are not restricting ourselves here to groups for individual problem solving but also refer here to all groups, including committees, task forces, and so on.

REFERENCES

Fraser, M. F. (2003). Intervention research in social work: A basis for evidence-based practice and practice guidelines. In A. Rosen & E. K. Proctor (Eds.), *Developing practice guidelines for social work interventions: Issues, methods, and research agenda*. New York: Columbia University Press.

Gambrill, E. (1999). Evidence-based practice: An alternative to authority-based practice. *Families in Society: The Journal of Contemporary Human Services*, 18(3), 341–350.

Gambrill, E. (2003). Evidence-based practice: Sea change or the emperor's new clothes? *Journal of Social Work Education*, *39*(1), 3–23.

Papell, C., & Rothman, B. (1980). Relating the mainstream model of social work with groups to group psychotherapy and the structured group approach. *Social Work with Groups*, *3*(2), 5–23.

Toseland, R. W., & Siporin, M. (1986). When to recommend group treatment: A review of the clinical and the research literature. *International Journal of Group Psychotherapy*, *36*(2), 171–201.

Part I

Theoretical and Philosophical Foundations

Group workers draw from a number of theoretical and philosophical frameworks in developing their practice principles. It would take a volume in itself to present all of these in depth. We have chosen, therefore, to highlight the main components of these frameworks in enough detail for the reader to understand these foundations and to assess the adequacy of practice paradigms in terms of their attention to relevant theories, propositions, empirical findings, and concepts.

The first two chapters of this book present theoretical material from somewhat different standpoints. Chapter 1 presents important information from the field of group dynamics. This chapter discusses many of the theories that are used to understand the processes and other conditions that occur *within* groups, such as group development, the ways members influence one another, communication patterns, and various group structures. Chapter 2 seeks to place the group within the broader sphere of the organizations and other systems that surround the group. This kind of understanding is necessary, as all groups influence their social environments and are, in turn, influenced by them.

The next three chapters in this section present important value-related and other philosophical considerations that group workers should heed. One chapter on ethics and values of importance to group work portrays the ethical principles that distinguished social work practice with groups throughout its history (Chapter 5). This chapter also considers issues that were not anticipated by group work pioneers, issues that grow out of such contemporary phenomena as the current legal environment and the use of modern technological inventions. A very important contemporary principle is that group work should be empowering, as members take on the challenge of changing oppressive conditions. We, therefore, commissioned a chapter exclusively devoted to empowerment issues in group work (Chapter 4).

We recognized that knowledge and philosophy are very much responsive to the locale and the concomitant cultural context in which group work is practiced. Consequently, we have included a chapter that examines group work practice and education as it occurs around the world and that portrays some of the similarities and differences in group work in different nations with different needs, languages, and cultures (Chapter 3).

11

Chapter 1

Group Dynamics

RONALD W. TOSELAND
LANI V. JONES
ZVI D. GELLIS

This chapter focuses on group dynamics. We review group dynamics in five domains and examine group dynamics within the context of group development.

There are many theories about the development of group dynamics, but fundamental to all of them is the notion of groups as social systems. A system is composed of elements in interaction. When group members interact with each other, they form a social system, with attendant group dynamic processes. Group dynamics are the forces that emerge and take shape as members interact with each other over the life of a group. These dynamic forces are the product of both the here-and-now interactions of group members and what members bring to the group from the larger social environment.

THE IMPORTANCE OF GROUP DYNAMICS

An understanding of group dynamics is essential for effective practice with any type of task or treatment group. Failure to pay careful attention to group dynamics can lead to unproductive meetings and dissatisfied members. In extreme cases, such as the mass suicide at Jonestown, group dynamics gone awry can have serious consequences for individual members or the group as a whole (Galinsky & Schopler, 1977; Smokowski, Rose, & Bacallao, 2001; Smokowski, Rose, Todar, & Reardon, 1999). Moreover, with the increasing multicultural diversification of this society, these dynamics are likely to remain a major concern for group workers (Jones, 2000). Groups that do not consider racial, ethnic, and cultural variables may present significant consequences for racially and ethnically diverse members. Therefore, throughout this chapter we consider the impact of racial, ethnic, and cultural variables on group dynamics.

To practice effectively with groups, social workers should be able to (1) understand group dynamic processes as they emerge during the ongoing interaction of group members, (2) consider the impact of these dynamics on members from different racial/ethnic and socioeconomic backgrounds, (3) assess the impact of emerging dynamics on current and future group functioning, and (4) guide the development of group dynamics that facilitate member participation and satisfaction while simultaneously enabling the group to achieve its goals.

CONCEPTUALIZING GROUP DYNAMICS

Group dynamics can be conceptualized as falling within the following five domains: (1) communication processes and interaction patterns, (2) interpersonal attraction and cohesion, (3) social integration and influence, (4) power and control, and (5) culture. A conceptual framework of group dynamics is an important heuristic device for workers seeking to assess and understand how any group works. A conceptual framework enables workers to identify and understand group dynamics as they emerge during interaction. Since the 1940s, many scholars have attempted to conceptualize and categorize group dynamics. Some of the most notable include Bales and colleagues (Bales, 1950; Bales, Cohen, & Williamson, 1979), Cartwright and Zander (1968), Forsyth (1999), Hare, Blumberg, Davies, and Kent (1995, 1996), Lewin (1951), McGrath (1984), Nixon (1979), Olmstead (1959), and Parsons (1951). The conceptualization of group dynamics presented in this chapter is based on the work of Toseland and Rivas (2001), but it also draws heavily on the work of these scholars. The chapter gives special attention to racial and ethnic variations so that group work practitioners can develop and lead effective multicultural groups. Because group dynamics are not static over the life of the group, they change as the group develops; thus this chapter also includes a section on models of group development.

COMMUNICATION PROCESSES AND INTERACTION PATTERNS

Communication processes and interaction patterns are fundamental group dynamics. They are the components of social interactions that influence the behavior and attitudes of group members. As a process, communication involves the transmission of a message from a sender to a receiver. According to Toseland and Rivas (2001), communication includes (1) the encoding of perceptions, thoughts, and feelings into language and other symbols by a sender; (2) the transmission of language and symbols verbally, nonverbally, or virtually; and (3) the decoding of the message by the receiver.

Communication can be verbal, nonverbal, or virtual. Face-to-face group members experience both verbal and nonverbal communications, whereas members of telephone groups experience only verbal communications, and members of computer groups experience only virtual communication. Communication can also be synchronous (i.e., back and forth in real time) or asynchronous. Asynchronous communications occur in computer groups when members may respond to messages long after they are posted.

Whenever group members are communicating, they are sending messages that have meanings. Effective leaders listen hard for the meaning in messages. In face-to-face groups, members are always communicating, because even if they are not communicating verbally, their nonverbal behavior is observable and communicating something. In telephone and computer groups, nonverbal communication is absent. The greater anonymity due to the lack of face-to-face contact in telephone and computer groups has important implications for the way members communicate in these groups. For example, it has been pointed out that salience of race and socioeconomic issues is reduced and greater privacy is afforded to stigmatized individuals (Schopler, Abell, & Galinsky, 1998; Smokowski, Galinsky, & Harlow, 2001). A discussion of telephone and computer groups can be found in Toseland and Rivas (2001).

Although meaning is communicated in every message, it is important for workers to be aware that problems in sending or receiving messages and transmission problems can distort or obfuscate the intended meaning of messages. For example, the sender of a message may be unclear or ambiguous. The receiver of a message can suffer from selective perception or completely block out a message. Communication can also be distorted in transmission. Noise and other distractions within or outside of the meeting room (or on computers or telephones) can cause distortions.

Language barriers can sometimes interfere with effective communication in groups. Language often reflects social attitudes. It shapes thoughts and attitudes and guides thinking patterns and the expression of ideas. The roles that language plays in human interaction within the context of human diversity can encourage or discourage individual efforts and can influence whether groups and communities attain optimal health and well-being (Anderson & Carter, 2003). The use of standard English to communicate may unfairly discriminate against those from bilingual backgrounds. In particular, the bilingual backgrounds of many Asian Americans, Latinos, and Native Americans may lead to misunderstanding or alienation (Sue & Sue, 1999). For example, Gray-Little & Kaplan (2000) point out that white Americans had a significantly higher rate of verbal participation in groups than did Asian Americans, Native Americans, and Mexican Americans of similar educational background. Because higher levels of participation may reduce attrition, yield greater changes in self-esteem, and reduce questions about the value of involvement in groups, lower levels of verbal participation raise troubling questions about therapeutic outcomes for minority members of multicultural groups. When English is a second language, care should be taken to insure that members are able to understand what is being said in the group. In addition to accents and dialects that can sometimes interfere with clear communication, the meanings of many words are culturally defined. Thus care should be taken to clarify the meaning of messages in groups with members from different cultural and racial/ethnic backgrounds.

The most effective way to ensure that the meaning of the sender is understood by the receiver is for the receiver to provide feedback about that meaning he or she understood. Thus statements such as "Did I understand you correctly?" or "Let me make sure I understand what you are saying" help to prevent distortions in communication. Toseland and Rivas (2001) suggest that effective feedback should (1) describe the content of the communication as it is perceived by the member, (2) be given to the member who sent the message as soon as the message has been received, and (3) be expressed in a tentative manner so that it is clear that the feedback is intended to clarify the original message rather than confront or attack the sender.

Interaction patterns are also fundamental group dynamic processes. Some common interaction patterns include (1) the maypole, in which the leader is the central figure and most communication occurs from member to leader or leader to member; (2) the round robin, in which members take turns talking; (3) the hot seat, which features extended interaction between the leader and a member; and (4) the free-floating pattern, in which all members freely communicate. Although much of the group dynamics literature on interaction patterns focuses on the degree of centralization of communication, in most therapeutic social work groups, group-centered rather than leader-centered interaction patterns are valued because they help to insure the full participation of all members. It has been pointed out that, even in task groups such as teams, reciprocal interdependence often warrants decentralized communication networks (Stewart, Manz, & Sims, 1999).

Interaction patterns are affected by members' proclivity to communicate. Some members are more outgoing than others and take more opportunities to communicate. Interaction patterns are also affected by verbal and nonverbal cues. Praise and other supportive comments, eye contact, and other expressions of interest tend to elicit more communication. The status and power relationships within the group also affect interaction patterns. Higher status members tend to communicate more than lower status members. Interpersonal attraction and the emotional bonds that form between members also influence interaction patterns. For example, members of subgroups tend to interact more with each other than with other group members. The size of the group also affects interaction. In general, the smaller the group, the more chance there is for each member to communicate. Physical arrangements can also have an important impact on interaction patterns. Many factors, such as how chairs are arranged, whether a conference table is used, the size of the room, and whether the environment is comfortable and private should be considered.

Workers may want to reduce communications from talkative members or encourage reserved members to talk. Pointing out interaction patterns is often sufficient to bring about change, but other methods may also be used. For example, reserved group members may benefit from go-rounds because they are expected to speak when it is their turn. Selective attention, clues, and reinforcement also can be used to change interaction patterns. By acknowledging and praising selected communications, workers can draw out reserved members. By directing communication to others, workers can reduce the communication of dominant members. Giving members specific roles or tasks, changing seating arrangements, and asking members to break into subgroups are other methods that can be used to change interaction patterns.

Subgroup formation occurs naturally in all groups, because members do not all interact with equal valence. Interpersonal attraction, emotional bonds, and interest alliances are stronger among some members than others. Subgroups can take the form of dyads, triads, or cliques. Also, there can be isolates, who are not attached to subgroups, and scapegoats, who receive negative attention and criticism from the group. Subgroups usually are not a problem in groups unless such a strong alliance is formed among subgroup members that it threatens to supersede their allegiance to the group as a whole.

An important process in group work is changing the way individuals accept and interact with each other. This change can be accomplished by helping members to increase their personal honesty and to become more aware of their own attitudes and feelings toward people who are different from them. Groups can be structured so that minority members feel comfortable without having their values ignored, minimized, or challenged. Developing norms that celebrate and embrace diversity are one way to accomplish this objective (Han & Vasquez, 1995).

INTERPERSONAL ATTRACTION AND COHESION

Interpersonal attraction contributes to subgroup formation and to the level of cohesion of the group as a whole. Several factors contribute to interpersonal attraction. Proximity increases interaction among people, which, in turn, often increases attraction. Therefore, just the physical act of meeting together helps to form bonds among members. However, proximity alone is usually not sufficient for interpersonal attraction to occur. In research done al-most half a century ago, Newcomb (1960, 1961, 1963) showed that interpersonal attraction is fostered by similarity (i.e., we tend to like people who are similar to us). We can also be attracted to people who are dissimilar to us if they complement our personal qualities in some way (Forsyth, 1999).

Other factors also contribute to interpersonal attraction—for example, acceptance and approval. Thus, group members who are accepting and positive and those who praise others for their contributions tend to be viewed as interpersonally attractive. Reciprocity also fre-quently operates in these situations, so that positive accepting behavior begets positive, ac-cepting responses.

Compatibility in member expectations also tends to promote interpersonal attraction. Members are often attracted to those who engage in group interactions that meet their ex-pectations. For example, if high disclosure is expected, a member who discloses deeply is more likely to be found to be interpersonally attractive than a member who is reserved. Sim-ilarly, members who fulfill the unmet needs of others in the group will also frequently be found to be interpersonally attractive. For example, if the group desires a strong leader, the member who demonstrates strong leadership capacities is generally viewed as interperson-ally attractive by the other members of the group.

Group cohesion is the sum of all the forces that are exerted on members to remain in the group (Festinger, 1950). Interpersonal attraction is just one of the building blocks of group cohesion. In addition to interpersonal attraction, other factors contributing to cohe-sion include (1) satisfaction of members' needs for affiliation, recognition, and security; (2) resources and prestige that members believe will be garnered through group participation; (3) expectations about the beneficial consequences of the work of the group; and (4) positive comparison of the group with previous group experiences (Cartwright, 1968).

Groups satisfy members' needs for affiliation, recognition, and security in many ways. Individuals who are lonely or isolated, for example, often find that groups provide opportu-nities for socialization that are unavailable to them in other contexts. People are also at-tracted to groups that recognize their accomplishments, that foster their sense of compe-tence, and that build their self-esteem. Similarly, when members' contributions are valued and when they feel that they are well liked by the other members of the group, they are more likely to place a high value on participating in the group. For example, leaders may provide an overwhelmed African American single father with culturally relevant parenting informa-tion or referrals. Here, the sharing of relevant cultural information validates unique multi-cultural parenting needs, informs mutuality, and reinforces cohesion of the group.

Access to resources and prestige also tends to make groups cohesive. Groups that give members access to resources they might not otherwise have are attractive. Members may de-velop new contacts with high-status members who might also help them outside of the group. Being a part of a group that has the power to make important decisions can raise member's status and prestige within the sponsoring organization. Cohesion is enhanced when members feel that they are working on important issues that they can influence. Con-versely, when members feel that their input is being ignored or that it is ineffectual, they are not likely to feel strongly connected to the group or the people in it.

Members tend to compare their experiences in a group with their experiences in other groups. When studying cohesion in groups, Thibaut and Kelley (1959) found that members' continued desire to stay in a group was based on the satisfaction derived from participating in the group compared with other alternatives, what they called the "com-parison level for alternatives." Thus members who are satisfied with a group and who do not think that they will be more satisfied participating elsewhere will tend to remain committed to the group.

Members' reasons for being attracted to a group affect how they act in it. For example, members who are attracted to a group primarily because of the prestige it brings to them are not likely to initiate controversial or difficult topics that might affect their status in it. Similarly, members who join a group primarily for the opportunity it provides for social interaction tend to engage in more off-task conversations than those who join a group because of the important work it is charged to accomplish.

The level of cohesion in a group also influences members' behaviors in many different ways. After reviewing the clinical and research literature, Toseland and Rivas (2001) noted that high levels of cohesion have been associated with many beneficial group-member behaviors, such as greater (1) perseverance toward group goals, (2) willingness to take responsibility for group functioning, (3) willingness to express feelings, (4) willingness to listen, and (5) ability to use feedback and evaluations.

High levels of group cohesion have also been associated with positive outcomes. These include (1) greater satisfaction with the group experience; (2) higher levels of goal attainment by individual group members and the group as a whole; (3) greater commitment to the sponsoring organization; (4) increases in members' feelings of self-confidence, self-esteem, and personal adjustment; and (5) higher levels of meeting attendance and an increased length of participation.

Despite the many beneficial aspects of high levels of group cohesion, it can also have some negative consequences. For example, high levels of cohesion can lead to dependence on the group. This can be a particular problem in support and therapy groups in which members have severe mental health or substance abuse problems and poor self-images. Cohesion can also lead to a level of conformity that detracts from the work of the group. For example, members may remain silent rather than share helpful information, ideas, and thoughts because they believe these may be contrary to what the majority wants to hear.

Conformity can become pathological when members' fears of losing status or being ostracized prevent them from voicing innovative but unpopular ideas or from raising the possibility that negative consequences may result from actions being contemplated by the group. Janis (1972, 1982), for example, noted that pathological cohesion is one ingredient of groupthink. The members' striving for unanimity and acceptance within the group can become so great that it overrides their motivation to think independently and to realistically appraise alternative courses of action (Janis 1972, 1982). Thus, while promoting group cohesion, workers should strive to preserve members' individuality. Workers can do this by guiding groups to develop norms that encourage the free and open expression of ideas and opinions and that value the expression of divergent opinions and ideas.

SOCIAL INTEGRATION AND INFLUENCE

Social integration refers to how members fit together and are accepted in the group. Norms, roles, and status are group dynamics that promote social integration by influencing how members behave. These dynamic processes set out members' places within the group. They lend order and familiarity to group processes, helping to make individual member's behaviors predictable and comfortable for all. Norms, roles, and status help groups to avoid excessive conflict and unpredictability, which can, in turn, lead to chaos and the disintegration of the group. Groups cannot function effectively without a fairly high level of social integration of members. Social integration helps to build unanimity about the purposes and goals of the group, helping the group move forward in an orderly and efficient manner to accomplish work and achieve its goals.

Many years ago, Deutsch and Gerard (1955) postulated two forms of social influence: normative influence and informational influence. *Normative* influence is the desire to meet other people's expectations and to be accepted by others. *Informational* influence is accepting and being persuaded by information provided by others.

Too much conformity and compliance, resulting from the strong social influences of norms, roles, and status hierarchies, can also lead to groupthink. This can have negative consequences for group productivity because members' individual creative and intellectual contributions are suppressed. At the same time, a certain amount of predictability, conformity, and compliance is necessary to enable members to work together to achieve the goals of the group. Thus it is important for group workers to understand and manage the norms, roles, and status hierarchies that are associated with social integration and influence so that a balance can be achieved between too little and too much conformity.

Norms are shared beliefs and expectations about appropriate ways to behave in social situations, such as a group (Toseland & Rivas, 2001). Norms are rules about what constitutes valued, preferred, and acceptable behavior within the group. Norms can be overt and explicit or covert and implicit. A group leader who states that the group will begin and end on time and then follows through on that rule each week is developing an explicit group norm in an overt fashion. In contrast, a covert, implicit norm might develop for members of a couples group to avoid any discussion of their sexual satisfaction with their partner or of infidelity. The norm is "we don't talk about those kinds of things in this group."

Norms also vary by the extent to which they are perceived to be binding on all members of the group. When a norm is highly binding, violating it often means severe sanction. Norms also vary by degree of salience for individual members. Some members may perceive norms whereas others may not perceive them at all, and some members may perceive that a particular norm is more binding than other members do.

Norms develop slowly in the group as members experience what is valued and preferred behavior through group interaction. Therefore, it is important for workers to be cognizant of the development of norms, especially in the beginning, and to help the group avoid developing norms that will reduce member satisfaction or prevent the group from achieving its goals. Workers can share perceptions about group norms and suggest ways in which norms could be changed to promote the growth of the group and its members. Roles are shared expectations about the functioning of individual members of the group. Whereas norms are shared expectations about appropriate and valued behavior by all members of the group, roles define how individual members are expected to perform with respect to the work of the group. Roles help to insure a division of labor when working on group goals. Members can take on many different roles in a group. Many years ago, Benne and Sheats (1948) developed a typology of group roles that included (1) task roles, such as the coordinator and the information seeker; (2) socioemotional roles, such as the encourager and the harmonizer; and (3) individual roles, such as the aggressor and the help seeker.

Special attention should be given to norm development in culturally diverse groups. Especially when minority members are significantly underrepresented, conscious and unconscious group dynamics of mainstreaming and devaluation of differences can undermine needed therapeutic work (Han & Vasquez, 1995). Being the only racial/ethnic minority, gay, or female can be isolating and may make it difficult to relate to others in the group. Minority members may question their own judgment. They may also feel inferior or pressured to agree with the majority. For these reasons, minority members may derive less benefit from the group (Fenster, 1996).

It is helpful for the group to have some members who take on roles that facilitate task accomplishment and other members who take on roles that meet members' socioemotional needs. Thus members who keep the group on task, who are empathic, and who inject humor all help the group develop in a positive fashion. Members who take on other roles, such as monopolizers, jesters, scapegoats, or aggressors, can be problematic for the effective functioning of the group. Leaders should take the time to analyze the roles that members play in the group and help members to take on roles that promote social integration and that support effective group functioning.

Status refers to the ranking of importance of members of the group relative to each other. Status is determined by the prestige, power, position, and expertise members bring with them to the group and by the contributions members make to the work of the group. Because a group member's status is measured in relationship to other members, it may change when other members join or leave the group. Status is also determined by the situation. Members' status may change depending on the extent of their contributions to various aspects of the work of a group. For example, when a group is focused on health issues, the status of a group member who happens to be a nurse may increase.

Status hierarchies have a good deal of influence on social integration within groups. For example, low-status members are the least likely to conform to group norms and to perform up to role expectations because they have less to lose by deviating from expected behavior. Therefore, low-status members have the potential to be disruptive of productive group processes. The leader should provide opportunities for low-status members to contribute to the group so that they can become more socially integrated and achieve a higher status. Medium-status members tend to conform to norms and roles so that they can retain their status or achieve a higher status. High-status members generally conform to norms and role expectations when they are establishing their position, but they have more freedom to deviate from established norms once their high-status positions are established. Thus high-status members can be an important force in changing norms that are counterproductive for achieving group goals.

Norms, roles, and status are important components of the social influence that groups have on members. The well-known early studies by Sherif (1936), Newcomb (1943), and Asch (1952, 1955, 1957) clearly demonstrated that the views of individual group members are influenced by majority opinion. Members with minority points of view, however, can also influence the majority. In a series of experiments, Moscovici and colleagues, for example, showed that a small number of vocal and persistent confederates were able to have some influence on the views of the majority who held differing opinions (see, e.g., Moscovici, 1985, 1994; Moscovici & Lage, 1976; Moscovici, Lage, & Naffrechoux, 1969).

Forsyth (1999) has pointed out that those with minority opinions are more likely to be heard if they (1) offer compelling and consistent arguments, (2) are assertive about the importance of listening to their opinion, (3) appear confident rather than rigid or close-minded, (4) are flexible and able to grant small concessions to the majority, and (5) confront majorities that are not certain about their positions. Therefore, members with minority opinions can have an important voice when their arguments are well reasoned and persuasive, especially in groups in which open-mindedness is a valued norm.

POWER AND CONTROL

Power and control are often uncomfortable subjects for social workers, who frequently prefer to talk about their work in terms of empowerment, facilitation, mediation, mutual aid, partnership, or relationship building. Despite this, the power of the designated leader of a group is undeniable. There are at least two types of power, attributed power and actual power. Attributed power comes from the perception of people within and outside the group about the worker's ability to be an effective leader. Attributed power comes from such sources as professional status, education, organizational position experience, boundaries between worker and member roles, fees paid for group participation, and so forth. Actual power refers to a worker's resources for changing conditions within and outside the group.

French and Raven's (1959) classic analysis suggests that leaders can draw on seven power bases: (1) connection power—the ability to draw on the resources of influential people and organizations; (2) expert power—having the knowledge to help the group achieve a particular goal; (3) information power—possessing information that is needed by the group; (4) legitimate power—holding an official position and the authority, rights, and privileges that go with that position; (5) reference power—being liked and admired by group members; (6) reward power—the ability to offer social or tangible rewards; and (7) coercive power—the ability to sanction, punish, or deny access to resources, rewards, and privileges.

The power and control of group leaders are especially visible in early group meetings, when members direct most of their communications to the leader rather than to each other. Still, the power of leaders should not be underestimated at any point in the life of a group. In a series of laboratory experiments, Milgram (1974) showed that people will follow orders given by authority figures even after they are given cues that following orders might cause harm. Although questions have been raised about the validity of Milgram's experiments (Forsyth, 1999), a good deal of evidence from other research supports his pioneering findings.

Attention should also be paid to the roles of power and powerlessness in multicultural groups. In the multicultural encounter, leaders must be aware of how they manage feelings, perceptions, and attitudes about power and authority in relation to their own group status. A lack of personal and group understanding of power dynamics on the part of the leader can affect group process and outcome. This absence may provoke certain feelings of alienation and anxiety for minority group members and send a message that they are not competent to join in the group process. It is important that group leaders not only develop self-awareness but also promote empowerment and self-empathy to reduce the internalization of feelings of a devalued and powerless ethnic identity for all members (Hopps & Pinderhughes, 1999; Jones, 2000).

A certain amount of power and control is needed in groups to maintain orderly and efficient group meetings and motivated members. Leaders, for example, can use power and control constructively by helping the members to overcome motivational problems. Members can lose motivation for many reasons, but three of the better known reasons are social loafing, free riding, and the sucker effect (Levi, 2001). "Social loafing" is a term used to describe a reduction in individual motivation and contributions when working in a group rather than alone (Latané, Williams, & Harkins, 1979). Those who think their contributions are not important and who know they will receive their share of the rewards regardless of their level of input have been called "free riders" (Sweeney, 1973).

There is also the "sucker effect," in which good performers slack off so as not to be taken advantage of by those who are less talented or less motivated (Johnson & Johnson,

2000). Leaders can set up incentive systems and use other power and control mechanisms to help avoid these motivational problems. For example, social loafing and free riding can be avoided or undone by increasing a member's personal stake in the group. To do this, leaders can help members to perceive the meaningfulness of the task, how they will personally benefit from being actively engaged, and how their active engagement will benefit others. Making the group smaller, clarifying group rules, setting high standards, being a role model, helping members to believe that their fellow group members are capable and willing to contribute, and helping the group as a whole to feel that it is efficacious are some other ways to reduce social loafing and free riding.

Power and control are often associated with the designated leader, but to insure the active involvement and commitment of members, it is essential for designated leaders to share power and control as the group progresses. This principle recognizes that members also can have power and control over each other. Toseland and Rivas (2001) suggest that this can be done by (1) encouraging member-to-member rather than member-to-leader communications, (2) insuring that members have input into the agenda for group meetings and the direction the group will go in future meetings, (3) supporting indigenous group leaders as their attempts at leadership emerge during group interaction, and (4) encouraging attempts at mutual sharing and mutual aid among group members. Members can also be empowered by encouraging them to take on leadership roles in subgroups that work on specific tasks between meetings, by recognizing their special skills and talents, and by praising and rewarding them for their active involvement in the work of the group.

Early studies of group leadership emphasized the benefits of democratic leadership as compared with autocratic and laissez-faire leadership (Lewin & Lippitt, 1938; Lewin, Lippitt, & White, 1939). Over the years, leadership studies have become more sophisticated. Transactional models of leadership that emphasize rewards, punishments, cost–benefit ratios, and the coercive power of the "carrot and the stick" were developed. These models have largely been replaced with charismatic and transformational leadership models (Bass, 1995; Conger & Kanungo, 1998; House & Aditya, 1997; Shamir, House, & Arthur, 1993). The components of transformational leadership include (1) vision, (2) inspiration, (3) role modeling, (4) intellectual stimulation, (5) meaning-making, (6) appeals to higher order needs, (7) empowerment, (8) setting of high expectations, and (9) fostering collective identity (Conger, 1999).

Transformational leadership models emphasize the role of the leader as a charismatic role model who helps members to overcome self-interest and perceive larger group and organizational goals (Alimo-Metcalfe & Alban-Metcalfe, 2001; Bass, 1985; Bass & Avolio, 1994). Transformational leaders encourage member autonomy and individuality in pursuing group and organizational goals. They encourage members to question assumptions, to approach problems and old solutions in new ways, to reframe problems as opportunities, and to be creative and innovative problem solvers (Alimo-Metcalfe & Alban-Metcalfe, 2001). Transformational leaders use their power bases, but they do so while inspiring members with visionary leadership as to what is possible and appealing to members' altruistic motives to transcend their own self-interests for the good of the group and the organizational sponsor (Bass & Avolio, 1994). They are focused on inspiring and empowering members rather than on inducing compliance (Conger, 1999). A recent study of 47 work groups suggests that transformational leadership is associated with empowerment of members, cohesiveness, and perceived group effectiveness (Jung & Sosik, 2002). Other literature suggests that the most effective leaders are charismatic individuals who promote safe, welcoming group environments that avoid the extremes of aggressive confrontation of members or passive abdication of leadership to aggressive group members (Kivlighan & Tarrant, 2001; Smokowski, Rose, & Bacallo, 2001).

CULTURE

The culture of a group is defined by the values, beliefs, customs, traditions, and preferred ways of doing business that are implicitly understood and shared by all group members. Deeply held beliefs and assumptions that define a group culture emerge through interaction over time. The values, preferences, and interpersonal styles of individual members that come from their ethnic, cultural, and racial heritage, previous life experiences, and genetic disposition have to be blended together before a group culture develops. As members meet, they explore their value systems and interpersonal styles, searching for a common ground on which to relate to each other. Valuing members from diverse backgrounds involves facilitating an exploration of their ethnic and racial heritages and experiences, their attitudes about themselves, and how these attitudes and feelings affect their functioning. It also involves leaders' actively generating a set of group norms that are consonant with the cultural values and perspectives of all group members (Tsui & Schultz, 1988). As a result of this process, a common set of assumptions, values, and preferred ways of doing business emerge, forming the group's culture.

Levi (2001) views culture as having three levels of depth. On the surface level are symbols and rituals that display the culture of the group. At a deeper level, culture is displayed in the styles and approaches that group members use when interacting with each other. For example, the way conflict or competition is handled in a group says much about its culture. The deepest level of culture consists of core ideologies, values, and beliefs held in common by members of the group (Levi, 2001).

The culture of a group is also determined, in part, by the sponsoring organization, the community, and the larger society. Groups take on some of the dominant values and traits of these larger social systems. The influence of these systems depends on the nature and extent of their interactions with the group. When a group is dependent on an organization for its sanction and its resources, it is particularly likely to take on the dominant culture of the organization. For example, a team or a governance committee is more likely to take on the culture of an organization than is a self-help group sponsored by the same organization. Similarly, a sports team sponsored by a neighborhood community center is more likely to take on the cultural values of the larger society than is a gang that meets in a private location.

Multicultural differences are also salient interpersonal factors that have significance for the group culture. Traditionally, group processes have reflected the European and American values of individualism, independence, competiveness, and achievement. These values are different from the values of humility and modesty that are dominant in some other cultures. A potential consequence is the worker's insensitivity to group members with other racial/ ethnic backgrounds. This insensitivity has the potential to negatively affect group dynamic processes in the whole group.

Racially and ethnically diverse groups tend to have their own cultural attributes, values, and experiences because of their unique histories. Cultural experiences of group survival, social hierarchy, inclusiveness, and ethnic identification influence the way members interact with one another in the group. Members' expectations and goals in a multicultural group vary widely. They significantly influence the dynamics of the group (Hopps & Pinderhughes,

1999; Matsukawa, 2001). To be effective with all group members, the group leader should be sensitive to racial/ethnic and socioeconomic differences, should understand the effect of these differences on group dynamics, and should translate this knowledge into culturally sensitive modes of program development and service delivery (Davis, Galinsky, & Schopler, 1995).

A distinct culture tends to emerge more quickly in groups that are homogeneous. When members share similar values and life experiences, their unique perspectives blend more quickly than in groups with diverse membership. For example, a caregiver support group made up of the spouses of frail veterans tends to form a distinct culture more quickly than does a caregiver support group made up of both spouses and adult children who are caring for frail older persons who have not all shared military service. Conversely, heterogeneous groups include multiple opportunities to provide and receive diverse feedback (Merta, 1995), to develop more knowledge and understanding of oneself and others (Avila & Avila, 1988), and to develop the skills needed to relate to people with different backgrounds (Fenster, 1996). However, if facilitated inappropriately, heterogeneous multicultural groups run the risk of reenacting oppressive dynamics of invalidation, disempowerment, lack of empathy, and mutuality (Han & Vasquez, 1995). Therefore, it is important that group leaders be informed, attuned, and adept at processing the roles of race, culture, ethnicity, and power (Pinderhughes, 1989).

Once a culture has developed, members who endorse and share in the group culture feel at home, but those who do not feel isolated and alienated. For the isolated member, the group is not a very satisfying experience. Isolated members are more likely to leave the group because it does not meet their socioemotional needs. Feeling misunderstood and left out is demoralizing and depressing. More extreme feelings of alienation can lead to rebellious, acting-out behavior. For subgroups that are not part of the dominant culture, feelings of isolation are often equated with feelings of oppression. Subgroups that feel repressed are likely to rebel in various ways against the norms, roles, and status hierarchies that have been established in the group. By providing individual attention to isolated members and by stimulating all members to consider values that transcend individual differences, leaders can foster the full participation and integration of all group members into the life of a group.

GROUP DEVELOPMENT

As groups develop over time, group dynamic processes evolve. Many attempts have been made to conceptualize these changes in stage models of group development. There is, for example, the well-known model by Tuckman (1963): (1) forming, (2) storming, (3) norming, and (4) performing. There is also the widely used model by Garland, Jones, and Kolodny (1976): (1) preaffiliation, (2) power and control, (3) intimacy, (4) differentiation, and (5) separation. For a more complete list of some of these models, see Toseland and Rivas (2001).

Beginning stages of group development are characterized by the formation of group dynamics. At first, members interact tentatively, establishing norms, roles, and status hierarchies, and a group culture slowly emerges through interaction. Before cohesion can develop, social integration of members must occur. At first, the interaction is tentative and cautious, with little conflict. Then, as members become more comfortable and emboldened, conflict and resistance can occur. Members want to become a part of the group but at the same time maintain their own identity and independence. While becoming socially integrated, members explore and test roles, and they challenge developing norms and status hierarchies. Encountering some conflict is normal, and dealing with it is an important skill for a group worker. Conflict resolution strategies can be found in many sources (see, for example, Forsyth, 1999, or Toseland & Rivas, 2001). For instance, if racism is perceived in the early stages of group development, cross-cultural issues can be frightening to explore. Anxiety experienced by group members often fosters stereotypical thinking and ego states that are representative of less mature development. Group members often look to the group leader to resolve the group's discomfort. In this case, group leaders should promote interpersonal skills in ways that build mutual connection and create norms that facilitate an exploration of these difficult issues.

The middle stages of groups are characterized by an emphasis on work. Energy devoted to developing cohesive group functioning and comfortable norms and productive roles in earlier group meetings gives way to productive interaction during the middle stage of the life of a group. Words such as intimacy, performance, and problem solving are frequently used in models of group development to convey the emphasis in the middle stage on work and goal achievement.

The ending stages of group development focus on the completion of remaining tasks. Evaluations of the work of the group are conducted, and ending ceremonies are planned. Task groups finish their business, make decisions, and produce the results of their efforts. Therapeutic groups help members to reduce their emotional attachment to the group. They also focus on methods for maintaining positive changes made during the group after the group ends. While accomplishing these tasks, norms and roles may change, and the group's culture matures.

Stage models of group development are helpful in providing guidance to workers about what might occur as a group develops. At the same time, each group is unique. Many factors affect a group's development. Structural characteristics, such as whether a group is time limited or has an open or closed membership, have an important impact on development (Galinsky & Schopler, 1989). Similarly, the capabilities of group members and the support of the sponsoring organization can also affect group development. Therefore, workers should not assume that all groups follow the same developmental pattern. Stage models of group development are good heuristic devices for understanding how group dynamics may evolve over time, but the actual unfolding of group dynamics in a particular group can only be ascertained by careful observation or by using one or more of the measures described in the following section.

MEASURING GROUP DYNAMICS

The measurement of group dynamics is essential in understanding the behavior of individuals and of the group as a whole. Over the past two decades, several reviews have critically examined group process and outcome instruments (Delucia-Waack, 1997; Fuhriman & Barlow, 1994; Fuhriman & Packard, 1986). These instruments have been described as useful in analyzing group therapy processes, group climate and therapeutic dimensions, and interactions among group members. In this section, we present a brief sample of group dynamics measures to acquaint group leaders and researchers with currently available standardized procedures for understanding group process. Our selected descriptions are intended to be introductory, thus permitting readers to choose measures, review them in further detail, and apply the most suitable instrument for their group work needs.

Forsyth (1999) describes a variety of observational methods available to the group work practitioner. Some practical measurement methods that involve observing and record-ing of individual and group behaviors include participant observation and structured obser-vational measures. One useful measurement system is interactional process analysis (IPA), developed by Bales (1950). IPA is a structured coding system for classifying behaviors among group members and is delineated by task and socioemotional activities. Forsyth (1999) notes that IPA is valuable because it reports the frequency of occurrences of behavior of group members and "makes possible comparisons across categories, group members, and even different groups" (p. 33).

Group cohesion, engagement, and level of trust can be measured with the Group Cli-mate Questionnaire (MacKenzie, 1983), a brief 12-item measure consisting of three scales: Engagement, Differentiation, and Individuation. The Group Cohesiveness Scale (Budman, Soldz, Demby, Davis, & Merry, 1993) explores group connectedness and openness to self-disclosure and consists of six subscales (Withdrawal, Interest, Trust, Cooperation, Ex-pressed Caring, and Focus) and one global scale (Cohesiveness). Another recently developed instrument is the Groupwork Engagement Measure (Macgowan, 1997, 2000). It consists of a 37-item scale composed of seven dimensions: group member attendance, contributions, relations to members and to worker, contracting, and working on own and other members' problems.

There are also tools to measure therapeutic group factors and group session outcomes. The Therapeutic Factor Scale (Butler & Fuhriman, 1983), for example, examines the exis-tence of therapeutic factors across group sessions. It is based on the work of Yalom (1995), a leading scholar in group psychotherapy. Important group therapeutic factors delineated in this model include catharsis, insight, interpersonal learning, and cohesion, all essential di-mensions of group dynamics. Other scales for measuring group outcomes include the Group Sessions Rating Scale (Getter, Litt, Kadden, & Cooney, 1992), practical for assessing the use of various therapeutic interventions by both group members and facilitators of counseling and psychoeducational groups; the Individual Group Member Interpersonal Process Scale (Soldz, Budman, Davis, & Demby, 1993), for analyzing group interactions along 21 group process dimensions; and the Interpersonal Relations Checklist (Shadish, 1986), a 66-item self- or observer-related behavioral checklist that assesses group members' knowledge and skills in understanding emotions, thoughts, and behaviors.

A variety of comprehensive scales measure a range of group dynamic processes simulta-neously. These include the Group Emotionality Rating System (GERS; Karterud & Foss, 1989), the Hill Interaction Matrix (HIM; Hill, 1977), the Member–Leader Scoring System (Mann, Gibbard, & Hartman, 1967), the Hostility/Support Scale (Beck, 1983), the Client and Therapist Experiencing Scales (Klein, Mathieu-Coughlan, & Kiesler, 1986), and the Sys-tematic Multiple Level Observation of Groups Scale better known as SYMLOG (Bales et al., 1979). The GERS is a coding system for group functioning based on the work of Bion (1961). GERS includes five rated group dimensions of emotionality: Fight, Flight, Depend-ency, Pairing, and Neutral. The GERS is a conceptually driven rating system with high reli-ability and validity, though its utility is questionable in deriving a detailed process analysis of one session when used alone. It has been recommended in combination with qualitative methods such as hermeneutics.

The HIM is a behavioral coding scheme that measures the therapeutic quality of ex-changes among group members (Hill, 1965). The HIM comprises four process instruments, including the HIM-SS (statement by statement), HIM-A and B (predicting an individual's behavior in a group), and HIM-G (examining group interaction). Another group dynamics assessment package, the Member–Leader Scoring System, is used to code the verbal interactions of group leaders and members in small groups. It has been used to understand the leader-to-member and member-to-leader exchanges in therapy, educational, and training groups (Cytrynbaum & Hallberg, 1993). The main focus of this group process system is on how group members relate to authority.

The Hostility/Support Scale is a group process analysis measure designed to assess whether statements made in the course of group interaction are negative or supportive toward the person being addressed. The instrument was developed to identify changes from group periods of tension, criticism, and conflict to ones of mutual support and encouragement in psychotherapy groups. In conjunction with the Hostility/Support Scale, the Client and Therapist Experiencing Scales measure both therapist and group member exchanges, including engagement and involvement in the group process and facilitative responses made by group therapists toward group members.

A well-known group dynamics assessment system is SYMLOG, a measurement method for assessing norms, roles, and other dimensions of group as a whole (Bales, 1980; Bales et al., 1979). This measurement system allows for graphical representation and quantification of group observation data. SYMLOG can be used as a self-report measure or as an observational measure. Polley, Hare, and Stone (1988) have developed a group practitioner's handbook with examples of applications of SYMLOG for educational and therapy settings. For a more comprehensive discussion of methods to measure group dynamics, see the previously described review articles or books by Forsyth (1999) and Toseland and Rivas (2001).

CONCLUSION

In this chapter, we have presented a conceptual framework to help guide, organize, and refine thinking about group dynamics in social work practice with treatment and task groups. We have conceptualized these dynamics as falling into five domains: (1) communication processes and interaction patterns, (2) interpersonal attraction and cohesion, (3) social integration and influence, (4) power and control, and (5) the overall group culture.

Although an understanding of group dynamics is essential for effective practice with individuals and communities, it is our belief that focused attention to the dynamic processes that occur in groups is what distinguishes group work from other forms of social work practice. In the case of treatment groups, it is also important to remain cognizant that group work is not just working with a collection of individuals within a group context.

We hope that this chapter has highlighted the power that group dynamics have to change the lives of people. Neglecting the therapeutic power of group dynamics greatly diminishes the ability of the worker to help members achieve their goals. Similarly, task groups, such as committees, teams, and boards of directors, are not merely collections of individuals. The synergy that is created when people come together to work in these groups transcends the collection of individual efforts. The group takes on a life of its own, and the group dynamic processes that result have an impact far beyond what the collection of individuals working alone could accomplish by themselves.

Looking to the future, we believe that more attention will be paid to group dynamics in virtual groups. It is becoming easier and less costly for people to meet over the telephone using teleconferencing capabilities and through chat rooms, bulletin boards, and other forms of computer-mediated groups. (See Meier, Chapter 28, this volume, for detailed information on this subject.) Because there are no visual cues in telephone or computer groups, and because communication may be asynchronous in computer groups, dynamic processes are somewhat different in these groups than in face-to-face groups. Although some work has already been done to elucidate the dynamic processes in virtual groups, more work is needed as these groups continue to become more popular in our culture.

It is clear that culture, ethnicity, and race affect the dynamic processes that develop and evolve in groups. In this increasingly multicultural society, it is imperative to examine in greater depth the impact of culture, ethnicity, and race on the groups in which we all participate. This priority is in keeping with a long and rich tradition within social group work practice of bringing together and fostering understanding and mutual respect among people from different backgrounds.

REFERENCES

Alimo-Metcalfe, B., & Alban-Metcalfe, R. J. (2001). The development of a new transformational leadership questionnaire. *Journal of Occupational and Organizational Psychology, 74*, 1–27.

Anderson, J., & Carter, R. W. (Eds.). (2003). *Diversity perspectives for social work practice: Constructivism and the constructivist framework*. New York: Pearson Allyn & Bacon.

Asch, S. E. (1952). *Social psychology*. Englewood Cliffs, NJ: Prentice-Hall.

Asch, S. E. (1955). Opinions and social pressures. *Scientific American, 193*(5), 31–35.

Asch, S. E. (1957, April). An experimental investigation of group influence. In *Preventive and Social Psychiatry*. Symposium conducted at the Walter Reed Army Institute of Research, Washington, DC.

Avila, D. L., & Avila, A. L. (1988). Mexican Americans. In N. A. Vacc, J. Wittmer, & S. DeVaney (Eds.), *Experiencing and counseling multicultural and diverse populations* (2nd ed., pp. 289–316). Muncie, IN: Accelerated Development.

Bales, R. (1950). *Interaction process analysis: A method for the study of small groups*. Reading, MA: Addison-Wesley.

Bales, R. (1980). *SYMLOG: Case study kit*. New York: Free Press.

Bales, R., Cohen, S., & Williamson, S. (1979). *SYMLOG: A system for the multiple level observations of groups*. New York: Free Press.

Bass, B. M. (1985). *Leadership and performance beyond expectations*. New York: Free Press.

Bass, B. M. (1995). Theory of transformational leadership redux. *Leadership Quarterly, 6*, 463–478.

Bass, B. M., & Avolio, B. J. (1994). *Improving organizational effectiveness through transformational leadership*. Thousand Oaks, CA: Sage.

Beck, A. P. (1983). A process analysis of group development. *Group, 7*(1), 19–26.

Benne, K. D., & Sheats, P. (1948). Functional roles of group members. *Journal of Social Issues, 4*(2), 41–49.

Bion, W. (1961). *Experiences in groups*. London: Tavistock.

Budman, S., Soldz, S., Demby, A., Davis, M., & Merry, J. (1993). What is cohesiveness? An empirical examination. *Small Group Research, 24*, 199–214.

Butler, T., & Fuhriman, A. (1983). Level of functioning and length of time in treatment variables influencing patients' therapeutic experience in group psychotherapy. *International Journal of Group Psychotherapy, 33*, 489–504.

Cartwright, D. (1968). The nature of group cohesiveness. In D. Cartwright & A. Zander (Eds.), *Group dynamics: Research and theory* (3rd ed., pp. 91–109). New York: Harper & Row.

Cartwright, D., & Zander, A. (Eds.). (1968). *Group dynamics: Research and theory* (3rd ed.). New York: Harper & Row.

Conger, J. A. (1999). Charismatic and transformational leadership in organizations: An insider's perspective on these developing streams of research. *Leadership Quarterly, 10*(2), 145–179.

Conger, J. A., & Kanungo, R. N. (1998). *Charismatic leadership in organizations*. Thousand Oaks, CA: Sage.

Cytrynbaum, S., & Hallberg, M. (1993). Gender and authority in group relations conferences: So what have we learned in fifteen years of research? In S. Cytrynbaum & S. A. Lee (Eds.), *Proceedings of the 10th Scientific Meeting of the A. K. Rice Institute (pp. 63–73). Jupiter, FL: A. K. Rice Institute.

Davis, L. E., Galinsky, M. J., & Schopler, J. H. (1995). RAP: A framework for leading multiracial groups. *Social Work, 40*(2), 155–165.

Delucia-Waack, J. (1997). Measuring the effectiveness of group work: A review and analysis of process and outcome measures. *Journal for Specialists in Group Work, 22*(4), 277–293.

Deutsch, M., & Gerard, H. (1955). A study of normative and informational social influence upon individual judgement. *Journal of Abnormal and Social Psychology, 51*, 629–636.

Fenster, A. (1996). Group therapy as an effective treatment modality for people of color. *International Journal of Group Psychotherapy, 46*(30), 399–416.

Festinger, L. (1950). Informal social communication. *Psychological Review, 57*, 271–282.

Forsyth, D. (1999). *Group dynamics* (3rd ed.). Belmont, CA: Brooks/Cole-Wadsworth.

French, J. R. P., Jr., & Raven, B. (1959). The bases of social power. In D. Cartwright (Ed.), *Studies in social power* (pp. 150–167). Ann Arbor, MI: Institute for Social Research.

Fuhriman, A., & Barlow, S. (1994). Interaction analysis: Instrumentation and issues. In A. Fuhriman & G. Burlingame (Eds.), *Handbook of group psychotherapy: An empirical and clinical synthesis* (pp. 191–222). New York: Wiley.

Fuhriman, A., & Packard, T. (1986). Group process instruments: Therapeutic themes and issues. *International Journal of Group Psychotherapy, 36*(3), 399–425.

Galinsky, M., & Schopler, J. (1977). Warning: Groups may be dangerous. *Social Work, 22*(2), 89–94.

Galinsky, M. J., & Schopler, J. H. (1989). Developmental patterns in open-ended groups. *Social Work with Groups, 12*(2), 99–114.

Garland, J., Jones, H., & Kolodny, R. (1976). A model of stages of group development in social work groups. In S. Bernstein (Ed.), *Explorations in group work* (pp. 17–71). Boston: Charles River Books.

Getter, H., Litt, M., Kadden, R., & Cooney, N. (1992). Measuring treatment process in coping skills and interactional group therapies for alcoholism. *International Journal of Group Psychotherapy, 42*, 419–430.

Gray-Little, B., & Kaplan, D. (2000). Race and ethnicity in psychotherapy research. In C. Snyder & R. Ingram (Eds.), *Handbook of psychological change*. New York: Wiley.

Han, A. Y., & Vasquez, M. (1995). Group interventions and treatment with ethnic minorities. In J. Aponte, R. Rivers, & J. Wohl (Eds.), *Psychological interventions and cultural diversity* (pp. 109–127). Boston: Allyn & Bacon.

Hare, A. P., Blumberg, H. H., Davies, M. F., & Kent, M. V. (1995). *Small group research: A handbook*. Norwood, NJ: Ablex.

Hare, A. P., Blumberg, H. H., Davies, M. F., & Kent, M. V. (1996). *Small groups: An introduction*. Westport, CT: Praeger.

Hill, F. (1965). *Hill Interaction Matrix* (rev. ed.). Los Angeles: University of Southern California, Youth Studies Center.

Hill, F. (1977). Hill Interaction Matrix (HIM): The conceptual framework, derived rating scales, and an updated bibliography. *Small Group Behavior, 8*(3), 251–268.

Hopps, J. G., & Pinderhughes, E. B. (1999). *Group work with overwhelmed clients*. New York: Free Press.

House, R. J., & Aditya, R. N. (1997). The social scientific study of leadership: Quo vadis? *Journal of Management, 23*, 409–473.

Janis, I. L. (1972). *Victims of groupthink*. Boston: Houghton Mifflin.

Janis, I. L. (1982). *Groupthink: Psychological studies of policy decisions and fiascos* (2nd ed.). Boston: Houghton Mifflin.

Johnson, D., & Johnson, F. (2000). *Joining together: Group theory and group skills* (8th ed.). Boston: Allyn & Bacon.

Jones, L.V. (2000). *Enhancing psychosocial competence among black women through an innovative psycho-educational group intervention*. Ann Arbor, MI: UMI Bell & Howell.

Jung, D., & Sosik, J. (2002). Transformational leadership in work groups: The role of enpowerment, cohesiveness, and collective efficacy on perceived group performance. *Small Group Research,* *33*(3), 313–336.

Karterud, S., & Foss, T. (1989). Group Emotionality Rating System: A modification of Thelen's method of assessing emotionality in groups. *Small Group Behavior, 2,* 131–150.

Kivlighan, D., & Tarrant, J. (2001). Does group climate mediate the group leadership–group member outcome relationship? A test of Yalom's hypotheses about leadership priorities. *Group Dynamics: Theory, Research, and Practice, 5*(3), 220–234.

Klein, M., Mathieu-Coughlan, P., & Kiesler, D. (1986). The Experiencing Scales. In L. S. Greenberg & W. M. Pinsof (Eds.), *The psychotherapeutic process: A research handbook* (pp. 21–71). New York: Guilford Press.

Latané, B., Williams, K., & Harkins, S. (1979). Many hands make light the work: The causes and consequences of social loafing. *Journal of Personality and Social Psychology, 37,* 822–832.

Levi, D. (2001). *Group dynamics for teams.* Thousand Oaks: Sage.

Lewin, K. (1951). *Field theory in social science.* New York: Harper.

Lewin, K., & Lippitt, R. (1938). An experimental approach to the study of autocracy and democracy: A preliminary note. *Sociometry, 1,* 292–300.

Lewin, K., Lippitt, R., & White, R. (1939). Patterns of aggressive behavior in experimentally created "social climates." *Journal of Social Psychology, 10,* 271–299.

Macgowan, M. J. (1997). A measure of engagement for social group work: The Groupwork Engagement Measure (GEM). *Journal of Social Service Research, 23*(2), 17–37.

Macgowan, M. J. (2000). Evaluation of a measure of engagement for group work. *Research on Social Work Practice, 10*(3), 348–361.

MacKenzie, K. R. (1983). The clinical application of a group climate measure. In R. Dies & K. R. MacKenzie (Eds.), *Advances in group psychotherapy: Integrating research and practice* (pp. 159–170). New York: International Universities Press.

Mann, R., Gibbard, G., & Hartman, J. (1967). *Interpersonal styles and group development: An analysis of the member–leader relationship.* New York: Wiley.

Matsukawa, L. A. (2001). Group therapy with multiethnic members. In T. Wen-Sheng & J. Streltzer (Eds.), *Culture and psychotherapy: A guide to clinical practice* (pp. 243–261). Washington, DC: American Psychiatric.

McGrath, J. E. (1984). *Groups: Interaction and performance.* Englewood Cliffs, NJ: Prentice-Hall.

Merta, R. J. (1995). Group work: Multicultural perspectives. In J. G. Ponterotto, J. M. Casas, L. A. Suzuki, & C. A. Alexander (Eds.), *Handbook of multicultural counseling* (pp. 567–585). Thousands Oaks, CA: Sage.

Milgram, S. (1974). *Obedience to authority.* New York: Harper & Row.

Moscovici, S. (1985). Social influence and conformity. In G. Lindzey & E. Aronson (Eds.), *Handbook of social psychology* (3rd ed., Vol. 2, pp. 347–412). New York: Random House.

Moscovici, S. (1994). Three concepts: Minority, conflict, and behavioral styles. In S. Moscovici, M. Faina, & A. Maass (Eds.), *Minority influence* (pp. 233–251). Chicago: Nelson-Hall.

Moscovici, S., & Lage, E. (1976). Studies in social influence: 3. Majority versus minority influence in a group. *European Journal of Social Psychology, 6,* 149–174.

Moscovici, S., Lage, E., & Naffrechoux, M. (1969). Influence of a consistent minority on the responses of a majority in a color perception task. *Sociometry, 12,* 365–380.

Newcomb, T. M. (1943). *Personality and social change.* New York: Dryden.

Newcomb, T. M. (1960). Varieties of interpersonal attraction. In D. Cartwright & A. Zander (Eds.), *Group dynamics: Research and theory* (2nd ed.). Evanston, IL: Row, Peterson.

Newcomb, T. M. (1961). *The acquaintance process.* New York: Holt, Rinehart, & Winston.

Newcomb, T. M. (1963). Stabilities underlying changes in interpersonal attraction. *Journal of Abnormal and Social Psychology, 66,* 376–386.

Nixon, H. (1979). *The small group.* Englewood Cliffs, NJ: Prentice-Hall.

Olmsted, M. (1959). *The small group.* New York: Random House.

Parsons, T. (1951). *The social system.* New York: Free Press.

Pinderhughes, E. B. (1989). *Understanding race, ethnicity and power.* New York: Free Press.

Polley, R. B., Hare, A. P., & Stone, P. J. (Eds.). (1988). *The SYMLOG practitioner: Applications of small group research*. New York: Praeger.

Schopler, J., Abell, M., & Galinsky, M. (1998). Technology-based groups: A review and conceptual framework for practice. *Social Work, 43*(3), 254–267.

Shadish, W. R. (1986). The validity of a measure of intimate behavior. *Small Group Behavior, 17*, 113–120.

Shamir, B., House, R., & Arthur, M. B. (1993). The motivation effects of charismatic leadership: A self-concept based theory. *Organization Science, 4*, 584.

Sherif, M. (1936). *The psychology of social norms*. New York: Harper & Row.

Smokowski, P. R., Galinsky, M., & Harlow, K. (2001). Using technologies in groupwork: 2. Computer-based groups. *Group Work, 13*(1), 98–115.

Smokowski, P., Rose, S., Todar, K., & Reardon, K. (1999). Post-group casualty-status, group events and leader behavior: An early look into the dynamics of damaging group experiences. *Research on Social Work Practice, 9*(5), 555–574.

Soldz, S., Budman, S., Davis, M., & Demby, A. (1993). Beyond the interpersonal circumplex in group psychotherapy: The structure and relationship to outcome of the Individual Group Member Interpersonal Process Scale. *Journal of Clinical Psychology, 49*, 551–563.

Stewart, G., Manz, C., & Sims, H. (1999). *Team work and group dynamics*. New York: Wiley.

Sue, D. W., & Sue D. (1999). *Counseling the culturally different: Theory and practice* (3rd ed.). New York: Wiley.

Sweeney, J. (1973). An experimental investigation of the free rider problem. *Social Science Research, 2*, 277–292.

Thibaut, J. W., & Kelley, H. H. (1959). *The social psychology of groups*. New York: Wiley.

Toseland, R. W., & Rivas, R. F. (2001). *An introduction to group work practice* (4th ed.). Boston: Allyn & Bacon.

Tsui, P., & Schultz, G. L. (1988). Ethnic factors in group process: Cultural dynamics in multi-ethnic therapy groups. *American Journal of Orthopsychiatry, 58*(1), 136–142.

Tuckman, B. (1963). Developmental sequence in small groups. *Psychological Bulletin, 63*, 384–399.

Yalom, I. D. (1995). *The theory and practice of group psychotherapy* (4th ed.). New York: Basic Books.

Chapter 2

An Ecological–Systems Perspective

JOHN E. TROPMAN

This chapter looks at the issues of ecological influence on groups and group practice. For these purposes, all kinds of groups might be considered, from therapeutic groups to performing groups to teams, among others (Andrews, 2001; Forte, 1994; Garvin, 1997; Toleman & Molidor, 1994).

AN ECOLOGICAL PERSPECTIVE

An ecological perspective uses group context—in particular, group characteristics, competencies, conditions, and change—to look at a group ecosystem. (I will say more about these five C's later.)

Originally a biological term, the "ecological" perspective is one that considers the relationship between a species and its environment. In a seashore ecosystem, for example, one might look at the crab population, what it affects, and what affects it. *Social ecology* came to mean the application of that biological term to human social interaction. Many environmental groups are specifically concerned about the relationship of humans to our world resources. More specifically, an ecological perspective in social work means looking at the interdependencies of a client or client system and other social systems in its environment.

Structural Influence

An *ecology of groups* considers the influences that *extragroup* variables have on group activity. Some of these variables are structural and deal with the influences that the position of the group has vis-à-vis other groups. Groups are, of course, embedded in larger and concurrent institutions and hence experience influence from their sociostructural location. The fact, for example, that we are members of so many groups creates the potential and the actuality of conflict between and among groups, which is one kind of ecological influence.

Sociocultural Influence

Other influences are cultural in nature and deal with the impact of extragroup beliefs and values on the structure and culture of the group itself. For example, groups within a social agency are influenced by the policy of that agency. That is structural influence. Groups within that same agency are also influenced by the values, beliefs, and norms of that agency. That is cultural influence. Those same intra-agency groups may experience influence from other groups in the community, as well as from the culture of the community. These, too, are ecological influences.

A SYSTEMS PERSPECTIVE

A *systems perspective* looks at the overall group as a real structure. Although it is made up of individual members at any point in time, the group is in (a) reality *sui generis* and has a history and evolution different from its current members or participants. By "in reality," I mean to emphasize that, although the group is in part the product of the elements that compose it and in part driven by the larger systems in which it nests (see Table 2.1), the group has a reality of its own that cannot be explained by its composition or context. (It is the context, or extragroup influences and resources, to be discussed momentarily, that form the crux of the ecological perspective.)

These realities of interaction and product can be productive or destructive, healthy or unhealthy. For example, in gangs, killing and vandalism may be the unhealthy product of group interaction, and group practitioners (gang workers) may be inserted into membership to change the nature of the interaction that leads to these unhealthy outcomes.

All systems, groups included of course, typically contain processes of flow, exchange, and transformation over time. *Flow* refers to influences such as resources, information, perspective, and energy that enter into or impinge on the group. Flow calls our attention, first, to the input phase, when resources enter the system; second, to their processing over time within the group system; and, third, to the output phase (which is usually input into another system).

Systems that deal with people are called *people processing systems*, and, if the goal is to change the people, we might call them *people changing systems* (Street, Vinter, & Perrow, 1966). *Exchange* refers to the use of the previously mentioned influences to attain some system goal.[1] *Transformation* addresses the change that resources and the system undergo as exchange takes place and calls attention to the product of the system. In people processing systems, we call this *outcome* (a changed state).

Many agencies talk about *outputs* instead, such as number of group meetings held and number of times people attended the group, among other things. It is important to remember that outputs are a system measure rather than a result. In other words, if an agency has group meetings about anger management, its report that 14 sessions were held is an output. That number does not tell us anything about outcomes—did the group members actually get better at anger management?

THE FIVE C'S PERSPECTIVE ON GROUP PRACTICE

As systems themselves embedded in an ecology of other, larger systems, groups have at least five properties that group practitioners can use to describe and change them and on which system influences may have an impact, intentional or random. These properties include group characteristics, group competencies, group conditions, group change, and group context. Let us consider each.

Group Characteristics

The property of group characteristics involves variables such as group composition (gender, race, ethnicity, age, other memberships, etc.). It also involves temperament of groups. Some groups are more task oriented and minimize process; others are more process oriented and have trouble getting to task. Some groups like to interact with participants outside the group; others value only the members. Group practitioners may influence groups by adjusting, changing, or working with issues of composition.

Group Competencies

Generally speaking, groups have competencies (knowledge plus skills) for dealing with certain kinds of issues, problems, and tasks. All groups do not have the same kinds of skills. For example, a cancer support group may be excellent at dealing with issues of cancer but not other kinds of issues. A string quartet may do well with Haydn but not Brahms. A football team may execute pass plays well but not running plays. Decision-making groups may do well with some kinds of decisions but not others. Group practitioners may need to teach members skills the members do not have or assist them in unlearning skills that the group is overapplying (as in the phrase, when you are a hammer, everything is a nail!).[2]

Group Conditions

Conditions address issues of group structure and culture. Structure refers to the way in which the group is organized, both formally and informally (though informal structure comes close to culture). The group may have a formal structure, with officers and other appointed, assigned, or elected roles, or it may be more loosely structured, with rotating roles. (In my grandson Jared's co-op play school, for example, he gets to be the leader when his mom or dad are on for their "day"; mom or dad are helpers, and they better not forget it.)

Group culture addresses the norms and values of how the group works. Norms are group behavioral guidelines. Values—ideas to which feeling is attached—are concepts held to be vital by the group. For example, some groups encourage open participation, in which members or participants say what they think as they wish, whereas in others, newer members (or older ones) may speak first; there may be other rules of participation. How a group handles criticism of members is another issue. Some cultures allow very direct criticism, whereas others prefer more muted disagreement.

Group values are also important. Most groups like members or participants to be committed to the same kinds of things. Groups are entitled to have their values, but they must also recognize diversity and respect the values of others—both group members who hold different values and other groups that have different values. Group practitioners often work with the structure and culture of groups to assist the group in its functioning.

Group Change

Group change has several foci. One refers to the development of a group over time, as in the stages of group development identified by one writer (Bruce Tuckman)[3] as "forming, storming, norming, and performing" (Schopler & Galinsky, 1995, p. 10).

Group goals are another area in which change can occur. Groups can pick goals to pursue and achieve (both outcomes and outputs). They may be formalized in a strategic plan, or they may be less formal than that. In production groups, whose very purpose is to create some result—such as a decision, a piece of music, or a meal—change occurs as information, musical ideas, or ingredients that move into the group at the input stage are transformed and come out of the group as a finished product.

In *throughput*, the inputs are combined and remade or assembled into a final output, such as a decision, a performance, or a meal. This example further illustrates the difference between outputs and outcomes. In this case, the output goal is the decision, the performance, or the meal. However, another goal for the outcome is to produce a *good* decision, a *good* performance, or a *good* meal. Even further, a more encompassing goal might be to have the good decision implemented, to have the audience enjoy the good performance, and to have the diners enjoy the good meal.

To assist groups in achieving these outputs and outcomes, group practitioners may alter change processes (velocity, sequence, handling, etc.) to create different outputs or outcomes. For example, processes of becoming a group member may take too long and need to be shortened; alternatively, termination or processes of "unbecoming" a group member may take too long. Each of these issues might be addressed by a group practitioner.

Group Context

Groups exist and are embedded in milieus. Four types of contexts are important: other groups, organizational contexts, community contexts, and societal contexts. Of course, there are world contexts for some groups, but I touch on that only briefly. Each of these entities, systems in themselves, is part of an ecology that shapes and steers groups in ways that the group does not always understand or appreciate. It is this focus that is the core of the chapter.

AN ECOLOGICAL–SYSTEMS PERSPECTIVE FOR GROUP PRACTICE

As a way of approaching the issue of group ecology and assisting us to focus on this system model, we consider the following six levels: the person, the group (our focus here), the organization, the community, the society, and the world. Each system level or client system has two elements: the source of problems or issues and the target of intervention. That is, problems can occur at the individual, the group, the organization, the community, the society, or the world levels. Each problem or issue may be dealt with at a variety of levels, or several at once.

Direct intervention means that the problem is addressed at the level at which it is mani-

TABLE 2.1. Relationships among Six System Levels as Sources of Problems/Issues and Targets of Intervention

Source system level for problem/issue (independent variable)	"Target" system (dependent variable)					
	Individual	Group	Organization	Community	Society	World
Individual	D(1)	Usi(2)	Usi(3)	Usi(4)	Usi(5)	Usi(6)
Group	Dsi(7)	D(8)	Usi(9)	Usi(10)	Usi(11)	Usi(12)
Organization	Dsi(13)	**Dsi(14)**	D(15)	Usi(16)	Usi(17)	Usi(18)
Community	Dsi(19)	**Dsi(20)**	Dsi(21)	D(22)	Usi(23)	Usi(24)
Society	Dsi(25)	**Dsi(26)**	Dsi(27)	Dsi(28)	D(29)	Usi(30)
World	Dsi(31)	**Dsi(32)**	Dsi(33)	Dsi(34)	Dsi(35)	D(36)

Note. Target system, the system that is the target of change (effect); source system, the system that is the source of the impetus for change; *D*, direct system connection—that is, the target and source system are on the same level [*D(1, 8, 15, 22, 29,* and *36*)]; hence, a group problem of issue has a group-level intervention; Usi, upward system influence (compositional), where interventions through the components of a system level are used to change the system level; Dsi, downward system influence (contextual), where supraordinate systems influence their components; **Dsi**, downward influence on groups, the subject matter of this chapter [**Dsi** (14, 20, 26, and 32)].

fest (e.g., individual-level problems are addressed at the individual level). But that is not the only choice, as Table 2.1 makes clear.

Compositional intervention is possible. This approach is called "compositional" because it looks "below" the system levels at which the problem occurs and seeks to change subsystem components.

When a problem occurs at the group level, group practitioners may seek to intervene at the individual level. When a problem occurs in an organization, practitioners may wish to intervene at the group or individual level, and so on.

Some examples may help. If an individual has a problem or issue and the practitioner intervenes at that level (individual adjustment and change), that would be a direct strategy. So, if an individual is depressed and is individually treated, that would be a direct strategy. If that individual joins a group with others who have similar issues, that would be downward system influence (cell 7). If a problem exists at a group level (e.g., "Queen Bee" junior high girls abusing "Wannabe" other girls in the school, then working with both groups directly would be a direct intervention (cell 8). An attempt to change policies in the school and to increase acceptance of diversity would be an organizational intervention (cell 14). An attempt to change culture in the community of the school, to involve parents, and so forth, would be a community intervention (cell 20).

Alternatively, *contextual* strategies are also appropriate (Tropman & Richards-Schuster, 2000). Here, the group practitioner might focus on systems that encompass the target system. Hence, if a problem occurs at the group level, the practitioner may wish to work at the organizational, community, societal, or world level in which the group is embedded. Ecologically speaking, this is the focus of this chapter. What might be the influences of organizational location, community location, societal location, or world location on the group and group practice in question?

Table 2.2 gives a completely described set of the intersections at which influence can occur. Each of the superordinate systems can influence the group and group practice, as well. Groups exist, and group practice occurs, in organizational, community, societal, and world contexts. Each context may influence groups and group practice, and groups and group practice may experience influence from one or all of those systems.

TABLE 2.2. Illustrative Grid of the Influence of "Suprasystem" Structure and Culture on Group Variables and Practice

Context	Group characteristics	Group competencies	Group conditions	Group change	Group practice
Organizational	1	2	3	4	5
Community	6	7	8	9	10
Societal	11	12	13	14	15
World	16	17	18	19	20

Obviously, every influence "cell" cannot be considered here—there are 40 of them, not counting, of course, the possibility of multiple influences just mentioned. But readers can see the flow and add examples themselves as well. The sheer size and complexity of the ecology, however, explains why workers might be tempted to give little more than lip service to the ecological perspective. There is a lot to think about. For our purposes here, we can see that each system level "above" the group has a structure and a culture (or really many structures and cultures). These structures and cultures can and do influence the C's that I discussed before (group characteristics, group competencies, group conditions, group change, and group context). They can also influence the things that the group practitioner needs.

But as a start, let's look at cells 1, 2, 3, 4, and 5 in Table 2.2. For example, in cell 1, an agency (organizational context for a group) might influence whom the group values as a member (e.g., domestic violence victims but not domestic violence perpetrators), and they might actually restrict membership as well. In cell 2, agency policy and practice influence what skills they teach group participants (e.g., fight vs. flight skills for victims). In cell 3, the agency also influences elements of group structure (when the group can meet, how often) and group culture (appropriate norms and values). Cell 4 represents the influence of an agency on forming and disbanding the group. The group, of course, reciprocally influences these things as well. Similar examples of influence come from the community, the society, and the world.

The concept of "influence" is not all of a piece, either. Let us assume that contextual influences fall into two large categories: structural and cultural forces. In other words, context can influence groups and group practice through values and beliefs (and other "soft" controls) or through rules, regulations, and other physical structures (and other "hard" controls). Either or both can operate to influence both groups themselves and group practice.

As mentioned before, structural elements are the "hard" side of society—laws, regulations, money, equipment, population, workers, members, and so forth. In general, these are the things that Karl Marx and B. F. Skinner (Cowling, 1999; Nye, 1996) felt to be dominant. On the other hand, the "soft" side of systems—cultures and subcultures—deals with attitudes, norms, beliefs, and values, which are harder to see and track. In general, these are the kinds of variables that Max Weber and Sigmund Freud (Nye, 1996; Tropman, 2002; Weber, 1956) thought mattered.

THE FLOW OF INFLUENCE

Group Characteristics

Groups are limited by whom they can draw on as members and participants. This influence obtains both in terms of numbers and types of people. Apart from "raw" numbers, ecological influences create openings for and barriers to group membership. Years ago, for example, when Boy Scout troops were primarily organized within a church/synagogue framework, the troops used to favor membership of those from their own faith and suggested that potential members from other faiths join their own faith-based troop.

Communities also influence groups through racial, ethnic, and religious segregation (usually housing based) and accepted prejudicial norms and values. Communities also exist within regions that vary greatly in size and diversity. In America, there are the New England or Yankee community, the somewhat broader eastern community, the midwestern community, the southern (and perhaps southwestern) community, the West, and of course, the Far West, including California, Oregon, and Washington. The Washington community includes Vancouver, which sees itself more connected to the Pacific Rim than to Canada. Each of these regions has structures and values that can sometimes lay dormant for years, appearing suddenly and unexpectedly on certain occasions, like a giant Internet pop-up advertisement. These structures and values influence group characteristics (not only in the Boy Scouts, but in all kinds of groups, including boards of directors, self-help groups, camping groups, character-building groups, therapeutic groups, etc.).

Looking at societal influences, "macro values" of a state certainly influence group participation. American society, for example, is well known for its participative, voluntaristic orientation, something that makes voluntary organizations more a part of the American landscape than is true elsewhere in the world (De Tocqueville, 1835/1945). On the other hand, there is evidence that this participative trend is declining. Harvard political scientist Robert Putnam (2000), in his book *Bowling Alone*, has pointed out that in many sectors, volunteer participation in community groups is declining.

But perhaps this trend is not so surprising after all. For, on the one hand, America is known for its volunteerism; on the other hand, it is also known for its individualism. Culture in the West celebrates the mountain man much more than the wagon train. And even in social work itself, group work has had a harder time than social casework, which focuses more on the individual. And then there are world elements that affect group membership and characteristics.

For all of its problems, the United States seems to be the place people worldwide want to come to. It is both a testimony to that observation and a huge sadness that people are literally dying to get to America. But the number of ethnicities and religions in the United States is staggering. Group practice needs not only to be aware of these trends and situations but also to develop the cultural competence to work with the greatest diversity of group members.

Group Competencies

Competence can be defined as knowledge plus skill. Involved in the competent group are raw and synthesized knowledge, as well as the ability to reorganize and apply that knowledge to group task and process issues. Groups and individuals seem to do best when they are at the intersection of challenge and skill, as suggested in Figure 2.1.

When a group's challenge exceeds its skill, the group becomes anxious and frenetic (A4); when a group's skill exceeds its challenge, the group becomes bored (A2). When challenge and skill are in harmony (A1, A3), groups are in the flow channel and performing well. Group practitioners need, overall, to work at increasing both the challenges and the skills (competencies) of groups, because neither groups nor individuals remain static. They

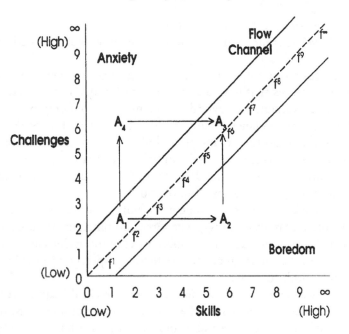

FIGURE 2.1. Going with the flow: Why the complexity of consciousness increases as a result of flow experiences. Adapted from Csikszentmihalyi (1991, p. 74). Copyright 1991 by HarperCollins. Adapted by permission.

are either moving up the flow channel or to one or the other side. Most typical is that skills increase faster than challenges, thus leading to group and member boredom (Csikszentmihalyi, 1991).

Moving up involves a "staircase" of competence, from the novice to the beginner to the journeyperson to the expert to the master. Simply stated, the novice is one who is just beginning and paying a lot of attention to rules. Performance is slow and jerky. The beginner is one who has learned the basics and is not attending to patterns not mentioned in rules. At the end of the beginner phase, *rule fade* begins—that situation in which we begin to operate more automatically. Performance is quicker and smoother.

The journeyperson is one for whom rule fade has become mostly complete, and performance is standard in terms of speed and smoothness. The expert is one who knows many of the nuances and special features. Performance is rapid and sure. The master is one whose performance seems effortless and unerring, as well as innovative and creative.

The flow chart displayed in Figure 2.1 illustrates this progress. For example, in terms of location in the flow channel, the novice could be at 22, perhaps, the beginner at 33, the journeyperson at 44, the expert at 66, and the master at 99.

These differences can of course be applied to members or participants of the group. Group practitioners have to work skillfully to integrate memberships of different levels of personal competency. These designations can be applied to the group itself. Indeed, groups, teams, and boards are rated along these lines. For example, teams with lots of individual experts and masters do not necessarily perform well as a unit.

Context influences and affects both challenge and skill. Challenge usually comes from context, though in its raw form, challenge can arrive in undifferentiated pulses of varying amounts. It therefore needs to be managed (organized, structured) so as to be sufficiently stimulating yet not overwhelming when the pulses are large and "boosted" when the pulses are low.

Context influences the supply of competence in groups in several ways. From an organizational perspective, teams that have a complement of experts and masters and that function well are desirable assignments, rewards in themselves from employees of the organization (Ancona, Kochan, Van Maanen, Scully, & Westney, 1999). However, there are only so many experts and masters, so the organizational allocation of these resources is always an issue.[4] Organizations also, conversely, may find the suggestions of "top teams" irritating and weird. Organizations in general tend to the pedestrian rather than the innovative, in spite of lots of talk about organizational innovation.

One of the hallmarks of the very competent group is that it may pursue the "road not taken," which usually threatens existing procedures and patterns of influence in the organization. Similar perspectives prevail with respect to community, societal, and world influences. The very skills of the top team may cause these perspectives to be threatening to community, societal, or world interests.

Musical groups and sports teams do not necessarily have the same problems as organizational groups and teams. In both cases, their working interaction is episodic and time limited. Further, there are fairly well accepted standards of performance. Oddly, then, it is easier for top-performing musical or sports groups to gain acceptance. Coaches and maestros may, in a way, be thought of as group practitioners, as well as subject matter experts.

With respect to competency, the goal of the group practitioner is to blend different competency levels as needed to assist the group to grow in competency as a group over time and to integrate the performance of groups with very competent members (experts and masters) such that their performance can be greater than the sum of the parts—not, as is so often the case, less.

One final point about competency needs stressing. Groups have a real potential to perform many tasks better than individuals, if they are run right (Hackman, 1990, pp. 479ff.).[5] There is always subject matter knowledge of the engineering problem, the therapeutic problem, the musical piece, or the pass play.

However, there is one mechanism that all groups use at some point in their work: the meeting. Skills in effective meeting structure are essential for group practitioners and groups themselves. As readers know, the meeting is one area of American society (and the world, for that matter) that seems to have a universally problematic reputation. Group practitioners can help their groups through practicing and teaching excellent meeting management skills (Tropman, 2003).

Group Conditions

Groups must live in an organizational, community, societal, and world milieu. They must find some way to relate or connect to that milieu for their own survival and prosperity. And it is likely to be the case that the following proposition applies: Fissures and cleavages that separate and affect the organization, community, society, and world are likely to affect the groups within those entities. More particularly, I offer the following principles:

- *Principle 1*—the principle of structural isomorphism. Specifically, I argue that the structure of the group will be optimized by the group to fit or articulate with the structures of its important organizational, community, societal, and world connections. If the external environment is complex, then the structure of the group is likely to be complex as well. Otherwise it will have difficulty dealing with the environment on which it depends.

- *Principle 2*—the principle of substantive isomorphism. Specifically, the substantive nature of the group's organization will tend to match that of its environment.[6] Hence, if the group needs resources from, say, the United Way, it will tend to have someone (or a subcommittee) affect that connection.
- *Principle 3*—the principle of values. In general, groups will move toward adopting the same values held by those on whom they depend for resources. (Resources here can mean space to meet, cash for programs, members, staff, or simple permission to exist, among others.)[7]

Of course, it is not as simple as this. Some groups will take the opposite tack and become specifically counterstructural or countercultural, or they will seek other environmental locations in which their behaviors and values will be welcomed. The group practitioner here needs to be aware of the issues of "resource dependency" and assist the group in developing appropriate intragroup structures and values, within ethical limits, that will optimize its interactions with extragroup environments.

Group Change

Groups, like other forms of social organization, tend to avoid change. When change occurs, it is usually problematic. Some changes, as in the forming, storming, norming, and performing stages, are built into the group structure itself and seem to be natural elements in group development. For this kind of change, group practitioners need to assist groups in awareness of the cycle and the need to move through it. To move through it, the group must not become stuck in one cycle or endlessly repeat the cycle each time the group convenes. Of course, this work is made more difficult because new members who are "off cycle" are continually entering the group.

Another kind of change is suggested by the flow chart in Figure 2.1. As I mentioned, groups are in a dynamic field, not a static one, a point Csikszentmihalyi (1991) stresses. Being "in the flow channel" requires that the group continually undertake more complex tasks—move up the staircase of competence, as it were. The dynamism of the developmental situation means that groups cannot stand still. They either move "up" the flow channel or move into anxiety or boredom.

Thus the values and structures of any group need, at minimum, small adjustments over time. If done proactively, these adjustments (transactional change or evolution) allow the group to remain current and "ahead of the curve." The general rule is that the environment (mentioned in the previous section) is slowly changing all the time. For groups, the rule is that the rate of change within the group should be slightly greater than the rate of change in the environment, or the group may begin, slowly, to die.[8]

But slow changes are not always the answer. Sometimes social groups need to make fundamental shifts in their purpose and mission. We call this kind of change "transformational" change or revolution (Tichy & Devanna, 1986). It may be a board changing the purpose of the agency, a string quartet taking on a whole new repertoire, a therapeutic group altering its fundamental focus, or other changes. These are among the most difficult changes to make, and groups often do not negotiate them successfully.

One particular kind of transformational change that is very common and very difficult deserves mention here. It is the transition from "group" to "organization." I think it is fair to say that most social agencies started as small groups of concerned volunteers. For a while, they operated as a group, then they became a "quasi-organization" with a small/limited budget and a "working board" (usually the founders who have renamed themselves as a board and gotten a few more friends to help).

At some point, however, the quasi-organization needs to move into formal organizational status. It often gets grants, a budget, and a professional executive. It is at this point that the camaraderie of the founding period seems to disappear. Founding group members are often "fired" from the organization (Flamholtz & Randle, 2000). Transformational change does mean that different members win and lose. Often, though, groups are not able to take this step and remain in a sort of perpetual adolescence, with a problematic blend of informal funding structures and more formal group structures.

The role of the group practitioner here is to work with the group as a whole and with the individual members to assist in appropriate transitions. Often that means that founders must move on.

Group Context

The "flow" approach—and indeed my approach in this chapter—suggests that context influences groups, and no one would seriously disagree. It is important to note, though, that groups influence context as well. A touching article about a hospitalized terminally ill child in a family group reveals that "Hannah" would not let a large team of residents examine her. Rather, they had to come in smaller groups of two or, at the most, three. Also, they had to tell the 3-year-old Hannah their "real" names—Dr. Tony was the first. Soon all the doctors knew Hannah's routine and abided by it. Shortly after that, they applied her precepts to all their work with children, to great success. Though Hannah died, her "upward influence" affected her context (and a medical context at that) in a powerful and helpful way (Housden, 2002).

CONCLUSION

Obviously, the contextual influences are many and varied. The purpose of this discussion is one of sensitization and awareness enhancement. There is a system in which groups exist that has elements of flow, exchange, and transformation. We can look as well at the way that the five C's—characteristics, competencies, conditions, change, and context—affect group structure and culture. It needs to be understood as well—and group practitioners know this intuitively—that structure and culture, which need to support each other, do not change at the same rate and hence are the focus separately of group practice efforts.

An ecological approach to group practice tries to be somewhat more specific about context, which is, after all, rather large. I have outlined here a "periodic table" of sorts, which at least specifies the structure of influence. Group practitioners can use it as a sort of checklist when they are working with groups to get a more detailed perspective on the kinds of influences that an ecological perspective might provide. All too often the ecological perspective is used as a synonym for "everything and anything out there" that might "be important." The purpose of this work is to provide greater specification.

NOTES

1. "Effect" implies an intended use of influences; one might also note that "influences" affect systems operations and goals.
2. Typically, one teaches skills to individual members. Conceptually, though, it is possible to think of teaching the group a skill, especially when the group needs to perform qua group, as in a sports team or musical ensemble.
3. See *http://www.businessballs.com/tuckmanformingstormingnormingperforming.htm.*
4. It is also worth noting that organizations are frequently bad at identifying the experts they do have and often misidentify "compliance" as "expertise."
5. Hackman (1990) identifies several different types of work groups, including top management groups, one-shot project groups, professional support groups, performing groups, human service groups (taking care of people), customer service groups, and production groups, among others.
6. Conant and Ashby (1970) had a similar idea, though I was unaware of it until recently. They offer the "Law of Requisite Variety," which states that organizations (we could say groups) should be as "messy" as the surrounding environment.
7. Another example of this approach is called the "stakeholder model" in organizational work. See Ancona et al. (1999), Figure 9.3, and the associated discussion in that volume.
8. This phenomenon has come to be called the "boiled frog" effect. If you put a frog in cold water and slowly heat it, the frog does not notice that it is getting hotter and boils to death. When the "just noticeable difference" in environmental change outside the group is small, groups do not notice it (Tichy & Devanna, 1986).

REFERENCES

Ancona, D. G., Kochan, T., Van Maanen, J., Scully, M., & Westney, E. (1999). *Managing for the future: Organizational behavior and procedures* (2nd ed.). Cincinnati: South-Western.

Andrews, J. (2001). Group work's place in social work: An historical analysis. *Journal of Sociology and Social Welfare, 28*(4), 45–65.

Conant, R., & Ashby, R. (1970). Every good regulator of a system must be a model of that system. *International Journal of Systems Science, 7*(2), 89–97.

Cowling, M. (Ed.). (1999). *The Communist Manifesto: New interpretations.* New York: New York University Press.

Csikszentmihalyi, M. (1991). *Flow: The psychology of optimal experience.* New York: HarperCollins.

De Tocqueville, A. (1945). *Democracy in America* (H. Reeve, Trans.; F. Bowen & P. Bradley, Eds.). New York: Knopf. (Original work published 1835)

Flamholtz, E. G., & Randle, Y. (2000). *Growing pains: Transitioning from an entrepreneurship to a professionally managed firm.* San Francisco: Jossey-Bass.

Forte, J. (1994). Around the world with social group work. *Social Work With Groups, 17*(1, 2), 143–162.

Garvin, C. (1997). *Contemporary group work.* Boston: Allyn & Bacon.

Hackman, J. R. (Ed.). (1990). *Groups that work (and those that don't): Creating conditions for effective teamwork.* San Francisco: Jossey-Bass.

Housden, M. (2002). *Hannah's gift.* Retrieved July 21, 2003, from: *http://www.hannahsgift.com.*

Nye, R. (1996). *Three psychologies: Perspectives from Freud, Skinner, and Rogers.* Pacific Grove, CA: Brooks/Cole.

Putnam, R. D. (2000). *Bowling alone.* New York: Simon & Schuster.

Schopler, J., & Galinsky, M. (1995). Boundary spanning and group leadership functions: The third dimension. *Social Work with Groups, 18*(4), 3–17.

Street, D., Vinter, R., & Perrow, C. (1966). *Organization for treatment.* New York: Free Press.

Tichy, N., & Devanna, M. A. (1986). *The transformational leader.* New York: Wiley.

Toleman, R., & Molidor, C. (1994). A decade of social group work research: Trends in methodology, theory, and program development. *Research on Social Work Practice, 4*(2), 143–159.

Tropman, J. (2002). *The Catholic ethic and the spirit of community*. Washington, DC: Georgetown University Press.

Tropman, J. (2003). *Making meetings work: Achieving high quality group decisions* (2nd ed.). Thousand Oaks, CA: Sage.

Tropman, J., & Richards-Schuster, K. (2000). The concept of system levels in social work. In P. Allen-Meares & C. Garvin (Eds.), *The handbook of social work direct practice* (pp. 65–84). Thousand Oaks, CA: Sage.

Weber, M. (1956) *The Protestant ethic and the spirit of capitalism* (T. Parsons, Trans.). New York: Scribner.

Chapter 3

Social Group Work
in a Global Context

NAZNEEN S. MAYADAS
REBECCA SMITH
DOREEN ELLIOTT

The purpose of this chapter is to identify the international component and global issues in social group work and to raise the question, Is social group work socially constructed? If so, are there any global commonalities? Is it possible to have an international conception of social group work? Thus historical developments in social group work are briefly reviewed, the importance of the cultural context is discussed, and findings from reviews of the literature are presented. The chapter further reports findings from a worldwide study of group work in social work education. The results of this study are discussed in the context of professional imperialism, international knowledge transfer, and electronic communication.

INTERNATIONAL INFLUENCES
IN THE DEVELOPMENT OF SOCIAL GROUP WORK

Social group work, as we know it today, had its origins in international influences and exchanges. Canon Samuel Barnett founded the first Settlement House based on principles of community, participation, and democracy at Toynbee Hall in London, England, in 1885. That same year, the first transatlantic visitor, a theological student from the United States, arrived, followed by many, including Jane Addams, who first visited in 1887. Visits were reciprocated, and Henrietta Barnett, wife of Canon Barnett, was appointed president of the United States Federation of University Settlements in 1920 (Reinders, 1982). It is ironic that, despite the inconvenience and expense of travel and communication at the time, there was much more interaction and mutual transatlantic influence in those early days, maybe even more than at the present time. The settlement movement grew out of the dire social conditions created by industrialization, and, in contrast to the Charity Organization Society, it was identified with a social rather than an individual response to those conditions, thus providing a beginning for the development of group work. The settlement house movement, on the one hand, leaned toward social reform and, on the other, utilized the power of the group to provide education, training, and skills of daily living directed toward emancipation of the poor (in England) and new undereducated immigrants (in the United States). This emphasis on social reform and human empowerment changed in the second decade of the 20th century, when the emphasis moved toward recreational and service programs, with an activity orientation geared to serve the troops returning from World War I. Later, the second wave of international influence on group work saw the impact of psychoanalysis from Europe, and social group work extended itself to incorporate group treatment and therapy in its already extensive *modus operandi* (Coyle, 1948; Konopka, 1949; Shaffer & Galinsky, 1989). This development was reinforced by the mental health needs of soldiers in Britain and the United States returning from World War II and the limited resources for treatment. New models of group work emerged in psychiatry and influenced social group work to become treatment oriented (Bion, 1961; Foulkes & Anthony, 1957). Refugees from a Europe challenged by the rise of national socialism, such as Gisela Konopka and Fritz Redl, made seminal contributions to the development of group work with children and adolescents. Thus the early history of social group work reflects two strands of development: activity-, recreation-, and education-oriented groups, reflected in the work of the settlement houses and organizations such as the YMCA; and the mental health and treatment focus coming from the medical/psychiatric service delivery sector.

A GLOBAL PERSPECTIVE ON SOCIAL GROUP WORK TODAY

In seeking a global context for social group work, one has but to take cognizance of the single common thread that binds all humankind, the gregarious nature of the human race, which, from the very inception of the species, has led humans to organize themselves in groups and collectivities. This tendency in humans to gravitate toward living, functioning, and interacting in groups, from dyads to clans, reinforces the concept of groups as the natural and desirable habitat of humankind. If groups serve as the cradle of social strength, human growth, and development, then it stands to reason that groups must provide some gains to humans. To understand what these gains are, attributes of groups—such as roles, functions, structure, and process—have been identified, examined, and utilized in an organized and systematic way to maximize human well-being and, in turn, the well-being of the society in which they live. That all people interact and function in and through groups in a given society is a universally recognized condition; that these interactions may differ from one region to another is determined by the cultural context of the interaction (Okum, Fried, & Okum, 1999).

This contextual difference has been researched by North American proponents of social group work. The disciplines of sociology and social psychology have undertaken extensive studies of groups and the various processes associated with group activities, group phases and development, structure, and goals (Cartwright & Zander, 1968; Forsyth, 1999). The applied science/art of social work has utilized and adapted these findings to develop both professional interventions and methods of social group work in work with task, process, and educational groups (Coyle, 1959; Forsythe, 1999; Garvin, 1997; Hartford, 1972;

Northen, 1988; Vinter, 1967; Wilson & Ryland, 1949). The question arises, Are these structures, processes, functions, roles, and skills—identified by this substantial body of North American social work literature—equally evident and recognizable in other countries?

Whereas group work in Western industrialized countries essentially takes the form of small group interventions in task and process groups, in many countries of the global south (i.e., less industrialized and less technologically advanced countries), it takes on different ideologies that relate to larger systems and that may be more politically radical. For example, conscientization and liberation theology have influenced practice in South America (Friere, 1973). Social development incorporates economic and social factors in the attempt to empower constituencies and communities to participate in decision making with the goal of structural change (Elliott & Mayadas, 1996; Estes, 1992; Mayadas & Elliott, 1995; Midgley, 1995). There are other forms of social group work that are age old and that have evolved naturally; for example, the village-level local councils in India (*panchayats*), which are based on the ideology of internal political self-governance within the context of the country's central government. Other ideologies that use basic group work strategies and that are applied globally are community organization and community development (Regan & Lee, 1992). With so many worldwide applications of social group work, one may well raise the question of whether social group work is a socially constructed concept of the Western world.

CULTURAL CONTEXT AND GROUP WORK

Can one surmise that there is a culture-specific orientation to groups held by respective societies around the world? This stance might best be determined by viewing, on a continuum, the relationship of individuals to groups and vice versa, on which at the one extreme, the locus of social control lies with the person, and at the other, the group is regarded as the unit of social control.

A doctrine of individualism suggests that the cultural milieu in societies tends to attribute primary significance to the individual vis à vis the group. Individuals function within the context of the group but maintain their social identities. The individuation of the person supersedes the power of the group identity. Groups within this orientation are entities designed to enhance individual well-being. For example, in the North American and European tradition the methodology and interventions of social group work are specifically designed for the betterment of the individual, whether the goal is therapeutic change, social enhancement, interpersonal competence, skill acquisition, or self-help and support (Edwards & Edwards, 1984). Similarly, task and decision-making groups are designed to increase organizational efficiency through concerted group effort to improve service delivery to clients, customers, and patrons. Groups in individual cultures serve as instruments of change for human well-being. Individual-oriented cultures are, by and large, associated with Western

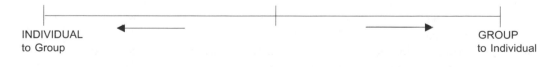

INDIVIDUAL   GROUP
to Group   to Individual

FIGURE 3.1. Locus of social control.

industrialized and technologically advanced nations, in which the competitive philosophy of self-enhancement has already disintegrated the bonding of natural groups (extended families, close communities, and agrarian households in which individuals, of necessity, had depended on the group for survival). With the decrease in dependency on the natural group, the need for groups as an integral part of the human environment has become only more evident and has taken the shape of professional services through the medium of planned group interventions. Because groups are admittedly acknowledged as a medium of change in individualistic societies, the role of the group worker, at any level of task or process groups, remains overt, clearly delineated, mutually acknowledged, and directly focused on the techniques and knowledge that are recognized as the expertise needed to achieve the desired outcome. This lack of role ambiguity and presence of task clarity leads to brevity of time expended on the task and results in relatively uncomplicated and open communication patterns, attributes of social interaction that are valued by the individual-oriented society.

The group-oriented society, on the other hand, focuses on the group maintaining social control through the group ego, to which individuals surrender their respective identities. Individual differences are minimized, if not ignored, and personal preferences, values, attributes, and characteristics are relegated to a *persona non grata* status (Chu & Sue, 1984). Assertion of individuality is seen as an act of sedition against the group, the ultimate price for which could be total ostracism. Thus, within cultures in which the group is sacrosanct and the individual merely a cog in the wheel, "outsiders" such as professional social workers are viewed with suspicion as interlopers and their presence regarded as an intrusion. Group-oriented cultures behave as closed systems with esoteric norms, traditions, rituals, and values that all members of the group must adhere to or lose face with the group (Sue & Sue, 1999). Most countries of the global south profess a group ego. Japan, even though technologically an advanced nation that beare greater resemblance to the global north in its material productivity, shares the concept of group ego with its more traditional neighbors. The group-oriented cultures primarily value the group and individuals only to the extent to which they conform and abnegate their own interests in the overarching interest of the group.

On the surface, it would appear that in cultures in which the concept of group is so deeply imbedded and in which social control has been with the group since the beginning of history, the techniques of social group work would be easily incorporated and applied toward desired social and behavioral change. However, the experience of professional group workers has demonstrated otherwise (Okum et al., 1999; Pearson, 1991). The direct methods of interventions associated with social group work from its professional inception, practiced in individual-oriented low-context cultures, are questioned and rejected. Sharing personal concerns with strangers is seen as betrayal of the group. The integrity of the group requires "trust." Why should one place one's faith in strangers who advocate the "unnatural" formation of groups as decision makers and change agents when the community has, in its opinion, managed society for centuries through its own deeply embedded group structure (Lee, Juan, & Hom, 1984)? The universal practice of group work as it is understood in the global north, if applied to the global south, is fraught with difficulties and requires an inordinate amount of expended time. It may take a year, or perhaps more, for a high-context culture to allow the "strangers" to share their views and for the community to actually listen. This prolonged testing period, so alien to the service provider educated in the global north, ends in frustration, failure, and a stalemate situation (Mistry & Brown, 1997).

Although no one culture would fall into the extreme on either end of the individual–group continuum, the natural proclivity of cultures to lean toward one or the other affects the nature of group work interventions if cultural disparity exists between clients and professionals. Put another way, successful group work interventions on a global level are shaped by and are contingent on how well these interventions dovetail with the cultural expectations of the country.

GROUP WORK AND INTERNATIONAL INFLUENCES

To cope with cultural variance, a global perspective is necessary for professionals to be sensitively alert to differences and aware of the repercussions of these differences on practice. A global perspective removes the cobwebs and dispels the mirage, showing us that, although the assumptions we hold regarding universal truth or ethical behavior or a problematic situation may indeed be justifiable for us, they may have very different connotations for other cultures. Moreover, service delivery systems in various parts of the world are differently designed and constructed according to their own perceived needs; hence, methods of practice, to be effective, also need to match the existing service systems of a given culture.

As Garvin (1984) has stated, group work is significantly influenced by its contexts, including political and economic structure, social norms, and the service delivery systems within which the social work profession operates. One would expect, therefore, that significant differences would be evident in the practice of social group work across the world. For example, in countries in which social workers are mainly government or local government employees, such as the United Kingdom, the role of mandatory social work may play a larger part. This may occur not only in the form of social control of certain populations, such as delinquents, but also in the statutory requirement of that government body to provide certain services for some populations, for example, home-based services.

Another illustration of the political influences on group work practice is shown by Brown (1990), who argues that group work is based on principles of shared responsibility, collective solutions to problems, mutual aid, and empowerment. As a consequence of the conservative trend in British politics during the administrations of Prime Ministers Margaret Thatcher and John Major, group work was polarized into social control and social action. Hence during that period group work with offenders, child abusers, substance abusers, and delinquents became more evident, while at the same time there was a reactive and opposite polarity of social action groups, in which members focused on goals external to the group at the expense of internal dynamics. The cooperative movement in Canada for profit sharing and distribution of everyday goods and the kibbutz movement, a social experiment in group living in Israel, are further examples of group work reflecting political arrangements in a different way. These examples also reflect the social construction of social group work (Shapiro, 1990).

Forte (1994) undertook a content analysis of the journal articles on group work from four countries: Israel, Great Britain, Canada, and Australia. In total in this study, 271 published articles represented 17 countries outside the United States. The rank order of countries in terms of productivity was Canada, Great Britain, Australia, and Israel. Family and clinical welfare settings represented 21% of the articles, with corrections (12%) and mental health (11%) preceding medical social work (6.6%) and geriatrics (6.3%). Most authors were social workers.

Regarding content of the international literature on social group work, Forte's (1994) study confirmed the findings of earlier analyses by Silverman (1966) and Feldman (1987) that the majority of articles (39.1% in the Forte, 1994, study) were not researched based but were descriptions of practice with only elementary data analysis; 47.1% of the research articles used descriptive statistics, and a further 26.5% used only simple bivariate analysis.

Forte (1994) asserts that these articles did not build on previous literature, nor did they use qualitative or quantitative research methods to document and evaluate practice. This presents an area of concern noted by Forte, as it suggests little contribution to the knowledge base of social group work. Only 12.6% of articles were considered to be in the research and survey category, and 19.9% were in the innovations in practice theory category. No experimental or single-subject designs were reported. However, the descriptive accounts of international group work give a good picture of the state of the art. They showed that the international groups bore some similarities to and some differences from group work in the United States as reported by Tolman (1989). Similarities included weekly meetings, a preference for closed-ended groups, length of meetings, and a comparable number of sessions. Forte (1994) further noted that differences occurred in the theory base preferred by international group workers, who favored self-help, group psychotherapy, feminist theory, and social goals as theoretical models among a very broad range reported. International groups did not focus primarily on services to children. These groups focused on adults and the elderly, as well as adolescents. Leading areas of focus were problems with family, aging, and health. Forte (1994) points out that the range seemed broader than the range of American group work reported by Tolman (1989).

In summary, Forte reports that Australia published more research-based articles, that Canadian group work was based on more traditional theoretical roles, and that British group work represented newer models (e.g., Mullender & Ward, 1991). For Britain, Canada, Israel, and Australia, the major focus of group work was on adults.

Rice (1999) compared group work in the United States and Australia with a survey of students in 12 schools of social work and practitioners in 30 agencies in Australia and with a survey of 230 family and field coordinators in the United States. Models of group work practice reported were, in the same rank order for both countries: (1) education and psychoeducation, (2) therapeutic and personal growth-oriented groups, (3) problem-solving and task groups, and (4) skills training groups. Rice reports that there was a stronger emphasis on educational and psychoeducational groups in Australia, although the rank order in the two countries was the same.

CURRENT STATUS OF GROUP WORK ACROSS THE GLOBE: AN EMPIRICAL STUDY

Today there are numerous conceptualizations of social group work; however, if commonalities were to be extrapolated from these and presented in one integrated framework, they would consist of a comprehensive understanding of group dynamics, a recognition of processes and interventions as they shape the group structure, a systemic perspective for the analysis of all social exchanges within the group, and, finally, evaluation of group intervention outcome (Garvin, 1997; Schopler & Galinsky, 1995; Toseland & Rivas, 2001). These principles are common to all orientations of social group work in the United States and in those parts of the globe where American social group work has been exported, but are they also prevalent in countries in which group work may have had a different origin? This research question prompted a survey of schools of social work across the globe to assess the current situation with regard to international social group work. A recent survey of social group work content in doctoral programs in the United States suggested that social group work has a low priority in the doctoral curricula of Canadian and U.S. schools of social work (Mayadas, Smith, & Elliott, 2001). Low availability of social group work courses and low enrollment in them, as well as low priority status ascribed to social group work, was evident in the majority of the responding programs. These findings raised concern that social work educators were not being prepared to teach group work. Yet, in the field of practice, social workers are consistently confronted with work in groups, such as committees, task groups, peer groups, cliques, and coalitions. The focus on a study of group work in social work education as opposed to practice was based on the rationale that if group work was to have any place in social work practice in a particular country, then it must start with academic training and education of professionals. The assumptions of the researchers were that group-oriented cultures would place a greater curriculum emphasis on the study of task and support groups, whereas individual-oriented cultures would emphasize both but might lean more toward process groups.

This international study is a follow-up study of the North American survey to see if the same factors existed internationally. Other, specific goals of the study are to explore whether social group work:

- Is included in the curricula of professional schools at the master's level
- Is ranked equally with other social work intervention methods in the curriculum
- Forms a major concentration of study in the program
- Has identifiable models of group work used in teaching
- Has specific teaching methods associated with its education and training

Methodology

A survey was sent to 443 schools in 32 countries that are listed as members of the International Association of Schools of Social Work. A Spanish version was sent to Spanish-speaking countries; the remainder were in English. One hundred thirty-five surveys (response rate 30.5%) were returned, representing schools from Africa, Asia, Australia, Europe, North America, and South America.

The survey instrument consisted of 30 items. Demographic data on the schools, the social work programs, and the social work faculty were obtained. Information on group work included courses offered in group work, group work content in other social work courses, the main focus of group work content, theoretical orientation, group work in the practicum, and group work as a component of thesis and/or dissertation.

Findings

Of the 135 schools responding to the survey, 37% were in Europe, 35.6% were in North America, 10.4% were in Asia, 6.7% were in Africa, 5.9% were in South America, and 4.4% were in Australia (Table 3.1). The majority of the responding schools (82.6%) were in urban settings, with 12.1% being located in suburban areas and 5.3% in rural areas. Most of the responding social work programs were located in larger universities: 52.6% had enrollments of 8,000 students or more; 25.2% had enrollments between 1,000 and 8,000 students; and 14.8% had enrollments of fewer than 1,000 students.

These 135 institutions with social work programs represent 41,495 social work students and 2,497 social work faculty members, a 16:1 student-to-faculty ratio. Thirty percent of the institutions required a doctoral degree for teaching, 56% required the master's in so-

TABLE 3.1. Universities Responding to Survey

Location of responding schools	n	%
Africa	9	6.7
Asia	14	10.4
Australia	6	4.4
Europe	50	37.0
North America	48	35.6
South America	8	5.9
Total	135	100

cial work (MSW) and 14% accepted other social science degrees. The requirement for a PhD was most prevalent in North America, whereas the MSW was most prevalent in Europe as the terminal degree for teaching.

The degrees awarded by the reporting institutions varied. Doctoral degrees were awarded by 38.5% of the schools, MSW degrees were awarded by 63.7%, bachelor's in social work (BSW) degrees were awarded by 61.5%, and 15.6% of the schools awarded other degrees or certificates in the field of social work. In reference to part-time social work programs, 29.6% of doctoral programs, 43.7% of MSW programs, 28.1% of BSW programs, and 11.9% of other social work education programs could be completed on a part-time basis. Australia reported the largest number of part-time programs in all categories.

The 135 responding schools reported that 174 social work faculty members were trained instructors and were teaching in group work courses. As noted previously, the total number of social work faculty represented was 2,497. Therefore, only 7% of social work faculty in this study are group work specialists.

The area of expertise among group work faculty varied. Of the faculty teaching group work, 39.2% have expertise in direct practice or clinical work, 36.5% list group work as their primary area of expertise, 22.7% focus on administration or community practice, and 1.6% have an "other" orientation, not specified.

Of the 174 group work faculty members, 47.7% have more than 10 years of experience, 28.7% have 6–10 years of experience, 21.8% have 1–5 years of experience, and 17.2% have less than 1 year of experience (Table 3.2). The correlation between faculty trained in group work and faculty experienced in group work is statistically significant ($p = .001$). Only 7% of faculty are trained in group work, and the majority of these are long-time faculty members, indicating an expected decline in the number of trained group work faculty members as the more experienced retire.

The survey revealed that social group work is taught both as a separate course and as

TABLE 3.2. Group Work Faculty Experience in Group Work Practice

Years of experience	n	%
0–1	3	17.2
1–5	38	21.8
6–10	50	28.7
10+	83	47.7

content in generic courses. The 135 schools reported 131 separate group work courses (Table 3.3). North America was the only area reporting more than one course in some schools. South America and Asia reported one course per school. The remaining locations reported fewer courses in group work. Because group work courses may be taught in other departments, enrollment in those courses was investigated; 54.9% of the schools reported that students were not allowed to enroll in group work courses in departments other than social work, with Europe accounting for 45% of the "no" responses. Students in 45.1% of the schools were allowed to take group work courses outside of the social work department, with North America accounting for 62% of the "yes" responses. In addition to the specialized group work courses, the 135 schools reported 158 generic courses with group work content. The majority of these courses were at the undergraduate level, 40.5%, with 38.0% being offered at the graduate level, 9.5% at the postgraduate level, and 12.0% at the certificate level.

Both graduate and undergraduate programs placed equal emphasis on specialized group work courses, with 41.2% of programs in each case having specialized courses in social group work. At the postgraduate level, only 5.3% of programs had specialized courses. At other levels, such as certification and continuing education, 12.2% of programs had specialized group training.

Schools were asked to identify the main focus of the group work content in their courses. A compilation of study data resulted in a group work approach for each of the geographical areas relating to focus of content. Eight foci of group work content included therapy, support, self-development, education, research, administration, community practice, and social action. The schools were asked to prioritize group work content in their programs as high, low, or not a priority (Table 3.4). The highest rankings were from South America and Africa, with 87.5% of schools listing a high priority. This was followed by Europe at 68.1%, North America at 53.0%, and Asia and Australia at 50.0%, with an overall ranking of group work as a high priority at 62.7%.

Summary of Main Findings

The main findings of the study may be summarized as follows:

- Only 7% of social work faculty in universities worldwide are considered to be social group work specialists.
- Of these social group work specialists, 36.5% list social group work as their *primary* area of expertise.

TABLE 3.3 Group Work Courses Offered by Location

Location	Number of schools	Number of group courses
Africa	9	10
Asia	14	14
Australia	6	5
Europe	50	38
North America	48	56
South America	8	8
Total	135	131

TABLE 3.4. Foci of Group Work Content, Rank Ordered by Continent

Rank order	Africa	Asia	Australia	Europe	North America	South America	Global model
1	Support	Self-dev.	Support	Support	Support	Comm. prac.	Support
2	Therapy	Support	Therapy	Self-dev.	Therapy	Soc. act.	Comm. prac.
3	Comm. prac.	Therapy	Educ.	Comm. prac.	Comm. prac.	Res.	Self-dev.
4	Self-dev.	Comm. prac.	Comm. prac.	Soc. act.	Educ.	Self-dev.	Therapy
5	Educ.	Educ.	Soc. act.	Educ.	Self-dev.	Educ.	Soc. act.
6	Res.	Soc. act.	Self-Dev	Therapy	Soc. act.	Support	Educ.
7	Soc. act.	Admin.	Res.	Admin.	Admin.	Admin.	Res.
8	Admin.	Res.	Admin.	Res.	Res.	Therapy	Admin.

- Those who are identified as group work faculty are well experienced: 76.4% have more than 6 years experience, with 47.7% having more than 10 years of experience.
- South America and Africa were foremost in listing group work courses as high priority.
- Global approaches to group work were, with the exception of South America, focused on those that seem to emphasize individual needs, such as support, therapy, and self-development.

Limitations of the Study

This study looks at the worldwide spread of social group work and attempts to investigate whether social group work has a common language and shared approaches to practice. Though the survey responses are subjective, they draw attention to possible trends and open up heuristic possibilities for more rigorous studies. For example, issues for further investigations would need to address ways of assessing comparability of course content.

A confounding trend in the survey is the consistency with which schools across the globe gave primary importance to support groups, with only Asian and South American schools leaning more toward self-development and community practice, respectively. This finding may be attributed to a limitation of the survey in that terms were not made explicitly operational and thus may reflect cultural variance in interpretation, according to the country's understanding of the language. For example, self-development could be interpreted as economic self-reliance, a model frequently used in countries of the global south in community development projects to empower groups for socioeconomic interdependence and self-sufficiency. Taking the findings at face value, one could conjecture that, because support groups most closely approximate one's social reality—that is, we are attracted to and find comfort in conditions familiar to us—it stands to reason that this model of social group work practice has the most widespread appeal. In this model, members who share a common concern get together either with or without a professional facilitator to pool and evaluate their subjective experiences, provide mutual understanding and consolation through burden sharing, and allay their apprehension of isolation and despair (Schopler & Galinsky, 1993). When looked at in this context, it is understandable that support groups have a universal appeal.

A total of 7% of faculty were experienced in and were identified as teachers of social group work, and 47.7% of these had more than 10 years of experience. These findings suggest that these individuals represent a small and older cohort of faculty and are consistent with findings in the North American study, as reported earlier (Mayadas et al., 2001). The questions that arise from this study are: Are a sufficient number of new faculty being trained in social group work? Are new faculty being trained adequately, or are they being trained at all? If they are not being appropriately trained, yet students continue to practice social group work in their internships and practitioners conduct groups in practice, is social work education giving way to the apprenticeship/anecdotal model of group work training? This view might very well seem to be supported by the fact that the group work literature is dominated by anecdotal and descriptive accounts of practice. This apparent crisis in the training of social group work service providers and educators occurs at a time when, in the Western world, the cost–benefit issues of insurance companies are insuring the popularity of the group paradigm.

Table 3.4 lists the rank order of group work approaches prevalent across continents. The striking similarity in approaches suggests a global linkage in the literature and academic and scholarly exchange. Most of the approaches are focused on the psychosocial approach, and it would be safe to say with Midgley (1981) that "professional imperialism" has spread American literature, values, ethics, and practice models across the globe through a predominantly one-way transfer of knowledge.

FUTURE TRENDS

What is the future of the international perspective in social group work? As in North America, it seems that there is an imperative for training. As demonstrated by the literature, there is an imperative for theory building and a move to build research on group work practice, as social work progresses to evidence-based practice. There is also an imperative for the development of indigenous models in different parts of the world that depart from the established psychosocial model. Finally, the rapid growth in technology has opened new areas of practice for international social group work. An operational measure of internationalism is the existence of linkages or channels of communication between groups, organizations and societies. The term "globalization" demonstrates these linkages through multilevel cross-national exchanges. Social group work, which has historically been shaped by globalization, now finds a new dimension with virtual reality added to its international exchange repertoire. Web-enhanced, Web-mediated, Web-based groups have proliferated in recent years. They serve similar functions of support, education, and task to traditional groups. However, they transcend time and space and make group benefits constantly available to members. These groups provide assistance and community to those who cannot travel to a meeting place: women with young children, people who are physically sick, physically challenged people, and people living in rural areas all benefit from such groups. Many of these groups are also international in membership: They are truly diverse, not bounded by the barriers of race, religion, age, class, or nationality. They are focused on their concern and mutual need for learning and support. For example, many medical groups (for example, the Association of Cancer Online Resources, *www.acor.org*), exchange information and support on a worldwide basis. These groups are not time limited and offer convenience of participation. Research has shown that participation increases with anonymity. Weinberg, Schmale, Uken, and Wessel (1995) discuss the advantages and disadvantages of computer-mediated support groups. Although we are moving toward this group work approach, very little is known about interactions. Mostly, these groups have grown outside the profession of social work and with no social group work expertise on the part of list owners/moderators. There is opportunity for social service agencies, medical hospital social work departments, and psychiatric services to develop such lists as part of their regular service to clients. Group work skills adapted to operating in a virtual group are required of the leader or the mediator. Communication without face-to-face interaction is different in nature. Delayed responses and delayed feedback may present other problems. Access to technology can be a problem sometimes in some countries. Nevertheless, this is a new field that has great potential for international social group work practice and that is wide open for theory development and research.

REFERENCES

Bion, W. R. (1961). *Experiences in groups*. London: Tavistock.

Brown, A. (1990). British perspectives on group work: Present and future. *Social Work with Groups*, *13*(3), 35–40.

Cartwright, D., & Zander, A. (1968). *Group dynamics: Research and theory* (3rd ed.). New York: Harper & Row.

Chu, J., & Sue, S. (1984). Asian Pacific Americans and group practice. *Social Work with Groups*, *7*(3), 23–36.

Coyle, C. (1948). *Group work with American youth*. New York: Harper & Row.

Coyle, G. (1959). Group work in psychiatric settings: Its roots and branches. *Social Work*, *4*(1), 74–81.

Edwards, E. D., & Edwards, M. E. (1984). Group work practice with American Indians. *Social Work with Groups*, *7*(3), 7–16.

Elliott, D., & Mayadas, N. S. (1996). Social development and clinical practice in social work. *Journal of Applied Social Sciences*, *21*(1), 32–39.

Estes, J. J. (1992). Group work in international perspective: The professional agenda. In D. F. Fike & B. Rittner (Eds.), *Working from strengths: The essence of group work* (pp. 122–145). Miami: Center for Group Work Studies.

Feldman, R. A. (1987). Group work knowledge and research: A two decade comparison. *Social Work with Groups*, *9*(3), 7–13.

Forsyth, D. R. (1999). *Group dynamics* (3rd ed.). Pacific Grove, CA: Brooks/Cole.

Forte, J. A. (1994). Around the world with social group work: Knowledge and research contributions. *Social Work with Groups*, *17*(12), 143–162.

Foulkes, S. H., & Anthony, E. J. (1957). *Group psychotherapy: The psychoanalytic approach* (2nd ed.). Middlesex, England: Penguin Books.

Freire, P. (1973) *Education for critical consciousness*. New York: Seabury Press.

Garvin, C. D. (1984). The changing context of social group work practice: Challenge and opportunity. *Social Work with Groups*, *7*(1), 3–19.

Garvin, C. D. (1997). *Contemporary group work* (3rd ed.). Boston: Allyn & Bacon.

Hartford, M. (1972). *Groups in social work*. New York: Columbia University Press.

Konopka, G. (1949). *Therapeutic group work with children*. Minneapolis: University of Minnesota Press.

Lee, P. C., Juan, G., & Hom, A. B. (1984). Group work practice with Asian clients: A sociocultural approach. *Social Work with Groups*, *7*(3), 37–48.

Mayadas, N. S., & Elliott, D. (1995). Developing professional identity through social group work: A social development systems (SDS) model for education. In M. D. Feit, J. H. Ramey, J. S. Wodarski, & A. R. Mann (Eds.), *Group work in the 21st century: Capturing the power of diversity* (pp. 89–107). Binghamton, NY: Haworth Press

Mayadas, N. S., Smith, R., & Elliott, D. (2001). Social group work in doctoral programs: Implications for social work practice and education. *Journal of Teaching in Social Work*, *21*(1/2), 175–194.

Midgley, J. (1981) *Professional imperialism: Social work in the third world*. London: Heinemann.

Midgley, J. (1995). *Social development: The developmental perspective in social welfare*. Thousand Oaks, CA: Sage.

Mistry, T., & Brown, A. (Eds.). (1997). *Race and group work*. London: Whiting & Birch.

Mullender, A., & Ward, D. (1991). *Self-directed group work: Users take action for empowerment*. London: Whiting & Birch.

Northen, H. (1988). *Social work with groups* (2nd ed). New York: Columbia University Press.

Okum, B., Fried, J., & Okum, M. L. (1999). *Understanding diversity*. Pacific Grove, CA: Brooks/Cole.

Pearson, V. (1991). Western theory, Eastern practice: Social group work theory in Hong Kong. *Social Work with Groups, 14*(2) 45–58.

Regan, S., & Lee, G. (1992). The interplay among social group work, community work and community action. *Social Work with Groups, 15*(1) 35–50.

Reinders, R. (1982). Toynbee Hall and the American settlement movement. *Social Service Review, 56*(1) 39–54.

Rice, A. H. (1999). Crossing boundaries: Comparing group work in the United States and Australia. *Social Work with Groups, 22*(2/3) 159–178.

Schopler, J. H., & Galinsky, M. J. (1993). Support groups as open systems: A model for practice and research. *Health and Social Work, 18*, 195–207.

Schopler, J. H., & Galinsky, M. J. (Eds.). (1995). Group practice overview. In R. L. Edwards & J. G. Hopps (Eds.), *Encyclopedia of social work* (19th ed., Vol. 2, pp. 1129-1142). Washington, DC: NASW Press.

Shaffer, J., & Galinsky, M. D. (1989). *Models of group therapy* (2nd ed.). Englewood Cliffs, NJ: Prentice-Hall.

Shapiro, B. Z. (1990). Social group work and the challenge of the future: Canada and Israel. *Social Work with Groups, 7*(1), 3–19.

Silverman, M. (1966). Knowledge in group work: An overview of the literature. *Social Work, 11*(3), 59–62.

Sue, D. W., & Sue, D. (1999). *Counseling the culturally different: Theory and practice* (3rd ed.). New York: Wiley.

Tolman, R. M. (1989, May). *A decade of social group work research: A methodological overview*. Paper presented at the Fifth Annual Symposium on Empirical Foundations of Group Work, Ann Arbor, MI.

Toseland, R. W., & Rivas, R. T. (2001). *An introduction to group work practice* (4th ed.). Boston: Allyn & Bacon.

Vinter, R. D. (1967). *Readings in group work practice*. Ann Arbor, MI: Campus Publishers.

Weinberg, N., Schmale, J. D., Uken, J., & Wessel, K. (1995). Computer-mediated support groups. *Social Work with Groups, 17*(4), 43–54.

Wilson, G., & Ryland, G. (1949). *Social group work practice*. Boston: Houghton Mifflin.

Chapter 4

An Empowerment Perspective

MARGOT BRETON

The word "empowerment" is ubiquitous, and it is given drastically different meanings. These meanings range from the extreme left, radical Marxist one—which postulates that the whole system must be overthrown before the people can be empowered—to the equally extreme right-wing, trickle-down-economics meaning—which assumes that if we give more to the rich and powerful, more will trickle down to the poor and disempowered, who will then become empowered.

There is, however, agreement, in social work and related fields, that empowerment involves both a process and a goal whereby people gain mastery and control over their lives and become active participants in efforts to influence their environments (Rappaport, 1987).

The process in question is one of consciousness raising, or, more accurately, conscientization, in which people become aware of (1) the interconnections between issues and the ways in which personal issues are linked to interpersonal and to political, social, economic, and cultural issues and (2) how the interconnections between the personal and the political manifest themselves in specific power arrangements in the world around them. They go from a naïve consciousness of interconnections to a critical awareness of the workings of power (Freire, 1970/1993). The goal is to gain access to needed resources through collective action on the environment. It is important to stress that change at the personal–interpersonal level without change at the social–political level does not lead to empowerment (see Breton, 1994a; DuBois & Miley, 1999; Gutiérrez, 1994; Lee, 2001).

The cognitive and psychological shift resulting from the process of conscientization is a *necessary* condition for people to move from being disempowered and having no control over what happens to them to being empowered—but it is not a *sufficient* condition. To become empowered, people must act on their cognitive and psychological discoveries, on how they have come to think and feel about themselves and their world, to try to change that world (Freire, 1970/1993). "Without exercising the power to act, the awareness of personal strengths and competence may give people a *sense* of empowerment (Riger, 1993) and lead them to think and feel that they have more power and are more in control—it does not mean that they have more power and are more in control" (Breton, 2002, p. 26).

Lest the idea of empowerment be diluted into an "everything bucket" (Pernell, 1986, p. 13), it is important to stress that empowerment is directly related to oppression (Ward & Mullender, 1991). The disempowered are individuals burdened with a stigmatized collective identity (Solomon, 1976).

This chapter begins by clarifying issues of purpose and of the means of attaining purpose in empowerment-oriented groups. It then analyzes the components of group practice from an empowerment perspective. Philosophical and conceptual foundations for this practice are examined next. The concluding section focuses on trends and future directions.

THE PURPOSE OF GROUP WORK
FROM AN EMPOWERMENT PERSPECTIVE

In light of the meaning just given to empowerment, the overall purpose of groups, from an empowerment perspective, is to change oppressive cognitive, behavioral, social, and political structures or conditions that thwart the control people have over their lives, that prevent them from accessing needed resources, and that keep them from participating in the life of their community.

Cognitive structures are oppressive when people see themselves and the world in such a way that they automatically blame themselves for their situations. Fanon (1968), Memmi (1965), and Freire (1970/1993) discuss the phenomenon of the oppressed internalizing the opinions oppressors hold of them. Oppressive cognitive structures can also lead individuals to perceive their situations as inevitable, either the will of God or the result of destiny or fate. Thus individuals may fail to seek out or to effectively use social services, consequently being labeled by professionals as "unmotivated," "resistant," or "hard to reach" (see Breton, 1985; Holmes & Saleebey, 1993). Finally, oppressive cognitive structures may lead individuals to perceive their situations as hopeless and themselves as helpless. Seligman (1975) notes that as a result of "learned helplessness," individuals believe that nothing they do will affect the outcome of events. Oppressive cognitive structures, whatever form they take, create oppressive behavioral structures (ways of thinking lead to ways of behaving). Individuals abdicate their competence—they do not make use of their strengths, skills, and abilities—and give up trying to influence their environment (Breton, 1994b).

Oppressive social structures, which include oppressive institutional and organizational structures, are the arrangements, sanctioned by society and embodied in policies and procedures that exclude individuals from participating in the decisions that affect their lives and keep them from accessing the resources they need to have decent lives. Policies and procedures are the result of value orientations. Public policies that affect how society's resources are distributed derive from the beliefs held by that society. When those beliefs are colored by racism, colonialism, sexism, ageism, and other discriminatory and exclusivist ideologies— such as a market-oriented philosophy that holds that governments should leave social welfare and health matters to the market—the public policies that result will hurt all but the wealthy and powerful members of that society (see Haynes & Mickelson, 1997).

Organizational and professional policies and procedures are also affected by value orientations. The penchant for paternalism prevalent in social work (Reamer, 1983) has, among other things, influenced the hierarchical bureaucratic arrangements that characterize many social work organizations, tending to reduce the independence and professional autonomy of social workers. Similarly, valuing the medical paradigm at the expense of so-cial change paradigms has led to the view of the professional as the expert who knows best what people need and, consequently, to discounting the opinions and wishes of people, to neglecting their strengths, and to overlooking their abilities to assess their situations and to make decisions regarding these situations (see Hartman, 1993; Holmes & Saleebey, 1993; Weick, 1983). It has also led to the ever-growing popularity of "clinical" practice and the relative inattention to social justice issues (see Specht & Courtney, 1994).

In democracies, oppressive political structures refer to institutions, policies, and prac-tices that systematically exclude citizens from participating in the normal responsibilities and benefits of a free and open society. When, for example, voting arrangements are such that the poor, or members of other marginalized groups, are unable to exercise their elec-toral responsibility, those arrangements are oppressive. Practices and policies that deny the right of individuals and groups to participate in public protests and demonstrations or that make the exercise of that right onerous constitute another type of oppressive political struc-tures. A recent study points to the existence of such structures within social work (Andrews & Reisch, 2002).

To change oppressive cognitive and behavioral structures, a combination of cognitive restructuring and behavioral unlearning and relearning is required. In empowerment-oriented groups, this means facilitating a consciousness-raising process aimed at surmount-ing internal blocks (negative self-evaluations) and at connecting personal and interpersonal situations to the socioeconomic context. This work must be accompanied by work at the behavioral level, that is, opportunities must be provided within the safety of the group for members to experience new ways of acting and interacting based on their new ways of per-ceiving themselves and their world.

To change social and political structures requires groups to mobilize and organize to take collective action. Action aimed at bringing about societal change (surmounting external blocks) will have a better chance of succeeding if groups do not have to "go it alone." It therefore pays to create partnerships between empowerment-oriented groups and communi-ties and to connect groups to community resources, thereby establishing support, as well as information networks. Establishing connections with the community is, from an empower-ment perspective, more than a means of attaining specific social change goals. It provides group members opportunities to begin to see themselves as members of a community and eventually to fully participate in the life of that community. In that sense, community work, whereby people collaborate to build supportive communities for themselves, goes hand-in-hand with empowerment work (McKenzie, 1999).

Finally, to attain their purpose, empowerment-oriented groups, like all groups, have to contend with the institutional and organizational structures in which they operate. Empow-erment work requires ensuring the support of the administrators and managers of social ser-vices organizations and confronting organizational structures when they prevent groups from fully participating in decisions that affect them (Bartle, Couchonnal, Canda, & Staker, 2002; Gutiérrez, GlenMaye, & DeLois, 1995).

INTERVENTION/COLLABORATIVE ACTION

From an empowerment perspective, which posits an equalitarian frame of reference, it is more accurate to conceptualize the work that takes place as collaborative action rather than "intervention"—the latter conveys the idea that experts intervene or act, while ordinary people are intervened with, or acted upon (Breton, 1992). In empowerment work, this collaboration takes place from the very beginning, that is, from the planning stage, through the conscientization stage, the collective action stage, and the postgroup stage of embeddedness in the community.

Planning

In an empowerment-oriented group, it is imperative that everyone who will be involved in the group has the opportunity to share the power to define what the group will be about and what it will do. Before the formal start of a group seeking the empowerment of African American custodial grandparents, for example, informal discussions to explore topics that would be interesting and useful to participants were held between potential members and group leaders (Cox, 2002; Cox, 1988; Gutiérrez, 1990). In other words, the "identification of needs" component of classic group planning (Kurland, 1978) is seen, in empowerment work, as the initial occasion for members to have a say, acquire a voice, and name their world. To share the power to shape the group requires that social workers trust the potential group members, respect their views, and acknowledge that they know best their own situation (Mullender & Ward, 1991).

Planning also involves deciding who will be in a group. This can be done in a more or less democratic fashion, from the worker choosing individuals and inviting them to join a group to announcing, in one form or another (e.g., ads in local papers, flyers, posters, word of mouth), that there is an intention to set up a group to holding a public pregroup meeting to which people can choose to come for the express purpose of sharing ideas about the prospective group. The more democratic the selection of members, the more empowering the selection process is for the potential members. Participating in that process also establishes that decision making in the group will be democratic and that group members will be expected to voice opinions and make responsible choices—liberating behaviors that are necessary components of empowerment.

Sharing ideas about the overall purpose of the group means, from an empowerment perspective, that workers and potential members recognize that the work of the group will involve both personal and social change. The specifics of these change goals will develop as the group develops, but the general notion that the group will involve not only thinking and talking about issues but also doing something about them has to be acknowledged from the beginning. The idea of praxis (Freire, 1970/1993) is introduced, even if only in an indirect and very general way, from the inception of the group, in addition to the idea of social justice.

In order to make the case for both personal and social change goals, workers must be clear in their own minds about the values on which empowerment work is based. Social justice is central to empowerment and needs to be identified as such by everyone. Concern about just and unjust social conditions has to inform the discussion of what the group will be about, even though it will do so in a precursory fashion at this stage.

Another point that needs to be touched on is that pursuing social change and social justice goals entails risk taking of a different nature—more public, involving more wide-range environmental side effects or externalities—than the usually more private risks attendant to personal change goals. Workers need to introduce the idea of risk taking as a group norm that members will have the opportunity to uphold in the group. Publicly recognizing that aversion to risk taking is a natural motivation (Breton, 1985) can help workers and potential members alike to confront their reservations about social change efforts (Wohl, 2000).

At this early stage, workers and potential members will also recognize conflict as a standard group feature from which they can learn. Confronting and dealing constructively with the interpersonal conflict bound to occur in the planning stage is a first step in preparing the group to eventually confront oppressive social structures and policies.

Clarifying the kinds of roles to be expected in an empowerment-oriented group is also part of the planning stage. As in any mutual-aid group, roles such as enabler and advocate are shared between all group participants. Remembering that negotiating skills are important to empowerment (Garvin, 1997), workers and potential members will take the opportunity provided in the planning stage to begin to negotiate roles and the meaning of shared responsibility for role taking.

Empowerment is not something achieved quickly. This means that, from the start, the organization, the workers, and the potential members recognize that supporting or participating in an empowerment-oriented group requires a significant commitment in terms of time. Without that commitment, the group will be set up for failure.

A successful planning stage involves preliminary but careful consideration of all these issues. This prepares the group to engage productively in the next stages.

Consciousness Raising/Conscientization

In this stage, collaborative action begins with the group engaging as a system of mutual aid. The mutual-aid dynamic of exchanging personal information or stories is the means through which members first discover that they can help each other (see Steinberg, 1997). In empowerment-oriented groups, the dynamic will also be used deliberately as the medium through which members either discover that they have voices, acquire voices if opportunities to be heard have always been denied them, or repossess their voices if they have been silenced. That is the beginning of discovering that they have a say and that they can influence others.

When the stories exchanged are received with respect and recognized as "legitimate knowledge" (Weick, 1992, p. 23), opportunities are created to explore and substantiate the members' competence and strengths (often simply as survivors, to begin with). Recognizing that they have something to say that is of genuine interest and help to others and that they have some degree of competence facilitates the cognitive restructuring process of challenging their negative self-images and self-evaluations, an initial part of consciousness raising.

To eventually lead to empowerment, however, consciousness raising cannot be conceptualized as a strictly personal process of cognitive restructuring whereby views of oneself and the world change. Consciousness raising must also involve an awareness that negative views of self are connected to social, economic, and political forces. That awareness is promoted when group members see the common patterns in their individual stories.

Consciousness of the interconnections between issues, though essential, is only a first step (a "naïve" awakening to reality, as Freire, 1970/1993, points out). It must be followed by an awareness of both the internal and external blockages that keep people from having control of their lives and the consequent need for change at the personal, interpersonal, and sociopolitical levels (Cox, 1991; Du Bois & Miley, 1999; Gutiérrez, 1994; Lee, 2001). In other words, consciousness raising that leads to empowerment is not only a personal process of cognitive restructuring but a politicization and liberation process that creates a demand for sociopolitical or systemic restructuring. That is the essence of conscientization. The difference between consciousness raising and conscientization may offer a clue as to why a study would conclude that "even the linkage of personal to political issues . . . has fostered a renewed emphasis on individual rather than collective solutions to social issues (Reisch, 1998)" (Andrews & Reisch, 2002, p. 7).

Going through the conscientization process, members begin to identify themselves as citizens—political beings—who, in a democracy, have the right and responsibility to participate on the sociopolitical scene, to be heard, and to influence policies so that they can access the resources they need. This situates them in a position from which they can move to the next stage of empowerment work, that of taking collective action to change their situation of disempowerment.

Social/Collective Action

As Rappaport (1981, p. 13) put it: "Having rights but no resources and no services is a cruel joke." This is why empowerment work cannot stop at the stage of conscientization. The challenge of this next stage is to build on new perceptions of self and society in order to bring about targeted, specific changes that will permit access to needed resources.

As it is natural for group members and facilitators alike to experience some trepidation at the idea of getting politically involved, groups must first mobilize and prepare to take action. At this point, the "strength-in-us" dynamic of mutual aid can be channeled to act as a motivator ("we are all in this together") and as a reality test ("let's see how we can use our collective voice").

Once mobilized, groups decide on the action(s) to be taken. This step is crucial, for taking action will lead to empowerment only when the people involved in the action have had a say in deciding what action will be taken and have weighed the costs, in terms of energy, time, possible conflicts, and consequences of taking a particular action (Breton, 1995; Garvin, 1991). It is only then that action becomes responsible and autonomous.

As part of evaluating these costs, groups will question whether they have the support of the communities to which they belong. Creating community alliances is an effective means of getting that support and of lowering the costs of taking action (Breton, Cox, & Taylor, 2003). It is also a means of creating long-term solidarities between group members and their communities, which will eventually affect how the newly empowered become embedded in society.

The types of action taken will depend on the sophistication, skills, and abilities of the group members. Actions may include taking part in demonstrations; giving interviews to newspaper, radio, or television reporters; participating in town hall meetings; leading or coleading seminars; and writing letters to the editor or newspaper articles. These undertakings should also be geared to leading the public and government policy makers (civil servants and politicians) to begin their own process of conscientization (Breton & Breton, 1997).

To be empowering, any action must be followed by reflection; it must involve what Freire (1970/1993) calls "praxis," that is, a constant movement from reflection to action back to reflection. It is through assessing the results of their action that group members acquire an increasingly critical consciousness of the workings of power in their environment and society. As Breton (1994a, p. 25), following Freire (1970/1993) and Longres and McLeod (1980), has argued: "Action without reflection is not autonomous and authentic action, but rather a *reaction* to others' ideas, while reflection without action is, for the disempowered, mere teasing or provocation, akin to adding insult to injury."

As they reflect on the action they have taken, groups must decide whether they are satisfied that they have been heard or whether they need to take more radical action to be heard. In the latter instance, they will design and adopt strategies that will elicit attention and "force" the community and politicians to listen. Such strategies often involve some form of confrontation, as when a group of homeless women and men pitch a tent on a courthouse lawn (Sacks, 1991).

Having got the attention of the public and policy makers, the group's action now shifts to lobbying in an organized fashion and to formulating precise demands for legislation, policies, and services. Applying focused pressure is a skill that the disempowered need to develop to become empowered. It will be more easily acquired if members, from the earliest stages of the group, have learned to formulate as precisely as possible what they want, what means they are ready to take to get what they want, what costs they are prepared to pay, and so forth. As the members gain experience in seeing their requests attended to seriously, and as they begin to participate in earnest in the democratic political process, they become empowered.

This does not mean that they will obtain everything they demand; participating in the democratic process does not, nor should it, guarantee this. It does mean, however, that their actions have the same probability of succeeding as those of other groups in society who are seeking their fair share of resources.

Embeddedness in the Community

Empowerment-oriented groups, though long-term groups, eventually come to an end. As for all groups, the end phase is associated with the question of how best to insure that the gains achieved through the group will endure. Once the group terminates, ex-group members cannot protect, consolidate, and build on these achievements if they are socially isolated; they need a supportive environment. They need, just like any empowered person, to be embedded in a community. Embeddedness is taken here in its original sense of rootedness and interdependence and does not connote the subservience and dependence with which the word became associated when reporters were attached to military units in the 2003 invasion of Iraq. Being rooted in, or being part of, a community is a safeguard against the social marginalization that plagues the disempowered.

All means of becoming embedded in a community require some degree of participation in the affairs of that community. To consolidate and build on the gains made in empowerment-oriented groups, a typical strategy is for ex-members to join or be incorporated into the organizations that hosted the groups. This may mean that they become employees of the organizations; that they become volunteers, peer supporters or coleaders of groups; that they become spokespersons for the organizations at conferences or trainers in educational programs (Cox, 2002); or that they get elected to boards of directors (Cohen, 1994). Another typical strategy is for ex-members to become active in other community institutions or organizations or make use of community resources, such as community colleges. The affirmation and testing of strengths and abilities provided through empowerment-oriented groups often act as the trigger that releases the energy and courage of ex-members to go back to school—thus safeguarding themselves against the economic marginalization that so often goes hand in hand with lack of schooling. Ex-members can also consolidate gains made at the political level by joining existing lobbies or advocacy organizations. Cox (2002, p. 52) writes about a grandparent who, having graduated from an empowerment training group program, spoke up at a public meeting on changes in social services agency priorities and "demanded to be placed on an advisory board so that she could have direct involvement in policy."

CONCEPTUAL FOUNDATIONS OF EMPOWERMENT

As Gil (1998, p. 1) has pointed out, "Social workers and social policy professionals have always been involved with victims of injustice and oppression." This involvement, however, has not necessarily translated into confronting injustice and oppression directly. Such confrontation, it is fair to say, is not at the core of the practice models most favored by the profession. It is at the core of empowerment-oriented group practice.

Social Movements

One can trace some of the philosophical bases of empowerment-oriented group work to the three social movements that were seminal influences on the development of social group work: the *settlement house movement*, the *progressive education movement*, and the *recreation movement* (Breton, 1990). The first of these movements categorically stood for professionals throwing their lot with the people they wanted to help, sharing their lives, refusing to distance themselves from the people, refusing to separate personal issues and problems from social, economic, and political issues and problems, and getting involved in community and neighborhood concerns in an immediate and concrete fashion. These professionals "chose to perceive people not only as individuals but as members of social groups and cultures affected by the social, economic and political conditions in which they live" (Breton, 1990, p. 22). They believed that when these conditions were unjust, the people themselves should get involved in efforts to change the conditions, and they facilitated that involvement. They shared the view of contemporary liberation movements that it is not good enough to learn about different groups and cultures; one has to learn *from* different groups and cultures.

The progressive education movement was influenced by Dewey's (1922) philosophical positions on ideal forms of government and his views on citizenship. It led group workers to perceive the small group as an experience that prepared members to participate in the democratic affairs of the community. Providing opportunities for people to learn to become citizens and to learn the importance of citizenship was a central preoccupation of group work pioneers such as Jane Addams, Mary Parker Follet, Eduard Lindeman, and Grace Coyle (Shapiro, 1991). Their thinking is relevant to a contemporary practice perspective that is diversity based and multicultural. As Shapiro (1991, p. 9) notes, "A distinctive aspect of their ideas was an emphasis on the role of groups and voluntary associations in a pluralistic society. Groups would provide an arena within which individual interests and differences might be 'socialized' (to use Jane Addams' term) and mediated."

As the settlement and progressive education movements drew attention to the social and political self, the recreation movement directed group workers to pay attention to the whole self. That is a focus that, in its emphasis on the "deep delight available in the mutual interactions of a democratic and creative group" (Coyle, 1947/1955, p. 96), anticipated the strengths perspective, for it recognized the innate potential of human beings and their immense capacity for growth when not stigmatized with labels or stuck in sick roles. Groups were structured "so that the whole person in each member [was] invited to participate, [not only] the troubled, or broken, or hurt part" (Breton, 1990, p. 27).

The influence of the conceptual and philosophical premises of the early social movements of the 20th century on empowerment-oriented group work has been followed by that of contemporary liberation and other social movements. These movements include:

1. *The critical/radical practice movement* (Galper, 1980; Gil, 1998; Longres, 1996), which emphasizes institutional and social change and redefines the client–professional relationship as a partnership and expertise as a shared resource—not the exclusive property of the professionals.
2. *The self-help movement*, which points up the iatrogenic effects of the helpee's role and the obverse beneficial effects of the helper's role (Gartner & Reissman, 1984; Reissman, 1990).
3. *The feminist movement*, with its insights into gendering processes, the workings of privilege and oppression to the detriment of women, and the conceptualization of power not as hierarchical but as collective (see Butler & Wintram, 1991; Garvin & Reed, 1995; Pollio, 2000; Saulnier, 2000; Weick, 1982).
4. *The critical consciousness and radical pedagogy movement* (Freire, 1970/1993, 1990; Kieffer, 1984), which engages people's ability to critically perceive their relationships with the world in which they live, as well as their ability to critically act on that world, and sees the education process as a dialogue—as opposed to the "banking notion" of education, in which the ones who know deposit that knowledge into empty vessels.
5. *The multicultural and diversity movement*, which calls attention to the special strengths of ethnic, cultural, and other distinct groups and eschews paternalistic approaches (McKenzie & Morrissette, 1993; Spencer, Lewis, & Gutiérrez, 2000).
6. *The community-building movement*, which shifts the emphasis from community organizing led by professionals to community building led by members of the community—thereby highlighting both participation *and* accountability by treating community members as equal partners in social enterprises (Ewalt, Freeman, & Poole, 1998; Weil, 1996; Zippay, 1995).
7. *The strengths perspective*, which is implied in all the above movements (Saleebey, 1997; Weick, Rapps, Sullivan, & Kisthardt, 1989). It is built on the premise that individuals and communities have strengths and resources. As Swenson (1998, p. 530) put it succinctly, "Without a strengths perspective, social workers are left with theories that pathologize, emphasize deficits, and 'blame the victim.'"

Major Themes

Many common themes emerge from the ethics or moral philosophy that underlies the preceding social movements, young and old. The themes all relate to empowerment-oriented group work, for they all ensue from the moral precept to fight oppression and social injustice. Because of space limitations, only a few selected themes are discussed here.

Power

Essential to understanding empowerment is confronting questions such as: Where does power come from? How is it used by social work professionals and organizations? Can it be shared?

In their influential work on the sources of social power, French and Raven (1960) identify and analyze five of the most common and important bases of power. These are: reward power, coercive power, legitimate power, referent power, and expert power. Their analysis can be used to shed light on empowerment-oriented group practice.

The first point to note, because it is relevant to cognitive restructuring and the consciousness-raising process, is that French and Raven (1960) hypothesize that power is exerted on a person because that person *perceives* that the one exerting the power has either the ability to mediate rewards (reward power); the ability to mediate punishment (coercive power); the legitimate right to prescribe behavior (legitimate power); or some special knowledge or expertise (expert power). Referent power is based on a person's identification with the one exerting power, a psychological mechanism that calls to mind the "oppressor within" construct.

To signal the importance of perception in power relationships does not imply that consciousness raising (which involves a change in perception) leads to ignoring the real power that people or organizations possess because they control critical resources or because they have abilities, knowledge, and socially, politically, or culturally sanctioned statuses and rights. What consciousness raising does is get people who previously thought of themselves as powerless to realize that they, too, have power because they, too, control resources and they, too, have abilities, knowledge, and rights. Through the process of consciousness-raising, the disempowered broaden their perception of power to include their own heretofore unacknowledged power. In that sense, empowerment is a matter of equalizing or rectifying power imbalances. It is not a takeover of power; it does not require disempowering those who are already empowered; it means sharing that power by becoming empowered.

To argue that the disempowered have resources may seem to contradict the very notion of oppression unless the distinction is made between positive and negative sources of power (Wax, 1971). When people have insufficient positive sources of power, such as the ability to reward, they can use negative sources of power. The main source of negative power is the ability to withhold consent, support, or participation. Withholding does not imply passive behavior. It often involves some form of confrontation, such as the use of obstruction to influence the relative costs of projects (c.f. O'Sullivan, Waugh, & Espeland, 1984).

The second point to be drawn from French and Raven's (1960) theory relates to referent power. The importance of understanding and using mutual-aid dynamics in empowerment-oriented practice has been mentioned previously. What can be derived from the analysis of the bases of power is that a mutual-aid group per se has the essential elements to become a significant referent group for its members (Shapiro, 1990; Sherif & Sherif, 1964). When a reference group is also empowerment oriented and addresses the issue of the "oppressor within," it has the opportunity to substitute for that internalized oppressor a group of peers perceived as equal partners striving and helping each other to gain control over their lives.

Power issues exist in any empowerment-oriented group facilitated by professional social workers. Hasenfeld (1987), discussing power as an integral and neglected component of social work practice, argues that the main source of social workers' power is that they are members of an organization that controls critical resources and services needed by clients. Members of empowerment-oriented groups know this, as do the social workers who facilitate such groups. The organization can withhold rewards and mete out punishments to both. But then group members and staff can withhold consent, support, and participation in the organization's operations and programs; they have and can use negative power. As this use of power will probably entail confrontation, the attendant risks must at least be acknowledged, as mentioned earlier, from the beginning of the group.

Self-determination, that hallowed social work construct, is by definition connected to power and control issues and therefore is highly relevant to empowerment. Haynes & Mickelson (1997) have argued that because self-determination is perceived in social work at the micro, as well as at the macro, level as an absolute, it is largely irrelevant in terms of real practice and power relationships, both of which involve compromise. To be serious about empowerment, the social work profession needs to rethink and reevaluate self-determination so as to make it a truly applicable and honestly applied value.

Social Justice

Philosophers such as Rawls (1971) and Sen (1999) have made major contributions to theories of social justice, and social work theorists have identified and analyzed core issues in terms of the application of social justice concepts (see Swenson, 1998; van Soest, 1995). Heffernan, Shuttlesworth, and Ambrosino's (2001) proposition that social and economic justice includes fairness and equity in regard to basic civil and human rights, protections, resources and opportunities, and social benefits encompasses the concerns of empowerment-oriented group practice. The proposition helps to explain why social justice is being considered as the organizing value in social work (Wakefield, 1988).

There is a paradox in that consideration, for social policy receives relatively little of the profession's attention. "Yet social injustices cannot be dealt with in any significant way without dealing with the policies that create or exacerbate them, nor can social justice be pursued effectively without promoting just social policies" (Breton et al., 2003). The paradox is related in part to social work history. In the process of becoming a profession, social work decided in essence to favor psychology and psychiatry as foundational knowledge. That decision was a costly one, as it resulted in the neglect of sociology, economics, and political science, which are important to understanding and assessing social and economic policy and to engaging in policy making.

In order to work effectively toward the implementation of just and equitable social policies, social workers and members of empowerment-oriented groups need to be able to contextualize problems in terms of their social and economic origins and their ramifications in a specific social and economic environment. Contextualizing socioeconomic problems does not require the ability to use the tools of economics. It does require understanding an economic approach to problems and being able to make sense of and to criticize interpretations of raw data on such things as affordable housing or unemployment or poverty in a given metropolitan area. Inability to contextualize socioeconomic problems—because it leads to inadequate assessment of these problems and therefore to arbitrary and poorly conceived efforts at policy making—will tend to relegate social justice to the status of a revered but nonoperationalized value.

Radical Pedagogy

Radical pedagogy has been referred to previously; its importance to empowerment warrants further elucidation. Paulo Freire (1973/1993), the foremost exponent of this pedagogy, sees education as the practice of freedom—freedom from the culture of silence in which oppressed people live, freedom for people to have their say, freedom to name the world. He rejects conventional education, which he identifies as a taming process through which people learn to conform and are assimilated into the prevailing system.

On the contrary, radical pedagogy presumes that educators enter into a dialogue with "educands," become partners, and act as problem posers, not problem solvers. Freire assumes further that educators must acknowledge and respect the "knowledge of living experience"—and in this he antedated the narrative approaches so popular today (see White & Epston, 1990), as well as the strengths perspective. He cautions, however, that that knowledge is not the *only* knowledge people have a right to access. It is in this context that Freire assumes that educators should present their "dream" to people, who all have a vocation to "be more," to be subjects who act on and transform the structure of oppression.

Based on these assumptions, Freire (1973/1993, p. 55) develops his theory of conscientization as a process through which the oppressed, who are "beings for others," become "beings for themselves" and his complementary theory of praxis, in which reflection and action belong to the oppressed themselves. As he put it (1973/1993, p. 60), "Liberation is a praxis: the action and reflection of men and women upon their world in order to transform it." Freire is uncompromising in his position on the need for both reflection and action. Twenty years after writing *Pedagogy of the Oppressed*, he scathingly observes that when consciousness raising produces change "only in the interiority of awareness [and] the world is left untouched," it produces "nothing but verbiage" (Freire, 1994, p. 104). That the oppressed must be the agents of their own liberation is the central hypothesis of all liberation theories and *ipso facto* of empowerment theory.

Liberation Theology

Boff and Boff (1987, p. 3) write: "Liberation theology was born when faith confronted the injustice done to the poor." They add (p. 14) that it is "a broad and variegated phenomenon [which] encompasses a wide range of ways of thinking the faith in the face of oppression" or simply that it is "faith confronted with oppression" (p. 12). In this theology, the word "liberation" is taken for what it is: "the concept of a historical reality, the reality of the social emancipation of the oppressed" (Boff & Boff, 1984, p. 81).

Liberation theologians assume that liberation presupposes a commitment to the poor and oppressed: "Commitment is the first step" (Segundo, 1976, p. 81). Early on, they recognized that this commitment required them to confront a powerful institution and its vested interests. They also assumed that both a commitment to the oppressed and a challenge to the institutional status quo meant being ready to use "the mighty weapon" of politics (Boff, 1977/1986, p. 43). They assumed in effect that there can be no liberation theology without a liberation praxis, that is, without taking actions that lead to the liberation of the poor and oppressed.

Following Freire—they acknowledge owing much to his pedagogy *of* the oppressed and not *for* the oppressed—they insist that it is the oppressed themselves who must become the primary agents of their own liberation. Liberation is not occupation: The powerful cannot occupy or take over from the oppressed the task of becoming enfranchised, liberated, or empowered.

Thus the liberation theologians' challenge to institutional power involves a challenge to the power of clerics, that is, professionals, to speak for the people. As Boff (1977/1986) observes, when people have the opportunity to have a say, the monopoly of experts on speech is over. Insisting that the oppressed speak for themselves assumes that they have resources that can be mobilized to begin a process of change. An "assistentialist" stance of helping people in need is to be replaced by a partnership stance of working with people who have not only needs but also resources and rights. It is not a question of ignoring needs. On the contrary, Segundo (1976, p. 41) stresses that liberation theology arises out of "the urgent problems of real life." Those problems, however, "are definitely not tackled on a plane of certain knowledge ... science [cannot] provide any ready-made option in advance" (Segundo, 1976, p. 76). Scientists, experts, professionals, are not in possession of incontestable knowledge that allows them to speak for the oppressed.

The change advocated by liberation theologians is not reform but transformation of the system. They assume that reformism, synonymous with timid measures, is insufficient in the long term and counterproductive in achieving a genuine transformation (see Breton, 1989). They are aware that the transformation of the system will not necessarily bring about a richer society but a more just, fraternal, and participatory society (Boff, 1985). Finally, liberation theologians assume and caution that liberation involves long-term work: "a journey of resistance and struggle, not of facile enthusiasm" (Boff, 1977/1986, p. 43).

Mutual Aid Groups and Organizations

In order to develop a sound theory of empowerment, some assumptions about mutual aid groups and about organizations must be added to those about power, social justice, education, and liberation. It is widely assumed that empowerment is facilitated through membership in an empowerment-oriented mutual aid group housed in a supportive organization (see Bartle et al., 2002; Gutiérrez et al., 1995 Home, 1991; Lee, 2001; Longres & McLeod, 1980).

In terms of groups, the following assumptions can be made:

1. When a group becomes a system of mutual aid, the power imbalances between professional facilitators and group members are significantly reduced because everyone becomes a helper.
2. There is, in groups, a better chance of seeing how private troubles and public issues are connected. When private troubles become shared troubles, their structural (i.e., nonpersonal) sources can be more easily identified.
3. The realization that one belongs to a particular class comes more naturally in mutual aid groups, in which one is face-to-face with others who are identified as being "in the same boat."
4. The disempowered or disenfranchised need a context in which to realize that they have a voice and a say, and the optimal context for this is a group in which they share their stories, debate issues, and make decisions.
5. Although it is possible to create such a context in a one-on-one situation, the outcome of individuals asserting their voices among a group of peers is that they develop that essential component of empowerment that Kieffer (1984) called "participatory competence"—the ability to participate in a common enterprise.
6. Mutual aid groups facilitate the action phase of empowerment work (Cox, 1991; Lee, 2001; Shapiro, 1991) through the mutual aid dynamic referred to as "the strength in us," which makes it easier for group members to mobilize for and take action. (See Gitterman, Chapter 6, this volume for a detailed discussion of the mutual aid approach.)

Assumptions about organizations that are relevant to a theory of empowerment can be derived from the research literature (see Bartle et al., 2002; Gutiérrez et al., 1995). They include the following:

1. As empowerment involves sharing power, and therefore challenges established power structures within organizations, organizational barriers to empowerment are to be expected.
2. As one of the organizational barriers to empowerment concerns the expectations of funding sources, organizations have to be ready to work around the rules of funders (see Bartle et al., 2002).
3. Practitioners who regularly interact with many organizations will hesitate to refer people to one that is hostile to the empowerment approach or that is simply very conservative and traditional (because they know it is service users who bear the costs of inconsistencies in approaches); this will tend to isolate empowerment-oriented organizations.
4. To fight isolation, empowerment-oriented organizations need to network and support one another.
5. Three types of organizational support are crucial to empowerment-oriented work: staff development, a collaborative or team-like approach, and administrative leadership and advocacy (Gutiérrez et al., 1995).
6. Because empowerment looks different in different contexts and even settings (Rappaport, 1985; Saleebey, 1997), organizations have to be innovative and open as to the form empowerment will take in their own settings.

FUTURE DIRECTIONS AND CONCLUSION

It is clear from this discussion that changes in the delivery of social work services would help to consolidate an empowerment approach in group work. In order to put social justice at the center of group work—addressing social policy issues and engaging in social action as normal, not exceptional, practice—the boundaries between levels of practice must be opened up (Breton et al., 2003; Cohen & Mullender, 1999). What Reid (2002) identifies as a trend toward multilevel intervention or integration needs to develop into a commonplace reality. This would lead to more systematic engagement of social work groups with the communities in which they operate. In that sense, the trend toward community-based practice dovetails with an empowerment-oriented group approach in that both stress the importance of partnerships with and within communities (Ewalt et al., 1998; Weil, 1996; Zippay, 1995). So too does the trend toward mandated collaboration between social services and communities (Bailey & McNally Koney, 1996).

Another change that is of the essence relates to power-sharing arrangements within social work organizations. Though conditions for the establishment of empowering organizational practices have been spelled out and examples documented (Gutiérrez et al., 1995; Shera, 1995), evidence of power sharing is still scarce. This may be due in part to the prevailing educational culture within schools of social work, a culture that would benefit from integrating a strengths perspective and creating an empowering environment (Breton, 1999).

The trend toward establishing consumer rights in social and mental health services has helped to foster, and is bound to help maintain, an empowerment perspective in these services (Staples, 1999). It is crucial to emphasize that a device such as a bill of rights for group members must have an enforcement mechanism if it is to be empowering. Without institutional measures guaranteeing its implementation, a bill of rights may make group members *feel* empowered or have a *sense* of empowerment; it will not mean that they have more control over what happens to them in a given institution. If it is not enforced, it may lead to disillusionment, disappointment, and further disempowerment.

Finally, the recognition and acceptance of participatory research is an indication of growing professional respect for the contribution of service users and has the potential, when used appropriately, to strengthen empowerment-oriented group practice (see Alvarez & Gutiérrez, 2001; Cox & Parsons, 2000).

This brief look at future directions has been, on the whole, optimistic. It would be misleading, however, not to mention at least one negative trend that is gaining ground in the social services and that could seriously threaten empowerment-oriented practice. That is the trend toward managed care and all forms of divestment of public, not-for-profit services onto the private for-profit sector. It has been stated more than once throughout this chapter that empowerment is achieved after a usually lengthy process of conscientization that leads to usually lengthy participation in a collective/social action. Empowerment work is not suited for short-term intervention that produces quickly reached goals. And it is obviously not suited to the preservation of the sociopolitical, organizational, or institutional status quo. Those who want to engage in empowerment-oriented group practice need to come to terms with these realities.

REFERENCES

Alvarez, A. R., & Gutiérrez, L. M. (2001). Choosing to do participatory research: An example and issues of fit to consider. *Journal of Community Practice, 9*(1), 1–20.

Andrews, J., & Reisch, M. (2002). The radical voices of social workers: Some lessons for the future. *Journal of Progressive Human Services, 13*(1), 5–30.

Bailey, D., & McNally Koney, K. (1996). Interorganizational community-based collaboratives: A strategic response to shape the social work agenda. *Social Work, 41*(6), 602–611.

Bartle, E. E., Couchonnal, G., Canda, E. R., & Staker, M. D. (2002). Empowerment as a dynamically developing concept for practice: Lessons learned from organizational ethnography. *Social Work, 47*(1), 32–43.

Boff, L. (1985). *Church: Charism and power.* New York: Crossroad.

Boff, L. (1986). *Ecclesiogenesis: The base communities reinvent the Church* (R. Barr, Trans.). Maryknoll, NY: Orbis Books. (Original work published 1977)

Boff, L., & Boff, C. (1984). *Salvation and liberation: In search of a balance between faith and politics.* Maryknoll, NY: Orbis Books.

Boff, L., & Boff, C. (1987). *Introducing liberation theology.* Maryknoll, NY: Orbis Books.

Breton, M. (1985). Reaching and engaging people: Issues and practice principles. *Social Work with Groups, 8*(3), 7–21.

Breton, M. (1989). Liberation theology, group work, and the right of the poor and oppressed to participate in the life of the community. *Social Work with Groups, 12*(3), 5–18.

Breton, M. (1990). Learning from social group work traditions. *Social Work with Groups, 13*(3), 21–34.

Breton, M. (1992). Clinical social work: Who is being empowered? In D. F. Fike & B. Rittner (Eds.), *Working from strengths: The essence of group work* (pp. 81–85). Miami, FL: Center for Group Work Studies.

Breton, M. (1994a). On the meaning of empowerment and empowerment-oriented practice. *Social Work with Groups, 17*(3), 23–37.

Breton, M. (1994b). Relating competence-promotion and empowerment. *Journal of Progressive Human Services, 5*(1), 27–44.

Breton, M. (1995). The potential for social action in groups. *Social Work with Groups, 18*(2/3), 5–13.

Breton, M. (1999). Sharing power. *Journal of Progressive Human Services, 10*(1), 33–51.

Breton, M. (2002). Empowerment practice in Canada and the United States: Restoring policy issues at the center of social work. *Social Policy Journal, 1*(1), 19–34.

Breton, M., & Breton, A. (1997). Democracy and empowerment. In A. Breton, G. Galeotti, P. Salmon, & R. Wintrobe (Eds.), *Understanding democracy: Economic and political perspectives* (pp. 176–195). New York: Cambridge University Press.

Breton, M., Cox, E. O., & Taylor, S. (2003). Social justice, social policy, and social work: Securing the connection. *Social Policy Journal, 2*(1), 3–20.

Butler, S., & Wintram, C. (1991). *Feminist group work.* London: Sage.

Cohen, M. B. (1994). Overcoming obstacles to forming empowerment groups: A consumer advisory board for homeless clients. *Social Work, 39*(6), 742–749.

Cohen, M., & Mullender, A. (1999). The personal in the political: Exploring the group work continuum from individual to social change goals. *Social Work with Groups, 22*(1), 13–31.

Cox, C. B. (2002). Empowering African American custodial grandparents. *Social Work, 47*(1), 45–54.

Cox, E. O. (1988). Empowerment of the low income elderly through group work. *Social Work with Groups, 14*(4), 111–125.

Cox, E. O. (1991). The critical role of social action in empowerment oriented groups. *Social Work with Groups, 14*(3/4), 77–90.

Cox, E. O., & Parsons, R. J. (2000). Empowerment-oriented practice: From practice value to practice model. In P. Allen-Meares & C. Garvin (Eds.), *The handbook of social work practice* (pp. 113–129). Thousand Oaks, CA: Sage.

Coyle, G. L. (1955). Group work as a method in recreation. In H. B. Trecker (Ed.), *Group work: Foundations and frontiers* (pp. 91–108). New York: Whiteside and William Morrow. (Original work published 1947)

Dewey, J. (1922). *Human nature and conduct.* New York: Random House.

Du Bois, B., & Miley, K. K. (1999). *Social work: An empowering profession* (3rd ed.). Boston: Allyn & Bacon.

Ewalt, P. L. Freeman, E. M., & Poole, D. L. (Eds.). (1998). *Community building: Renewal, well-being, and shared responsibility.* Washington, DC: NASW Press.

Fanon, F. (1968). *The wretched of the earth.* New York: Grove Press.

Freire, P. (1993a). *Education for critical consciousness.* New York: Continuum. (Original work published 1973)

Freire, P. (1993b). *Pedagogy of the oppressed.* New York: Continuum. (Original work published 1970)

Freire, P. (1994). *Pedagogy of hope: Reliving pedagogy of the oppressed.* New York: Continuum.

French, J. R. P., & Raven, B. (1960). The bases of social power. In D. Cartwright & A. Zander (Eds.), *Group dynamics: Research and theory* (2nd ed., pp. 607–623). New York: Harper & Row.

Galper, J. H. (1980). *Social work practice: A radical perspective.* Englewood Cliffs, NJ: Prentice-Hall.

Gartner, A., & Reissman, F. E. (Eds.). (1984). *The self-help revolution.* New York: Human Sciences.

Garvin, C. D. (1991). Barriers to effective social action by groups. *Social Work with Groups, 14*(3/4), 65–76.

Garvin, C. D. (1997). *Contemporary group work* (3rd ed.). Boston: Allyn & Bacon.

Garvin, C. D., & Reed, B. G. (1995). Sources and visions for feminist group work: Reflective processes, social justice, diversity, and connection. In N. Van Den Bergh (Ed.), *Feminist visions for social work* (pp. 41–69). Silver Springs, MD: NASW Press.

Gil, D. G. (1998). *Confronting injustice and oppression.* New York: Columbia University Press.

Gutiérrez, L. M. (1990). Working with women of color: An empowerment perspective. *Social Work, 35*(2), 149–153.

Gutiérrez, L. M. (1994). Beyond coping: An empowerment perspective on stressful life events. *Journal of Sociology and Social Welfare, 21*(3), 201–219.

Gutiérrez, L. M., GlenMaye, L., & DeLois, K. (1995). The organizational context for empowerment practice: Implications for social work administration. *Social Work, 40*(2), 249–258.

Hartman, A. (1993). The professional is political. *Social Work, 38*(4), 365–366, 504.

Hasenfeld, Y. (1987). Power in social work practice. *Social Service Review, 61*, 469–483.

Haynes, K. S., & Mickelson, J. S. (1997). *Affecting change: Social workers in the political arena* (3rd ed.). White Plains, NY: Longman.

Heffernan, J., Shuttlesworth, G., & Ambrosino, R. (2001). *Social work and social welfare.* Belmont, CA: Brooks/Cole.

Holmes, G. E., & Saleebey, D. (1993). Empowerment, the medical model, and the politics of clienthood. *Journal of Progressive Human Services, 4*(1), 61–78.

Home, A. (1991). Mobilizing women's strengths for social change: The group connection. In A. Vinik & M. Levin (Eds.), *Social action in group work* (pp. 153–173). New York: Haworth Press.

Kieffer, C. H. (1984). Citizen empowerment: A development perspective. In J. Rappaport, C. Swift, & R. Hess (Eds.), *Studies in empowerment: Steps toward understanding and action* (pp. 9–36). New York: Haworth Press.

Kurland, R. (1978). Planning: The neglected component in group development. *Social Work with Groups, 1*(2), 173–178.

Lee, J. A. B. (2001). *The empowerment approach to social work: Building the beloved community.* New York: Columbia University Press.

Longres, J. (1996). Radical social work: Is there a future? In P. Raffoul & C. A. McNeece (Eds.), *Future issues for social work practice* (pp. 229–239). Boston: Allyn & Bacon.

Longres, J. F., & McLeod, E. (1980). Consciousness raising and social work practice. *Social Casework, 61*(5), 267–276.

McKenzie, B. (1999). Empowerment in First Nations child and family services: A community-building process. In W. Shera & L. M. Wells (Eds.), *Empowerment practice in social work* (pp. 196–219). Toronto, Ontario, Canada: Canadian Scholars' Press.

McKenzie, B., & Morrissette, L. (1993). Cultural empowerment and healing for aboriginal youth in Winnipeg. In A. Mawhiney (Ed.), *Rebirth: Political, economic and social development in First Nations* (pp. 117–130). Toronto, Ontario, Canada: Dundurn Press.

Memmi, A. (1965). *The colonizer and the colonized.* New York: Orion Press.

Mullender, A., & Ward, D. (1991). *Self-directed group work: Users take action for empowerment,* London: Whiting & Birch.

O'Sullivan, M. J., Waugh, N., & Espeland, W. (1984). The Fort McDowell Yavapai: From pawns to powerbrokers. In J. Rappaport, C. Swift, & R. Hess (Eds.), *Studies in empowerment: Steps toward understanding and action* (pp. 73–97). New York: Haworth Press.

Pernell, R. (1986). Empowerment and social group work. In M. Parnes (Ed.), *Innovations in social group work: Feedback from practice to theory* (pp. 107–117). New York: Haworth Press.

Pollio, D. E. (2000). Reconstructing feminist group work. *Social Work with Groups, 23*(2), 3–18.

Rappaport, J. (1981). In praise of paradox: A social policy of empowerment over prevention. *American Journal of Community Psychology, 9*(1), 1–25.

Rappaport, J. (1985). The power of empowerment language. *Social Policy, 16*(2), 15–21.

Rappaport, J. (1987). Terms of empowerment/exemplars of prevention: Toward a theory for community psychology. *American Journal of Community Psychology, 15,* 121–145.

Rawls, J. (1971). *A theory of justice.* Cambridge, MA: Harvard University Press.

Reamer, F. G. (1983). The concept of paternalism in social work. *Social Service Review, 57,* 254–271.

Reid, W. J. (2002). Knowledge for direct social work practice: An analysis of trends. *Social Service Review, 76*(1), 6–33.

Reisch, M. (1998). The socio-political context and social work method, 1890–1950. *Social Services Review, 72*(2), 161–181.

Reissman, F. (1990). Restructuring help: A human services paradigm for the 1990s. *American Journal of Community Psychology, 18*(2), 221–230.

Riger, S. (1993). What's wrong with empowerment. *American Journal of Community Psychology, 21*(3), 279–292.

Sacks, J. (1991). Action and reflection in work with a group of homeless people. *Social Work with Groups, 14*(3/4), 187–202.

Saleebey, D. (Ed.). (1997). *The strengths perspective in social work practice.* New York: Longman.

Saulnier, C. F. (2000). Incorporating feminist theory into social work practice: Group work examples. *Social Work with Groups, 23*(1), 5–29.

Segundo, J. L. (1976). *The liberation of theology* (J. Drury, Trans.). Maryknoll, NY: Orbis Books.

Seligman, M. (1975). *Helplessness: On depression, development and death*. San Francisco: Freeman.

Sen, A. (1999). *Development as freedom*. New York: Knopf.

Shapiro, B. Z. (1990). The social work group as social microcosm: Frames of reference revisited. *Social Work with Groups, 13*(2), 5–21.

Shapiro, B. Z. (1991). Social action, the group and society. *Social Work with Groups, 14*(3/4). 7–21.

Shera, W. (1995). Empowerment for organizations. *Administration in Social Work, 19*(4), 1–15.

Sherif, M., & Sherif, C. W. (1964). *Reference groups*. New York: Harper & Row.

Solomon, B. B. (1976). *Black empowerment: Social work in oppressed communities*. New York: Columbia University Press.

Specht, H., & Courtney, M. (1994). *Unfaithful angels: How social work abandoned its mission*. New York: Free Press.

Spencer, M., Lewis, E., & Gutiérrez, E. (2000). Multicultural perspectives on direct practice in social work. In P. Allen-Meares & C. Garvin (Eds.), *The handbook of social work direct practice* (pp. 131–149). Thousand Oaks, CA: Sage.

Staples, L. H. (1999). Consumer empowerment in a mental health system: Stakeholder roles and responsibilities. In W. Shera & L. M. Wells (Eds.), *Empowerment practice in social work* (pp. 119–141). Toronto, Ontario, Canada: Canadian Scholars' Press.

Steinberg, D. M. (1997). *The mutual-aid approach to working with groups: Helping people help each other*. Northvale, NJ: Aronson.

Swenson, C. R. (1998). Clinical social work's contribution to a social justice perspective. *Social Work, 43*(6), 527–537.

van Soest, D. (1995). Peace and social justice. In R. L. Edwards (Ed.), *Encyclopedia of social work* (19th ed., Vol. 3, pp. 1810–1817). Washington, DC: NASW Press.

Wakefield, J. C. (1988). Psychotherapy, distributive justice, and social work: 1. Distributive justice as a conceptual framework for social work. *Social Service Review, 62,* 187–210.

Ward, D., & Mullender, A. (1991). Empowerment and oppression: The indissoluble link. *Critical Social Policy, 32,* 21–30.

Wax, J. (1971). Power theory in institutional change. *Social Service Review, 45*(3), 274–288.

Weick, A. (1982). Issues of power in social work practice. In A. Weick & S. T. Vadiver (Eds.), *Women, power, and change* (pp. 173–185). Silver Spring, MD: NASW Press.

Weick, A. (1983). Issues in overturning a medical model of social work practice. *Social Work, 28*(6), 467–471.

Weick, A. (1992). Building a strengths perspective for social work. In D. Saleeby (Ed.), *The strengths perspective in social work practice* (pp. 18–26). New York: Longman.

Weick, A., Rapp, C., Sullivan, W. P., & Kisthardt, W. (1989). A strengths perspective for social work practice. *Social Work, 34*(4), 350–354.

Weil, M. (1996). Community building: Building community practice. *Social Work, 41*(5), 481–499.

White, M., & Epston, D. (1990). *Narrative means to therapeutic ends*. New York: Norton.

Wohl, B. J. (2000). The power of group work with youth: Creating activists of the future. *Social Work with Groups, 22*(4), 3–13.

Zippay, A. (1995). The politics of empowerment. *Social Work, 40*(2), 263–267.

Chapter 5

Ethics and Values
in Group Work

HELEN NORTHEN

Social workers with groups have a long history of embracing a set of social values. Only recently, however, has there been an increase of interest in translating these values into ethical principles that govern the conduct of practitioners in their relationships with individuals and groups. Codes of ethics have been developed by professional organizations, but they do not specify special applications to work with groups. In this chapter, I attend to selected ethical issues concerning groups: group relationships, multiculturalism, empowerment, confidentiality, self-determination, and professional competence. Attention is also given to ethical dilemmas that require workers to choose from among alternative principles. Concern with ethics is integrally related to the use of knowledge and skills in practice.

Social group work is defined as a method of social work whose purpose is the enhancement of the psychosocial functioning of individuals and improvement of their environments. According to findings from a survey by Turner (1979), the term "psychosocial" has been used since 1930 to refer to the feelings, attitudes, and behaviors of persons in their relationships with others. Coyle (1947) emphasized that the term also refers to the social conditions and situations in the environment that influence the well-being of people. Enhancement of functioning includes both prevention and treatment. The small group is the appropriate modality of practice when a person's needs can be met through interaction with others, as distinguished from help in a one-client-to-one-practitioner situation.

Values are abstract propositions about what is right, desirable, or worthwhile. Ethics are the rules of conduct governing a particular group. According to Loewenberg and Dolgoff (1988, p. 21), "Ethics are generally defined as that brand of philosophy that concerns itself with human conduct and moral decision making. . . . Morality consists of principles of conduct which define standards for right behavior." In a profession, the values are translated into ethical principles of practice.

The National Association of Social Workers (NASW) has a Code of Ethics (1996) that sets forth standards for professional conduct. According to the code, "broad ethical princi-ples are based on social work's core values of service, social justice, dignity and worth of the person, importance of human relationships, integrity, and competence. These principles set forth ideals to which all social workers should aspire" (p. 1). Little attention, however, was given to the use of these principles in social work practice with groups. That is true also for major books on social work, for example, Levy, 1976; Loewenberg and Dolgoff, 1988; Reamer, 1999; and Rhodes, 1986. These books contain almost no references to group work.

Social workers are bound by the ethical principles set forth in codes of ethics, but, when working with groups, they need also to understand and differentially apply these principles. Hartford (1976, p. 60) noted that "ethical commitments based on knowledge are particu-larly crucial in an area of work where the group can be used so powerfully to modify beliefs and behavior, for "brain washing," or even for the destruction of an individual's self image, personality, and feelings of competency." Knowledge of groups can be used for destructive as well as constructive purposes (Galinsky & Schopler, 1977; Schopler & Galinsky, 1981). The use of ethical principles is complicated in services to groups, owing to the larger number of persons involved and the nature and quality of the relationships and communications among them. The basic values of group work deal with relationships.

BASIC VALUES

Dignity and Worth

A primary value of group work is belief in the inherent worth and dignity of each person. If this value is accepted, then certain ideas follow about individuals in relation to society. All persons should be accepted as they are and their special strengths recognized. They should be treated with respect, regardless of their similarities and differences in relation to other persons and population groups. They should have freedom to express themselves without fear of negative sanctions. They should have the right to privacy, with information treated confidentially unless their informed consent has been obtained.

Social Justice

Social justice is a closely related value. Everybody has the right to civil liberties and equal opportunity without discrimination as to race, ethnicity, religion, social class, gender, sexual orientation, health, and capacities. They should have access to resources that are essential to meet their basic needs. They have the right to self-determination, that is, to make their own personal decisions and to participate in making group, family, or organizational decisions within the limits imposed by the individual's culture and status and with regard for the rights of others. A delicate balance exists between individual and societal welfare.

Mutual Responsibility

The value of mutual responsibility is based on the conviction that people are interdependent for survival and fulfillment of their needs. They are capable of helping one another. Mutual aid is the process whereby the reciprocal relations among people are used for helping each other (Lee & Swenson, 1994; Steinberg, 1997). As individuals interact with others in the en-vironment, they both influence and are influenced by each other. That is a democratic con-cept. Group work builds on this interdependence, a major reason that groups can become potent forces for development and change. Each member carries a contributing, as well as a receiving, role. Stimulation directed to enhancing psychosocial functioning arises from the network of interpersonal influences in which all members participate. The social worker is one important influence, but so too is each member of the group (Northen & Kurland, 2001). The worker is responsible for helping members to develop patterns of communication and norms of behavior that foster mutual aid.

THE IMPORTANCE OF HUMAN RELATIONS

Relationships among individuals are of crucial importance in groups. The ethical principle, according to the Code of Ethics, is that "Social workers recognize the central importance of human relationships. They engage people as partners in the helping process, seek to strengthen relationships among people in a purposeful effort to promote, restore, maintain, and enhance the well-being of individuals, families, social groups, organizations, and communities" (pp. 3–4). That is what happens in group work. Konopka (1992, p. 109) has eloquently reminded us that "all lives are connected to other lives. . . . It is the vital interrelationship of human beings that is the heart of social group work."

The Professional Relationship

The social worker's relationships with members and other persons in their behalf is an important component of practice. It is based on trust and used only for the benefit of clients (Kutchins, 1991). Practitioners are expected to demonstrate acceptance, empathy, and genuineness in their relationships with the persons they serve. They are expected to respect all members, regardless of their personal and cultural characteristics, interests, and capacities. They demonstrate trust through their attitudes and behavior. To be able to do this, the worker needs reflective self-awareness about his or her biases, prejudices, and moral preferences. Workers must recognize that each member has a particular psychological meaning for them; for example, some members may trigger reactions of fear, hostility, affection, or overprotection (Northen & Kurland 2001, p. 294). Workers need to learn to deal with these reactions so they do not interfere with the worker–group relationship.

Social workers are authority figures with professional power. They do not use this power to deceive, exploit, have sexual contacts with, or otherwise harm members. Shaffer and Galinsky (1989) discuss ways that practitioners may use their power to influence the emotions or actions of members unfairly. Serious injustice to clients' autonomy may occur when they are pressured into making decisions or performing tasks that are against their values or capacities.

Honesty and openness are crucial in the development of effective worker–group relationships. Withholding important information from the group creates difficulties in communication and may be unethical. A frequent example concerns the lack of honesty in informing members about the agency's purpose for the group. Social workers may not intend to deceive, but they may fail to present simply and clearly the purpose for which the group was formed. They may be fearful of negative responses or that prospective members will decide not to join the group. When workers present clearly the hoped-for outcomes and the means for achieving them, members often are relieved, and their interest in the group is enhanced (Kurland & Salmon, 1998). When there is disparity between the stated and hidden purposes, trust has been violated. Sneaking in a different purpose is not congruent with the qualities of acceptance, empathy, and genuineness. It is unethical practice. The principle is, "if the practitioner cannot say it to clients, then the practitioner has no right to try to do it" (Northen & Kurland, 2001, p. 179).

Group Relationships

The nature and quality of interpersonal relationships in the group have great impact on the meaning and value of the group to its members. People are interdependent; they have responsibilities toward each other. It is a fact that, as John Donne wrote a long time ago, "No man is an island entire of itself; every man is a piece of the continent, a part of the main." More recently, many social workers, particularly those interested in groups, identify with Ryan's (1985, p. 338) concern for a "world that would de-emphasize the exaltation of the individual as some kind of disconnected, omnipotent being and that would accept the reality that human accomplishments are the result of the actions of many persons working together." Falck (1995) is concerned about the focus on individuals, rather than on mutual aid through which members teach each other to meet their needs through a democratic group process. As Humphreys (1989) said, "There is something stronger than each of us individually and that is all of us together."

As members of groups, people engage in mutual aid, learning to receive from and give to others to the extent of their capacities and the opportunities that are available to them. Democratic attitudes, according to Phillips (1957, p. 26) "are not acquired by coercion, but through experience in democratic process." And Lindeman (1939, p. 50) wrote that "the democratic way of life rests firmly upon the assumption that means must be consonant with ends." Group work offers an experience in democratic participation in achieving agreed-upon goals.

Social workers have an ethical responsibility to help members to develop accepting and mutually helpful relationships. As noted earlier, a democratic philosophy places values on justice, dignity and worth, and mutual responsibilities. Social workers, then, make efforts to accept all members, regarding them as being worthy of respect, who come into the group with their varied customs and traditions based on their religious, ethnic, racial, and social class identifications. "It is an attitude that transcends tolerance: it is a positive acceptance of the values and differences among human beings, of their right to be different one from another" (Wilson & Ryland, 1949, p. 88).

Fundamental to group work values is the right of people to be different in a society in which each person has an equal right to membership and a responsibility for the common good. Maier (1997, p. 15) wrote that practitioners need to have "a decisive commitment to values for participatory interaction, mutual aid, and for a strong reliance on membership power." When these values are present, relationships tend to be maintained. Members need opportunities, both to provide and receive support.

The development of a contract—a working agreement with, not for, the group—is a means for assuring that the relationship between the worker and members will be based on mutual understanding. It involves both workers and clients in participating in decision making that results in mutual commitment and responsibility. It is through the process of contracting that members give their informed consent to participate in the group, with understanding of what that entails. Contracts clarify ethical issues and accountability. They encourage commitment and involvement (Seabury, 1976).

MULTICULTURALISM

Multiculturalism, according to Chau (1990), is becoming a professional ethic. He said that "the ethics of cultural pluralism is epitomized by accepting cultural differences and respecting the strengths inherent in these differences. . . . Cultural sensitivity in responding to the ethnic realities of our clients is the sine qua non for effective group work in multicultural contexts" (p. 10), and Walker and Staton (2000) agree that multiculturalism is a guiding principle of "virtuous practice." It is a belief about how people should be understood and treated, rather than a category of objective facts. These writers view it as an ethical principle that directs social work practice, and they discuss how treating multiculturalism as a body of knowledge, rather than as a value, promotes unintended stereotyping.

Social workers need to respect diversity and simultaneously focus on what human beings have in common. Understanding of shared values enhances respect for diversity, as Siporin (1982) pointed out. And "unity in diversity" was a major value in the philosophy of one of the profession's great founders, Jane Addams.

EMPOWERMENT

Empowerment is both a value and a goal (Hirayama & Hirayama, 1986). In the first social work book on the subject, Solomon (1976, p. 6) defined it as "a process whereby persons who belong to a stigmatized social category throughout their lives can be assisted to develop and increase skills in the exercise of interpersonal influence and the performance of valued social roles." She described groups as opportunity systems that can be used in a wide variety of efforts to empower clients. She said that work with groups and communities provides a richer opportunity system for reducing powerlessness than do one-worker-to-one-client approaches (p. 323). In groups, according to Simon (1994, p. 9), members derive "a sense of personal and interpersonal power from the collectivity that is able, to some degree, to reduce the structural power imbalance between the social worker and his or her clients." Social workers have an ethical responsibility to assist clients to achieve appropriate power.

Writing specifically about groups, Pernell (1986) described empowerment as an enabling process through which members are provided with the knowledge and opportunity to achieve their goals. "Power," she wrote, "is simply the ability or capacity to act or perform effectively. . . . It is the capacity to influence the forces which affect one's life space for one's own and others' benefit" (p. 117). She presented information about the potential of social group work to help members to develop such power. Gutiérrez and Lewis (1999) agreed with that and reminded readers that power may also be used to block opportunities and to exclude and control other persons. (See Mayadas, Smith, & Elliott, Chapter 3, this volume, for a detailed discussion of the idea of empowerment.)

CONFIDENTIALITY AND PRIVACY

Confidentiality refers to the degree of control that people have about the release of information about themselves. Members of groups have the right to a reasonable expectation of confidentiality (Skolnik & Attinson, 1978). The Code of Ethics states that "social workers should seek agreements among the parties involved concerning each individual's right to confidentiality and obligation to preserve the confidentiality of information shared by others." But implementing the principle is complicated, especially in groups.

Groups vary in their purposes, structures, and composition. The need for strict confidentiality, therefore, varies. For example, confidentiality is seldom an issue in educational groups with a stable structure and program plan. But it is crucial in therapeutic groups in which members have sensitive problems and are expected to disclose their feelings, ideas, and problems. Workers can, by word and deed, demonstrate that they can be trusted to keep confidential what they know about members, with certain exceptions that are explained to, and discussed by members. These exceptions include the duty to warn a third party about a client who is dangerous to self, others, or property when disclosure can prevent the threatened danger (Houston-Vega & Nuehring, 1997; Polowy, 1996). In 1976, the California Supreme Court in its Tarasoff decision stated that mental health practitioners have a responsibility to protect victims of violent clients. In a study by Weil and Sanchez (1983), the results clearly indicated that social workers recognized that responsibility but that they placed greater weight on professional and personal ethics than on legal mandates. The conclusion was that "the Tarasoff decision is an instance of good laws supporting responsible professional practice" (p. 123). The duty to warn other people conflicts with the duty to maintain confidence.

In groups, confidentiality is not limited to the social worker's behavior, because members acquire information about each other. The worker cannot guarantee that members will protect each other's privacy. Respect for privacy and maintenance of confidentiality depends on the extent to which a norm of confidentiality can be developed within the group. Such a norm ought to specify the nature, extent, and limits of confidentiality. Members need to decide what kind of information they will keep to themselves and what can be shared with family and friends (Northen, 1998). After all, if members are having a good experience, it is natural and appropriate to tell other people about it, without revealing sensitive material about other members. An issue is how the worker's interventions can help the members to protect confidentiality without unduly limiting self-determination.

One important ethical issue concerns the use of records about individuals or the group that contain sensitive information (Kagle, 1990). In general, members have the right to know what the records contain about them. One task of the profession is to find ways to keep essential records that will minimize the risks to each member when records are released for various purposes. If a record is used to obtain information about an individual, as in a team meeting or court hearing, data about other members are revealed. The same is true of audio or video recordings. Confidentiality is more likely to be protected if records are kept on each member rather than including that information in a group record.

Guidelines for promoting confidentiality in groups have been published by Congress and Lynn (1997) and Rock and Congress (1999). In essence, these include having correct information about policies and laws, avoiding the imposition of one's own values on other people, being explicit in contracting with members on issues of confidentiality, assessing the level of confidentiality appropriate for the particular group, helping the group to develop a norm of confidentiality, and exploring the issue in early meetings. The nature of the discussion needs to be appropriate to the type of group and the characteristics of members, including their capacities and problems. With groups of children and adolescents, it is often important to discuss the issue with parents or legal guardians.

SELF-DETERMINATION

Self-determination has long been viewed as a fundamental social work value. Barker (1991) defined it as "an ethical principle in social work which recognizes the rights and needs of clients to be free to make their own choices and decisions" (p. 210). The NASW Code states, "Social workers respect and promote the right of clients to self-determination and assist clients in their efforts to identify and clarify their goals" (p. 5). The Code does not, however, apply the principle to groups.

There are limitations to individuals' rights to make their own decisions and behave as they desire. In some cases, certain individuals do not have a choice about attending a group. Attendance is required, for example, as a condition of probation or by school assignment. The principle of informed consent is violated. An agent of the community has decided that help in a group is necessary. The issue of authority needs to be dealt with openly. "The demand that they face the problem is the beginning of the helping process," according to Shulman (1992, p. 371). Such members have the right to know the reason for the decision and to decide how they will participate in the group within the agreements in the group's contract.

Siporin (1982) has emphasized, for example, that self-determination deals with rights to socially responsible self-direction. Ewalt and Makuau (1995) provide evidence that the values of many cultures emphasize the collective, with individuals taking into account the welfare of the group in making their decisions. Similarly, Daly, Jennings, Beckett, and Leashore (1994) note that in African cultures humanity is viewed as a collective, expressed as shared concern and responsibility for the well-being of all. These value perspectives are in harmony with the emphasis in group work on interdependence, mutual aid, group problem solving, and respect for human diversity.

Congress and Lynn (1997) discuss the tension between the rights of members to self-determination and the need to develop a consensus. The skilled use of the worker's authority (power) is required to help the group to explore ideas, goals, and feelings and to set appropriate limits. The right of members to make their own choices does not deter the worker from intervening in ways that Schwartz (1961) called "lending a vision" to the members. Workers may use the term "self-determination" inappropriately as a rationale for failing to intervene (Kurland & Salmon, 1990). An example is of a graduate student who was forming a group for parents of children with special needs. She made a home visit to Mrs. C, whose son was complaining about his mother's strictness and was having difficulties in his relationships at the center. The visit was very brief. The student told Mrs. C about the group and invited her to attend. Mrs. C said she was not interested. The student said she should think about it and left. Mrs. C was not helped to understand how her participation could be of value both for her and for her son. It was not an informed decision. In reaching a group decision, the choices of individuals need to be modified in order to resolve the conflict and reach the agreed-upon goals.

The issue of social workers' power is central to ensuring the rights of members to make their own choices to the extent possible in a given situation. Long ago, Wilson and Ryland (1949) recognized the need for different degrees of direction by social workers, depending on the members' capacities to make informed decisions. They presented a chart that indicated six degrees of direction by the worker, ranging from controller to enabling observer. Similarly, and more recently, Rothman, Smith, Nakashima, Peterson, and Mustin (1996) conducted research that found that practitioners use a range of gradations of direction with an individual or group. These are: (1) reflective, involving exploration of a problem with an individual or group, without offering any direction; (2) suggestive, involving exploration in which the worker gives a mild or tentative preference for a solution; (3) prescriptive, involving consideration of a direction in which the worker clearly indicates a specific course of action; and (4) determinative, involving the use of an independent action by the worker on behalf of a client or group without their awareness or acquiescence. All four levels of direction were judged to be ethically suitable, depending on the situation.

Judgment about the appropriate degree of direction by workers requires, in addition to placing value on the clients' rights, knowledge about the capacities of clients, stages of group development, and limits posed by laws and environmental circumstances. Ethical practice is that in which social workers enable the group to take responsibility for itself as soon as possible. The right of the group to make its own decisions within its contract is based on the principle that it is important for people to learn to govern their own lives. Workers release responsibility to the members as they become able to assume it. Gradually, most power shifts from the worker to the group. Ethically, social workers do have authority, with its concomitant responsibility for the welfare of the group.

PROFESSIONAL COMPETENCE

Clients have a right to competent help. They have a right to expect that service will be provided in a manner that is consistent with ethical principles and standards of practice (Reamer, 1990). The rule is, "Do only what you know how to do."

The absence of professional competence, that is, having adequate ability to do something, is an ethical issue. The NASW Code of Ethics states that "social workers practice within their areas of competence and develop and enhance their professional expertise" (p. 5). It is unethical to perform a service when one is not competent to do it reasonably well. According to Levy (1976), practitioners are ethically accountable for what they do, the way they do it, and the results. They are ultimately responsible for the nature and quality of the services that they provide. In the final analysis, it is competence that counts. Values, knowledge, and skills need to be translated into effective performance.

The use of any approach to practice needs to be appropriate to the culture, characteristics, problems, and strengths of prospective members. Competent practitioners are aware of their own personal and cultural values and the ways these are similar to, or different from, those of their clients, those espoused by the organization that employs them, and those expressed by dominant segments of the community. They are knowledgeable about professional ethics and evaluate their own behavior in relation to them. They need to be able to respond respectfully to people of varied races, religions, ethnic backgrounds, sexual orientations, and socioeconomic status in a manner that recognizes and affirms their worth. They appreciate the importance of multiculturalism (Chau, 1990; Davis, 1984; Durst, 1994; Tsang & Bogo, 1997; Tsui & Schultz, 1988).

Konopka (1978, p. 126) described the tendency of group workers "to grab on" to models of group work that were developed outside the profession. These include marathons, Gestalt therapy, behavior modification, and computer counseling. Malekoff (1997) proposed a principle concerning new approaches. He wrote, "Group workers who decide to adopt approaches that are rising in popularity, whatever these approaches might be, must not lose sight of the core principles of group work"(p. 41).

Certainly, knowledge about varied models can provide new ideas or techniques to strengthen practice. Much has been learned, for example, from Carl Rogers's (1957) research on the qualities of relationships that positively influence outcomes. That knowledge has been integrated into most social work approaches to practice. There is need to be clear about which clients these types of practice are effective with and the value system on which they are based.

Social workers should determine whether or not they have the skills to make adequate use of specific approaches that will benefit the group. Being acquainted with theory is not enough. The theory must be transformed into action. Ethical practice and legal duty require workers to provide a reasonable standard of service. Social workers with groups should use interventions that are new to them only after acquiring in-depth understanding of the theory and being trained and supervised to use them competently (Thyer & Myers, 1999). It is clear that verbal interventions or activities that deceive members or that harm them are not ethical. Furthermore, workers may be held liable for the actions of members who violate ethics (Houston-Vega & Nuehring, 1997). Casualties do occur, and workers are responsible for preventing them to the extent that is humanly possible. A study by Schopler and Galinsky (1981) identified reasons that some members were hurt by groups. Smokowski, Rose, Todar, and Reardon (1999) also studied the dynamics of damaging group experiences. Being in the casualty group was associated with the members' perceiving the group leader as the perpetrator of a stressful event, having an intense emotional reaction to an event, and being discouraged from pursuing additional help. A key factor was that members perceived that they were being betrayed and humiliated. The quality of relationships is crucial to good practice.

ETHICAL DILEMMAS

Ethical dilemmas are perplexing situations that require a practitioner to choose from among alternative actions. They concern obligations to protect the rights and welfare of clients. They include issues of social policies, equal opportunity, termination of services, differences in values, and use of records of members.

A frequent dilemma for group workers is how to adapt or change organizational policies so that they meet the needs of clients. Through research, Conrad (1988) found that most ethical conflicts were those between professional values and policies that interfered with the provision of effective services to clients. In groups, such conflicts are common. An example is from a group of young adults in which the social worker explained that the group could meet for up to 8 weeks. One member said, "Oh, no, I was in a group that lasted only six weeks. We had just gotten to know and not be afraid when 'pow!' our leader pulled the rug from under us and left us out in the cold to live with all of the hang-ups we had when we first came to the group." Other members chimed in, protesting that it was unfair not to have the group last as long as they needed it. Based on preliminary assessment of the capacities and problems of the members, the worker also did not favor the imposed time limit. What choices did the worker have in attempting to solve this problem? Based on the use of the problem-solving process, the worker's decision might be to advocate for extension of the time limit with the director; to continue by ignoring agency policy based on a conviction that the needs of clients have priority; to extend the number of sessions per week within the time limit; or to enable the group to select limited goals that might be achieved within the time limit,

The basic value of human justice means that equal opportunities should be provided for individuals to receive appropriate services to meet their needs (NASW, 1986). That principle may create a dilemma for workers with groups. The principles of group formation may limit who is selected for membership from among the individuals who were referred to or applied for membership and who met the criteria set by the worker or agency policies (Glassman & Kates, 1986). The dilemma is the conflict between the rights of an applicant for services and the need for a group's composition, including its size, to be suitable to its purposes. A related dilemma is that members of ongoing groups may oppose the entry of new members, claiming it is their right to make that decision, thus denying a necessary service to the prospective member. In other situations, some members may try to force another member out of the group, which would deny the ousted member the right to be helped and deny the group the opportunity to learn how to deal with conflicts in relationships.

A principle of practice is that groups should end when the goals have been achieved or when it becomes clear that the group is unable to meet the members' needs. In terminating a group or one of its members, ethical dilemmas occur. For example, if a majority of members are ready to leave the group, what happens to those who need more time? What happens when a worker resigns or has been reassigned to other duties and there is no replacement? In such instances, members may feel abandoned, sometimes realistically so. Abandonment is a "legal concept that refers to instances in which a professional is not available to a client when needed" (Reamer, 1999, p. 151). Numerous malpractice suits have resulted from clients' feelings of abandonment before their goals have been achieved (Houston-Vega & Nuehring, 1997).

One ethical issue for social workers concerns making decisions when differences in values between worker and members or among members and their families prevent the group from developing its program. Open discussion is difficult when cultural values include the belief that personal matters should not be aired in public or that they should remain within the family. For example, members may need to deal with issues of sexual behavior or birth control that conflict with beliefs that talking about such issues is taboo.

An example concerns a group of adolescent girls. Lydia entered the room a little late and announced that she had just seen her doctor and learned that she is pregnant. "I'll just have to find a way to get rid of it," she said. The worker knew that the girls had a need and were ready to deal with the issues of pregnancy and abortion. She knew also that discussion of sex was taboo. What can the worker do to resolve the issue? The worker decided to discuss the dilemma with the group, referring to Lydia's situation and the need of all girls to have adequate information. She suggested that discussion in the group could be helpful, but their parents thought that such matters belonged only at home. The consensus of the members was, "we want to do it here." The worker suggested that she could talk to their parents or that the group could have a meeting that included the parents and asked for other suggestions. The girls decided to invite their parents to a meeting, and plans for such a meeting were made. With increased understanding of the members' interest and their confidence in the worker's leadership, the parents consented, and they even felt relieved that, as one said, "you will help us, too."

Many other ethical dilemmas face social workers and members of their groups. These include clients' access to their records; the release of records to others; conflict between the duty to aid and personal values over such issues as child abuse, birth control, or sexual misconduct; the duty to report illegal acts; and determining whose needs take priority in conflict situations. Dilemmas are resolved through use of the problem-solving process, with special attention to self-awareness, knowledge of ethical principles and relevant laws, consideration of alternatives, priorities for meeting needs of individual versus group versus society, and the use of consultation with experts (Congress & Lynn, 1997; Rock & Congress, 1999).

In studies of values and ethics, Reamer (1999, p. 118) asserts that there are two major orientations. The first is grounded in social work's enduring concern about the similarities and differences in values between social workers and their clients and significant others. The emphasis is on making ethical decisions and resolving conflicts of values. The purpose is to enhance ethical practice for the benefit of clients. That is the orientation used in this chapter.

The second orientation is a defensive one; its focus is on protecting practitioners from accusations of malpractice. The concern is to avoid liability for violation of laws and regulations. "Malpractice" is defined in *Black's Law Dictionary* (Black, 1979, p. 864) as "any professional misconduct, unreasonable lack of skill or fidelity in professional or fiduciary duties, evil practice, or illegal or immoral conduct." All social workers may be subject to the risks of malpractice and, therefore, need to become acquainted with guides for managing risks (Houston-Vega & Nuehring, 1997). The best defense against litigation is accurate documentation of practice decisions and interventions and, above all, competent ethical practice.

THE FUTURE

Changes in technology that make it possible to hold groups by telephone or computers enhances ethical dilemmas for social workers. A review of relevant literature by Schopler, Abell, and Galinsky (1998) suggests that such groups are beneficial in meeting the needs of a variety of clients who find it difficult to attend meetings of groups, but there also are disadvantages. These include problems in maintaining confidentiality and privacy, lack of equality of access to the technology, and limits to the extent that adequate ongoing assessment of individuals and groups can be achieved when one's understanding is based only on verbalization or written words.

The major ethical issue, however, is one of professional competence. Such work is, according to Smokowski et al. (1999), very different in many ways from work with groups in which the worker and members are together. To use computer or telephone groups successfully, both the worker and members need to have adequate knowledge and skills in the use of technology. They need to understand and adapt to the differences in the composition and structure of such groups, the variations in communication and problem solving, the frequent withdrawal of members, and means of evaluating outcomes.

Another major trend in social work is an increase in allegations of malpractice. The growing body of knowledge about malpractice in social work does not deal with the special risks involved in practice with groups. Dealing with issues of malpractice is beyond the scope of this chapter, but group workers need to understand the legal issues involved in malpractice (Houston-Vega & Nuehring, 1997). The best defense against litigation is, of course, ethically competent practice. If social work with groups is to meet the needs of diverse clients, knowledge of the interrelatedness of ethics with knowledge and skills needs to be accelerated.

Dolgoff and Skolnik (1996) reviewed textbooks on group work to discover what attention was given to the topic of ethics. The conclusion was that "there has been no detailed examination of ethical dilemmas from a social group work perspective and no assessment of the pertinence of the NASW Code of Ethics for group work" (p. 100). Similarly, in a study of teaching group work, Strozier (1997) found that only a small number of syllabi of courses on group work included ethics and values as a major topic. Isn't it strange that, in light of the early emphasis on democracy in group work, more studies of ethics have not been conducted? Arlien Johnson wrote in 1955 that in the United States the basic concepts of social work are expressions of a democratic philosophy, including the importance of group effort. She emphasized that there is a need to formulate standards of "what is good and honorable" in practice (p. 126). The time is now!

In closing our book (Northen & Kurland, 2001), Roselle Kurland and I quoted Ben Orcutt (1990, pp. 56–57), who suggested that "competence evolves out of commitment, curiosity, and the thirst for knowledge—a creative, imaginative search to know." Social workers with groups have a responsibility to practice within the realm of the accumulated theoretical base, tested interventions, and ethical principles.

REFERENCES

Barker, R. L. (1991). *The social work dictionary* (4th ed.). Washington, DC: NASW Press.

Black, H. C. (1979). *Black's law dictionary* (5th ed.). St. Paul, MN: West.

Chau, K. (1990). Social work groups in multicultural contexts. *Group Work, 3*(1), 8–21.

Congress, E. P., & Lynn, M. (1997). Group work practice in the community: Navigating the slippery slope of ethical dilemmas. *Social Work with Groups, 20*(3), 61–74.

Conrad, A. (1988). Ethical considerations in the psychosocial process. *Social Casework, 69*(10), 603–610.

Coyle, G. (1947). *Group experience and democratic values.* New York: Woman's Press.

Daly, A., Jennings, J., Beckett, J., & Leashore, B. (1994). Effective coping strategies of African Americans. *Social Work, 40*(2), 240–248.

Davis, L. (Ed.). (1984). Ethnicity in social work practice [Special issue]. *Social Work with Groups, 7*(3).

Dolgoff, R., & Skolnik, L. (1996). Ethical decision making in social work with groups. *Social Work with Groups, 19*(2), 49–66.

Durst, D. (1994). Understanding the client-social worker relationship in a multicultural setting: Implications for practice. *Journal of Multicultural Social Work, 3*(4), 29–42.

Ewalt, P., & Makuau, N. (1995). Self determination: Pacific perspectives. *Social Work, 40*(2), 168–176.

Falck, H. S. (1995). Central characteristics of social work with groups: A sociocultural analysis. In R. Kurland & R. Salmon (Eds.), *Group work practice in a troubled society* (pp. 63–72). New York: Haworth Press.

Galinsky, M., & Schopler, J. (1977). Groups may be dangerous. *Social Work, 22*(2), 89–94.

Glassman, U., & Kates, L. (1986). Developing the democratic-humanistic norms of the social work group. In M. Parnes (Ed.), *Innovations in social group work: Feedback from practice to theory* (pp. 49–72). New York: Haworth Press.

Gutiérrez, L., & Lewis, E. A. (1999). *Empowering women of color.* New York: Columbia University Press.

Hartford, M. E. (1976). Group methods and generic practice. In R.W. Roberts & H. Northen (Eds.), *Theories of social work with groups* (pp. 45–74). New York: Columbia University Press.

Hirayama, H., & Hirayama, K. (1986). Empowerment through group participation: Process and goals. In M. Parnes (Ed.), *Innovations in social group work: Feedback from practice to theory* (pp. 119–131). New York: Haworth Press.

Houston-Vega, M. K., & Nuehring, E. M. (1997). *Prudent practice: A guide for managing malpractice risks.* Washington, DC: NASW Press.

Humphreys, G. (1989). *Valedictory address.* Address given at the University of Southern California, School of Social Work, Los Angeles, CA.

Johnson, A. (1955). Educating professional social workers for ethical practice. *Social Service Review, 29*, 125–136.

Kagle, J. (1990). *Social work records* (2nd ed.). Belmont, CA: Wadsworth.

Konopka, G. (1978). The significance of social group work based on ethical values. *Social Work with Groups, 1*(2), 123–128.

Konopka, G. (1992). All lives are connected to other lives: The meaning of social group work. In M. Weil, K. Chau, & D. Southerland (Eds.), *Theory and practice in social group work* (pp. 108–115). New York: Haworth.

Kurland, R., & Salmon, R. (1998). Purpose: A misunderstood and misused keystone of group work practice. *Social Work with Groups, 24*(3), 5–17.

Kurland, R., & Salmon, R. (1990). Self-determination: Its use and misuse in group work practice. In D. Fike & B. Rittner (Eds.), *Working from strengths: The essence of group work* (pp. 105–121). Miami, FL: Center for Group Work Studies.

Kutchins, H. (1991). The fiduciary relationship: The legal base for social workers' responsibilities to clients. *Social Work, 36*(2), 106–111.

Lee, J. A. B., & Swenson, C. R. (1994). The concept of mutual aid. In A. Gitterman & L. Shulman (Eds.), *Mutual aid groups, vulnerable populations, and the life cycle* (2nd. ed., pp. 412–430). New York: Columbia University Press.

Levy, C. (1976). *Social work ethics.* New York: Human Sciences Press.

Lindeman, E. (1939). Group work and democracy: A philosophical note. In J. Lieberman (Ed.), *New trends in group work* (pp. 47–53). New York: Association Press.

Loewenberg, F. M., & Dolgoff, R. (1988). *Ethical decisions in social work practice* (4th ed.). Itaska, IL: Peacock.

Maier, H. W. (1997). Social group work and developmental care: Retrospect and prospect for both. In A. Alissi & C. Corto Mergins (Eds.), *Voices from the field* (pp. 11–21). New York: Haworth Press.

Malekoff, A. (1997). *Group work with adolescents: Principles and practice.* New York: Guilford Press.

National Association of Social Workers. (1996). *Code of ethics.* Washington, DC: Author.

Northen, H. (1998). Ethical dilemmas in social work with groups. *Social Work with Groups, 21*(1/2), 3–17.

Northen, H., & Kurland, R. (2001). *Social work with groups* (3rd ed.). New York: Columbia University Press.

Orcutt, B. A. (1990). *Science and inquiry in social work practice.* New York: Columbia University Press.

Pernell, R. B. (1986). Empowerment in social group work. In M. Parnes (Ed.), *Innovations in social group work: Feedback from practice to theory* (pp. 107–118) New York: Haworth Press.

Phillips, H. U. (1957). *Essentials of social group work skill.* New York: Association Press.

Polowy, C. (1996, September). Client confidentiality and privileged communication. *NASW Newsletter, Washington State Chapter,* p. 5.

Reamer, F. G. (1999). *Social work values and ethics* (2nd ed.). New York: Columbia University Press.

Rhodes, M. L. (1986). *Ethical dilemmas in social work practice.* London: Routledge.

Rock, B., & Congress, E. (1999). The new confidentiality for the 21st century in a managed care environment. *Social Work, 44*(1), 253–262.

Rogers, C. (1957). The necessary and sufficient conditions of therapeutic personality change. *Journal of Consulting Psychology, 21*, 95–103.

Rothman, J., Smith, W., Nakashima, J., Peterson, M. A., & Mustin, J. (1996) Client self-determination and professional intervention: Striking a balance. *Social Work, 41*(4), 396–406.

Ryan, A. S. (1985). Cultural factors in casework with Chinese Americans. *Social Casework, 66*(6), 337–340.

Schopler, J., Abell, M., & Galinsky, M. (1998). Technology-based groups: A review and conceptual framework for practice. *Social Work, 43*(3), 254–268.

Schopler, J., & Galinsky, M. (1981). When groups go wrong. *Social Work, 25*(5), 424–429.

Schwartz, W. (1961). The social worker in the group. In National Conference of Social Work (Eds.), *The Social Welfare Forum* (pp. 145–171). New York: Columbia University Press.

Seabury, B. (1976). The contract: Uses, abuses, and limitations. *Social Work*, 21(1), 16–21.

Shaffer, J., & Galinsky, M. D. (1989). *Models of group therapy* (2nd ed.) Englewood Cliffs, NJ: Prentice-Hall.

Shulman, L. (1992). *The skills of helping individuals, families, and groups* (3rd ed.). Itasca, IL: Peacock.

Simon, B. L. (1994). *The empowerment tradition in American social work*. New York: Columbia University Press.

Siporin, M. (1982). Moral philosophy in social work today. *Social Service Review*, 56(4), 516–538.

Skolnik, L., & Attinson, L. (1978). Confidentiality in group work practice. *Social Work with Groups*, 1(2), 165–174.

Smokowski, P. R., Rose, S., Todar, K., & Reardon, K. (1999). Post group-casualty status, group events, and leader behavior: An early look into the dynamics of damaging group experiences. *Research on Social Work Practice*, 9(5), 555–571.

Solomon, B. B. (1976). *Black empowerment: Social work in oppressed communities*. New York: Columbia University Press.

Steinberg, D. M. (1997). *The mutual aid approach to working with groups*. Northvale, NJ: Aronson.

Strozier, A. L. (1997). Group work in social work education: What is being taught? *Social Work with Groups*, 20(1), 65–78.

Thyer, B. A., & Myers, L. L. (1999). On science, anti-science, and the client's right to effective treatment. *Social Work*, 44(2), 109–114.

Tsang, A. K. T., & Bogo, M. (1997). Engaging with clients cross-culturally: Toward developing research based practice. *Journal of Multicultural Social Work*, 6(3/4), 73–91.

Tsui, P., & Schultz, G. (1988). Ethnic factors in group practice: Cultural dynamics in multiethnic therapy groups. *American Journal of Orthopsychiatry*, 58(1), 136.

Turner, F. J. (Ed.). (1979). *Social work treatment: Interlocking theoretical approaches* (2nd ed.). New York: Free Press.

Walker, R., & Staton, M. (2000). Multiculturalism in social work ethics. *Journal of Social Work Education*, 36(3), 449–462.

Weil, M., & Sanchez E. (1983). The impact of the Tarasoff decision on clinical social work practice. *Social Service Review*, 57(1), 112–124.

Wilson, G., & Ryland, G. (1949). *Social group work practice*. Boston: Houghton Mifflin.

Part II

Group Practice Models: Principal Foundations

Initially, when group work was first conceptualized as a social work practice method, group workers presumed that they were using a common set of assumptions and seeking common purposes. As group work evolved, it became clear that group workers were diverging from one another by conceiving of group purposes in different ways, seeing the group worker's role differently, and utilizing somewhat different theories and practice principles. This is not to imply that theories were completely different. The kinds of social psychological terms presented in Chapter 1, for example, are likely to be found in the language of most, if not all, group workers. Several authors sought to analyze the group work models that were emerging. Papell and Rothman (1968), for example, described three models they termed "social goals," "remedial," and "reciprocal." A few years later, Roberts and Northen (1976), as editors, asked a group of writers whom they believed had created distinct group work approaches to present their ideas. These writers also met together to discuss each other's work, and Roberts and Northen, in their book, performed a comparative analysis of these approaches.

We chose in this book not to seek to update or repeat the work of Papell and Rothman or of Roberts and Northen. We believe that practice has become too eclectic to permit a neat typology of group work models. Rather, we sought to rely on each of our contributors to portray the models most pertinent to their topics. We did not, on the other hand, choose to relegate the issue of practice theory differences solely to these authors. We selected two perspectives to present in this section that represent different emphases that are often cited. One influential tradition is referred to as the "mutual aid model." This material draws heavily on principles of mutual aid, democratic decision making, and the importance of understanding the quality of member-to-member interactions, and Chapter 6 presents this set of ideas.

Another influential tradition has emerged from an emphasis on member goal achievement, the ways members and workers influence each other, and the cognitive-behavioral concepts that explain member influences and achievements. Chapter 7 explicates these ideas.

We do not believe that any of the current models of group work practice are mutually exclusive. Many practitioners draw upon several, even though there are differences in the terminology and assumptions of various ways of thinking that may, at times, seem contradictory. Nevertheless, some writers, such as Galinsky and Schopler (1989), have sought to reconcile differences.

We recognize that there are different emphases in group work in clinical than in macro settings, and some writers have sought to provide a conceptualization of macro group practice (Ephross & Vassil, 1988; Fatout & Rose, 1995). This aspect of group work is rapidly expanding, and for this reason we have undertaken to portray emerging models in Part V rather than in this part of the book.

REFERENCES

Ephross, P., & Vassil, T. (1988). *Groups that work*. New York: Columbia University Press.

Fatout, M., & Rose, S. (1995). *Task groups in the social services*. Thousand Oaks, CA: Sage.

Galinsky, M. J., & Schopler, J. (1989). The social work group. In J. Shaffer & D. Galinsky, *Models of group therapy* (2nd ed., pp. 18–40). Upper Saddle River, NJ: Prentice-Hall.

Papell, C. P., & Rothman, B. (1966). Social group work models: Possession and heritage. *Journal of Education for Social Work, 2*, 66–77.

Roberts, R., & Northen, H. (Eds.). (1976). *Theories of social work with groups*. New York: Columbia University Press.

Chapter 6

The Mutual Aid Model

ALEX GITTERMAN

The mutual aid model is embedded in group work's historic social goals tradition. William Schwartz, its major proponent, elaborated and refined the social goals' philosophical and value base by proposing a bold conception of social work function, phases of helping, mutual aid, and professional methodology. This chapter traces the historical context of the mutual aid model and Schwartz's distinctive contributions to its formulation. It presents his ideas and those of others, particularly in the conceptualization of a unique social work function, the specification of mutual aid processes, and the identification of specialized group work methods and skills. The chapter concludes with a practice illustration of mutual aid at work.

HISTORICAL CONTEXT

The history of group work and the mutual aid model are inextricably interwoven. In contrasting group work history to that of casework's one-on-one approach, Schwartz (1983/1986) wrote:

> A second direction has been to help needy people in their own milieu, surrounded by their peers and working in an atmosphere of mutual aid. Here the effort is to find, in the people's own conditions of life, the energy and resources with which they can help each other to act on common problems. People are brought together for many reasons: to organize themselves for action on special interest and common concerns; to help each other face difficult problems; to learn new skills with which to enrich the quality of their lives . . . experiences are communicated among the members . . . and the worker is surrounded by a host of surrogate helpers, each claiming a share of the supportive function. The lines of communication are intricate, and the worker's authority is diffused in the network of relationships that goes to make up the pattern of mutual aid. This is the direction we came to know as social group work. (pp. 7–8)

Social group work emerged from the settlement, recreation, and progressive education movements (Gitterman, 1979). These movements articulated two primary functions for small-group experiences. Some leaders emphasized using the small group to socialize members, whereas others emphasized using the small group to maintain a democratic society (Reid, 1991, p. 24).

From the settlements, group work derived its institutional base. Settlement leaders deeply believed in democratic group processes for the development of responsible citizenship, mutual aid, and collective action (Lee & Swenson, 1994). They divided their attention between developmental and citizenship experiences and environmental reform. They also used small-group experiences to build character and teach social skills. Group leaders were expected to model social values (Addams, 1910, 1930; Wald, 1915).

From the recreation movement, group work gained its interest in the value of play, activities, movement, and action. Initially, recreation and play were primarily used to fill leisure time and recreational needs. Later, activities were used to socialize members, build their "character," and instill a sense of competence and mastery (Lee, 1931). Camping stressed the importance of interaction with the natural environment, its appreciation and effective uses (Lieberman, 1931). The settlement and community center leaders incorporated recreational methods and programs into their services.

From progressive education, group work acquired a heuristic philosophical base (Dewey, 1916, 1938; Kilpatrick, 1940). Dewey emphasized the use of group process—peer learning—in the classroom. Dewey believed that participation and experience in democratic groups was the most effective means for learning and perpetuating democracy. His philosophy of education drew on the democratic ideal, reflecting the inspirations and visions of the settlements. The writings of Follett (1924, 1926) and Lindeman (1924, 1926) also provided group work with its philosophical base.

In the late 1930s, the settlement and community center, recreation, and adult education movements flourished. Practitioners from the various settings identified common interests and visions and formed the American Association for the Study of Group Work (AASGW). In its early development, a few distinctive characteristics differentiated group work from casework. Reid (1991, p. 27), citing Pernell (1986), identifies these differences:

> the emphasis on member versus clients; doing with versus doing for; doing versus talking about doing; activity and others as primary agents in the helping process versus the worker alone as the primary agent; personal and social development and social contribution as legitimate professional foci versus a remedial and rehabilitative focus; health and strength versus sickness and breakdown.

Professional differences in emphases were not limited to casework and group work. Among group workers, the practice of group work had different meanings and visions. In the 1940s and 1950s, group work practitioners and educators attempted to define the boundaries and functions of group work and to develop a conceptual base. The number of schools of social work with a group work specialization increased and resulted in the "method" becoming more "generic" and less setting bound.

Using ideas and research findings from sociology, social psychology, and group dynamics, a common core knowledge base began to emerge in the group work literature (Coyle, 1930, 1937). Related to this was an ongoing struggle to make sense of the diverse and competing demands placed on the burgeoning "method." Some leaders perceived group work as a social movement; others defined group work as a field of practice, identifying agencies with a common practice base. Still others began to define group work as a distinct process and method. To incorporate the varied definitions and interests, the boundaries and functions of group work were defined quite broadly: (1) the growth and development of the individual; (2) the development of the group; (3) the development of a democratic society. The writers searched for the elusive link between the needs of the individual and the needs of society, individual health and social participation, individual responsibility and democratic society. To fulfill this elusive but interrelated link, various educational, cultural, socialization, and social action functions were elaborated (Papell & Rothman, 1966). Broad premises and goals were in the foreground; professional methodology remained in the background.

In 1946, AASGW members voted to become the American Association of Group Workers (AAGW), a professional organization. And, in 1956, AAGW was incorporated into the National Association of Social Workers (NASW). Integration of AAGW with NASW brought group work fully into the profession. During the same period, group work practice expanded into clinical settings. These settings required "new psychological insights and understanding on the part of group workers" (Alissi, 1980, p. 7). As group work practice became more diverse, the Committee on Practice of the Group Work Section of the NASW assumed responsibility for developing working definitions and for establishing a frame of reference for social group work practice. A number of practitioners and educators were invited to prepare statements on these subjects; 10 were published (Hartford, 1964). Although participants were unable to agree on a common definition and frame of reference, the discussions renewed interests and identified critical knowledge gaps—particularly an underdeveloped professional methodology. Group work scholars further advanced the "method's" knowledge base, but professional group work methods and skills continued to be underdeveloped (Coyle, 1947, 1948; Konopka, 1949, 1954; Phillips, 1951; Trecker, 1955, 1956; Wilson & Ryland, 1949). It is important to note that during this period McCarthyism led to a general suspicion of group participation (Andrews & Reisch, 1997).

In the early 1960s, the writings of Vinter and Schwartz received wide attention and interest because of their common concern and commitment to the development of a professional methodology. Vinter (1967) moved toward the paradigm used by caseworkers of social study, diagnosis, and treatment. The group represented a context for the treatment of individuals with difficulties in social functioning. Vinter's emphases on individual behavioral change and professional methodology supported group work's integration into casework agencies and departments and into greater acceptance by the professional community.

Schwartz, whose approach is a major focus of this chapter (1961, 1962), shared Vinter's primary concern for the development of a professional methodology. He proposed a bold and ambitious paradigm through which he attempted to elaborate and refine the social goals tradition rather than move toward the casework paradigm (Gitterman, 1979). His "reciprocal model" is referred to as the "interactional model" and, more recently, as the "mutual aid model." The idea of "reciprocal" captures the mutually dependent relationship that exists among members within a group and between the group and its social environment.

Schwartz used the term "interactionist approach" to emphasize the interaction between people and external systems. Schwartz was probably the first to introduce the term "mutual aid" into social work scholarship and was its major proponent (Steinberg, 1997, p. 1). Shulman (1986, p. 51) states that of the many scholarly contributions Schwartz made to social work, "none has been as important as his conceptualization of social work groups as enterprises in mutual aid." Thus this chapter is titled "The Mutual Aid Model."

MEDIATING FUNCTION

Schwartz (1961) used systems theory to develop his conception of a mediating function for the profession of social work. He suggested that the concept of function "implies the existence of an organic whole, a dynamic system, in which the worker performs certain movements, in relation to the movements of others" (p. 151). He went on to say that a functional statement must "reflect the activity of the social worker as it affects, and is affected by, the activity of others within the system . . . to see the system as one within which relations determine the properties of its parts" (p. 152). Schwartz (1976) further suggested that within the social system the individual possesses a natural impetus "toward health, growth and belonging" and a similar natural impetus of society to "integrate its parts into a productive and dynamic whole" (p. 1258). He viewed the existence of a "symbiotic" relationship between individual and social needs[1]: "A relationship between the individual and his nurturing group . . . can be described as symbiotic . . . each needs the other for its own life and growth and each reaches out to the other with all possible strength at a given moment" (1971b; p. 1259).

In a highly complex society, the symbiotic relationship becomes obscure, obstructed, diffuse, and tenuous, as "people are weakened in their reach to the system and the system is too clumsy to incorporate the people it needs to serve" (Schwartz, 1994, p. 114). Therefore, the profession of social work is required to deal with all the strains that develop between people and their social systems: "it works with the individual to use his system and it works with the systems to reach its people" (Schwartz, 1994, p. 115). The obstacles to reciprocal individual and societal need fulfillment provide social work with a distinctive professional function: namely, to mediate the transactions between the group and societal institutions and between individual members within a group. In other words, groups face two primary challenges to their elaboration and survival: (1) to deal with external, environmentally induced stressors and (2) to deal with internal, interpersonally induced stressors. Consequently, the worker's primary function is to help a group and its members to establish and maintain a favorable interchange with the environment and a mutual aid system among its members. When successful in these twin challenges and tasks, a group may be said to be in adaptive balance.

External Mediation

To actualize this conception of a mediating function, social workers represent their groups and members, as well as their employing organization. They identify with their common need to engage each other rather than with one over the other. If social workers align themselves solely with their group members and disown their employing agencies, they will diminish their credibility and ability to help group members obtain agency resources. Similarly, if social workers align themselves with the employing agencies and "become" their organizations, they lose their credibility with group members. The professional task is to represent the employing organization without becoming or disowning it (Gitterman, 1986). The focus is on improving the fit between members' needs and agency services. In doing so, "the practitioner is required neither to change the system, nor to change the people, but to change the ways in which they deal with each other" (Schwartz, 1969, p. 41).

Internal Mediation

In dealing with environmental pressures and internal group processes, members encounter interpersonal tensions and obstacles. Dysfunctional communication and relationship patterns are generated in the system, hindering mutual aid processes. Withdrawal, factionalism, alliances, and scapegoating are illustrative of these dysfunctional patterns (Berman-Rossi, 1993; Bogdanoff & Elbaum, 1978; Brown & Mistry, 1994; Galinsky & Schopler, 1994; Germain & Gitterman, 1996; Gitterman, 1989; Malekoff, 1997; Shulman, 1999; Steinberg, 1996, 1999). To mitigate these maladaptive patterns, the worker must identify the pattern and encourage members to change their behaviors. Usually, members are reluctant to change an entrenched and comfortable pattern because it protects them from dealing with painful material and issues related to interpersonal intimacy. Scapegoating, for example, may stave off difficulties in the group while promoting difficulties in the scapegoated member (Antsey, 1982; Shulman, 1967). The worker must be direct and persistent in challenging dysfunctional patterns and be comfortable in dealing with avoidance, as well as conflict. By relating to negative feelings and thoughts, the worker conveys a faith in group members' abilities to confront difficult issues. During these difficult discussions, group members require support and credit for their willingness to struggle and to risk themselves.

PHASES OF HELPING

Schwartz (1971a) placed the mutual aid processes within four interrelated helping phases: preparation, or "tuning in," in which the worker prepares him- or herself to move into the group experience; development of a mutual agreement, or "contract," in which the worker helps group members to develop a common focus; the actual "work," in which members deal with group tasks and any obstacles that impede mutual aid processes; and termination, in which members separate and the group ends or the worker leaves.

In the preparation phase, the worker acquires essential organizational sanctions and supports; formulates group purpose; composes the group (or, at least, considers the implications of an externally composed group); pays attention to time, size, space, and recruitment factors; and anticipates members' possible reactions to the first meeting (Gitterman, 1994; Kurland, 1978; Northen & Kurland, 2001). In the second phase, contract, the worker helps members to reach a common agreement about what they will work on and how they plan to go about it. Essentially, the worker's task is to help the group develop a clear and mutual agreement about group purpose and respective responsibilities (Garvin, 1969, 1997; Germain & Gitterman, 1996; Gitterman, 1986; Kurland & Salmon, 1998; Shulman, 1999; Toseland & Rivas, 2001). According to Schwartz (1971a), "The contract, openly reflecting both stakes, provides the frame of reference for the work that follows, and for understanding when the work is in process, when it is being evaded, and when it is finished" (p. 8).

Members require a clear understanding about the group's purpose in order to evaluate appropriateness and suitability. Informed members are less likely to fear a hidden agenda and more likely to be receptive to an offer of help than uninformed members. The worker must also invite members' reactions to the offered group services. There are potentially differing perceptions among the agency, the worker, and the group members. For example, children referred by a teacher for being "troublemakers" will resist such an offer of service. In contrast, a statement that takes into account the youngsters' perceptions—"I sense that the school hasn't been much fun and that you may feel teachers and other kids pick on you"—will more likely be positively received. Taking into account members' perspectives on their life issues encourages mutually supportive behaviors rather than mutually exploitative behaviors. Group members also need to know that they are meeting with a social worker and have some idea about what social workers do. Children in a school group, for example, will use their teachers as role models for expected adult behaviors. With discrepant expectations, mutual aid can be inhibited.

In the work phase, Schwartz (1971a, p. 16) identified four major tasks for the group worker:

1. Finding, through negotiation, the common ground between the requirements of the group members and those of the systems they need to negotiate.
2. Detecting and challenging the obstacles to the work as these obstacles arise.
3. Contributing ideas, facts, and values from his or her own perspective when he or she thinks that such data may be useful to the members in dealing with the problems under consideration.
4. Defining the requirements and limits of the situation in which the client–worker system is set.

The subsequent sections of this chapter describe and illustrate the skills required to carry out these tasks. The ending phase makes specific demands on the group members and the worker. These demands include dealing with the feelings aroused by the ending, processing various termination phases, planning for the future, and reviewing and evaluating the group experiences. Like the initial phase and the ongoing phases of practice, the ending phase requires the worker's sensitivity and range of professional skills (Germain & Gitterman, 1996; Irizarry & Appel, 1994; Nadelman, 1994; Shulman, 1999).

MUTUAL AID

Schwartz (1961) perceived the social work group as:

> an enterprise in mutual aid, an alliance of individuals who need each other, in varying degrees, to work on certain common problems. The important fact is that this is a helping system in which the clients need each other as well as the worker. This need to use each other, to create not one but many helping relationships, is a vital ingredient of the group process and constituted a common need over and above the specific task for which the group was formed. (p. 19)

An agency-formed group is composed of individuals who come together under the agency auspices to work on common life issues, interests, and tasks. If members quickly develop a sense of common purpose, they will begin to share common experiences and concerns. Initially, group members present safer and less threatening issues to feel out the worker's and each other's trustworthiness and genuineness. And through a testing process—sometimes quite overt, at other times much more subtle—group members begin to develop and reinforce mutual bonds and alliances as they process the roles of each member and the worker in the group's interpersonal system. When members experience collective support and individual comfort, they develop an increased willingness to risk more personal and sometimes taboo concerns (Gitterman, 1986, 1989).

Hearing others' life issues often helps group members to experience their difficulties and stressors as being less unique and deviant. From these exchanges, members feel less isolated, stigmatized, and pathologized. Learning to share and to reach out to each other, members experience a "multiplicity of helping relationships," with all members invested and participating in the helping process rather than the worker alone assuming that function and role (Schwartz, 1961, p. 18). Because they may have had similar life experiences, they are often receptive to each other's views and suggestions. The group experience itself is a microcosm of members' interpersonal self-presentations and therefore serves as a rich arena for members to examine their respective adaptive, as well as maladaptive, perceptions and behaviors. From these exchanges members are helped to develop and practice new interpersonal and environmental strategies and to receive feedback on such efforts (de Jong & Gorey, 1996; Gottlieb, 2000; Gregory & Erez, 2002; Hopmeyer & Werk, 1994; Kinnevy, Healey, Pollio, & North 1999; Pepler, Catallo, & Moore 2000; Pomeroy, Rubin, Laningham, & Walker 1997; Springer, Lynch, & Rubin 2000; Tutty, Bidgood, Rothery, & Bidgood 2001).

Groups also provide the impetus for members to act and gain greater control and mastery over their environments. Collective action achieves greater organizational and community attention, increases the likelihood of success, and mitigates individual isolation and reprisals. The opportunity to participate in a group and to influence one's environment provides a sense of competence and efficacy. Mutual aid provides groups their energy, drive, and momentum.

Shulman (1986, 1999) divides mutual aid into distinct processes evident in effective groups. Group members have accumulated varied life experiences. Through the processes of sharing of relevant data, members serve as a significant resource to each other. As members share their perspectives on life issues and concerns, a dialectical process takes place through which members discuss, challenge, argue, and, through the give-and-take, develop greater clarity and personal synthesis. For mutual aid to deepen, members learn to explore taboo concerns. They find their voices and courage to explore buried material. Listening to each other's troubles, members experience the "all in the same boat" phenomenon. They discover that they are not alone in their experiences, reactions, and coping efforts. This realization has a special healing value: "Guilt over 'evil' thoughts and feelings can be lessened and self-destructive cycles broken when one discovers they are normal and shared" (Shulman, 1999, p. 306). Learning that others are in the "same boat" expands members' perspectives and helps members to universalize their life struggles. Oppressed and vulnerable populations often internalize societal stigmatization. Members raise their consciousness when they expand their perspective on their difficulties and take into account the external contexts for their troubles.

In sharing and universalizing common life issues, group members empathically understand each other's experiences and reactions in a deep and personal manner and are able to provide genuine mutual support. Group members' empathy and support allow members to "accept their own feelings in new ways" (Shulman, 1999, p. 308). Members provide each other mutual support not only through expressions of caring but also through mutual demands for them to "risk their real thoughts and ideas, listen to each other, put their own concerns aside at times to help another" (Shulman, 1999, p. 309). In helping another, the person becomes engaged in individual problem solving. By helping an individual solve a problem, group members are also helping themselves to deal with similar issues. A particular form of problem solving is rehearsal, through which group members try out new behaviors in a safe environment. And when the focus is on collective rather than individual problem solving, the group provides a "strength in numbers" that increases courage and lessens risks.

To actualize these mutual aid processes, Gitterman (1989) identifies essential professional group work tasks, methods, and skills. Early in a group's life, members usually speak to and through the worker. To facilitate mutual aid processes, the worker directs members' transactions to each other. Initially, members may talk at each other rather than to each other. The worker helps members to build on each other's contributions by linking their comments to each other. The worker identifies and focuses on salient group themes. Common salient group themes are the "glue" that bind members together as they help each other with mutual concerns and issues.

In previous groups, members may have learned to compete with, withdraw from, and/or exploit each other. To mitigate these dysfunctional patterns, the worker encourages and reinforces cooperative mutual support norms. Primarily, the worker who models, teaches, and credits their expression achieves these norms. As another method for creating mutual support norms, the worker may help group members examine their interpersonal system of rewards and punishments—their system of sanctions. These include implicit and explicit statements of approval through praise and recognition, disapproval, and stronger sanctions, as well as interpersonal punishment that may range from mild rebukes and teasing to more extreme responses, such as scapegoating and ostracism. The worker helps group members to develop clearer behavioral guidelines and greater interpersonal acceptance. "When members are clear about what behaviors are preferred, permitted, proscribed and prohibited, they are likely to be less anxious and more available to each other" (Gitterman, 1989, p. 13).

Encouraging group members to participate in collective activities also facilitates mutual aid processes. Participation in role play, sports and games, arts and crafts, and music and dance, as well as in social action, requires members to interact and communicate, to plan and make decisions, and to differentiate roles and tasks. The worker and group members (when possible) must assess their readiness and motivation to undertake collective activity. By encouraging collective activities and by experiencing collective successes, the group's mutual aid processes are further elaborated. So that they may participate effectively in collective activities, the worker clarifies members' tasks and role responsibilities. Specification of tasks and role assignments facilitates mutual aid processes by integrating members and by reducing conflict and stress associated with ambiguity.

Some groups are disorganized, and members have difficulty with planning and decision making. Members require help learning such processes as achieving consensus and compromise. In these groups, the worker must, at least initially, structure planning and decision making. Gitterman (1989) offers an example of a group of disadvantaged older adolescent boys. They were unable to plan, to solve problems, or even to sustain a simple, focused discussion.

A member's comment would be immediately punctuated by another member's sneer or jeer about a girlfriend, mother, and so on. Chaos invariably followed! Since they had neither experienced nor learned the value of collaborative decision-making, they needed structure to facilitate collaborative processes. The worker developed an interactional sequence with them to use in planning any program or making any decision. 1) In a round robin fashion each member presented one idea at a time, the worker recorded each idea on a large master list. The round robin continued until all members' ideas were expressed (during this step no comments or alternative suggestions were allowed). 2) The worker limited discussion about each alternative to clarification and identification of potential problems. 3) After group members eliminated duplicate ideas and voluntarily withdrew impractical alternatives, members voted for the preferred plan or decision. The prescribed sequence provided a structure for decision-making and eliminated disabling criticisms and harshness. And as members learned to listen to each other, interpersonal support and competence replaced interpersonal exploitation and inadequacy. (p. 14)

The worker uses these professional tasks, methods, and skills to integrate members and to nurture mutual aid processes. Although strengthening collective functioning is essential to mutual aid, it is not sufficient. The worker must also be responsive to the needs of each individual member, as well as to the needs of the collectivity. This responsivity requires the worker to help each group member to negotiate his or her individual needs to be different and separate and not simply "fit in." The worker uses additional skills to help a group to develop a satisfactory balance between meeting the needs for group integration and individuation.

To meet the needs of individual members, the worker must be extremely careful not to stifle divergent perceptions and opinions. Premature consensus subverts mutual aid processes. The worker reaches for and pursues discrepant perceptions and opinions. By inviting and encouraging individual members to disagree, to have differing opinions and perceptions, the worker supports a group norm of accepting individual differences. As Gitterman (1989, p. 15) points out, "A collectivity is only as strong as its ability to allow and tolerate differences. Members can only be supportive of each other, if they feel sufficient comfort to state their thoughts and feelings openly."

For various reasons (discomfort with content or pace of conversation, shyness), some group members may have trouble participating. With caring and support, the worker invites and pursues the participation of the member who feels "outside" of the group process. This behavior conveys and models to all group members their individual importance. Often, more than one invitation is necessary; therefore, the worker demonstrates interest and caring through several invitations.

Group members desire different degrees of intimacy and distance and of group solidarity and individual distinctiveness. Some members need greater separateness and space than do others. The worker attempts to help group members to negotiate a comfortable balance and supports a member's need for greater emotional and physical space.

Essentially, as members feel more comfortable and less threatened, they become more invested in each other. They become willing to take chances and to lower their defenses when their individual styles and rhythms are respected and valued. Thus, for the worker, a critical professional task is to balance individual needs with group needs.

Relationship and communication obstacles are phenomena inherent in a group's life. Members usually have some ambivalence about intimacy, about being close to each other and to the worker. As members work out such issues, they become closer and more supportive and helpful to each other. Usually, with the worker's encouragement and professional skills, the interpersonal tensions diminish, and energies are released for the agreed-on tasks. When the worker ignores the obstacles or unskillfully deals with them, they become entrenched and threaten the group's existence. The worker thus has to have confidence in the members and in his or her abilities to deal with the maladaptive patterns. By meeting the challenge, members have the opportunity to gain greater self- and collective confidence and to learn about the quintessential meaning of mutual aid.

PRACTICE ILLUSTRATION

A social work intern led an educational group of at-risk 17- to 24-year-old gay males. They were sexually active, practiced unsafe sex with their friends and with anonymous partners, and were at high risk of HIV infection. The initial purpose of the group was to provide information about harm-reduction behaviors (Gitterman, 1999).

The group met weekly for 10 weeks. Seven members (3 white, 2 Latino, one African American, one Asian American) composed the group. Most members lived independently but were partially or fully financially supported by their parents. In screening interviews, members openly described their high-risk behavior as passive partners of anal intercourse without condoms or active partners of oral sex without condoms. Although they were aware of their risky behaviors, they presented as uninterested in changing them. However, they all agreed to try the group. In the fifth session, the intern records:

Jack stated, "I had a really rough day yesterday. I told my parents that I was not going back to school next semester and that I am going to take the semester off and they became really upset. They think I am lost or something. My mother was crying, and she never cries. It really upset them. I didn't expect it. They've been worried about me. They think my life is going nowhere. They told me that I am not the son they wanted me to be and that I had disappointed them." *I emphatically shook my head from side to side.* Jack went on, "I know they think I am not going to finish school because I am gay. Ever since I came out to them three years ago, they think my life has gone downhill. They think I have all of these negative influences in my life and that the negative influences made me decide not to return to school. I'm so pissed off at them, but it's hard because they have done so much for me." The room was silent. John, Mike, and Steve exchanged glances, indicated that they understood. I said, "*I see you guys nodding your heads. You know exactly what Jack is talking about?*"

Steve nodded yes and said, "I feel the same way." He looked at Jack and said, "I identify with you totally. I am so angry at my parents, but it is hard for me to be mad at them because they are doing so much for me, you know what I mean. I can't help it though. Whenever I am at home there is all this tension, and I know I am the cause of it. You know what I mean?" I asked, "*What do you think the tension is about, Steve?*" He answered, "I don't know, I mean, I guess I am tense because they don't really accept me. Like sometimes when we are all at home and watching some TV, a show comes on and there is the token gay character. You know what I mean?" We all laughed knowingly. Steve continued, "Well I always try to bring it up and talk about it. But they won't discuss it. I really try to talk about it, but they just won't. It's crazy. It's as if a wall comes down [Steve placed his hands out as if he was making a wall]. Sometimes, I push a little, but then they get really tense; so I stop. It makes me mad. I mean as far as the gay thing. Like, OK, so I am gay, but it's not like it's the end of the world. You know what I mean?" "*Yes, it really hurts not to have your parents accept who you are,*" I replied. Steve continued, "After I graduate, I am going to move into the city and be on my own and I won't have to deal with them."

Mike replied, "My parents are great, they really are, but I am mad at them, too. I treat them like shit. They have always been there for me, even when my lover died, and everything. I don't know why, but I am just a total bitch to them." I asked Mike, "*Any hunches what makes you so mad at them?*" "I don't know," he said. "I really don't. I can't help it. Do you know?" With that question all the members looked at me. I said, "*I am not sure, but on the one hand you are appreciative of the help your parents give you, but, on the other hand, you all feel different levels of acceptance about who you are, ranging from mild disappointment to total rejection.*" John agreed, "My parents pay for my apartment, my tuition, my living expenses, but I am not allowed to talk about being gay. It's a nonsecret secret!" "Yeah," Jack added, "In order to afford school, I had to live with my parents, and they are financially generous with me, but not in their acceptance of who I am—I always see the disappointment and hurt in their eyes." After a silence, I added, "*You know most guys your age go through a rough time separating from their parents, but being gay makes it much tougher, much more confusing. We grow up having our parents love us and then they find out we are gay and we become someone else. We are no longer the child they used to play with, protect, embrace. Their son is gay and for some, at least initially, they experience it as a terrible loss—a loss of their hopes and dreams. And we discover that some of their love is conditional. And then we too feel a powerful loss. What is it like for you when your parents make you feel that you are not the son they had hoped for?*"

Mike said, "It's awful—the pain shoots throughout my body." He looked down at the floor. John said, with tears welling in his eyes, "Terrible doesn't describe it—especially with my Mom. We used to be so close before I told her, and now she treats me as if I don't exist." A painful silence followed. Steve and Jack began to cry. Steve looked at me and said, "It really hurts, you know what I mean?" I said, "*I do know, Steve, I know what you mean and I know how it feels.*" John said, "I miss my Mom so much. She used to play with me and love me. It's really strange. She always had gay friends, but when it came to me, she couldn't accept it. Things have never been the same." John continued to wipe away his tears and asked me, "Does it ever get better?" I said, "*Yes, it does get better—we all find ways to heal. But what I worry most about is that you guys are acting out your pain in very self-destructive ways—like punishing yourself through unsafe sex—like my parents don't care about me, so why should I care about myself.*"

Steve responded, "You know right now I feel better than I have in a long time, I really do." John and Jack replied, "Me too! I am not alone with this pain." Mike agreed, "I feel much clearer—I didn't hear any of your lectures on safe sex. Today I heard you that you cared about me—about us."

This brief practice vignette poignantly illustrates some of the previously discussed mutual aid processes. Members share relevant facts and feelings, particularly about the complexity of their relationships to their parents and their profound feelings of rejection. For adults to express the devastating pain, alienation, and wounds from parental rebuff and their need for continued parental love and support opened the door for discussion of other taboos. Group members discover that they are not alone with their intense feelings and thoughts and experience the "all-in-the-same-boat" phenomenon. This experience expands their perspectives and helps them to externalize and universalize their life issues. Mutual support fuels their work. In subsequent meetings, they examine their self-destructive behaviors, confront avoidance and denial, engage in problem solving, and use role play to rehearse new behaviors.

As a gay man, the intern easily identifies with the suffering of these young adults. He has been there, walked in their shoes. He recognizes that they have been alone with their pain, alone in their transition from being gay adolescents to being gay young adults. Previously, they had confronted a tormenting dilemma: namely, to remain in or out of the closet in relation to their family members. If they decided to be true to themselves and their identity, they would inflict pain on those they loved. In sharing their sexuality, they probably received reactions from their parents that ranged from identifying their son's behavior as immoral and sinful to declaring that their son had a disease that needed to be treated to a milder view of a slight sexual imperfection and abnormality. At best, the members experienced reactions of hurt and disappointment and, at worst, rejection and abandonment.

These youngsters were adrift without essential supports and adult gay role models. The student helped them to find each other, and he served as an important gay adult role model who understood and accepted their realities. They had been previously exposed to safe-sex education but were unable to incorporate the information into their lives. As they explored their developmental pain, they began to make connections between unsafe sex and their low self-esteem and their search for love and acceptance. As one member explained his participation in unprotected sex, "I was afraid he wouldn't like me, and that he would ask me to leave." These youngsters internalized the dominant culture's oppression of homosexuals and turned the rage against themselves.

Providing information on safe sex, although important, is clearly not sufficient. How do we help gay and lesbian group members struggle with the existential question of "Who am I?" if their most loved ones do not know who they are, choose to act as if they are not who they are, or know but do not accept who they are? The group members must experience the worker's genuine caring and acceptance; otherwise, the worker's actions will seem to be a mechanical effort removed from the realities of their lives. Added to professional caring, the worker must have skills in group processes. For members to examine their risk-taking behavior and to consider changing these behaviors, the worker has to harness the constructive and healing power of mutual aid. Information combined with mutual aid might prevent much future suffering.

CONCLUSION

In conclusion, this chapter describes the historic context for the mutual aid model. Using the social goals philosophical and value base, Schwartz developed a distinct conception of social work function and an approach to group practice that emphasized the intrinsic value of mutual aid. He conceptualized phases of helping to describe a professional methodology. Others have added to the foundation he established by further specifying and illustrating mutual aid at work.

In contemporary practice, mutual aid is an essential process, whatever theoretical base is used. Mutual aid is provided to various vulnerable and resilient populations, such as survivors of AIDS (Amelio, 1993; Anderson & Shaw, 1994; Antle, 2002; De Ridder & Witte, 1999; Edell, 1998; Getzel, 1994, 1996; Getzel & Mahony, 1993; Hayes, McConnell, Nardozzi, & Mullican, 1998; Heckman et al., 1999; Meier, Galinsky, & Rounds, 1995; Pomeroy et al., 1997; Rittner & Hammons, 1992; Saparito, 2001; Subramanian, Hernandez, & Martinez, 1996); alternative sexual orientation (Galassi, 1991; Marrow, 1996; Peters, 1997; Saparito, 2001; Saulnier, 1997; Turrell & de St. Aubin, 1995); immigrants and refugees (Berger, 1999; Breton, 1999; Feinberg, 1996; Lopez, 1991); intimate partner violence (Gregory & Erez, 2002); sexual abuse (de Jong & Gorey, 1996; Schiller & Zimmer, 1994; Trimble, 1994; Tutty et al., 2001); homelessness (Brown, 1994; Cohen, 1994; Lee, 1994); and older elderly and their caregivers (Berman-Rossi, 1994; Brennan, Downes, & Nadler, 1996; Gottlieb, 2000; Kelly, 1999; Kelly & Berman-Rossi, 1999; Orr, 1994; Poole, 1999; Sistler & Washington, 1999). Mutual aid continues to be at the core of social action groups (Cohen & Mullender, 1999; Cox, 1991; Gutiérrez & Lewis, 1999; Mullender & Ward, 1991; Naparstek, 1999). For isolated and physically and emotionally challenged group members, mutual aid groups are offered via the Internet and telephone (Bowman & Bowman, 1998; Heckman et al., 1999; Kaslyn, 1999; Meier, 1997; Meier, Galinsky, & Rounds, 1995; Rittner & Hammons, 1992; Rounds, Galinsky, & Stevens, 1991; Schopler, Galinsky, & Abell, 1997; Weiner, 1998).

Until recently, mutual aid processes have received insufficient empirical attention. In a review of 54 studies, for example, Tolman and Molidor (1994) found that cognitive-behavioral groups dominated the research literature. Only four studies systematically measured any aspect of group process. Although several studies acknowledged the importance of group process, "only two attempted statistical analysis to examine the impact of small group differences" (p. 155). More recently, mutual aid processes are being studied in various fields of practice. In the area of sexual abuse, for example, Gorey, Richter, and Snider (2001) explored the impact of group work intervention on female survivors' feelings of guiltlessness, affiliation, and hopefulness. In the area of HIV/AIDS, Pomeroy et al. (1997) studied a 6-week psychoeducational group intervention to alleviate stress, depression, and anxiety. In the area of corrections, Springer, Lynch, and Rubin (2000) studied the impact of a mutual aid group intervention for children of incarcerated parents. In the area of intimate partner abuse, Tutty et al. (2001) evaluated 15 treatment groups for male batterers; Pandya and Gingerich (2002) provided a microethnographio study of a group intervention for male batterers; and Pepler et al. (2000) evaluated a peer counseling program for children exposed to domestic violence. In gerontology, Gottlieb (2000) reviewed the literature on process and outcomes of health-related self-help and support groups for older adults. In future studies, researchers could use, for example, Macgowan's (2000) measure of members' engagement in the group process. The measure offers potential for more effective examination of mutual aid processes.

A significant challenge for the mutual aid model is the lack of group work education in schools of social work. Social work students receive limited exposure to group work theory, methods, and skills related to forming groups, contracting, supporting mutual aid in phases of group life, building mutual aid group structures and cultures, and dealing with blocks to mutual aid. Without sufficient exposure to group work history, theory, and practice traditions of commitment to democratic values of partnership, mutuality, and social justice, graduates do not fully appreciate the potential of mutual aid and lack sufficient group work skills (Kurland & Salmon, 2002). Thus what remains unclear is where the future educators, administrators, practitioners, and researchers will learn the art and science of mutual aid processes. The Association for the Advancement of Social Work with Groups (*www.aaswg.org*) is attempting to assure the survival and growth of social group work practice.

NOTE

1. Schwartz (1961) acknowledges Kropotkin (1925), Mead (1934), Sherif (1936), and Murphy (1958) for providing the rationale for the symbiotic perspective.

REFERENCES

Addams, J. (1910). *Twenty years at Hull House*. New York: Macmillan.

Addams, J. (1930). *The second twenty years at Hull House*. New York: Macmillan.

Alissi, A. (1980). Social group work: Commitments and perspectives. In A. Alissi (Ed.), *Perspectives on social group work practice: A book of readings* (pp. 5–33). New York: Free Press.

Amelio, R. (1993). An AIDS bereavement support group: One model of intervention in a time of crisis. *Social Work with Groups, 16*(1/2), 55–72.

Anderson, D. B., & Shaw, S. L. (1994). Starting a support group for families and partners of people with HIV/AIDS in a rural setting. *Social Work, 39*(1), 135–138.

Andrews, J., & Reisch, M. (1997). The legacy of McCarthyism on social group work: An historical analysis. *Journal of Sociology and Social Welfare, 24*(3), 211–235.

Antle, B. (2002). No longer invisible: Group work with children and youth affected by HIV and AIDS. In T. Kelly, T. Berman-Rossi, & S. Palombo (Eds.), *Group work: Strategies for strengthening resiliency* (pp. 101–117). Binghamton, NY: Haworth Press.

Antsey, M. (1982). Scapegoating in groups: Some theoretical perspectives and case record of intervention. *Social Work with Groups, 5*(3), 51–63.

Berger, R. (1999). Group work with adolescent immigrant groups: Issues, obstacles, and principles. In H. Bertcher, L. Kurtz, & A. Lamont (Eds.), *Rebuilding communities: Challenges for group work* (pp. 141–150). New York: Haworth Press.

Berman-Rossi, T. (1993). The tasks and skills of the social worker across stages of group development. *Social Work with Groups, 16*(1/2), 69–92.

Berman-Rossi, T. (1994). The fight against hopelessness and despair: Institutionalized Aged. In A. Gitterman & L. Shulman (Eds.), *Mutual aid groups, vulnerable populations and the life cycle* (pp. 367–409). Itasca, IL: Peacock.

Bogdanoff, M., & Elbaum, P. L. (1978). Role lock: Dealing with monopolizers, mistrusters, isolates, helpful Hannahs and other assorted characters in group psychotherapy. *International Journal of Group Psychotherapy, 28*(2), 247–262.

Bowman, R. L., & Bowman, V. E. (1998). Life on the electronic frontier: The application of technology to group work. *Journal for Specialists in Group Work, 23*(4), 428–435.

Brennan, F., Downes, D., & Nadler, S. (1996). A support group for spouses of nursing home residents. *Social Work with Groups, 19*(2), 17–34.

Breton, M. (1999). The relevance of the structural approach to group work with immigrant and refugee women. *Social Work with Groups, 22*(2/3), 11–29.

Brown, A., & Mistry, T. (1994). Group work with 'mixed membership' groups: Issues of race and gender. *Social Work with Groups, 17*(3), 5–21.

Brown, J. (1994). Agents of change: A group of women in a shelter. In A. Gitterman & L. Shulman (Eds.), *Mutual aid groups, vulnerable populations, and the life cycle* (pp. 273–296). New York: Columbia University Press.

Cohen, M. (1994). Who wants to chair the meeting? Group development and leadership patterns in a community action group of homeless people. *Social Work with Groups, 17*(1/2), 71–88.

Cohen, M. B., & Mullender, A. (1999). The personal in the political: Exploring the group work continuum from individual to social change goals. *Social Work With Groups, 22*(1), 13–31.

Cox, E. O. (1991). The critical role of social action in empowerment oriented groups. *Social Work with Groups, 14*(3/4), 77–90.

Coyle, G. L. (1930). *Social process in organized groups.* New York: Smith.

Coyle, G. L. (Ed.). (1937). *Studies in group behavior.* New York: Harper.

Coyle, G. L. (1947). *Group experience and democratic values.* New York: Women's Press.

Coyle, G. L. (1948). *Group work with American youth.* New York: Harper & Brothers.

de Jong, T. L., & Gorey, K. M. (1996). Short-term versus long-term group work with female survivors of childhood sexual abuse: A brief meta-analytic review. *Social Work with Groups, 19*(1), 19–27.

De Ridder, N. F., & Witte, S. S. (1999). "Positive feelings": Group support for children of HIV-infected mothers. *Child and Adolescent Social Work Journal, 16*(1), 5–21.

Dewey, J. (1916). *Democracy and education.* New York: Macmillan.

Dewey, J. (1938). *The theory of inquiry.* New York: Holt, Rinehart & Winston.

Edell, M. (1998). Replacing community: Establishing linkages for women living with HIV/AIDS—A group work approach. *Social Work with Groups, 21*(3), 49–62.

Feinberg, R. I. (1996). Use of reminiscence groups to facilitate the telling of life stories by elderly Russian Jewish immigrants. *Smith College Studies in Social Work, 67*(1), 39–51.

Follett, M. F. (1924). *Creative experience.* New York: Longmans, Green.

Follett, M. F. (1926). *The new state: Group organization, the solution of popular government.* New York: Longmans, Green.

Galassi, F. (1991). A life review workshop for gay and lesbian elders. *Journal of Gerontological Social Work, 16*(1/2), 75–86.

Galinsky, M. J., & Schopler, J. (1994). Negative experiences in support groups. *Social Work in Health Care, 20*(1), 77–95.

Garvin, C. D. (1969). Complementarity of role expectations in groups: The member-worker contract. In *National Conference on Social Welfare, Social Work Practice* (pp. 127–145). New York: Columbia University Press.

Garvin, C. D. (1997). *Contemporary group work* (3rd ed.). Boston: Allyn & Bacon.

Germain, C. B., & Gitterman, A. (1996). *The life model of social work practice: Advances in knowledge and practice* (2nd ed., pp. 241–278). New York: Columbia University Press.

Getzel, G. (1994). No one is alone: Groups during the AIDS pandemic. In A. Gitterman & L. Shulman (Eds.), *Mutual aid groups, vulnerable populations and the life cycle* (pp. 27–42). New York: Columbia University Press.

Getzel, G. (1996). AIDS and group work: Looking into the second decade of the pandemic. In B. L. Stempler, M. S. Glass, & C. M. Savinelli (Eds.), *Social group work today and tomorrow: Moving from theory to advanced practice* (pp. 33–44). New York: Haworth Press.

Getzel, G., & Mahony, K. (1993). Confronting human finitude: Group work with people with AIDS. *Social Work with Groups, 16*(1/2), 27–42.

Gitterman, A. (1979). *Group work content in an integrated method curriculum*. In S. Abels & P. Abels (Eds.), *Social work with groups: Proceedings 1979 symposium* (pp. 66–81). Louisville, KY: Committee for the Advancement of Social Work with Groups.

Gitterman, A. (1986). *The reciprocal model: A change in the paradigm*. In A. Gitterman & L. Shulman (Eds.), *The legacy of William Schwartz: Group practice as shared interaction* (pp. 29–37). New York: Haworth Press.

Gitterman, A. (1989). Building support in groups. *Social Work with Groups, 12*(2), 5–22.

Gitterman, A. (1994). Developing a new group service. In A. Gitterman & L. Shulman (Eds.), *Mutual aid groups, vulnerable populations and the life cycle* (pp. 59–77). New York: Columbia University Press.

Gitterman, A. (1999). AIDS education and group process. *Social Work with Groups Newsletter, 15*(3), 1–3.

Gorey, K. M., Richter, N. L., & Snider, E. (2001). Guilt, isolation, hopelessness among female survivors of childhood sexual abuse: effectiveness of group work intervention. *Child Abuse and Neglect, 25*(3), 347–355.

Gottlieb, B. H. (2000). Self-help, mutual aid, and support groups among older adults. *Canadian Journal of Aging, 19*(1), 58–74.

Gregory, C., & Erez, E. (2002). The effects of batterer intervention programs. *Violence Against Women, 8*(2), 206–232.

Gutiérrez, L., & Lewis, E. A. (1999). Strengthening communities through groups: A multicultural perspective. In H. Bertcher, L. Kurtz, & A. Lamont (Eds.), *Rebuilding communities: Challenges for group work* (pp. 5–16). New York: Haworth Press.

Hartford, M. E. (Ed.). (1964). *Working papers toward a frame of reference for social group work*. New York: National Association of Social Workers.

Hayes, M. A., McConnell, S. C., Nardozzi, J. A., & Mullican, R. J. (1998). Family and friends of people with HIV/AIDS support group. *Social Work with Groups, 21*(1/2), 35–47.

Heckman, T. G., Kalichman, S. C., Roffman, R. R., Sikkema, K. J., Heckman, B. D., Somlai, A. M., & Walker, J. (1999). A telephone delivered coping improvement intervention for persons living with HIV/AIDS in rural areas. *Social Work with Groups, 21*(4), 49–62.

Hopmeyer, E., & Werk, A. (1994). A comparative study of family bereavement groups. *Death Studies, 18*, 243–256.

Irizarry, C., & Appel, Y. (1994). In double jeopardy: Preadolescents in the inner city. In A. Gitterman & L. Shulman (Eds.), *Mutual aid groups, vulnerable populations and the life cycle* (pp. 119–149). New York: Columbia University Press.

Kaslyn, M. (1999). Telephone group work: Challenges for practice. *Social Work with Groups, 22*(1), 63–77.

Kelly, T. B. (1999). Mutual aid groups with mentally ill older adults. *Social Work with Groups, 22*(2/3), 119–138.

Kelly, T. B., & Berman-Rossi, T. (1999). Advancing stages of group development theory: The case of institutionalized older persons. *Social Work with Groups, 22*(2/3), 119–138.

Kilpatrick, W. H. (1940). *Group education for a democracy*. New York: Association Press.

Kinnevy, S. C., Healey, B. B., Pollio, D. E., & North, C. S. (1999). Bicycle WORKS: Task-centered group work with high-risk youth. *Social Work with Groups*, 22(1), 33–47.

Konopka, G. (1949). *Therapeutic group work with children*. Minneapolis: University of Minnesota Press.

Konopka, G. (1954). *Group work in institutions*. New York: Association Press.

Kropotkin, P. (1925). *Mutual aid: A factor of evolution*. New York: Knopf.

Kurland, R. (1978, Summer). Planning: The neglected component of group development. *Social Work with Groups*, 1, 173–178.

Kurland, R., & Salmon, R. (1998). Purpose: A misunderstood and misused keystone of group work practice. *Social Work with Groups*, 21(3), 5–17.

Kurland, R., & Salmon, R. (2002, October). Caught in the doorway between education and practice: Group work's battle for survival. Paper presented at the 24th Annual Symposium of the Association for the Advancement of Social Work with Groups, Brooklyn, New York.

Lee, J. (1931). *Play in education*. New York: Macmillan.

Lee, J. A. B. (1994). No place to go: Homeless women. In A. Gitterman & L. Shulman, (Eds.), *Mutual aid groups, vulnerable populations and the life cycle* (pp. 297–313). New York: Columbia University Press.

Lee, J. A. B., & Swenson, C. R. (1994). The concept of mutual aid. In A. Gitterman & L. Shulman (Eds.), *Mutual aid groups, vulnerable populations and the life cycle* (pp. 413–429)). New York: Columbia University Press.

Lieberman, E. (1931). *Creative camping*. New York: Association Press.

Lindeman, E. (1924). *Social discovery: An approach to the study of functional groups*. New York: New Republic.

Lindeman, E. (1926). *The meaning of adult education*. New York: New Republic.

Lopez, J. (1991). Group work as a protective factor for immigrant youth. *Social Work with Groups*, 14(1), 29–42.

Macgowan, M. J. (2000). Evaluation of a measure of engagement for group work. *Research on Social Work Practice*, 10(3), 348–362.

Malekoff, A. (1997). *Group work with adolescents: Principles and practice*. New York: Guilford Press.

Marrow, D. (1996). A coming out issues for adult lesbians: A group intervention. *Social Work*, 41(6), 647–658.

Mead, G. B. (1934). *Mind, self, and society*. Chicago: University of Chicago Press.

Meier, A. (1997). Inventing new models of social support groups: A feasibility study of an online stress management support group for social workers. *Social Work with Groups*, 20(4), 35–54.

Meier, A., Galinsky, M. J., & Rounds, K. A. (1995). Telephone support groups for caregivers of persons with AIDS. *Social Work with Groups*, 18(1), 99–108.

Mullender, A., & Ward, D. (1991). Empowerment through social action group work. *Social Work With Groups*, 14(3/4), 125–139.

Murphy, G. (1958). *Human potentialities*. New York: Basic Books.

Nadelman, A. (1994). Sharing the hurt: Adolescents in a residential setting. In A. Gitterman & L. Shulman (Eds.), *Mutual aid groups, vulnerable populations and the life cycle* (pp. 163–181). New York: Columbia University Press.

Naparstek, A. J. (1999). Community building and social group work: A new practice paradigm for American cities. In H. Bertcher, L. F. Kurtz, & A. Lamont (Eds.), *Building communities: Challenges for group work* (pp. 17–34). New York: Haworth Press.

Northen, H., & Kurland, R. (2001). *Social work with groups* (3rd ed.). New York: Columbia University Press.

Orr, A. (1994). Dealing with the death of a group member: Visually impaired elderly. In A. Gitterman & L. Shulman (Eds.), *Mutual aid groups, vulnerable populations, and the life cycle* (pp. 367–384). New York: Columbia University Press.

Pandya, V., & Gingerich, W. J. (2002). Group therapy intervention for male batterers: A microethnographic study. *Health and Social Work*, 27(February), 47–56.

Papell, C., & Rothman, B. (1966). Social group work models: Possession and heritage. *Journal of Education for Social Work, 2,* 66–77.

Pepler, D. J., Catallo, R., & Moore, T. E. (2000). Consider the children: Research informing interventions for children exposed to domestic violence. *Journal of Aggression, Maltreatment and Trauma, 3*(1), 37–57.

Pernell, R. (1986). Old themes for a new world. In P. Glasser & N. Mayadas (Eds.), *Group workers at work: Theory and practice in the 80's* (pp. 11–21). Totowa, NJ: Rowman & Littlefield.

Peters, A. (1997). Themes in group work for lesbian and gay adolescents. *Social Work with Groups, 20*(2), 51–69.

Phillips, H. (1951). *Essentials of social group work skill.* New York: Association Press.

Pomeroy, E. C., Rubin, A., Laningham, L. V., & Walker, R. J. (1997). "Straight talk": The effectiveness of a psychoeducational group intervention for heterosexuals with HIV/AIDS. *Research on Social Work Practice, 7*(2), 149–164.

Poole, J. (1999). Toward a community of care: The development of the family caregivers' support network. In H. Bertcher, L. F. Kurtz, & A. Lamont (Eds.), *Building communities: Challenges for group work* (pp. 17–34). New York: Haworth Press.

Reid, K. E. (1991). *Social work practice with groups: A clinical perspective.* Pacific Grove, CA: Brooks/Cole.

Rittner, B., & Hammons, K. (1992). Telephone group work with people with end stage AIDS. *Social Work with Groups, 15,* 59–72.

Rounds, K. A., Galinsky, M. J., & Stevens, L. S. (1991). Linking people with AIDS in rural communities: The telephone group. *Social Work, 36,* 13–18.

Saparito, J. W. (2001). Group work for heterosexual couples of mixed HIV status. In T. B. Kelly, T. Berman-Rossi, & S. Palombo (Eds.), *Group work: Strategies for strengthening resiliency* (pp. 181–202). New York: Haworth Press.

Saulnier, C. F. (1997). Alcohol problems and marginalization: Social group work with lesbians. *Social Work with Groups, 20*(3), 37–59.

Schiller, L., & Zimmer, B. (1994). Sharing the secrets: Women's groups for sexual abuse survivors. In A. Gitterman & L. Shulman (Eds.), *Mutual aid groups, vulnerable populations, and the life cycle* (pp. 215–237). New York: Columbia University Press.

Schopler, J. H., Galinsky, M. J., & Abell, M. (1997). Creating community through telephone and computer groups: Theoretical and practice perspectives. *Social Work with Groups, 20*(4), 19–34.

Schwartz, W. (1961). The social worker in the group. In *The social welfare forum* (pp. 146–177). New York: Columbia University Press.

Schwartz, W. (1962). Toward a strategy of group work practice. *Social Service Review, 36*(3), 268–279.

Schwartz, W. (1969). Private troubles and public issues: One job or two? In *The social welfare forum* (pp. 22–43). New York: Columbia University Press.

Schwartz, W. (1971a). On the uses of groups in social work practice. In W. Schwartz & S. Zelba (Eds.), *The practice of group work* (pp. 3–24). New York: Columbia University Press.

Schwartz, W. (1971b). Social group work: Interactionist approaches. In R. Morris et al. (Eds.), *Encyclopedia of social work* (pp. 1252–1262). New York: National Association Press.

Schwartz, W. (1986). The group work tradition and social work practice. In A. Gitterman & L. Shulman (Eds.), *The legacy of William Schwartz: Group practice as shared interaction* (pp. 7–27). New York: Haworth Press. (Original work published 1983)

Schwartz, W. (1994). The social worker in society. In T. B. Rossi (Ed.), *Social work: The collected writings of William Schwartz* (pp. 109–119). Itasca, IL: Peacock.

Shulman, L. (1967, April). Scapegoats, group workers, and pre-emptive interventions. *Social Work, 12,* 37–43.

Shulman, L. (1986). The dynamic of mutual aid. In A. Gitterman & L. Shulman (Eds.), *The legacy of William Schwartz: Group practice as shared interaction* (pp. 51–60). New York: Haworth Press.

Shulman, L. (1999). *The skills of helping: Individuals, families, groups, and communities* (4th ed., pp. 302–318). Itasca, IL: Peacock.

Sistler, A., & Washington, K. S. (1999). Serenity for African American caregivers. *Social Work with Groups*, 22(1), 49–62.

Springer, D. W., Lynch, C., & Rubin, A. (2000). Effects of a solution-focused mutual aid group for Hispanic children of incarcerated parents. *Child and Adolescent Social Work Journal*, 17(6), 431–442.

Steinberg, D. M. (1996). She's doing all the talking, so what's in it for me? *Social Work With Groups*, 19(2), 5–16.

Steinberg, D. M. (1999). The impact of time and place on mutual aid practice with short term groups. *Social Work with Groups*, 22(213), 101–118.

Steinberg, D. S. (1997). *The mutual-aid approach to working with groups: Helping people to help each other*. Northvale, NJ: Aronson.

Subramanian, K., Hernandez, S., & Martinez, A. (1996). Psychoeducational group work with low-income Latino mothers with HIV infection. *Social Work with Groups*, 18(2/3), 53–64.

Tolman, R. M., & Molidor, C. E. (1994). A decade of social group work research: Trends in methodology, theory, and program development. *Research on Social Work Practice*, 4(2), 142–159.

Toseland, R. W., & Rivas, R. F. (2001). *An introduction to group work practice* (4th ed.). Boston: Allyn & Bacon.

Trecker, H. (Ed.). (1955). *Group work foundations*. New York: Whitened, Marrow.

Trecker, H. (Ed.). (1956). *Group work in the psychiatric setting*. New York: Whitened, Morrow.

Trimble, D. (1994). Confronting responsibility: Men who batter their wives. In A. Gitterman & L. Shulman (Eds.), *Mutual aid groups, vulnerable populations, and the life cycle* (pp. 257–271). New York: Columbia University Press.

Turrell, S. C., & de St. Aubin, T. (1995). A relationship-focused group for lesbian college students. *Journal of Gay and Lesbian Psychotherapy*, 2(3), 67–83.

Tutty, L. M., Bidgood, B. A., Rothery, M. A., & Bidgood, P. (2001). An evaluation of mens battered treatment groups. *Research on Social Work Practice*, 11(6), 645–670.

Vinter, R. D. (Ed.). (1967). *Readings in group work practice*. Ann Arbor, MI: Campus.

Wald, L. (1915). *The house on Henry Street*. New York: Holt.

Weiner, L. S. (1998). Telephone support groups for HIV-positive mothers whose children have died with AIDS. *Social Work*, 43, 279–285.

Wilson, G., & Ryland, G. (1949). *Social group work practice*. Cambridge: Riverside Press.

Chapter 7

Cognitive-Behavioral Group Work

SHELDON D. ROSE

Cognitive-behavioral group work (CBGW) refers to a variety of different group approaches that take place within the context of a small group; such intervention consists of various combinations of behavioral, cognitive, and small-group strategies. It is, furthermore, an empirically based approach, because the combinations of techniques used in treatments have been evaluated in experimental research. The goals of intervention are behavioral, cognitive, and/or emotional change. More specifically, the approach aims at such concrete goals as the improvement of social skills, the reduction of stress responses, managing anxiety and depression more effectively, eliminating panic responses, reducing the frequency of bulimic behavior, losing weight, resolving phobic disorders, ameliorating agoraphobia, effectively managing chronic pain, improving general social functioning, abstaining from risky sexual activity, and reducing the frequency of drug and alcohol abuse.

Most groups treated by means of CBGW are homogeneous insofar as the clients in any given group typically work toward resolving only one or two of these presenting problems. One important step in the process of treatment is assessment of the presenting problems and of the resources the individual has for resolving them. In assessment, CBGW takes into consideration the environment in which the behavior and emotions occur. The cultural values, ethnicities, genders, and sexual preferences of the group members and the group workers are taken into account in the selection of goals and interventions designed to achieve them. In the model proposed in this chapter, the clients make use of the conditions of the group to enhance the clients' learning and motivation. Most CBGW models teach specific skills for coping with and resolving unique problem situations. In almost all cognitive-behavioral groups, extragroup tasks (homework) are negotiated with the clients as a means of trying out newly learned skills in the real world. The results of these tasks are monitored at a subsequent session. The group worker in CBGW, though presenting a highly structured program, in most cases involves the clients in many goal, task, and intervention decisions. Before I present CBGW in more detail, I examine a sample of the research related to this approach.

OUTCOME RESEARCH ON
COGNITIVE-BEHAVIORAL GROUP WORK

The research provides support for the effectiveness of CBGW in the treatment of a wide variety of overt and cognitive behaviors. ("CBGW" is used in all the studies described herein to represent the treatment described in this chapter, even though the authors may have used another acronym.) Several examples of the impact of CBGW on anxiety-related problems with both children and adults are described here. Only those outcome studies that used either a control or contrast group have been included. The first study also compared group and individual cognitive-behavioral treatment with a control group.

Flannery-Schroeder and Kendall (2000) compared group and individual cognitive-behavioral treatments for youth with anxiety disorders. Children ages 8–14 years with anxiety disorders were randomly assigned to cognitive-behavioral individual treatment, cognitive-behavioral group work or treatment (CBGW), or a wait-list control. Treatment outcome was evaluated using diagnostic status, child self-reports, and parent and teacher reports. Analyses of diagnostic status revealed that significantly more treated children (73% individual, 50% group) than wait-list children (8%) no longer met diagnostic criteria for their primary anxiety disorder following treatment. Other dependent measures revealed the superiority of both treatment conditions compared with the wait-list condition. However, a child report of anxious distress demonstrated only the individual treatment to effect significant improvement. Measures of social functioning failed to discriminate among conditions. Analyses of clinical significance revealed that a large proportion of treated cases were returned to nondeviant limits following treatment. Treatment gains were maintained at a 3-month follow-up.

The findings of Silverman and colleagues (1999) supported the effectiveness of CBGW in the treatment of anxiety disorders in children. The authors compared randomly selected clients with anxiety disorders in a CBGW group and a wait-list control condition. A randomized clinical trial evaluated the therapeutic efficacy of CBGW versus a wait-list control (WLC) condition to treat anxiety disorders in children. Their results indicated that CBGW, with concurrent parent sessions, was highly efficacious in producing and maintaining treatment gains. Children in CBGW showed substantial improvement on all the main outcome measures, and these gains were maintained at 3-, 6-, and 12-month follow-up. Children in the WLC condition did not show improvements from the pre- to posttreatment assessment points.

CBGW has received support in the treatment of drug and alcohol abuse. For example, Fisher and Bentley (1996) conducted a study looking at the effectiveness of two group treatment models, CBGW and a disease-and-recovery approach, along with a usual treatment comparison group. The CBGW condition consisted of interventions to enhance self-efficacy, to provide more realistic and appropriate expectations about the effects of the abused substance on symptoms of personality disorders, to increase adaptive coping skills, and to enhance relapse prevention capacity. The disease-and-recovery group approach consisted of interventions to develop an "alcoholic" or "addict" identity, to acknowledge a loss of control over the substance abuse and the effects of the personality disorder, and to accept abstinence as a treatment goal. It included participation in support group activities such as Alcoholics Anonymous (AA). Both experimental groups met for three 45-minute weekly sessions for 4 weeks. The usual treatment comparison group did not receive experimental interventions and met three times weekly in an open-ended group format. The analysis revealed that within the outpatient setting, the CBGW was significantly more effective than the disease-and-recovery group and the control group in reducing alcohol use, in enhancing psychological functioning, and in improving social and family relations.

A number of studies also provided some support for the effectiveness of CBGW in the treatment of eating disorders. For example, Telch, Agras, Rossiter, Wilfley, and Kenardy (1990) evaluated the effectiveness of CBGW in treating binge-eating disorders. Forty-four female patients who binged were randomly assigned to either CBGW (n = 23) for 10 sessions or to a wait-list control condition (n = 21). At posttreatment assessment, between-group comparisons revealed that participants in the intervention group reported significantly reduced binge-eating episodes compared with participants in the WLC group. CBGW participants continued to binge significantly less frequently than they had at baseline. However, bingeing was usually not eliminated entirely.

Tanco, Wolfgang, and Earle (1998) conducted a study evaluating the effectiveness of a cognitive group treatment program on morbidly obese women. Sixty-two obese women were randomly assigned to either the cognitive program (CBGW), a behavior therapy weight-loss program (BT), or a wait-list control condition (WLC). Both treatment groups consisted of eight 2-hour weekly sessions, with the WLC condition lasting 8 weeks. However, results revealed that scores for the CBGW group improved significantly across time, whereas those for the BT group and the WLC group did not. The CBGW group and the BT group, but not the WLC group, participants lost significant amounts of weight during the course of treatment. Analysis of body mass index (BMI) revealed decreases in both the CBGW group and the BT group. And finally, the proportion of participants in the CBGW group who exercised regularly increased significantly over the course of treatment. Six-month follow-up data suggested that all treatment benefits were maintained.

Avia and colleagues (1996) also examined the effectiveness of CBGW with hypochondriacal patients. Seventeen participants were assigned to either the CBGW groups or the WLC group. The CBGW condition consisted of six weekly 1½-hour sessions of general education that covered inadequate and selective attention, muscle tension and bad breathing habits, environmental factors, stress and dysphoric mood, explanations given to the somatic signals, practical exercises implementing educational material, and homework to practice skills related to topic areas. The two CBGW groups were identical except for the assigned group worker. The WLC condition did not receive any form of treatment for the duration of the experiment. Results suggested a significant difference between CBGW and the WLC condition in the reductions of physical symptoms, bodily preoccupation, symptom interference, the Illness Attitude Scale, and in dysfunctional health beliefs. One-year follow-up data reported that participants maintained their reductions in worry about illness and in reducing symptom interference.

Roffman and colleagues (1997) assessed the effectiveness of CBGW to prevent HIV transmission in gay and bisexual men. Approximately 159 men were matched and assigned to either receive the 17-session group counseling (n = 77) or remain in an 18-week WLC (n = 82) condition. The CBGW condition was based on a relapse prevention model. Early sessions emphasized building group cohesion (one of the few studies that explicitly did so), HIV education, motivational enhancement, and goal setting. Middle sessions focused on determining antecedents to risky behavior and developing appropriate coping strategies that included coping skills training in high-risk situations involving communication, cognitive activities, and behavioral strategies. Maintenance strategies for the preservation of safer behaviors were also included. This study utilized one specific dependent measure: abstinence from AIDS-risk sexual activity over the 3-month period prior to reassessment. Data reveal that men exposed to the treatment group had roughly 2.3 times the odds of success experienced by men assigned to the no-treatment control condition. Also, results indicate that the intervention appeared to be more effective with exclusively gay than with bisexual men. Similar findings were obtained by Lutgendorf et al. (1997).

A number of studies supported the effectiveness of pain management in groups. For example, Linton and Ryberg (2001) investigated the effects of a cognitive-behavioral program in a group of nonpatients with neck or back pain symptoms. A group of 253 people (ages 35–45 years) who had experienced four or more episodes of relatively intense spinal pain during the preceding year but who had not been out of work more than 30 days) were invited to participate. They were randomly assigned to either a cognitive-behavioral group intervention or a treatment in a usual comparison group. The experimental group received a standardized six-session program provided by a trained therapist. A significant overall analysis at the 1-year follow-up showed that the cognitive-behavioral group produced better results on 26 of the 33 outcome variables. Group comparisons indicated that the cognitive-behavioral group showed significantly better results with regard to fear-avoidance beliefs and number of pain-free days, as well as the key variable of sick leave. Participation in the cognitive-behavioral group reduced the risk for long-term sick leave during the follow-up by threefold. Thus, despite the strong natural recovery rate for back pain, the cognitive-behavioral intervention produced a significant preventive effect with regard to disability.

Sukhodolsky, Solomon, and Perine (2000) investigated the effectiveness of a 10-session weekly anger-control intervention for aggressive fourth- and fifth-grade boys. Thirty-three boys, ages 9–11, were referred by teachers and school psychologists for anger-related problems and were assigned to four to seven member groups, which received either cognitive-behavioral treatment or no treatment. All participants and their teachers completed a pre- and posttest battery, which included the Pediatric Anger Expression Scale, the Children's Inventory of Anger, and the Teacher Rating Scale. The treatment condition used cognitive-behavioral group training to help the students identify the experiences and control the expression of their anger. Compared with the control condition, participants in the treatment groups displayed a significant reduction on teacher reports of aggressive and disruptive behavior ($p < .02$) and a significant improvement on self-reports of anger control ($p < .05$).

In summary, the research lends some evidence for the effectiveness of CBGW with a wide variety of presenting problems using a wide variety of cognitive and behavioral procedures. However, there were a number of methodological problems in most of the research that evaluated small-group outcomes. Often the group phenomena was confounded with the cognitive-behavioral procedures. Although all of the previous examples included at least a no-treatment control group, in the absence of a best possible alternative, only the conclusion that CBGW was better than nothing was permitted. In the several studies in which contrast groups existed, differences occasionally occurred. A major problem was that in all cases the individual was the unit of analysis, in spite of the fact that the treatment was in groups, thus incurring both statistical and psychological dependency. Finally, there was little attention paid to the relevance of the group phenomena in group treatment, which should be focus of future research.

THE RELEVANCE OF THE GROUP
IN COGNITIVE-BEHAVIORAL GROUP WORK

Although most of the studies cited here do not explicitly include group interventions and group problems in their descriptions, at the very least all of them employed some form of group discussion and member interaction and some took steps to increase group cohesion. Unfortunately, the content and purpose of this discussion was not always made clear. This section describes the potential advantages, as well as the difficulties, created by working with clients as a group in a CBGW or any other group approach. Ways to deal with some of the difficulties inherent in groups are also suggested. Many of the assumptions stated have been drawn from clinical practice. (For more details for adult groups, see Rose, 1989, and for groups of children and adolescents, see Rose, 1998.)

Advantages of the Group

First, group membership commonly ends the sense of isolation many clients feel. It is difficult to maintain the feeling that you are the only person experiencing a particular problem when you are surrounded by other individuals who are dealing with similar issues. One of the potentially therapeutic factors in group treatment is the interaction with others who share common concerns. Yalom (1985, pp. 7–8) refers to this as "universality." Listening to others who describe and solve problems brings hope to the client that his or her problems are also manageable, a hope that Yalom (1985, pp. 6–7) also identifies as a curative factor. These group phenomena are supported by the group workers, who continuously encourage members to help each other and who create other conditions to increase the cohesion and work focus of the group. Helping others, a form of altruism, and group cohesion have also been labeled as curative factors by Yalom (1985, p. 3).

The group provides the client with a source of feedback about those behaviors that are irritating or acceptable to others and about those cognitions that can be viewed as distorted, self-defeating, and/or stress eliciting. At the same time, the feedback from others is a source of support for small and large achievements in the group. As a result, the group contributes to improved self-assessment for the individual client.

Another reason for using groups is the frequent and varied opportunity for mutual reinforcement. We have noted that clients find reinforcement from other group members more powerful than reinforcement from the group worker alone. Reinforcement is a highly valued commodity in interpersonal relationships. As clients increase the frequency with which they reinforce others, they note that they are reciprocally reinforced by others, and mutual liking increases (see Lott & Lott, 1965). Each client is given the chance to learn to improve his or her ability to mediate rewards for others in social interactive situations (with acquaintances, friends, family members, acquaintances in other groups, other group members, etc.). The group worker can create situations in which each client is given frequent opportunity, instructions, and rewards for reinforcing others in the group. Special group exercises have been designed to train clients in mutual reinforcement, and extragroup tasks (homework assignments) are used to encourage clients deficient in reinforcement skills to practice these skills in the real world. The completion of these tasks is monitored by other group members.

In groups, a client must learn to deal with the idiosyncrasies of other individuals. Clients must wait while other people explain their problems. They must learn to tolerate what they perceive to be inadequate or even inane advice. Clients may be required to tolerate major differences from other group members and, in some cases, to deal with them. They must learn how to offer other clients critical feedback and advice in a tactful and helpful manner. By helping others, clients are likely to practice a set of strategies for helping themselves and to learn a model of helping others that can be applied outside of the group. In this way, they are likely to improve their relationships with others.

Treatment groups simulate the real world of natural friendship groups more accurately than does individual therapy, if the group worker permits and even encourages such simulation. Individual therapy consists solely of a high-status social worker and a low-status client. Due to the greater similarity of the group to other social situations in the real world, the group setting facilitates transfer of newly learned behavior from the therapeutic setting to the community.

Groups create the opportunity for the group worker to use an abundance of therapeutic procedures that are either unavailable or less efficient in individual treatment. Among these procedures are the "buddy system," numerous group exercises (see for example, Rose, 1998, pp. vii–viii), multiple modeling, group feedback, group brainstorming, and mutual reinforcement. Groups also provide each client with a large number of diverse models, role players for overt and covert behavioral rehearsal, manpower for behavior monitoring, and partners for use in a "buddy system." By simulating the social world, the group provides a natural laboratory for learning, discussion, behavioral testing, and leadership skill development. All of these acquired skills are essential to forming good social relationships in any setting.

In the process of interaction in therapy groups, norms (informal agreements among members as to preferred modes of action and interaction in the group) often arise, which serve to control the behavior of individual members. If these norms are introduced and effectively maintained by the group worker, they serve as powerful therapeutic tools. Through discussion, the group pressures deviant members to conform to such norms as attending regularly, completing assignments, self-disclosing, analyzing problems systematically, and assisting peers with their problems. Of course, if the group worker is not careful, antitherapeutic norms also can be generated, such as members regularly coming late or group members inappropriately or prematurely confronting one another.

In addition to modifying the norms of the group, the group worker can facilitate the attainment of both individual and group goals by modifying such things as the cohesiveness of the group, the status pattern, or the communication structure in the group. Group problems are also dealt with and resolved when they arise. Much of the power that group therapy has to facilitate the achievement of therapy goals is lost if negative group attributes are permitted to fester.

Limitations of the Group as the Context of Therapy

Of course, groups are not without major disadvantages. As I mentioned previously, antitherapeutic norms occasionally develop and may be maintained if the group worker does not deal with them. Moreover, such phenomena as group contagion and mutual aggression can sometimes get out of hand in groups. Fortunately, strategies for dealing with such group phenomena are available.

A relevant limitation to be concerned with is that it is more difficult to individualize each client in the group than in individual therapy. For efficiency, the group worker is continually looking for common goals to pursue and may, therefore, overlook the unique needs of one individual. Within many complex group interactions, identifying the distinct needs of specific individuals requires a great deal of attention. Another threat to individualization is the fact that in order for everyone to have a chance to participate actively in every session, restraints must be placed on people who talk more than their share. These restraints are sometimes frustrating to the talkative client, but failure to limit excessive talking results in the frustration of other members. The use of exercises with built-in restrictions depersonalizes the giving of structure and usually makes it more acceptable.

Confidentiality is more difficult to maintain in groups than in the therapeutic dyad. Confidentiality, and the consequences of breaches in it, needs to be dealt with by the group worker in pregroup screening and early group sessions, so that all group members conform to appropriate standards of conduct. Nevertheless, the participants are not professionally trained, and abuses do occasionally occur. When revealed, they have to be dealt with in the group.

Finally, working with groups requires an extensive repertoire of skills and training to be minimally effective. Unfortunately, such training programs are not ubiquitously found in psychology, social work, counseling, psychiatry, or other professional training programs. However, training programs are available in the form of workshops. Exercises are available that can be used to develop in-service training (see, e.g., Rose, 1998, Ch. 17, pp. 461–474, for more details).

If the group worker is aware of these limitations, all of these potential problems can be avoided or, should they occur, dealt with. In the following sections the specific ingredients of CBGW are described. Because there are many models of CBGW, the focus is on the most eclectic approach, one that uses a wide variety of interventions and takes advantage of the group phenomena. How this model differs from other models is occasionally pointed out.

THE STRUCTURE OF THE GROUP
IN COGNITIVE-BEHAVIORAL GROUP WORK

Before the interventions and phases of treatment are described, a number of practical questions need to answered regarding number of participants, number and duration of sessions, number of group workers, and characteristics of members to be admitted to the groups.

Size of the Group

The size of a group depends on its purpose, its need for individualization, and practical considerations, such as available space, length of stay in an institution, and available staff. Because individualization within a group is highly valued, the outpatient groups with which this approach has been used usually range in size from three to eight members. Generally, however, six members makes it possible to involve everyone at every session. Having fewer than three members seems to lead to a loss of many of the beneficial group attributes discussed previously; having more than eight makes it difficult to allow every member to bring in a problematic situation at every meeting.

There are sometimes practical clinical reasons to modify this range. A limited number of staff members may be available when a need for a group has been established. In some agencies, groups of 12 or more clients have been run effectively, especially if all the clients share a common problem area or if two group workers can carry out the activities of the group in subgroups. If two experienced group workers are available, it would, based on my experience, be more efficacious to have two small groups than one large group. Often these larger groups have a didactic rather than a therapeutic purpose.

Institutional groups tend to be larger because they often overlap with the residential group. In order to facilitate greater individualization, the group may be divided into two subgroups, one led by the group worker and the other by the residential worker or family worker or even a supervisor. Another reason for having larger groups in institutions is that, as a rule, they meet much more frequently than outpatient groups. If a group meets every day, even if the group is large, each individual in the course of the several meetings a week will have the opportunity to focus on his or her problems.

Frequency, Length, and Duration of Group Sessions

Group size is also a function of the frequency, length, and duration of sessions. Most outpatient groups are time limited and meet for approximately 2 hours a week for 6 to 18 weeks. In our review of the literature, the modal number is 8, but most cognitive-behavioral group workers prefer 12 to 18 sessions in order to achieve most treatment goals. Regular weekly sessions, rather than the more variable schedule recommended herein, is the general pattern, primarily because of the personal or work schedules of the families, of the clients, and of the group worker rather than because of any particular therapy rationale. Some few have been able to follow eight weekly sessions with four monthly ones as a way of providing the clients with more gradual fading of the intensity of treatment.

The exact number of sessions for outpatient groups depends on the purpose of the group, its composition, and certain practical limitations. In heterogeneous groups (in which members have diverse presenting problems), in order to deal with a wide range of problems, fourteen to eighteen sessions are usually required to meet treatment goals. When a highly specific and limited goal is pursued, a fewer number of sessions may suffice. In general, however, assuming that major goals have been achieved after one set of therapy sessions, clients are referred to nontherapy groups, such as at the YMCA or YWCA, yoga classes, bridge clubs, or sports groups, to provide relatively safe opportunity to practice, unsupervised, what they have learned in therapy. Referral to individual therapy or support groups may also occur if clients have demonstrated increased motivation but are not yet ready to demonstrate their skills in the real world.

In institutions, transitional groups (groups that prepare the client to go back to the outside world) will meet from 1 to 3 hours daily from their onset until termination, which is usually about 3 to 6 weeks. Only modest research exists to point the way to differences in the number of sessions. In adult social anxiety groups, D'Alelio and Murray (1981) demonstrated that eight 2-hour sessions were significantly more effective in reducing social anxiety than four 2-hour sessions, perhaps because there is more extragroup time to practice what is learned in the group. In anger management groups for adolescents, Lochman (1985) demonstrated the greater effectiveness of 16 sessions over 8 in increasing the control of anger by the youth.

As I mentioned earlier, although most outpatient groups are closed, some are also are open-ended and have no set duration. In private practice especially, groups of indefinite length tend to be organized. When the clients provide evidence that goals have been attained and a plan for generalization has been designed, the clients are helped by the other members to plan to terminate. Of course, in such groups, termination of a given individual may also occur against the advice of the group worker as the attraction of the group fades for that individual without concurrent achievement of treatment goals.

In residential treatment, CBGW groups tend to meet every weekday or every other day for an hour and half while the clients are in the institution. Occasionally, clients will miss sessions for such practical reasons as illness, doctor's appointments, court appearances, psychological testing, and special programs. Some institutions use CBGW only 2 or 3 of the 5 days, using the other days for more traditional methods.

Number of Group Workers

As the number of group workers in any group increases, so does the cost to the client, to the agency, or to the community. There is no evidence that two experienced group workers are more effective than one, provided that the group worker is experienced and trained. Thus, in most cases, one worker is adequate and less costly than two or more. Moreover, when two group workers are with a group, one often seems to amplify what the other says, which limits the time available for the clients to participate. There are, however, several situations in which more than one worker is required: if one of the group workers is in training; if both group workers are learning the method for the first time; if the group is larger than 10 persons; and if there are several persons in the group who act out. If the gender of the group members is mixed, it is helpful to have a team of a male and a female therapist.

PHASES OF COGNITIVE-BEHAVIORAL GROUP WORK

Beginning the Group

The structure of interaction in most models of CBGW can be divided into phases. Each phase overlaps with other phases, but in each phase the group worker focuses somewhat more on one set of behaviors than another. All have a "beginning the group" phase, in which clients are oriented to the method and get to know each other and in which the cohesion of the group is developed. Orientation involves explaining to clients what they can expect from the group experience and what is expected from them. The group worker usually describes the larger picture in the beginning and gradually fills in the details as the group progresses or as a new intervention is introduced.

Cohesion refers to the mutual liking of members for each other and the group worker and their attraction to the program of the group. In our groups, the cohesion of the group can be enhanced by the use of group introductory exercises, in which members interview each other in pairs and partners introduce their partner to the group. It is also a safe way of increasing broad participation and is the first step in self-disclosure. Cohesion is also enhanced by creating opportunities for continued broad participation, by protecting members from premature and/or too harsh confrontation, by keeping the interaction for the most part positive, by using variation in the program, by occasional use humor, and by developing opportunities for choice and decision making by the members. The cohesion is continually monitored at the end of every session through a postsession questionnaire (see Figure 7.1, Question 5).

Motivational Enhancement Phase

In some models of CBGW, at the time the group begins and continuing into the later phases, the group worker focuses on increasing the motivation of the participants. When most clients enter a treatment group for the first time, they are often anxious, afraid of what others might think of them, and hesitant to expose their flaws to other people. They are often poorly motivated to work on the very problems that brought them to, or resulted in their being sent to, the group. This lack of motivation is particularly apparent in groups of involuntary clients, such as men who batter, prisoners, and those who suffer from addictions. However, even in voluntary groups, this ambivalence can often be detected. The type of behaviors often observed at the first session or even in the pregroup interview are a reluctance to speak, some anger about being in treatment, denial of any serious problems, setting themselves, apart from the others in the group, speaking only to the group worker, an unwillingness to disclose anything about themselves and an unwillingness to develop goals, treatment plans, or extragroup tasks.

Motivation has been operationally defined as the readiness of the client to participate actively in the treatment process (Miller & Rollnick, 1991, p. 14). Motivation can be assessed by the group worker's observations of the level of self-disclosure and other forms of participation or by a self-report checklist. Strategies for enhancing motivation should be implemented throughout the treatment process to maintain the clients' ever-changing commitment to change. Although Miller and Rollnick (1991) view motivation as an individual characteristic, one often observes in groups a phenomenon in which motivation of each mutually influences the motivation of others. There appears to be a shared or prevailing group level of motivation. Miller and Rollnick (1991, pp. 51–63) identify a number of principles to be considered in the process of enhancing motivation. Some of these principles include normalizing ambivalence, contrasting costs and benefits of changing or resolving problems, eliciting and reinforcing self-motivational statements, and removing barriers to treatment. In addition, the group worker carries out a set of interviewing principles, such as supporting self-efficacy, avoiding argumentation and early confrontation, providing clear advice, and delivering continued feedback to the client. In groups, the members are encouraged to respond in a similar fashion to each other.

Assessment Phase

Overlapping with cohesion building and orientation is the assessment phase. This actually begins with the client selecting a given group with a general theme in which she or he is interested or has major concerns (e.g., anxiety management, anger control, dealing with HIV infection) or being sent to a group with a given theme (men who batter). In the group and even in an intake interview, the particulars of the problem begin to be spelled out. Many practitioners make use of such paper-and-pencil tests as Beck's (1976) Depression Inventory, the Fear Survey Schedule, and the Fear Questionnaire (see, e.g., Evans, Holt, & Oei, 1991). Many other instruments are to be found in research summarized herein and depend on the initial complaint or the theme of the group. For practitioners, a qualitative procedure often used is some form of situational analysis. Members can be trained by means of group exercises and group worker modeling to identify and describe recent problematic or stressful situations in which they are dissatisfied with the responses. These situations are highly specific events that represent a sample of the more general complaint.

After the client provides a brief background, the situations are described in terms of what happened, where it happened, with whom it happened, and when it happened. Each client identifies a critical moment in the event and the behavioral, emotional, and cognitive response at the critical moment. (The "critical moment" is that instant in time that separates the triggering event from the response of the client.) The clients also state their level of dissatisfaction with the response and examine the long- and short-term consequences of their responses. In the assessment phase, the group members evaluate each other's presentations as to how well the description meets the criteria. Thus the group is active, with the members helping each other to formulate the problematic situation and client response.

> In a stress management group, Tom gave as a background to his situation that he has trouble getting along with people who attempt to dominate him and have no right, in his opinion, to do so. When asked to give a recent example of "not getting along," he said that yesterday (when) at work (where) Dave, his coworker (who) told him to go back to the lab and get some materials that Dave had forgotten (*What happened?*). This was the critical moment. Tom, who became angry, responded "get your own God damn materials." Tom was dissatisfied with the rudeness of his response and indicated he would like to act differently (*dissatisfied with own response*).

Goal setting is also part of the assessment phase. Both individual treatment and common treatment goals are developed by each client with the help of the other group members. Tom's general goal was to respond to what he perceived as the imposition of others in a calm, matter-of-fact manner in which he presented to the antagonist how he (Tom) felt in the situation and requested a change in behavior. As part of systematic problem solving, specific treatment targets or goals are concrete behaviors, sets of actions or identifiable cognitions that occur in response to a given specified problem situation. These behaviors and cognitions are specific to a given client and are identified in the interaction among members and in their description of problematic situations that they experience in their day-to-day social encounters.

Because goal attainment is future oriented, the group worker, group members, and each client together estimate a time frame for attaining the goal that is incorporated into the formulation of the goal. Although clients identify unique individual goals, in groups common goals are shared with some or all of the other group members. In Tom's group, several members indicated that they had problems with people who imposed on them. Common goals permit greater efficiency in terms of information to be provided, group exercises to be used, and problems to be solved. Most goals are developed over time, as members learn the language of therapy and begin to describe their problems using this highly specific terminology. When goals are not forthcoming from a given individual, the other members can "brainstorm" goals, based on earlier discussions, that might be considered by the reluctant client.

Group goals refer to a future change in interactive phenomena that occur in the group. An example of one group goal is "at the end of this session, all the members of the group will have actively participated in the role plays." Another is "by the end of the next session, the members all establish a norm that extragroup tasks will be completed, if agreed to at a prior session." A third example is "the attraction of the members to each other (as measured on a postsession questionnaire) will increase from the previous session to the end of this session." Although we urge formal goal setting as part of the treatment process, in some versions of CBGW the use of goals is more implicit than explicit. Group goals can sometimes be estimated by means of a postsession questionnaire (PSQ).

In the PSQ, participants rate their own response to various aspects of each group session. A variety of group problems and group goals can be formulated in terms of these scales that are in the form of 6–12 questions administered to all the members and the group worker at the end of every session. Figure 7.1 presents examples of commonly used PSQ items.

Means, discrepancies among the members, and discrepancies between the means of the members and the group worker's observations provide a rough estimate of some of the group phenomena as perceived by the members and group workers. These data and member comments are discussed at the beginning of the subsequent session.

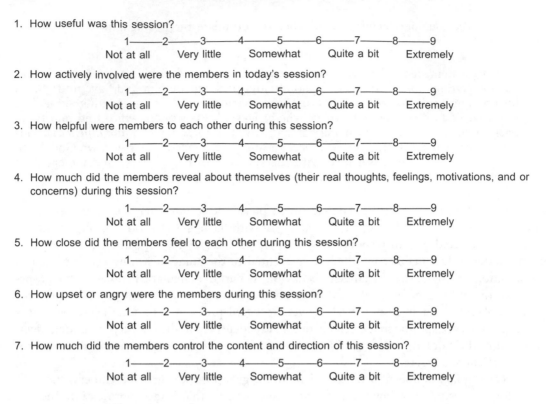

FIGURE 7.1. An example of questions and format of a postsession questionnaire.

As observed in some of the research summaries presented earlier, individual and common treatment goals in CBGW have included a wide range of targets, such as managing pain, stress, anger, depression or anxiety; reducing and/or eliminating use of drugs, alcohol, or cigarettes; eliminating violence toward one's spouse and children; improving parenting skills; reducing the frequency of bulimic behavior; increasing safe sex practices; increasing positive life experiences in the face of personal tragedies; building more satisfying experiences; and reducing negative or self-defeating self-statements or avoidance behavior. Most of these goals can be broken down into even more specific short-term goals to be achieved by the end of one or two subsequent sessions.

Intervention Phase

Situational analyses and goal setting become the foundation for the intervention phase, which may involve correcting cognitive distortions implied in the situation, providing corrective information, being exposed to the anxiety-producing object, systematic problem solving, modeling and rehearsing alternatives, reinforcing successful actions, and other interventions, most of which are carried out in the group with the help of the other group members. In the intervention phase, different models of CBGW tend to emphasize different sets of interventions. These include modeling techniques, problem-solving techniques, cognitive change procedures, guided group exposure, relaxation training, operant procedures, community change strategies, and small-group techniques, all of which are discussed in more detail in the following sections.

Systematic Problem Solving

Many models of CBGW make use of some form of systematic problem solving insofar as clients bring problems of concern to the group. The group, under the group worker's guidance, attempts to help find solutions to those problems. It is systematic insofar as the members follow specified steps that include orienting the members to the basic assumptions of problem solving, identifying and defining the problem and client resources for dealing with the problem, generating alternative solutions, evaluating and selecting the best set of solutions, preparing for implementation, implementing the solution outside the group, and evaluating the outcome with the other group members at a subsequent session (e.g., Heppner, 1978); we have added the intermediate step, called "preparation for implementation." In this preparation, modeling, cognitive restructuring, or information giving may be used, and a extragroup task is designed to be carried out prior to the next session. The tasks may involve small and gradually increasingly difficult steps toward performing the goal behavior.

Systematic problem solving is most effective as a group procedure because, in generating ideas for dealing with the problem, the group members are a rich resource for potential solutions. Moreover, in evaluating these ideas, the group members provide varied life experiences on which to support or reject some of the solutions generated. The group is also a source of reinforcement and support for carrying out the task.

In our earlier example, once Tom had decided what his goal was, the group members brainstormed what he might say and how he might say it. They wrote down their suggestions and one at a time shared them with Tom, who wrote them on the board. The group worker advised them that no one should evaluate until all the suggestions were made. After eliminating some of the ideas, Tom incorporated the others into a plan of how to respond when Dave or anyone else imposed on him. Tom indicated he would say, in a matter-of-fact tone of voice, that he too was busy and that he didn't appreciate being told rather than asked to be of help. Because Tom was not yet comfortable in doing this, he was trained through modeling and rehearsal to carry out the task.

Problem solving is also employed for more general problems. In one group, several members had recently lost jobs and needed some ideas about how to look for others. An expert was brought in to supplement the suggestions of the members. In another group, parents brainstormed different ways of dealing with a highly active 3-year-old when he appeared to be out of control. In a third group, adolescents discussed how they might improve their chances of getting into college and obtaining loans to help support themselves.

Modeling Methods

In my experience, symbolic modeling is one of the most effective strategies in group therapy. As I noted before, modeling by the group worker and the members for each other was an integral part of all of the other strategies described so far. Modeling strategies in groups have also been used in preventive and behavioral medicine with patients using the health care system (for examples, see Newton-John, Spence, & Schotte, 1995; Subramanian, 1991, 1994). It has also been used successfully with mentally ill patients with social impairments (Daniels & Roll, 1998; Van Dam Baggen & Kraaimaat, 1986) and with chronic alcohol-dependant inpatients (Vogel, Ericksen, & Bjoernelv, 1997). Modeling techniques are the central procedures in assertion training and play an important role in teaching clients how to cope with stress. In addition, because of the presence of many potential models and sources of feedback, modeling is especially useful in groups.

Symbolic modeling involves simulated demonstrations (role playing) by group members, the group worker, and/or special guests in the group. It may also include videotapes or audiotapes of actors or real clients. The advantage of symbolic modeling over real-life modeling is that simulated modeling can be focused and developed systematically by the group and group worker. It can be applied in simple situations with one critical moment, or eventually, in complex situations consisting of many critical moments. In symbolic modeling, the group worker can direct the action so that successful efforts can be reinforced and unsuccessful ones terminated and redeveloped. The small group is especially well suited to the use of symbolic modeling, as it affords a rich source of ideas as to what the model should do and multiple models and multiple sources of feedback to the person attempting to duplicate the role of the model. The techniques used in enhancing the modeling effects are drawn from the assumptions about and research on social learning theory (Bandura, 1977).

As in the preceding examples, most modeling is used solely by the group worker or another group member to demonstrate a given behavior or set of behaviors or interactive solutions to problematic situations. However, modeling may be used as a major intervention package. In that case the modeling sequence in its entirety makes use a number of steps:

1. The group worker orients the group to modeling and demonstrates the modeling steps (the first few times only).
2. Based on a situational analysis of an interactive situation, each client—one at a time—presents a situation for which he or she wants to have his or her behavior modeled. The client clarifies the roles of model, target person, significant others, and observers.
3. A model is selected who demonstrates the desired behaviors. The model may be the group worker, a group member, or a guest invited for that purpose.
4. The target person rehearses or practices what she or he has observed and, if necessary, with some coaching or assistance from others (rehearsal plus coaching). If coaching is used, the rehearsal is repeated without coaching.
5. The target person is provided with feedback from the other group members and the group worker.
6. The practice is repeated as many times as time permits until the target person is comfortable in his or her new set of behaviors. If necessary, additional practice may be carried out in pairs or triads within the group to save time or as extragroup tasks for partners.
7. With the assistance of the group or a partner, each client designs an extragroup task to perform the modeled behavior in the real world or to practice again outside of the group.

In Tom's case, after the plan was developed through systematic problem solving, Barry volunteered to play the role of Tom in telling Dave in a matter-of-fact tone of voice that he, too, was busy and that he didn't appreciate being told, rather than asked, to be of help. Another member played the role of Dave. After the modeling, the group worker asked Tom if he was ready to do the role play in his own role. The role play was repeated (behavioral rehearsal), and the group gave Tom feedback as to what he did well, first, and then feedback as to what he might consider doing differently. Tom repeated the role play and incorporated the suggestions of the group the second time. Tom decided that as an extragroup task, the next time anyone else attempted to impose on him, he would respond in a similar way and report back to the group what happened.

Several others in the group who had a similar concern also decided on a similar extragroup task.

Cognitive Change Methods

Because the method is referred to as cognitive-behavioral, the major strategies employed focus on correcting distorted cognitions and replacing them with coping thoughts. Specifically, it includes such techniques as cognitive restructuring and training in cognitive and behavioral coping skills.

The most commonly used form of cognitive restructuring in groups is derived from the work of Aaron Beck (1976). Bottomley, Hunton, Roberts, Jones, and Bradley (1996) used Beck's method of challenging dysfunctional thinking of clients. In groups, challenging may also be the responsibility of the other group members, as they learn the correct techniques. In addition, the clients are helped to develop alternative cognitive coping skills and some behavioral alternatives (e.g., relaxation, recreational skills, social skills). The cognitive coping responses are often practiced in the group in role plays (cognitive rehearsal). One technique, proposed by Beck and Emery (1985), that lends itself in particular to groups is "point counterpoint." In this technique, a target client argues why his or her position is distorted or illogical, while another member or the group worker tries to support the distorted position. The discussion is first developed in pairs and then later presented to the entire group. The group members may coach the target client in his or her new role. The danger is that sometimes the group is too aggressively confrontative. To avoid this, the group members are trained first through group worker modeling and explanation and a group exercise on how to deliver and receive critical feedback.

Another version of cognitive restructuring (Meichenbaum, 1977) that we employ most frequently (Rose, 1998, pp. 260–307) is characterized by a set of procedures used to change self-defeating or illogical patterns of thinking to self-enhancing or logical ones. It is the first step used in improving cognitive coping skills. It is assumed that in a given set of circumstances cognitions partially mediate overt behavioral responses. These cognitions include how one values oneself and one's actions and how one specifically thinks or responds covertly in a given situation. The clients are trained to identify self-enhancing and self-defeating thoughts in case examples or exercises. Later they learn to identify their own self-defeating thoughts and try to change these to self-enhancing thoughts. One exercise we commonly use to achieve these skills appears in Figure 7.2.

Group members should be warned that not all self-defeating statements readily lend themselves to substitution. Even if it sensitizes the client to the problem, frequent practice and self-monitoring may also be required to bring about a change. After all, most people have been practicing their self-defeating statements for a long time. In the case of some self-defeating statements, simply replacing the thought with a coping thought may be insufficient. Other strategies may be required as well. Often substituting coping cognition is merely part of a larger treatment package.

Guided Group Exposure

This technique has been primarily used in the treatment of agoraphobia (e.g., Hand, LaMontagne, & Marks, 1974), although some practitioners and researchers have used it with other phobic objects—usually in combination with cognitive restructuring and other

FIGURE 7.2. Identifying Self Defeating and Coping Statements

Rationale

Most clients make statements about themselves that are illogical, self-defeating, and distorted. These distortions often lead to anxiety, stress, depression, and anger. Much of treatment, regardless of its theoretical orientation, is aimed at correcting these distortions and replacing them with more functional evaluations, thoughts, or self statements. There are many strategies for accomplishing this. Based on the work of Meichenbaum (1977), this exercise represents a direct way of identifying those statements regarded as self-defeating and then replacing them with coping or self-enhancing statements. Most statements that are self-defeating meet several of the following criteria:

1. Does the person make an *absolute* judgment of him- or herself? (e.g., never, can't, always, won't, should, shouldn't)
2. Does the person need to *mind read* the thoughts of others to make the statement?
3. Does the person grossly *exaggerate* the conditions that are referred to in the statement?
4. Does the person make a *catastrophe* out of a difficult or uncomfortable situation?
5. Does the person leap to *conclusions* about self or situation without adequate evidence?
6. Does the person *overgeneralize* from one set of circumstances?
7. Does the person *put* him- or herself *down* or is the person overly critical of him- or herself?
8. Does the person *disregard* important aspects of situations while emphasizing other, more negative aspects?
9. Does the person *prophesy* the future without evidence?

The criteria for identifying coping or self-enhancing statements are the following (not all the criteria need be met):

1. Is the statement *realistic*, not overly optimistic or "Pollyannaish"?
2. Is the statement *positive* in content and intent?
3. Is the statement *instructive*? Is it guiding a behavior or set of behaviors?
4. Is the statement *appropriate* to the situation?
5. Is the statement *anxiety reducing*, and/or does it *reduce expectation of threat*?
6. Is the statement free of *self-defeating* elements? (See criteria for evaluating self-defeating statements.)

Purpose of exercise

By the end of this exercise the participant will have:

1. Identified his or her own most commonly used self-defeating statements and the conditions under which they occur
2. Identified more appropriate alternative self-enhancing or coping statements to replace the self-defeating statements
3. Differentiated among self-defeating statements and other statements indicating behavioral deficits or other behavioral problems
4. Identified at least five conceptual reasons why their own or the self-defeating statements of others are self-defeating
5. Demonstrated how to change self-defeating statements into more appropriate self-enhancing ones

Individual Task 1

In the following statements, each participant should identify which are self-defeating and which are self-enhancing statements. Indicate why a statement is self-defeating according to the criteria discussed in the "Rationale" of this exercise. Each participant should change the self-defeating statement to a coping statement by drawing upon the list of coping statements above (15 minutes or homework).

1. "I'll never be able to get that job, even if I am qualified."
2. "How can I ever have a decent interview when I know she (the interviewer) won't like me?"
3. "Sure it's complex, but what I can do is to take one thing at a time."
4. "I know I'm going to blow it with all those people looking at me."
5. "He (she) must really think I'm stupid."
6. "What if they think I'm imposing? Maybe I'm just wasting their time. I better not ask to see them."
7. "Why bother to ask her out? She probably won't like me anyway."
8. "I may not get the job, but I'll do my best in the interview."

(continued)

9. "It doesn't matter how hard I work, it will be just my luck to fail."
10. "Sure it's going to be a tough week, but if I plan my time well, I can get through it."
11. "It's been such a hectic day. I know I won't be able to sleep."
12. "They'll think I'm weird if I wear that sweater to the affair. No one will even talk to me."

Group Task 1

The group is divided into subgroups of four to five persons who will compare their responses in the above exercise. (Use criteria in the "Rationale" to evaluate whether a statement is self defeating.) (30 minutes)

Individual Task 2

Participants should add one self-defeating statement to the list that each has heard from a friend or client. (5 minutes)

Group Task 2

Participants will present their own self-defeating statement to the subgroup. Other members of the group will first give reasons why statements are self-defeating and carefully distinguish between self-defeating statements and statements of fact. Then the group should brainstorm alternative coping or self-enhancing statements. (40 minutes)

techniques. The guided exposure involves exposure of the client in groups to feared situations *in vivo*, first together with other group members and then, eventually, alone. For example, a group of clients who suffered from agoraphobia, after preparing by means of cognitive restructuring and the modeling sequence, went to a department store together. The first trial was in the morning when the store was almost empty; later they went at noon, when it was more crowded, and the third time, they went to the department store during a high-volume sale. Later, they tried out the same exercises with partners from the group, and eventually they performed them alone. Emmelkamp and Kuipers (1985) reviewed the commonly used procedures and the current research that lends support to these methods.

Relaxation Methods

Relaxation is a way of teaching clients to deal directly with such strong emotions as anxiety, stress, pain, or anger for which no external coping behavior is possible or for which cognitive coping behavior is insufficient, although the two procedures are often paired. In fact, it is used in almost all groups in which anxiety-related problems are described. This technique primarily involves teaching clients a modified version of the system developed by Jacobson (1929, 1978) in which various muscle groups are alternately tensed and relaxed. This is often referred to as neuromuscular relaxation. In later phases, the tensing of muscles is eliminated. After an initial demonstration by the group worker, the clients teach, monitor, and reinforce each other's efforts in the group for suitable performance and practice. Various alternatives uniquely suited to specific populations are also taught. Modest research support for the use of neuromuscular relaxation procedures for reducing anxiety and stress is to be found in studies by Stovya (1977) and by Lyles, Burish, Korzely, and Oldham (1982). Meditation and breathing exercises can be taught as alternatives to neuromuscular relaxation, depending on the preferences of the group members and the skills of the group worker. In order to make use of the group, the members are taught relaxation steps as a group. Then one person relaxes another person in the group, and then the process is reversed. The members are given tapes so that they can practice at home.

Operant Methods

These methods involve procedures in which the immediate consequences of a given behavior are followed in some systematic manner by a reinforcing event. It may also involve procedures in which the immediate conditions that lead to, or are parallel with, a given behavior are changed to create circumstances more amenable to the performance of a desired behavior. The latter is often referred to as stimulus control.

In groups, clients receive many kinds of reinforcement for the performance of prosocial group behavior and the completion of extragroup assignments or home tasks. With adults, this reinforcement takes the form of praise by the group worker or other group members. Occasionally, it takes the form of smiles, applause, approving nods, and delighted laughter. Reinforcers are withheld in response to undesirable behaviors. This process is referred to as "extinction," and it is an occasional response in groups toward someone who is frequently off task or complains a great deal. However, in groups, because so many people are involved, it is a difficult procedure to manage.

Operant procedures, especially reinforcement, lend themselves to be used in the group if the group worker trains and encourages members to reinforce each other and significant others outside of the group. Exercises such as the one in Figure 7.3 have been developed to train members in effective use of praise and constructive criticism as communication skills in their own right.

The feedback exercise is carried out throughout one entire session in which role playing modeling, and rehearsal are used. At the end of the session, the group worker provides positive feedback to the members on how well they adhered to the criteria.

Modifying the antecedent conditions, or stimulus control, was exemplified by a client in a weight-loss group who was urged by the others to eat only at a set table and with food that had been cooked. The group had a potluck dinner in which the behavior was modeled. Two college students in a study skill enhancement program developed a plan with each other in which they only studied at a clean desk and did nothing but study at that desk. They monitored each other. They removed the telephone and food from the study room. Success was followed by group approval and self-reinforcement.

Community Interventions

Community interventions are used as part of the generalization process. It involves the client in dealing with other organizations or social systems in which they might find social sup-

---

The purpose of this exercise is to train the members in giving and receiving feedback.

Steps in the exercise: Following each role play, the members are instructed to give feedback to the person who has rehearsed a new behavior. The members are instructed to adhere to the following criteria:

   All feedback should be specific. Examples should be given for general statements.
   Positive feedback is always given first.
   Initially the clients are asked to write down the feedback and read it to the target client.
   Feedback is given by one member at a time.
   Criticism should be formulated as suggested alternatives for the client to consider
   Feedback should eventually be summarized by the client receiving the feedback.

FIGURE 7.3. Giving feedback.

port, social recognition, and reinforcement. For example, a group of parents of intellectually challenged children organized a float in a local parade on which their children sat and waved to the public as a means of educating the public that they were not ashamed of their children. This same group developed a booklet for physicians on how to deal with the parents of special children and the children themselves (Kirkham, Schinke, Schilling, Meltzer, & Norelius, 1986) In working with clients with limited resources, referral to needed services may be considered. Ideas for community interventions may also come from the group.

Relationship Enhancement Methods

A number of skills have been identified as crucial to any helping relationship (Goldstein & Higgenbottom, 1991), whether or not this relationship is dyadic or within the structure of a small group. We have noted in our supervision of group workers that, in spite of high levels of technological skill, failure of group workers to possess these relational or clinical skills results in high dropout rates from groups, disinterest on the part of the clients, and high levels of group problems.

Many of these skills are to be found in the other methods described previously. For example, group workers who can comfortably and frequently provide their members with high levels of reinforcement and protect the clients from premature or abusive feedback tend to establish sound relationships with group members. Similarly, group workers who model self-disclosure (and all of the other skills that the members are expected to carry out) often discover that the indicators of group problems (high levels of conflict, low cohesion, low satisfaction, exclusive pairing off, low group productivity) seldom arise.

Some skills are unique to relationship building. For example, the use of humor with clients is not addressed in the foregoing methods. Yet successful group workers must be able to play and joke with clients. Involving clients and the group in their own therapy is a skill that is essential for achieving generalization of change. When they are comfortable with the other members and the group worker, clients become increasingly willing to take a chance in answering the questions of their fellow members, to make suggestions to each other for plans of action, to help each other to clarify the essential aspects of their problems, and to formulate appropriate goals. The process by which clients are involved is a vital relationship-building skill. Another skill is the ability to let clients make their own decisions as much as possible as to goals, extragroup tasks, and the extent of their participation, although encouragement and examples are provided. The more clients perceive themselves as deciding what happens to them, the more likely they will make use of interventions (similar to the ideas of Miller & Rollnick, 1991, p. 22).

Listening to clients is a skill that has not been covered here, yet the absence of careful listening often results in choosing wrong change targets. Effective listening does not necessarily require seeing the underlying implications of the client's words, but rather has to do with grasping the obvious meanings. While hastening to carry out the items on a group's given agenda, for instance, group workers might interrupt or ponder next steps while a client is still speaking. This can cut off important interpersonal messages.

Attending skills include competency in observing nonverbal responses, such as eye contact, body posture, and voice tone. Although these are nonspecific characteristics that are difficult to define, ratings by observers of group workers in action tend to indicate whether such skills are indeed operating.

Setting limits on disruptive or off-task behavior is another relational skill that must be considered if the goals of change are to be pursued in a safe environment. This is one of the more difficult of the relational skills and one of the most frequently needed. It is not always clear when to set limits and when to ignore disruptive behavior. Skill in reinforcement and developing interesting and attractive program content often protects the group worker from frequent application of limit setting.

Small-Group Procedures

We have already discussed the unique opportunities, as well as the limitations, offered in therapy in small-group settings. As mentioned earlier, interventions such as modeling, cognitive restructuring, relaxation, and so forth are administered in such a way as to encourage broad participation and high attraction among group members. In addition to the specific intervention strategies adapted from individual treatment, mentioned previously, there are some concrete group procedures that appear to contribute to helping clients move toward change. These group procedures include broad group participation, role playing, the buddy system, subgrouping, leadership skill delegation, group exercises, and sociorecreational procedures. These techniques are described here. Combinations of these procedures are often applied to attain group goals or resolve group interaction problems.

Broad group participation refers to client-to-client, as well as client-to-group-worker, interaction in which all members participate extensively. It is the essential element by which problems are laid out and considered, solutions are shared and evaluated, decisions are formulated and affirmed, values are deliberated, and friendships are made. Maximum involvement of all group members is essential for high cohesion and effective therapy. Broad group participation in the discussion is a necessary ingredient in the evaluation process in problem solving, in assessment as members respond to other persons' stories, and in providing feedback to each other. The worker promotes discussions but holds them to tight time constraints in time limited groups.

Role playing, in its most elementary form, can be defined as the practice of roles under simulated conditions. The group worker, by acting as a guide and structuring the role playing, contributes to the process and to the outcome achieved through role playing. If the group worker is clear about the purposes of role playing, this technique can prove highly beneficial in promoting change, broadening participation, and increasing cohesion. Role playing may be used in assessment to discover how clients actually handled a given situation. In the modeling sequence, role playing is used both to demonstrate specific skills and to practice them.

Role playing is also used to demonstrate and practice specific therapy skills, such as giving and receiving feedback or showing empathy to others. Role reversal is a form of role playing in which the client plays a significant person in his or her life and that person or another group member plays the client. It is a procedure aimed at giving insight in how it feels to be the other person. And, finally, role playing is used to practice generalization strategies evolved in the group. Some clients are initially reluctant to role-play; however, the activity appears to eventually gain the enthusiastic cooperation of almost all members if it is implemented in a supportive, nonthreatening atmosphere.

Subgrouping is a simple procedure for clients, working in pairs, triads, or other-size subgroups, to increase interaction among group members and provide them with an opportunity to work without the oversight of the group worker. It also may increase the amount of work that can be done in a given period of time. Subgrouping creates an opportunity for group members to practice leadership skills and affords them the opportunity to help others while being helped themselves. Care must be taken to constantly change the makeup of sub-groups in order to avoid the formation of negative cliques. Another danger of subgrouping is that the interaction occurs without the supervision of a group worker. In the group sessions, the group worker can sample the interaction by floating from subgroup to subgroup. Moreover, subgroup activities are usually highly structured with a specific task. The *buddy system* (see O'Donnell, Lydgate, & Fo, 1979) is a special subgrouping procedure for clients to work together outside of the group. In addition to the advantages mentioned, it contributes to the transfer of learning from the group to outside situations

Group exercises refer to the use of structured interactive activities as ways of teaching clients the skills that mediate the achievement of therapeutic goals. For example, an introduction exercise is used in which a client interviews and is interviewed by at least one other client in the group and then introduces the partner to the others. Another exercise is one in which the clients study a case and discuss how each of them is similar to or different from the person in that case. Other exercises involve teaching clients how to give and receive both praise and criticism to a partner in the group. Exercises, to be effective, are usually in writing, and the goals, as well as the activities, are stated.

The group worker must make sure that the exercise is understood before it is implemented. Usually, at least one group exercise is carried out in every session. Other interventions, in addition to subgrouping, may be embedded within group exercises. For instance, a "round robin" exercise uses modeling and rehearsal at a fast clip in order to provide multiple trials of new behavior. In teaching how to ask for help, Pete asks Don for help, then Don asks Robin for help, then Robin asks Jerry for help, and, finally, Jerry asks Pete for help. Other examples of exercises have been described earlier in this chapter and in Rose (1998).

Generalization Phase

In the generalization phase, which overlaps with the earlier phases, clients are prepared to transfer what they have learned in the group to the outside world and to maintain what they have learned in therapy beyond the end of therapy. In particular, extragroup tasks are designed for each member, usually at the end of every session, to be carried out in the workplace, school, playground, or home. Some of the other principles that are incorporated into treatment and that guide the planning for generalization are teaching the target behaviors in varied and multiple ways, finding opportunities for clients to teach what they have learned to others, encouraging clients to go public with their intervention plans and goals, gradually increasing the level of difficulty of expected behavior, preparing the clients for potential setbacks, having booster sessions following termination, and encouraging membership in support or social recreational groups following group therapy. In the following example, everyone in the group had a plan similar to Tom's.

> Tom, with the help of the other members of his group, planned to make use of the assertive skills he learned whenever a similar situation arose. He would report back to the group how it was handled and the result (multiple trials and going public). He would teach these same skills to his younger brother, who had a similar problem, with role-played modeling and rehearsal (teaching others). He told his friends that he was working on this and asked them to let him know if he succeeded or failed (going public and ongoing monitoring). He also agreed with a partner in the group, Rudy, to attend the booster session in a month and let the others know how he was doing.

Although the generalization phase occurs primarily in the last few sessions of treatment and beyond, the actions of the leaders take into account the principles of generalization throughout group treatment.

FUTURE PERSPECTIVES

In a recent survey of agencies in Madison, Wisconsin, I discovered that in 35% of the groups in the agencies sampled, behavioral or cognitive-behavioral procedures were the prominent interventions used. This represents a dramatic increase over the past 20 years, when it was almost impossible to find a group in which such interventions were used. In spite of this phenomenal growth, training in social work for CBGW is extremely limited. Almost no courses in group work from this orientation are available in schools of social work, although there is at least an increasing number of courses in cognitive-behavioral theory. Workshops are also available to practitioners who are interested in this approach. For this reason, agencies are turning to psychologists to lead cognitive-behavioral groups. If courses and field opportunity do not increase to meet the demand, social workers will eventually be squeezed out of this endeavor.

SOME CLOSING REMARKS

In this chapter, the process of using cognitive-behavioral and small-group strategies in the treatment of individuals in groups has been described. Where relevant literature was available, it was cited. However, I have also drawn on my own experience and that of other practitioners for examples and practice principles. This chapter has stressed the use of procedures commonly used by various helping persons *as they can be applied in groups*. It should be noted that this chapter has drawn from practice, research, and theoretical and clinical literature produced by psychologists, social workers, psychiatrists, and others in the helping professions and social sciences. The group workers exemplified in this chapter come from diverse professional backgrounds. The label used here has been cognitive-behavioral group work, although the name most commonly attributed to working with groups to achieve social-therapeutic goals has been "group therapy." In many cases, the labels "group treatment," "group work," "group training," or "group counseling" could have been used just as appropriately. We have also referred to the individual who leads the process as group worker—a label that cuts across all of the fields named. The group worker might just as readily be identified as group therapist, group leader, or group counselor, as the activities of each overlap the others considerably. We have used the words "clients" and "members" interchangeably to refer to the persons belonging to the groups.

As noted often, CBGW is not one approach but several similar ones. I have tried to point out some of the differences, as well as similarities. Some stress one intervention strategy, such as modeling, cognitive restructuring, reinforcement, or guided imagery, whereas others use a wide range of interventions. The particular model stressed in this chapter emphasizes the use of the group as means, as well as the context, of therapy, and a wide variety of both cognitive and behavioral procedures were presented. Other models are more didactic and less strictly involve the group actively in the treatment process. These are often referred to as psychoeducational groups.

Some social workers do not regard CBGW as part of social work. Yet CBGW shares the same value system as other approaches to social group work or theoretical models. The treatment goals mentioned previously toward which CBGW interventions are aimed, are compatible with the social values espoused by social work. In good practice, clients are not the subjects of interventions of which they are not aware and do not agree. In CBGW, clients are maximally involved in setting their own goals. In goal setting and intervention selection, the cultural background and the gender of the group members are given central consideration. Issues such as confidentiality are religiously adhered to. Clients are helped to enrich their own social networks if their original ones are deficient or faulty. In the group, cooperative behavior and mutually helping behavior is encouraged. One additional value is the tenet that all interventions in a given method should be based on empirical evidence that the method does what it claims to do. Ongoing data collection provides information as to whether the approach is succeeding or failing. Clients are protected from what can become merciless critical feedback without the given client's permission.

In conclusion, CBGW is closely linked to other goal-oriented approaches, such as problem-solving approaches, task-centered group work, and evidence-based practice. It is widely used, and it behooves social workers who are in clinical practice to become aware of its potential to serve their clients.

REFERENCES

Avia, M. D., Ruiz, M. A., Olivares, M. E., Crespo, M., Guisado, A. B., Sanchez, A., & Varela, A. (1996). The meaning of psychological symptoms: Effectiveness of a group intervention with hypochondriacal patients. *Behaviour Research and Therapy, 34*(1), 23–31.

Bandura, A. (1977). *Social learning theory.* New York: Holt, Rinehart & Winston.

Beck, A. T. (1976). *Cognitive therapy and the emotional disorders.* New York: International Universities Press.

Beck, A. T., & Emery, G. (1985). *Anxiety disorders and phobias.* New York: Basic Books.

Bottomley, A., Hunton, S., Roberts, G., Jones, L., & Bradley, C. (1996). A pilot study of cognitive behavioral therapy and social support group interventions with newly diagnosed cancer patients. *Journal of Psychosocial Oncology, 14*(4), 65–83.

D'Alelio, W. A., & Murray, E. J. (1981). Cognitive therapy for test anxiety. *Cognitive Therapy and Research, 5,* 299–307.

Daniels, L., & Roll, D. (1998). Group treatment of social impairment in people with mental illness. *Psychiatric Rehabilitation Journal, 21,* 273–278.

Emmelkamp, P. M. G., & Kuipers, A. C. M. (1985). Behavior group therapy for anxiety disorders. In D. Upper & S. M. Ross (Eds.), *Handbook of behavior group therapy.* New York: Plenum Press.

Evans, L., Holt, C., & Oei, T. P. (1991). Long-term follow-up of agoraphobics treated by brief intensive group cognitive-behavioral therapy. *Australian and New Zealand Journal of Psychiatry, 25*(3), 343–349.

Fisher, M. S., & Bentley, K. J. (1996). Two group therapy models for clients with a dual diagnosis of substance abuse and personality disorder. *Psychiatric Services, 47*(11), 1244–1250.

Flannery-Schroeder, E. C., & Kendall, P. C. (2000). Group and individual cognitive-behavioral treatments for youth with anxiety disorders: A randomized clinical trial. *Cognitive Therapy and Research, 24*(3), 251–278.

Goldstein, A. P., & Higgenbotham, H. N. (1991). Relationship-enhancement methods. In F. H. Kanfer & A. P. Goldstein (Eds.), *Helping people change: A textbook of methods* (Vol. 4, pp. 20–49). Elmsford, NY: Pergamon Press.

Hand, I., Lamontagne, Y., & Marks, I. (1974). Group exposure (flooding) in vivo for agoraphobics. *British Journal of Psychiatry, 124,* 588–602.

Heppner, P. P. (1978). A review of the problem-solving literature and its relationship to the counseling process. *Journal of Counseling Psychology, 25,* 366–375.

Jacobson, E. (1978). *You must relax.* New York: McGraw-Hill.

Jacobson, E. (1929). *Progressive relaxation.* Chicago: University of Chicago Press.

Kirkham, M. A., Schinke, S. P., Schilling, R. F., Meltzer, N. J., & Norelius, K. L. (1986). Cognitive-behavioral skills, social supports, and child abuse potential among mothers of handicapped children. *Journal of Family Violence, 1*(3), 235–245.

Linton, S. J., & Ryberg, M. (2001). A cognitive-behavioral group intervention as prevention for persistent neck and back pain in a non-patient population: A randomized controlled trial. *Pain, 90*(1–2), 83–90.

Lochman, J. E. (1985). Effects of different treatment lengths in cognitive behavioral interventions with aggressive boys. *Child Psychiatry and Human Development, 16,* 45–56.

Lott, A. J., & Lott, B. E. (1965). Group cohesiveness as inter-personal attraction: A review of relationships with antecedent and consequent variables. *Psychological Bulletin, 64,* 259–309.

Lutgendorf, S. K, Antoni, M. H., Ironson, G., Klimas, N., Kumar, M., Starr, K., et al. (1997). Cognitive stress management decreases dysphoric mood and simplex virus-type-2 antibody titers in symptomatic HIV-seropositive gay men. *Journal of Consulting and Clinical Psychology, 65,* 31–43.

Lyles, J. N., Burish, T. G., Korzely, M. G., & Oldham, R. K. (1982). Efficacy of relaxation training and guided imagery in reducing the aversiveness of cancer chemotherapy. *Journal of Counsulting and Clinical Psychology, 50,* 509–524.

Meichenbaum, D. (1977). *Cognitive-behavior modification: An integrated approach.* New York: Plenum Press.

Miller, W. R., & Rollnick, S. (1991). *Motivational interviewing: Preparing people to change addictive behavior.* New York: Guilford Press.

Newton-John, T., Spence, S., & Schotte, D. (1995). Cognitive-behavioral therapy versus EMG biofeedback in the treatment of chronic lower back pain. *Behavioral Research Therapy, 33,* 691–697.

O'Donnell, C. R., Lydgate, T., & Fo, W. S. (1979). The buddy system: Review and follow-up. *Child Behavior Therapy, 1,* 161–169.

Roffman, R. A., Downey, L., Beadnell, B., Gordon, J. R., Craver, J. N., & Stephens, R. S. (1997). Cognitive-behavioral group counseling to prevent HIV transmission in gay and bisexual men: Factors contributing to successful risk reduction. *Research on Social Work Practice, 7*(2), 165–186.

Rose, S. D. (1989). *Working with adults in groups: Integrating cognitive-behavioral and small group strategies.* San Francisco: Jossey-Bass.

Rose, S. D. (1998). *Group therapy with troubled youth: A cognitive-behavioral interactive approach.* Thousand Oaks, CA: Sage.

Silverman, W. K., Kurtines, W. M., Ginsburg, G. S., Weems, C. F., Lumpkin, P. W., & Carmichael, D. H. (1999). Treating anxiety disorders in children with group cognitive-behavioral therapy: A randomized clinical trial. *Journal of Consulting and Clinical Psychology, 67*(6), 995–1003.

Stoyva, J. (1977). Why should muscular relaxation be useful? In J. Beatty & H. Legewie (Eds.), *Biofeedback and behavior* (pp. 449–472). New York: Plenum Press.

Subramanian, K. (1991). Structured group work for the management of chronic pain: An experiential investigation and long-term follow-up of a structured group treatment for the management of chronic pain. *Research on Social Work Practice, 1,* 32–45.

Subramanian, K. (1994). Long-term follow-up of a structured group treatment for the management of chronic pain. *Social Work Practice, 4,* 208–223.

Sukhodolsky, D. G., Solomon, R. M., & Perine, J. (2000). Cognitive-behavioral, anger-control intervention for elementary school children: A treatment outcome study. *Journal of Child and Adolescent Group Therapy, 10*(3), 159–170.

Tanco, S., Wolfgang, L., & Earle, T. (1998). Well-being and morbid obesity in women: A controlled therapy evaluation. *International Journal of Eating Disorders, 23*(3), 325–339.

Telch, F., Agras, W., Rossiter, E., Wilfley, D., & Kenardy, J. (1990). Group cognitive-behavioral treatment for the nonpurging bulimic: An initial evaluation. *Journal of Consulting and Clinical Psychology, 58,* 629–635.

Van Dam Baggen, R., & Kraaimaat, F. (1986). A group social skills training program with psychiatric patients: Outcome, drop-out rate and prediction. *Behaviour Research and Therapy, 24*(2), 161–169.

Vogel, P., Eriksen, L., & Bjoernelv, S. (1997). Skills training and prediction of follow-up status for chronic alcohol dependent inpatients. *European Journal of Psychiatry, 11,* 51–63.

Yalom, I. D. (1985). *The theory and practice of group psychotherapy* (3rd ed.). New York: Basic Books.

Part III

Group Work Approaches Related to Purpose

Some group approaches have emerged that are related to the major foci of the group. These approaches cut across all fields of practice and are described in this section. The foci we have chosen are self-help and support, psychoeducation, and prevention.

The support and self-help focus seeks to help members who are coping with a broad variety of personal and social conditions, such as addictions, the stigma of mental illness, or oppression due to one's sexual orientation. These group members are typically not seeking therapy or broad personality change from the group in question, but, instead, to identify and use resources, overcome environmental obstacles, and find acceptance of themselves in a caring environment. Sometimes these groups have a professional leader, and we refer to these as "support" groups. At other times, these groups are facilitated by peers who are in the "same boat," and we refer to these as "self-help." Such services have become so widely used that we have devoted the first chapter in this section (Chapter 8) to this topic.

Another purpose is to provide what has come to be called "psychoeducation." This type of service recognizes that many people can be helped to function better and to solve problems if they learn new skills and acquire new information. Many techniques have been developed that can help social workers to offer this kind of group, an important part of professional knowledge; thus another chapter (Chapter 9) is devoted to this kind of group.

The third chapter in this section (Chapter 10) is devoted to groups created to *prevent* serious problems from emerging in people. Contemporary strategies can help group practitioners to identify "populations at risk." Individuals who may succumb to such risks can be helped to cope in ways that prevent problems at much less cost to themselves or the society than if severe breakdowns in functioning were to occur.

Chapter 8

Support and Self-Help Groups

Linda Farris Kurtz

Self-help[1] and support groups have become an integral part of mainstream culture, expressing a social philosophy that heralds individual empowerment and citizen involvement. Such groups are available for almost any situation or concern and are accessible to a growing number of people in the United States and around the world. They cost their beneficiaries nothing, and many can be joined without referral, application, or "red tape." Just before his death, Alfred Katz wrote:

> The values of cooperative self-organization and non-bureaucratic mutual helping methods exemplified by hundreds of organizations . . . have penetrated the general culture inescapably and irreversibly. Self-help is seen as a social resource so that people no longer have to suffer in isolation or feel despair that they can find no help in confronting and coping with their problems. (in White & Madara, 2002, p. 5)

These words were part of his Foreword to the seventh edition of *The Self-Help Group Sourcebook*, which listed over 1,100 national and international headquarters of self-help networks in the United States and Canada, many with branches throughout the world—a testimony to the significance of self-help/mutual aid in contemporary society. The *Sourcebook* defines a self-help group as one that provides mutual support, is composed of "peers," is primarily run by and for its members, and does not charge dues or fees (White & Madara, 2002, p. 29).

This chapter is about self-help *and* support groups. Though they are often lumped together, as ideal types self-help and support groups differ. A key difference between support and self-help groups involves their leadership. Professional facilitators often lead support groups, although this is not always so. At times professionals and members share leadership. Additionally, some support groups are led by members. Riessman and Carroll (1995) refer to support groups led by professionals as "quasi-self-help forms" (p. 2). A member of the group who shares the condition for which the group was formed, as the name implies, leads most self-help groups. Many, such as 12-step fellowships, have no official leadership; members rotate the meeting chairperson role. There are, however, exceptions among self-help groups that are not of the 12-step variety. Hybrid groups are self-help in character but have professional sponsors and member leaders (Parents Anonymous, 2001; Powell, 1987). There are other things that usually differentiate self-help from support groups.

Typically, support groups are sponsored by larger organizations, such as hospitals or foundations. They often are small, and their focus is more on emotional support and reassuring information and less on personal change or on advocacy and social action. Admission to membership is often controlled by the leader or social agency, rather than being open to anyone. Self-help groups are more often chapters of large federations of affiliated groups that are national and that espouse a program of either personal or social change (Kurtz, 1997; Powell, 1987). These associations typically welcome anyone who shares the concern of the group. One may refer to both types of group as "mutual help" groups, a term preferred by many (Silverman, 2002). A later section of this chapter provides illustrations of various types of self-help and support groups.

The purpose of this chapter is to provide a current review of the literature on practice involving self-help and support groups, including the use of groups on line and on the telephone, and to identify the various roles that social workers play with such groups. In addition, this chapter considers some of the significant issues and philosophical points that relate to the concept of self-help and summarizes research and theory on self-help and support groups. Examples illustrate various self-help and support group models. The chapter concludes with future projections related to self-help and support groups.

NUMBERS OF SELF-HELP AND SUPPORT GROUPS IN THE UNITED STATES TODAY

Wuthnow's (1994) study of the small-group movement in America estimated that there were 3 million such groups in the United States. He divided the various types of groups into four categories, including Sunday-school classes, Bible-study groups, self-help groups, and special interest groups. In his book he refers to all of these as support groups. He differentiates self-help groups using a definition provided in an early edition of *The Self-Help Sourcebook* (Madara & Meese, 1990).[2] He estimated that self-help groups numbered around 500,000, a figure that no doubt included many of what I define as support groups.

Some true self-help organizations—that is, the ideal type—have records of the groups they sponsor, and others offer educated estimates of how many members attend groups. Many, however, do not have such information available to the public. Self-help groups are generally nonbureaucratic and thus have few files and membership records. Websites of the most well-known and numerous 12-step fellowships show that Alcoholics Anonymous (AA) has 56,210 groups in North America and that several others (Al-Anon, Gamblers Anonymous [GA], Narcotics Anonymous [NA], Cocaine Anonymous [CA], Overeaters Anonymous [OA], Emotions Anonymous [EA]) added together number about 43,000 groups. AA reports another 2,531 groups in correctional facilities (AA World Services, 2002). A conservative estimate suggests that there are about 100,000 separate and individual 12-step "chapters" in North America. Twelve-step groups represent a majority of the ideal-type self-help groups.

Foundations such as the Alzheimer's and Related Disorders Association, the Parkinson's Foundation, and many others that serve people with chronic diseases sponsor large numbers of support groups throughout the United States and probably add many thousand to the number of self-help and support groups meeting throughout the country. Several studies have revealed that hospitals and health facilities are the most frequent sites for support group services (Lieberman & Snowden, 1994; Mok, 2001; Wituk, Shepherd, Slavich, Warren, & Meissen, 2000).

A reliable population survey in the middle of the last decade found that participants in self-help groups numbered 3–4% of the population, or between 7 and 10 million participants (Kessler, Mickelson, & Zhao, 1997). More than 1 million of these were North American members of AA (AA World Services, 2002). In 1989 Jacobs and Goodman (1989) predicted that the number of self-help members would grow to 10 million by 1999. Wuthnow's survey techniques suggested that 8 to 10 million Americans attend self-help groups (1994). These three sources arrived at their almost identical figures independently.

SELF-HELP ETHOS AND PHILOSOPHY

Frank Riessman introduced the concept of the "helper therapy" principle in 1965 (p. 27), but the ancient insight that one helps oneself in the act of helping others had already been rediscovered by the founders of AA 30 years earlier. In AA, the helping process begins when the participant tells his or her story of drinking and recovery to others; it was this singular act that characterized AA's legendary founding moment between Bill W. and Dr. Bob (Jensen, 2000; Riessman, 1965). The principle of "helper therapy" is one of the cornerstones of the self-help movement.

Self-help and independent support groups operate by assembling informally in agencies, churches, hospitals, and/or community rooms. There is usually an agenda through which participants learn something about their concerns and how to cope with them. Participants may also benefit from supportive discussion among themselves. Often there are refreshments and opportunities to become acquainted informally before, after, and in between meetings. Many groups, especially the 12-step variety, have a specific program to follow in the effort to change behavior, grow spiritually, or reduce the stress of everyday living. Professional treatments may be discussed but are not prescribed. Leaders discourage advice giving; participants are encouraged to speak from their own experience.

Riessman and Carroll (1995) help us understand that "self-help is not synonymous with individual help" (p. 3). Rather, the term is used to emphasize internal helping, whether the helping is internal to a person, a group, or a community. This is in contrast to "external interventions by teachers, experts, clergy, therapists or the state" (p. 3). Self-help interventions do not come from outside the entity; they come from within, and they share the "basic self-help philosophy"(p. 3). The self-help paradigm "views people with problems as potential help givers, as more independent than dependent" (p. 4). The self-help ethos emphasizes empowerment. Through a process of identifying the nature of the problem, joining with others, and educating themselves on how to achieve a solution, a person's initial "powerlessness" becomes transformed into empowerment.

PROFESSIONAL INTERVENTIONS
WITH SELF-HELP AND SUPPORT GROUPS

Professionals provide leadership and facilitation for support groups. However, professionals can play many other roles with both self-help and support groups. These include consulting with, linking to, and supporting groups in their efforts to get started; it may also include working to maintain helping factors in the group's process. At times negative factors interfere with the smooth functioning of groups whose leadership may come to a professional for consultation about the group. All open-ended groups need new members, and these come often from professional referrals. Sometimes groups decide to become Web-based and ask for professional assistance for mounting their discussion groups and information into a website.

This section reviews important aspects of professional and indigenous leadership of support groups. This review is followed by discussion of ways in which professionals can assist independent self-help groups.

Leading and Facilitating Support Groups

Unlike treatment groups, professionally facilitated support groups are less structured, and members are given more latitude in deciding on the content of meetings. Leaders act as motivators, organizers, and contacts for the group (King, Stewart, King, & Law, 2000). Leadership tasks include "phoning members, organizing and running meetings, finding speakers, maintaining records and documents for the group, dealing with correspondence and phone calls, organizing advocacy activities, planning social and/or fund-raising events, and acting as a contact person" (King et al., 2000, p. 230). It is essential for new support groups to decide what to focus on, how to structure the meetings, and how to divide the meeting time. Some members prefer to spend time discussing their situations, learning coping strategies, and hearing stories similar to their own. Others prefer informational meetings. The role of the facilitator differs depending on what the group decides is its focus.

Many support groups are co-led by a professional and a member. Leaders from within the regular membership conduct other groups, though often with professional consultation. When indigenous members take on leadership roles, burnout can be a problem (Chesler & Chesney, 1995; Medvene, Volk & Meissen, 1997). Groups often struggle to find ways to bring more people into leadership roles. Groups that flourish involve new members in leadership activities, maintain extensive community connections, and adapt activities to meet changing needs.

Professional leadership has some advantages over indigenous leadership because these groups are usually linked to social agencies and thus to the resources possessed by those agencies. Studies of successful groups have found that groups with relationships to either larger local or national organizations are healthier with respect to survival (Shepherd et al., 1999; Wituk, Shepherd, Warren, & Meissen, 2002). Agency resources help in the effort to keep the group afloat; this is particularly important in attracting new membership.

Consulting, Linking, and Supporting

Studies of self-help groups reveal a number of activities by professionals, in addition to group leadership and facilitation (Powell, Hill, Warner, Yeaton, & Silk, 2000; Wituk et al., 2000). For example, Powell et al. (2000) described a system of sponsoring new members into a group for bipolar disorder that substantially increased participation by newcomers. Wituk et al. (2000) were able to contrast successful and unsuccessful groups and to isolate the factors that correlated with success. They found that surviving groups were more connected to professional and community supports that fed new members to the group and provided practical, hands-on assistance. New members guarantee group survival; without them, groups will end. Some of the ways that groups maintain membership include furnishing between-meeting support, providing educational activity, advocating for members, and sponsoring other between-meeting activities. Between-meeting activities include telephone support, peer counseling, visitation and outreach, buddy systems, training seminars, and social events.

An examination of AA, probably the world's largest and most successful self-help fellowship, shows that, although no professionals are visible in meetings, an underlying professional support system in the alcoholism/drug treatment community sustains this 12-step fellowship (Kurtz, 1997, 2001). Professionals liberally supported AA during its founding and continued to do so throughout its 68-year history (Kurtz, 1979; White, 1998). A multitude of professional alcoholism treatment workers, administrators, educators, and scholars continue to link newcomers to AA, to involve aspects of the AA program in treatment centers, to attend open AA meetings, to study AA, and to participate in Al-Anon (Kurtz, 2001).

Maintaining Helping Factors

Much theoretical and empirical literature has focused on helping and change-inducing factors in self-help groups, some of which applies equally to support groups (Kurtz, 1997; Powell, 1987). Lieberman (1979) studied change mechanisms in a wide variety of groups, some of which were neither self-help nor support groups. He explored the extent to which change-induction factors found in studies of psychotherapy groups were also present in self-help groups. Lieberman concluded that self-help groups (his sample included one group that today would be seen as a support group) promote feelings of universality (similarity), support, and acceptance. Further, they have the capacity to generate a sense of belongingness and cohesiveness; they create a refuge for people who feel they are deviant in some way; and they provide a context for social comparison.

Levy's (1979) early study of helping processes and activities in self-help groups (his definition clearly excluded support groups as defined here) took a grounded-theory approach by first observing group processes and activities. Following this phase of his study, Levy and his research team constructed a questionnaire that listed 28 observed activities and asked members which of the observed processes occurred in their group. They found that the nine most frequently occurring activities were "empathy, mutual affirmation, explanation, sharing, morale building, self-disclosure, positive reinforcement, personal goal stating, and catharsis" (p. 264). Levy concluded that self-help groups focus their efforts on fostering communication, providing social support, and responding to members' needs. These are activities that "one might expect to find in any natural social setting," making them familiar and stress free (p. 265). How then do they induce change? They do so, Levy suggested, by providing empathy, mutual affirmation, advice, and feedback. This allows the participant to obtain the support necessary to change on his or her own terms.

Another important contribution to the literature on helping factors and change mechanisms came from Antze (1979), who examined group ideologies in AA, Synanon, and Recovery, Inc. According to Antze, the group's ideology is the feature that members take most seriously. The "group's teachings are their very essence" (p. 273). His work led to other studies of group ideologies in mental health groups and in groups for alcoholics and their families (Emerick, 1995; Humphreys, 1996).

A 1997 review of research on helping factors and change mechanisms in self-help groups found the following factors reported in support groups: group cohesiveness, instilling hope, universality, obtaining information and experiential knowledge, receiving support, having a sense of belonging, and learning methods of coping (Kurtz, 1997). In addition, more complex self-help associations provide change mechanisms such as identity transformation, empowerment, insight, and reframing (Kurtz, 1997). Recent studies of helping factors in self-help and support groups identify many of the same helping factors as those found by Kurtz (1997; Cheung & Sun, 2001; Cintron, Solomon, & Draine, 1999; Mok, 2001; Schiff & Bargal, 2000). Schiff and Bargal (2000), Israeli researchers, found that instillation of hope, universality, and emotional disclosure were most highly correlated with satisfaction with groups in Israel. An American study found that knowledge, information, and universality were found to be the most helpful factors reported (Cintron et al., 1999).

Two studies in Hong Kong provided opportunity for cultural comparison among self-help groups (Cheung & Sun, 2001; Mok, 2001). In one (Cheung & Sun, 2001), support and catharsis were the most predictive of member perception of benefits in the study, but universality, self-disclosure, and instillation of hope were more predictive of perceived helpfulness by their respondents. Cheung and Sun (2001) were surprised that catharsis was rated so highly in their study because Chinese people are not normally given to emotional display. They concluded, however, that these factors are helpful at different stages. Universality, self-disclosure, and instillation of hope are appropriate in beginning stages, when expression of feeling could be embarrassing. In later stages, support, encouragement, and catharsis are useful in helping members work through emotional blocks and in finding methods for coping. Mok's (2001) study in Hong Kong used survey questionnaires and in-depth interviews to ascertain the degree to which respondents agreed with a list of statements indicating how the group influenced changes in themselves. He found that social learning, acceptance of limitation, and enlarged social networks were the most common benefits seen by members.

Facilitators can influence groups in ways that support these factors through helping to provide information when needed, making sure that new members feel welcomed and accepted, advising the group to host speakers who can inspire hope to surmounting a difficult situation, and through maintaining a homogeneous group composition with regard to the condition the group addresses.

TECHNOLOGY-BASED GROUPS

Technology-based groups, including groups on the Internet and over the telephone, provide useful resources for people who are unable to find local face-to-face groups for their condition or who are not able or willing to travel to the sites where they meet (Galinsky, Schopler, & Abell, 1997; Schopler, Abell, & Galinsky, 1998). Such groups have distinctive individual, group, and environmental features. Individuals can participate anonymously, must be technologically savvy, and can control their self-presentation in ways not possible in face-to-face groups. On a group level, technology-based groups mask social cues and norms. The pace of communication is slower, but anonymity encourages more open expressions, leading to more rapid group cohesion. Anonymity may also lead to premature disclosure, making persons vulnerable to embarrassment and the insensitivity of others' responses. Salient environmental features include availability of technology resources, presence or absence of support, and lack of information about each participant's immediate context. In addition, computer technologies are complex and expensive, making them less accessible for some populations than the telephone.

Computer Groups

Virtually every large self-help association in existence has a Web page; further, it is possible to participate in many computer groups through "chat rooms," a type of "real time" discussion. In addition, newsgroups or discussion forums are available, in which discussion is asynchronous and runs "24/7." The ready availability and anonymity of computer-based groups makes them a medium that is rapidly growing in popularity. In 2002, 56% of the population in the United States was on line daily; 1% (610,000) was visiting an on-line support group, according to the Pew Internet and American Life Project (2002a). The project used on-line and telephone surveys of the population to "explore the impact of the Internet on children, families, communities, the work place, schools, health care and civic/political life" (Pew Internet and American Life Project, 2002b). According to the project, 9% of 109 million (close to 10,000,000) have participated in on-line support groups at some point in their lives. Ten percent of health seekers in fair or poor health consulted an on-line support group the last time they searched for health information (Pew Internet and American Life Project, 2002c).

Computer-based self-help groups overcome several obstacles that confront face-to-face groups. The prospective participant is not dependent on geographical location, nor does he or she need to be concerned about being seen in such a group. One can participate from home, office, a local library, or a community center. For persons who are incapacitated or whose time is limited, computers offer convenience, flexibility, and accessibility (Schopler et al., 1998). There are also challenges faced in the potential for confidentiality violation, insensitivity, and hostility among users.

Self-help on the Internet takes three primary forms (Madara, 1999–2000a). "Listservs" allow members to receive messages delivered to their e-mail addresses and to send messages to all on the subscription list. A second is through the USENET network that gives access to thousands of newsgroups, also referred to as discussion forums or conferences. "A newsgroup stores messages on a computer in a central location, which can be read and replied to by users" (Madara, 1999–2000a, p. 40). The third is through websites that provide interactive message boards or real-time chat meetings. Most or at least many of these websites also offer information.

Practitioners can make use of on-line groups for clients by simply helping the individual to gain access to a computer with connections to the Internet and showing them how to find relevant groups. Group workers can also start groups on line; however, readers should be cautious about this unless they are aware of the technicalities, ethics, and responsibilities that go with this endeavor. Madara (1999–2000b) suggests numerous ways that on-line groups can be started. Message boards or chat rooms can be placed onto existing websites, agencies can sponsor e-mail discussion on listservs, and newsgroups can be developed on sites such as those of Yahoo.com. For anyone interested in starting a new computer-based support group, Grohol's guide to on-line mental health resources gives needed details and instructions (Grohol, 2004). This guide tells you how to begin groups, set up websites, and locate a multiplicity of existing sites.

Salem, Bogat, and Reid (1997) and Finn (1999) have published two comprehensive examinations of on-line participation. Salem et al. coded the content of 1,863 postings by 533 participants over a 2-week period in a group for people suffering from depression; Finn analyzed 718 messages over a 3-month period to an unnamed on-line bulletin board system (BBS). In Salem et al.'s study, 13 response categories were subsumed under five subcategories: social support, help seeking and disclosure, affect responses, knowledge responses, and group structure and identification. Findings were compared with those of a face-to-face group. The users, of which more were male than female, did not differ significantly in their posts. Most frequently the postings were supportive and expressed positive feelings. The online group participants expressed less cognitive guidance and more self-disclosure than the face-to-face comparison groups.

Finn (1999) isolated 14 categories of messages from the BBS, including: expressing feelings, providing support, chitchat, universality, friendship expressions, extragroup relationships discussion, taboo topics, damaging statements, poetry and art thoughts, information asking, information stating, problem solving, computer talk, and group cohesion. He divided helping categories into two areas: socioemotional and task. The majority (55.3%) of the responses were socioemotional. Another large percentage revealed information provision and problem solving. Finn found little evidence of harmful communication and few messages that commented on the group itself, such as on universality or group cohesion.

Telephone Groups

Telephone groups are used with people who are unable to attend face-to-face groups due to lack of transportation, lack of time, or too much distance from others (Galinsky et al., 1997). Other reasons have to do with convenience or desire for anonymity. Telephone groups serve fewer people than computer groups. Practitioners are urged to keep the size of the group small, from three to six members, and to choose members carefully (Kaslyn, 1999; Kurtz, 1997; Schopler et al., 1998). Such groups must meet simultaneously, making them less flexible than computer groups.

After surveying practitioners who have used telephone groups, Galinsky et al. (1997) found that such groups have been used for support, education, organizational tasks, consultation team building, self-help, supervision, staff training, community organizing, crisis intervention, mediation and arbitration, and bereavement therapy. Most often the group selects a convenient time for a conference call. This can be expensive, with conference calls that last an hour costing as much as $150. The typical duration of closed, short-term groups is 6 to 12 weeks, although some groups meet for unlimited periods of time (Kurtz, 1997). Practitioners who use conference calls are urged to practice the process before introducing it to a group of clients. Comfort and confidence in the use of conference calling are critical to the leadership of such groups.

There are challenges in the use of telephone groups. An obvious one is the loss of nonverbal communication. Technological glitches can happen. Telephone conference calls can be expensive. Group process limitations occur, such as difficulty with a member bonding with the group. Galinsky et al.'s survey noted a number of other concerns about the use of technology-based groups, including problems in recognizing and dealing with potential suicide and safety issues, increased scheduling problems, and difficulties with billing for services (Galinsky et al., 1997). Another challenge for elderly people can be difficulty hearing each other (Kaslyn, 1999). Lack of participation is another challenge practitioners face. To deal with this, practitioners are urged to keep a checklist of who speaks. Unexpected interruptions can also impede the group process. Although group cohesion can develop rapidly over the telephone, bonds between members are not likely to extend after the group has ended (Kaslyn, 1999).

CHALLENGES IN SELF-HELP AND SUPPORT GROUPS

Practitioners need to be aware of challenges in face-to-face support groups, as well as in telephone and computer groups. Galinsky and Schopler (1994) have identified a number of ways in which support groups could be harmful to members. One is that the group will dispense misguided or inaccurate information. Another is that intense feelings expressed in a group's meeting may frighten some members. Members who express intense feelings in a meeting may also be harmed if there are not opportunities for follow-up support after the meeting.

For groups that serve people with potentially terminal illnesses, care must be taken not to mix members in early stages with members in late stages of illness. Furthermore, peer helpers are experts only on themselves and can only convey experiential knowledge to others (Borkman, 1999). Harm could occur if peer leaders attempt to administer guidance for which they are not prepared.

Psychotherapeutic interventions, such as probing questions, confrontations, and interpretations, are not appropriate activities in either self-help or support groups. Readers should, therefore, avail themselves of materials that assist professionals to work appropriately with support groups, such as White and Madara's (2002) *Self-Help Group Sourcebook: Your Guide to Community and Online Support Groups*.

In professionally facilitated support groups, the facilitator can establish norms preventing inappropriate advice giving, intrusive questioning, excessive negativity, and other harmful activities. Both support and self-help groups normally focus on solutions and coping methods. For example, a 12-step participant tells his or her story of recovery using the steps. A member of Recovery, Inc., gives an example of how he or she applied the Recovery method to a problem of everyday living (Low, 1950). Advice is replaced by stories of "how I did it," and this is often followed by "but your experience may differ." Another concern leveled at self-help groups is that they are either not effective for or inaccessible to some cultural groups in society. The concern over diversity is addressed in the next section of this chapter.

CULTURAL AND GENDER DIVERSITY

Self-help is an international phenomenon. This is evidenced in *The Self-Help Group Sourcebook* (White & Madara, 2002), which lists 33 separate clearinghouses for 23 different countries. Many of the large self-help associations in the United States are international and have groups throughout the world. Azaiza and Ben-Ari (1998) provide an illustration of why such diverse cultures accept the concept of self-help. The authors found that there is a natural fit between the Arab culture and self-help because "Arab professionals are raised within a society which emphasizes the empowering nature of the collective or the community" (p. 427). Arab professionals use self-help as one way to increase the resources available in their community.

That 12-step fellowships and other self-help groups can be molded to fit diverse cultures is inarguable. There are AA, NA, Al-Anon, and other 12-step groups in foreign countries that have different cultures, religions, and customs (Caetano, 1993; Mäkelä, 1996). AA reports groups in 150 countries outside the United States and Canada (AA World Services, 2002), with General Service Offices in 51 of those countries. These countries include Japan, Korea, the Russian Federation, Slovakia, and the Czech Republic.

AA is composed of many ethnic groups in North America, although its national membership is predominantly Caucasian (88%; AA World Services, 2003; Caetano, 1993). NA reports membership of 18% African American and 9% Latino (Narcotics Anonymous World Services, 2002). CA reports 27% African American and 4% Latino (Cocaine Anonymous World Services, 2001). Although the percentages of active minority members reported in these surveys is low for Latinos and Asians, AA's acceptability in these diverse communities is high, according to Caetano, who reviewed the literature on AA's adaptability and expansion among ethnic minority groups.

Omitting 12-step groups, Snowden and Lieberman (1994) examined minority group representation in California self-help groups and found them to be seriously underrepresented. However, a later study in Kansas found no difference in demographic factors among a broad range of groups in that state (Wituk et al., 2000). Numerous factors beyond ethnicity and race have been identified that could explain racial and ethnic differences in group retention (Heller, Roccoforte, & Cook, 1997; Humphreys & Woods, 1994; Luke, Roberts, & Rappaport, 1994; Mankowski, Humphreys, & Moos, 2001). These factors include language, lack of transportation, "group fit," prior exposure to treatment and to the group, and personal- and group-belief compatibility. Heller et al. (1997) found that African American and Hispanic groups participated in family groups when those groups served meals, provided transportation, and had Spanish-speaking members. Several studies have found some evidence that "group fit" (a new member resembles the membership of the group) increased attendance by African Americans (Humphreys & Woods, 1994; Luke et al., 1994).

Women are generally seen as more likely to attend self-help and support groups than men; membership statistics of large self-help associations support that generalization. There are, however, important differences in gender makeup depending on the type of problem addressed (Luke et al., 1994; Wituk et al., 2000). Fellowships that serve traditionally male populations, such as AA, CA, and NA, have fewer women members, both because there are fewer women addicts and because the group's male culture may make some women uncomfortable. For example, AA's membership is 67% male (AA World Services, 2003), Cocaine Anonymous is 68% male (CA World Services, 2001), and NA's membership is 56% male (NA World Services, 2002). Groups with traditionally high female memberships include Al-Anon Family Groups, Overeaters Anonymous, Recovery, Inc., Parents Anonymous, Candlelighters, Alzheimer's Disease and Related Disorders Association support groups, and Compassionate Friends (Kurtz, 1997).

What is of primary importance is communication of the availability and existence of self-help groups to those who need them. It was for this reason that self-help clearinghouses were developed in most states. Unfortunately, these services are losing their funding. Professional practitioners can fill this void by informing themselves about groups and helping to start new chapters, by helping existing groups make their services accessible to all sectors of society, and by referring all those in need of service.

SELF-HELP AND SUPPORT GROUP RESEARCH

Research reveals support and self-help groups to be effective in reducing the need for more costly and unnecessary professional services, improving quality of life, and many other benefits (Humphreys & Moos, 2001; Kurtz, 1997). This section relies on a summary of 44 outcome studies by Kyrouz, Humphreys, and Loomis (2002). According to these authors, much of the research on effectiveness of self-help and support groups blurs the boundaries between the two types of groups. For this reason, they limited their review of the effectiveness research on self-help groups to studies of groups that are truly self-help in character rather than those groups that are led by professionals (the latter fits the category of "support groups"). The authors also "focused primarily on studies that compared participants to non-participants and/or gathered information repeatedly over time" (p. 71), thus eliminating single-group cross-sectional surveys that reflected how members felt when they were currently involved in their group.

The summarized investigations were all published between the years of 1977 and 2001. Included were 44 outcome studies representing the following types of groups: addiction-related groups (16 studies), bereavement groups (5 studies), cancer groups (2 studies), caregiver groups (4 studies), chronic-illness groups (5 studies), diabetes groups (2 studies), groups for elderly persons (1 study), mental health groups (8 studies), and weight-loss groups (2 studies).

The research designs among these 44 studies predominantly (73%) compared outcomes of the same respondents before and after the intervention, compared respondents who followed through with participation with those that did not, or compared participants with matched samples of persons who did not have the problem. For example, a 1999 study (Cook, Heller, & Pickett-Schenk, 1999) compared the outcomes of parents of adult children with mental illness who attended National Alliance for the Mentally Ill (NAMI) support group meetings with nonattendees. The other 27% compared self-help participants with individuals who received an alternate form of intervention. For example, a study of bereaved parents who attended Compassionate Friends (CF) compared parents who attended the self-help group and parents who received psychotherapy (Videka-Sherman & Lieberman, 1985).

Outcome measures for all of these studies were varied. For the 16 addiction-related studies, outcome measures included, among others, number of days abstinent, measures of psychological factors such as anxiety and self esteem, improvements in relationships, size of social network, and costs of follow-up care. Outcomes assessed in the remaining 29 studies included things such as psychological distress, medical symptoms, caregiver burden, increased coping skills and strategies, increased satisfaction with life and with medical care, length of hospital stays, social adjustment, and weight loss. Overall, 39 (89%) of the studies found that self-help participation resulted in positive outcomes; when groups were compared with other interventions, the self-help condition was more effective and more cost efficient. Four studies, all of substance abuse groups, found that the self-help groups did not produce more favorable outcomes than no help at all or than an alternate form of help. Thus the majority of effectiveness studies of well-defined self-help groups, in which methodological rigor was at least partially achieved, found them to be effective in achieving their goals.

THEORETICAL APPLICATIONS TO SELF-HELP AND SUPPORT GROUPS

A summary of theoretical self-help literature includes social support, cognitive-behavioral, reference group, social comparison, social ecology, and empowerment theories. The following discusses some of the theories and concepts that have been applied to support and self-help groups.

Social support theory postulates that individuals in crisis are partially protected from the negative effects of stress if surrounded with human supports in the form of family, friendship networks, and/or fellow sufferers (Caplan & Killilea, 1976; Lieberman & Borman, 1979). Gerald Caplan proposed that "social support systems are attachments between individuals and between individuals and groups that promote mastery; offer guidance about the field of relevant forces, expectable problems, and methods of dealing with them; and provide feedback about behavior that validates identity and fosters improved competence" (Caplan, as quoted in Killilea, 1982, p. 177). When friendship and family ties are weak, support groups of fellow sufferers offer substitutes for natural support systems; they also give specialized forms of experiential knowledge about the stressful condition (Borkman, 1999).

Cognitive-behavioral theory has been useful in understanding the ways in which some groups help members change thoughts and actions. Social learning principles can be found illustrated in both AA and Recovery, Inc., a group for persons with emotional and mental disorders (Kurtz & Powell, 1987). For example, in 12-step programs, new members find successful models in veterans who display their use of the steps and traditions. To induce cognitive change, group ideologies are codified; reframing strategies are taught and practiced. Recovery, Inc.'s, method of will training teaches participants to change their language, referred to as the "symptomatic idiom" and "temperamental lingo" (Low, 1950, pp. 19–20). In meetings, members present examples in which they were able to "spot" instances of symptomatic thinking and behaving and to substitute Recovery teachings. Recovery, Inc.'s, application of cognitive and social learning principles is one of the first known uses of cognitive methods as a mental health intervention (Kurtz, 1997; Lee, 1995; Low, 1950).

Reference group theory is another powerful conceptual tool that can be applied to both support and self-help groups (Powell, 1987). Such groups are highly cohesive, due in part to members having similar issues, for example, alcoholism, overeating, cancer. Thus their cohesiveness and their availability in a time of acute stress make their power as a reference group quite forceful. As Powell (1987) noted, "the greater the similarity between the individual and the group, the more likely the group will be a comprehensive, durable influence" (p. 75). As a result, participants' self-assessments evolve along with their growing identification with the group norm.

Social comparison theory provides another theoretical base from which to study self-help and support groups. This theory proposes that social behaviors can be predicted as individuals seek to maintain a sense of normalcy and accuracy about their world (Davison, Pennebaker, & Dickerson, 2000). When people are uncertain and under stress, affiliative behaviors increase as people seek others' opinions about what is happening to them. Basing their study on social comparison theory, Davison et al. (2000) identified the kinds of illness experiences that prompted patients in four metropolitan areas and in on-line forums to seek help through support groups. They questioned why professional treatment protocols for some illnesses include mutual support, whereas others do not. These researchers found that second to alcoholics, cancer patients exhibit the highest tendency to seek and offer support in groups. On the basis of their findings, they concluded that having an illness that is embarrassing, socially stigmatizing, or disfiguring leads people to seek the support of others with similar conditions; people with illnesses such as heart disease do not seek group support to the same extent.

Social ecology theory presents another conceptual framework for understanding mutual help and support groups (Humphreys & Woods, 1994; Luke et al., 1994; Maton, 1994; Moos, Finney & Maude-Griffin, 1993). Maton (1994) writes, "central to the social ecological paradigm is the assumption that social phenomena occur within and are shaped by a complex, interrelated network of factors that span multiple variable domains and levels of analysis" (p. 137). These variables include, but are not limited to, the importance of niche, group fit, group ideology, individual member characteristics, personal beliefs, existing support systems, social climate of the group, variations due to local conditions, and attitudes of professionals in the local area. For example, the concept of person–environment fit has been used in understanding who stays and who drops out of groups (Humphreys & Woods, 1994; Luke et al., 1994). Belief-system compatibility between the member and the group is another factor in person–environment fit (Kennedy & Humphreys, 1995; Mankowski, Humphreys, & Moos, 2001).

The concept of psychological empowerment has been used to explain mutual help processes (Zimmerman, 1995). Psychological empowerment refers to empowerment at the individual level of analysis, but organizational and community level empowerment build on the psychological level. Applied in the context of a mutual-help group, this theory directs one to examine whether individual problem solving and coping skill development lead to taking on leadership roles and getting involved in community activities. Maton and Salem (1995) have utilized this approach in an organizational case study of GROW, a mutual-help group for persons with mental illness. These authors found that empowering aspects of the GROW network were provision of a peer-based support system, availability of an opportunity role structure (that allows many individuals to take on meaningful roles), and inculcation of a belief system that inspires members to strive for mental health.

Interest in and scientific study of small groups have flourished over the past half century. Small community groups, such as self-help and support groups, offer a rich field for expanded research and theory. These groups have increased in number and developed into many varieties. The next section examines and attempts to categorize the various types of self-help and support groups.

ILLUSTRATIVE EXAMPLES OF SELF-HELP AND SUPPORT GROUPS

Support and self-help groups differ on so many dimensions that they almost defy categorization. Such groups can be international, national, or local in scope. They can be totally dependent on a professional agency or institution, part of a national foundation, or independent of other systems. They may have highly codified ideologies or be strictly focused on emotional support and information without teaching specific methods of coping or changing behavior. They may have no change orientation, may be interested only in behavioral change in members, or may be interested primarily in social change. Schubert and Borkman (1991) used organizational autonomy to come up with a self-help classification system. Their analysis found unaffiliated groups, groups that were federated into a loose national association without a central authority (such as 12-step fellowships), groups that were affiliated with a national central authority, managed groups (run by professionals hired by the national association or foundation), and hybrid groups that maintain a relationship with a professional and also have elements of being self-run.

In the past, I have categorized groups according to two factors: personal change orientation and dependence on professionals (Kurtz, 1997). Personal change orientation refers to the degree to which the organization is interested in changing its members' behavior or mood state. Such change is the primary purpose of some groups. Other groups are solely interested in changing social policy or advocating for individual cases. Support groups are typically not change oriented except in acquiring support and knowledge.

Using a classification system that pegs groups as professionally led or not and as change oriented or not, I have identified five different types of groups:

1. Type A: Groups that are change oriented and nonprofessionally led, such as AA.
2. Type B: Peer-led social change self-help groups that are primarily support, education, and advocacy groups, such as the National Alliance for the Mentally Ill.
3. Type C: Non-change-oriented, peer-led support groups that are part of national organizations, such as the Alzheimer's Foundation.
4. Type D: Smaller, local, professionally-led support groups that are held in social agencies.
5. Type E: Change-oriented groups that have peer leadership combined with professional involvement, either as an independent sponsor (such as Parents Anonymous) or as an agency-based co-leader.

Type A: 12-Step Fellowships—Life Changing, Peer-Led Self-Help Groups

12-step fellowships are the quintessential self-help groups. Although they rely on professionals for referrals and good will, 12-step traditions reject professional intrusions in meetings and in fellowship-related services to the membership. They also reject formal alliances with other organizations. The mission of all 12-step fellowships is to help the individual who still suffers from the condition served by the fellowship, whether it is drugs, compulsive sex, or gambling. Relationships with professionals are cordial, and fellowships are dependent on professional referrals for new membership. These fellowships maintain an individual change orientation with a well-defined program of steps and traditions that are codified in books, pamphlets, and brochures. The larger fellowships also maintain workbooks, videos, audiotapes, and other materials for groups to disseminate.[3]

Type B: National Alliance for the Mentally Ill—Support/Educational/Advocacy Groups

The National Alliance for the Mentally Ill (NAMI) is dedicated to the eradication of mental illnesses and to the improvement of the quality of life of all whose lives are affected by these diseases" (National Alliance for the Mentally Ill, 2003, para. 1). NAMI is a nonprofit, grassroots, self-help, support and advocacy organization of consumers, families, and friends of people with severe mental illnesses, such as schizophrenia, major depression, bipolar disorder, obsessive–compulsive disorder, and anxiety disorders. Its goals include dissemination of information about mental illness, improved public understanding of the biological bases of mental illness, incorporation of current research in treatment of persons with mental illness, and allocation of increased government resources for research and treatment.

These goals are pursued largely by the national organization, although local affiliates also engage in dissemination of information and advocacy on the local level. NAMI defines "self-help" as the support and education part of its program, separate from its advocacy activities. Three main elements of self-help—emotional support, self-education, and practical advice—remain chiefly the function of local affiliates. Local affiliates typically sponsor educational meetings open to the public and smaller support groups that are often closed meetings for those who have the problem of a relative with mental illness or are themselves diagnosed with a mental illness. NAMI is a self-help group because it is self-led by members and has a complex program with numerous goals, including advocacy for social policy change.[4]

Type C: Alzheimer's Disease and Related Disorders Association—Foundation-Sponsored Support Groups

The Alzheimer's Association, a national network of chapters, is the largest national voluntary health organization committed to finding a cure for Alzheimer's and helping those affected by the disease (Alzheimer's Association, 2003). The Alzheimer's Association's national network of chapters provides programs and services to persons with Alzheimer's disease, their families and caregivers, and health care professionals. Support groups are a part of the association's mission. Local chapters educate victims, their families, professional caregivers, and the general public. The chapters provide a variety of local services, including meetings, newsletters, help lines, and speakers' bureaus. In addition, some chapters provide respite care, day care, and case management. Professionals, mainly social workers and nurses, staff approximately half of the affiliated chapters and either lead or co-lead many of the support groups. These groups differ from Type D groups because they are part of a large, national association with a high degree of volunteer support and activity. They are not self-help groups like Type A groups because they do not seek behavioral changes in members and they do permit professional facilitation. Affiliated chapters meet standards drawn up by the national association.[5]

Type D: Life after Loss—A Small, Local, Professionally Led Support Group

Life after Loss is a support group for adults experiencing grief after the death of a loved one. It is a small support group facilitated by a staff member of a local hospice in a small midwestern city. Members share experiences and participate in activities that allow them to remember their loved ones and help them to move on with their lives. The group meets once a week for 8 consecutive weeks in the offices of the hospice. This small group is typical of local agency-based support groups. It has no national affiliation. The members meet for support and information. Groups of this type may be open or closed to new members and may have a limited number of meetings. They are representative of this category because they are facilitated by a staff member and do not seek behavioral change, although they do assist members to transition to life without the lost loved one.

Type E: Parents Anonymous—A Hybrid Group

Both professionals and parent members (Parents Anonymous, 2001) lead Parents Anonymous (PA) groups. Despite its name, it is not a 12-step fellowship. PA's mission is (1) to help parents learn how to discipline and care for their children without being abusive and (2) to help those who were abused as children. In addition, PA seeks to establish programs that prevent child abuse through public education. Both peer leaders and professional facilitators are PA-trained volunteers. During meetings, parents receive education, as well as emotional support, and learn skills for better parenting. PA fits the category of "hybrid group" because leadership is shared with a professional. It is not a support group because it does seek behavioral change in members and because it is national, with affiliated chapters throughout the United States.[6]

FUTURE DIRECTIONS FOR SELF-HELP
AND SUPPORT GROUP PRACTICE

U.S. society over the next decade faces numerous critical concerns for social and human services. Current societal trends and conditions, such as the lack of national health insurance coupled with the high cost of health care, will influence the development and continuance of self-help and support groups in the near future. Several factors suggest that such groups will increase. These include: the influence of managed care that limits available professional services, thus creating a larger need for self-help and support group alternatives; groups on the Internet and other forms of technology that make participation more feasible; and increased recognition that self-help groups save health care costs. Other factors, however, endanger the numbers and growth of self-help and support groups. These include reductions in funds for state self-help clearinghouses and fewer professional services that provide linkages to available self-help and support groups.

Managed care organizations should promote increased use of self-help and support groups over time in order to save on costs while providing needed follow-up services. However, a recent survey of managed care directors and providers indicates that self-help groups were the least used among a variety of types of group (problem focused, psychoeducational, process oriented, short-term, and self-help; Taylor et al., 2001). Managed care directors were more familiar with and positive about self-help groups than providers were; however, it is not clear whether these directors will influence greater use of such groups. Mental health practitioners lacked training in the use of self-help groups and were pessimistic about their potential effectiveness. The authors noted, nevertheless, that group modalities, used as a supplement to other treatments, will likely increase over time. In order for this to happen, however, practitioners must learn more about self-help groups. They need training and education. In addition, research on effectiveness needs to continue and to be disseminated to practitioners.

Groups on the Internet seem destined to increase as more people equip themselves with computers, Internet browsers, and e-mail addresses (Gary & Remolino, 2000). It is difficult to control the quality of Internet resources; therefore, practitioners will need to offer support and assist clients who wish to supplement professional service with on-line support. As the computer-literate population ages, health information and experiential knowledge from others with similar conditions will be in demand, and on-line websites and support groups will meet much of this need. Cain and Mittman (1999) predicted that on-line support groups for patients with specific diseases and the people who care for them will develop rapidly. They stated that patients participating in the groups will feel more in control and have better outcomes, but "there will be points of strain . . . between patients and some physicians who feel a loss of control over their patients' care" (Cain & Mittman, 1999, para. 17).

A combination of population increases in older age brackets and reductions in funding for medical services will mean that there are more people with chronic and acute illnesses who need the information and support provided by self-help and support groups. At least one study has shown that such groups are more efficient because they reduce the use of professional services and the costs associated with those services without sacrificing positive outcomes (Humphreys & Moos, 2001). More research is needed on cost effectiveness of self-help and support groups. At this point, government support for enlarging the critical mass of self-help and support group resources has decreased. This is demonstrated in decreasing funds for state self-help clearinghouses in the United States (Ed Madara, personal communication, July 11, 2002). These clearinghouses, when funded, refer potential members to groups, facilitate development of groups, and foster interdisciplinary working relationships among professionals and members of self-help groups (Meissen & Warren, 1994). If groups like this are truly a cost-effective means of distributing needed health care information, public policy in support of them should increase.

Earlier in this chapter, I discussed the linking roles played by professionals with self-help and support groups. Professional treatment services are at the front line in treating physical and mental health disorders; when those services are reduced, efforts to stabilize clients following formal treatment are limited or omitted, thus reducing professional referrals to self-help and support groups. Evidence of this can be found in the reduction in the number of people in existing AA groups over the past decade as the number of treatment centers has decreased (AA World Services, 1998; AA World Services, 2002). AA reported 73,352 fewer members in 2002 than they reported in 1998. This trend could be due to reductions in substance abuse services over the past decade as funds for treatment have decreased (White, 1998). This trend, along with the demise of clearinghouses, could severely reduce the availability of groups in the community.

CONCLUSION

This chapter began with a commentary on the significance and growth of the self-help/support group movement over the past 20 to 30 years. It ends by suggesting that the self-help phenomenon, while more needed than ever, is experiencing decreasing support because of government policy intent on reducing professional and human services. Although the nature of professional roles differs in self-help and support groups, professional relationships with both self-help and support groups are critical to their existence and well-being. Face-to-face groups may decrease in number and importance as the fast pace of society impels people toward the instantaneous gratification of the Internet rather than the more leisurely companionship found in church basements. Professional roles with Internet-based groups will need to evolve.

Research on effectiveness, as well as theoretical investigations, of group processes and outcomes in these kinds of groups needs to continue. Dissemination of these findings will be important in determining the extent of public support for them. Practitioners and policy makers must gain more understanding and awareness of the power of such group resources and of their potential to offer solutions to our rapidly aging population. A working knowledge of self-help and support groups will thus become more and more necessary and useful for practitioners and professionals of all types.

NOTES

1. The term "self-help" is used interchangeably with "mutual help."
2. Wuthnow used the self-help group definition by Madara and Meese (1990): "groups that provide mutual support . . . are composed of peers who share common experiences or situations, are run by and for their members, and operate on a voluntary, nonprofit basis" (Wuthnow, 1994, p. 71).

3. AA's website can be found at: *www.aa.org.*
4. Individual support groups and chapters can be found on the NAMI website: *www.nami.org.*
5. For information, contact the website at: *www.alz.org.*
6. Information on Parents Anonymous can be found on their web site: *www.parentsanonymous.org.*

REFERENCES

Alcoholics Anonymous World Services. (1998). Estimates of groups and members as of January 1, 1998. *Box 459, 44*(3), 3.

Alcoholics Anonymous World Services. (2002, June/July). Estimates of groups and members as of January 1, 2002. *Box 459, 48*(3), 3.

Alcoholics Anonymous World Services. (2003). *Alcoholics Anonymous 2001 membership survey.* Retrieved March 5, 2003, from: *http://www.aa.org.*

Alzheimer's Association. (2003). *About us.* Retrieved March 7, 2003, from: *http://www.alz.org/aboutus/respite.htm.*

Antze, P. A. (1979). The role of ideologies in peer psychotherapy groups. In M. A. Lieberman & L. Borman (Eds.), *Self-help groups for coping with crisis* (pp. 272–304). San Francisco: Jossey-Bass.

Azaiza, F., & Ben-Ari, A. T. (1998). The self-help concept among Arab professionals in Israel. *International Social Work, 41*(4), 417–430.

Borkman, T. J. (1999). *Understanding self-help/mutual aid: Experiential learning in the commons.* New Brunswick, NJ: Rutgers University Press.

Caetano, R. (1993). Ethnic minority groups and Alcoholics Anonymous: A review. In B. S. McCrady & W. R. Miller, *Research on Alcoholics Anonymous: Opportunities and alternatives* (pp. 209–232). New Brunswick, NJ: Rutgers Center of Alcohol Studies.

Cain, M., & Mittman, R. (1999). The future of the Internet in health care: A five-year forecast. Retrieved July 9, 2002, from: *http://www.informatics-review.com/thoughts/future.html.*

Caplan, G., & Killilea, M. (Eds.). (1976). *Support systems and mutual help: Multidisciplinary explorations.* New York: Grune & Stratton.

Chesler, M. A., & Chesney, B. K. (1995). *Cancer and self-help: Bridging the troubled waters of childhood illness.* Madison, WI: University of Wisconsin Press.

Cheung, S., & Sun, S. Y. K. (2001). Helping processes in a mutual aid organization for persons with emotional disturbance. *International Journal of Group Psychotherapy, 51*(3), 295–308.

Citron, M., Solomon, P., & Draine, J. (1999). Self-help groups for families of persons with mental illness: Perceived benefits of helpfulness. *Community Mental Health Journal, 35*(1), 15–30.

Cocaine Anonymous World Services. (2001). Cocaine Anonymous membership survey. Retrieved March 6, 2003, from: *http://www.CA.org/.*

Cook, J. A., Heller, T., & Pickett-Schenk, S. A. (1999). The effect of support group participation on caregiver burden among parents of adult offspring with severe mental illness. *Family Relations, 48*(4), 405–410.

Davison, K. P., Pennebaker, J. W., & Dickerson, S. S. (2000). Who talks? The social psychology of illness support groups. *American Psychologist, 55*(2), 205–217.

Emerick, R. E. (1995). Clients as claims makers in the self-help movement: Individual and social change ideologies in former mental patient self-help newsletters. *Psychosocial Rehabilitation Journal, 18*(3), 17–35.

Finn, J. (1999). An exploration of helping processes in an online self-help group focusing on issues of disability. *Health and Social Work, 24*(3), 220–231.

Galinsky, M. J., & Schopler, J. H. (1994). Negative experiences in support groups. *Social Work with Groups, 20*(1), 77–95.

Galinsky, M. J., Schopler, J. H., & Abell, M. D. (1997). Connecting group members through telephone and computer groups. *Health and Social Work, 22*(3), 181–188.

Gary, J. M., & Remolino, L. (2000). *Online support groups: Nuts and bolts, benefits, limitations and future directions.* Retrieved July 9, 2002, from: *http://ericcass.uncg.edu/digest/200007.html.*

Grohol, J. (2004). *The insider's guide to mental health resources online* (2004/2005 ed.). New York: Guilford Press.

Heller, T., Roccoforte, J. A., & Cook, J. A. (1997). Predictors of support group participation among families of persons with mental illness. *Family Relations, 46*(4), 437–442.

Humphreys, K. (1996). Worldview change in Adult Children of Alcoholics/Al-Anon self-help groups: Reconstructing the alcoholic family. *International Journal of Group Psychotherapy, 46*(2), 255–263.

Humphreys, K., & Moos, R. (2001). Can encouraging substance abuse patients to participate in self-help group reduce demand for health care? A quasi-experimental study. *Alcoholism: Clinical and Experimental Research, 25*, 711–716.

Humphreys, K., & Woods, M. D. (1994). Researching mutual-help group participation in a segregated society. In T. J. Powell (Ed.), *Understanding the self-help organization: Frameworks and findings* (pp. 62–87). Thousand Oaks, CA: Sage.

Jacobs, M. K., & Goodman, G. (1989). Psychology and self-help groups: Predictions on a partnership. *American Psychologist, 44*(3), 536–544.

Jenson, G. H. (2000). *Storytelling in Alcoholics Anonymous: A rhetorical analysis*. Carbondale, IL: Southern Illinois University Press.

Kaslyn, M. (1999). Telephone group work: Challenges for practice. *Social Work with Groups, 22*(1), 63–77.

Kennedy, M., & Humphreys, K. (1995). Understanding worldview transformation in members of mutual help groups. In F. Lavoie, T. Borkman, & G. Gidron (Eds.), *Self-help and mutual aid groups: International and multicultural perspectives* (pp. 181–198). New York: Haworth Press.

Kessler, R., Mickelson, K. D., & Zhao, S. (1997). Patterns and correlates of self-help group membership in the United States. *Social Policy, 26*(3), 27–46.

Killilea, M. (1982). Interaction of crisis theory, coping strategies, and social support systems. In H. C. Schulberg & M. Killilea (Eds.), *The modern practice of community mental health* (pp. 163–214). San Francisco: Jossey-Bass.

King, G., Stewart, D., King, S., & Law, M. (2000). Organizational characteristics and issues affecting the longevity of self-help groups for parents of children with special needs. *Qualitative Health Research, 10*(2), 225–241.

Kurtz, E. (1979). *Not-God: A history of Alcoholics Anonymous*. Center City, MN: Hazelden.

Kurtz, L. F. (1997). *Self-help and support groups: A handbook for practitioners*. Thousand Oaks, CA: Sage.

Kurtz, L. F. (2001). Peer support: Key to maintaining recovery. In R. H. Coombs (Ed.), *Addiction recovery tools: A practical handbook* (pp. 257–272). Thousand Oaks, CA: Sage.

Kurtz, L. F., & Powell, T. J. (1987). Three approaches to understanding self-help groups. *Social Work with Groups, 10*(3), 69–80.

Kyrouz, E. M., Humphreys, K., & Loomis, C. (2002). A review of research on the effectiveness of self-help mutual aid groups. In B. J. White & E. J. Madara (Eds.), *The self-help sourcebook* (7th ed., pp. 71–85). Denville, NJ: St. Clare's Health Services.

Lee, D. T (1995). Professional underutilization of Recovery, Inc. *Psychiatric Rehabilitation Journal, 19*(1), 63–70.

Levy, L. (1979). Processes and activities in groups. In M. A. Lieberman & L. D. Borman (Eds.), *Self-help groups for coping with crisis: Origins, members, processes and impact* (pp. 234–271). San Francisco: Jossey-Bass.

Lieberman, M. A. (1979). Analyzing change mechanisms in groups. In M. A. Lieberman & L. D. Borman (Eds.), *Self-help groups for coping with crisis: Origins, members, processes and impact* (pp. 194–233). San Francisco: Jossey-Bass.

Lieberman, M. A., & Borman, L. D. (Eds.). (1979). *Self-help groups for coping with crisis: Origins, members, processes and impact*. San Francisco: Jossey-Bass.

Lieberman, M. A., & Snowden, L. R. (1994). Problems in assessing prevalence and membership characteristics of self-help groups. In T. J. Powell (Ed.), *Understanding the self-help organization: Frameworks and findings* (pp. 32–49). Thousand Oaks, CA: Sage.

Low, A. A. (1950). *Mental health through will-training*. Winnetka, IL: Willett.

Luke, D. A, Roberts, L., & Rappaport, J. (1994). Individual, group context, and individual–group fit predictors of self-help attendance. In T. J. Powell (Ed.), *Understanding the self-help organization: Frameworks and findings* (pp. 88–114). Thousand Oaks, CA: Sage.

Madara, E. (1999–2000a). From church basements to World Wide Web sites: The growth of self-help support groups on line. *International Journal of Self-Help and Self Care, 1*(1), 37–48.

Madara, E. (1999–2000b). How to start a new online computer mutual help group. *International Journal of Self-Help and Self Care, 1*(2), 181–188.

Madara, E. J., & Meese, A. (Eds.). (1990). *The self-help sourcebook: Finding and forming mutual aid self-help groups* (3rd ed.). Denville, NJ: St. Clare's Health Services.

Mäkelä, K. (1996). *Alcoholics Anonymous as a mutual-help movement: A study in eight societies.* Madison, WI: University of Wisconsin Press.

Mankowski, E. S., Humphreys, K., & Moos, R. H. (2001). Individual and contextual predictors of involvement in Twelve-Step self-help groups after substance abuse treatment. *American Journal of Community Psychology, 29*(4), 537–563.

Maton, K. I. (1994). Moving beyond the individual level of analysis in mutual-help group research: An ecological paradigm. In T. J. Powell (Ed.), *Understanding the self-help organization: Frameworks and findings* (pp. 136–153). Thousand Oaks, CA: Sage.

Maton, K. I., & Salem, D. A. (1995). Organizational characteristics of empowering community settings: A multiple case study approach. *American Journal of Community Psychology, 23*(5), 631–656.

Medvene, L. J., Volk, F. A., & Meissen, G. J. (1997). Communal orientation and burnout among self-help group leaders. *Journal of Applied Social Psychology, 27*(3), 262–278.

Meissen, G. J., & Warren, M. J. (1994). The self-help clearinghouse: A new development in action research for community psychology. In T. J. Powell (Ed.), *Understanding the self help organization: Frameworks and findings* (pp. 190–210). Thousand Oaks, CA: Sage.

Mok, B. H. (2001). The effectiveness of self-help groups in a Chinese context. *Social Work with Groups, 24*(2), 69–90.

Moos, R. H., Finney, J., & Maude-Griffin, P. (1993). The social climate of self-help and mutual support groups: Assessing group implementation, process, and outcome. In B. S. McCrady & W. R. Miller (Eds.), *Research on Alcoholics Anonymous: Opportunities and alternatives* (pp. 251–274). New Brunswick, NJ: Rutgers Center of Alcohol Studies.

Narcotics Anonymous World Services. (2002). *Facts about Narcotics Anonymous.* Retrieved March 5, 2003, from: *http://www.na.org.*

National Alliance for the Mentally Ill. (2003). *NAMI mission and history.* Retrieved March 7, 2003, from: *http://www.nami.org.*

Parents Anonymous. (2001). *About Parents Anonymous, Inc.* Retrieved March 7, 2003, from: *http://www.parentsanonymous.org/ABOUT.HTM.*

Pew Internet and American Life Project. (2002a). *Daily Internet activities.* Retrieved March 7, 2003, from: *http://www.pewinternet.org/reports/chart.asp?img=Daily_A8.htm.*

Pew Internet and American Life Project. (2002b). *Our mission.* Retrieved March 7, 2003, from: *http://www.pewinternet.org/about/about.asp?page=4.*

Pew Internet and American Life Project. (2002c). Daily and overall Internet activities. Retrieved March 7, 2003, from: *http://www.pewinternet.org/reports/chart.asp?img=Internet_A8.htm.*

Powell, T. J. (1987). *Self-help organizations and professional practice.* Silver Spring, MD: National Association of Social Workers.

Powell, T. J., Hill, E. M., Warner, L., Yeaton, W., & Silk, K. R. (2000). Encouraging people with mood disorders to attend a self-help group. *Journal of Applied Social Psychology, 30,* 2270–2288.

Riessman, F. (1965). The helper therapy principle. *Social Work, 10*(2), 27–32.

Riessman, F., & Carroll, D. (1995). *Redefining self-help: Policy and practice.* San Francisco: Jossey-Bass.

Salem, D. A., Bogat, G. A., & Reid, C. (1997). Mutual help goes on-line. *Journal of Community Psychology, 25*(2), 189–207.

Schiff, M., & Bargal, D. (2000). Helping characteristics of self-help and support groups: Their contribution to participants' subjective well-being. *Small Group Research, 31*(3), 275–304.

Schopler, J. H., Abell, M. D., & Galinsky, M. (1998). Technology-based groups: A review and conceptual framework for practice. *Social Work, 43*(3), 254–268.

Schubert, M. A., & Borkman, T. J. (1991). An organizational typology for self-help groups. *American Journal of Community Psychology, 19*(5), 769–787.

Shepherd, M. D., Schoenberg, M., Slavich, S., Wituk, S., Warren, M., & Meissen, G. (1999). Continuum of professional involvement in self-help groups. *Journal of Community Psychology, 27*(1), 39–53.

Silverman, P. (2002). Understanding self-help groups. In B. J. White & E. J. Madara (Eds.), *The self-help group sourcebook: Your guide to community and online support groups* (7th ed., pp. 25–28). Denville, NJ: St. Clare's Health Services.

Snowden, L. R., & Lieberman, M. A. (1994). African American participation in self-help groups. In T. J. Powell (Ed.), *Understanding the self-help organization: Frameworks and findings* (pp. 50–61). Newbury Park, CA: Sage.

Taylor, N. T., Burlingame, G. M., Kristensen, K. B., Fuhriman, A., Johansen, J., & Dahl, D. (2001). A survey of mental health care providers' and managed care organization attitudes toward, familiarity with, and use of group interventions. *International Journal of Group Psychotherapy, 51*(2), 243–263.

Videka-Sherman, L., & Lieberman, M. A. (1985). The effects of self-help and psychotherapy intervention and child loss: The limits of recovery. *American Journal of Psychotherapy, 55*(1), 70–82.

White, W. L. (1998). *Slaying the dragon: A history of addiction treatment and recovery.* Bloomington, IL: Chestnut Health Systems.

White, B. J., & Madara, E. (Eds.). (2002). *The self-help group sourcebook: Your guide to community and online support groups* (7th ed.). Denville, NJ: St. Clare's Health Services.

Wituk, S. A., Shepherd, M. D., Slavich, S., Warren, M. L., & Meissen, G. (2000). A topography of self-help groups: An empirical analysis. *Social Work, 45*(2), 157–165.

Wituk, S. A., Shepherd, M. D., Warren, M., & Meissen, G. (2002). Factors contributing to the survival of self-help groups. *American Journal of Community Psychology, 30*(3), 349–366.

Wuthnow, R. (1994). *Sharing the journey: Support groups and America's new quest for community.* New York: Free Press.

Zimmerman, M. A. (1995). Psychological empowerment: Issues and illustrations. *American Journal of Community Psychology, 23*(5), 581–599.

Chapter 9

Psychoeducational Groups

ROGER ROFFMAN

With both a broad array of possible contextual applications and a wide scope of potential participants, psychoeducational groups have a number of benchmark characteristics: issue specificity, goal directedness, a structured protocol that emphasizes learning, a high level of leader direction, an emphasis on skill acquisition, and a time-limited duration. In contrast to groups of a therapeutic nature that rely on the interactions of the group to guide members toward a "corrective emotional experience" (Yalom, 1995), psychoeducational groups are intended to enhance participant knowledge and behavior change through an emphasis on educational strategies akin to those used in a classroom. Just a few examples of the many applications for psychoeducational groups include:

- Loneliness in university students (McWhirter, 1995)
- Marijuana dependence in adults (Stephens, Roffman, & Simpson, 1994)
- Marital enhancement (Durana, 1996)
- Adjustment to divorce (Zimpfer, 1990)
- HIV prevention (Roffman, Beadnell, Ryan, & Downey, 1995)
- Perpetrators of domestic violence (Palmer, Brown, & Barrera, 1992)
- Adults with bipolar disorder (Bauer & McBride, 1996)
- Coping with AIDS (Heckman et al., 1999)
- Foster parents of children who have been sexually abused (Barth, Yeaton, & Winterfelt, 1994)
- Children whose parents have cancer (Taylor-Brown, Acheson, & Farber, 1993)
- Training opinion leaders (e.g., gay men in rural locales, women and adolescents in urban public housing developments) to widely disseminate HIV risk-reduction norms in a community (Kelly et al., 1997; Sikkema et al., 2002; Sikkema et al., 2000)

As the preceding list suggests, the targets of change may include the individual (e.g., the person living with AIDS), those in the individual's social network (e.g., caregivers of persons living with AIDS), and members of a larger community (e.g., gay men living in rural locales). The central theme and focus may include such issues as responding to developmental tasks and transitions across the lifespan (e.g., learning to study, effective parenting, preparing for midcareer vocational change, transitioning to retirement), prevention (e.g., stress reduction, avoiding HIV and other sexually transmitted diseases by adopting safer sex behaviors, coping with alcohol/drug relapse vulnerabilities) and dealing with illness or disability (e.g., living with cancer, managing psychiatric disorders). Psychoeducational groups may stand alone as the participant's single source of support or may serve as adjuncts to other, concurrent counseling modalities.

This chapter examines the purposes typically served by psychoeducational group work, the elements commonly found in the protocols for such groups, and the theoretical frameworks on which they are generally based. A heuristic model of a stage-sensitive typology of psychoeducational groups is presented, with examples selected to illustrate both their commonalities and unique features. Finally, the chapter concludes with speculation concerning the future for this type of group work.

THE PURPOSES OF PSYCHOEDUCATIONAL GROUP WORK

With varying emphases depending on the need, the purposes of psychoeducational groups focus on education, skill acquisition, and/or self-knowledge (Brown, 1998). When the priority is education, the protocol is predominantly composed of lecture and discussion, with the leader functioning primarily as a teacher. When skill acquisition is emphasized, the leader functions primarily as a trainer, and the protocol includes experiential learning involving mastery development through modeling, role playing, and feedback. Finally, groups that give priority to self-knowledge will likely have a closer resemblance to counseling, although the process remains predominantly educational and largely avoids encouraging participants to extensively self-disclose, work through resistance, and explore past relationships (Niemann, 2002). Although the specific function of a group may highlight one of these three purposes more than the others, it is common for such groups to be designed to meet all three (Brown, 1991).

Niemann (2002) underscores several qualities of psychoeducational groups that enhance their suitability and efficacy consistent with a wellness model of counseling:

1. *The client is empowered through preparation for informed decision making.* A key element in this model is supporting participants to better understand options open to them, to be prepared to make informed decisions among those options, and to become skillful in following through with their choices. Although participants may be grappling with disabling conditions, illnesses, and/or highly challenging barriers to change, the presumption underlying psychoeducational groups is that participants will benefit outside of the group from a within-group emphasis on enhancement of decision-making resources and capabilities. Garvin (1997) states that these groups support role attainment. He notes that the knowledge and skills taught enhance participants' learning of roles they currently occupy or aspire to fulfill (Garvin, 1997). Examples are study-skills groups for university students and groups that focus on infant care for soon-to-be parents.

2. *Group cohesion and focus are facilitated due to participants' shared concerns.* Be-

cause participants will select a group based on their needs vis-à-vis the group's goals, cohesion is likely to more quickly evolve with a shared sense of purpose. This homogeneity in participants' concerns also can be expected to reinforce and maintain group focus.

3. *Dissonance with incompatible cultural values is avoided.* Therapy, with its traditional emphasis on exploring personal issues, disclosing sensitive information, sharing difficult feelings, and interacting on a very personal level with other group members, is not perceived as an attractive and acceptable resource by many individuals, some of whose cultures would greatly discourage participation. The educational emphasis in psychoeducational groups, the implied "normalization" of the group's purpose for its members, the leader's authority made credible though his or her functioning as a teacher, and the existence of a clearly defined agenda that respects privacy makes this modality more culturally compatible and appropriate for many individuals.

4. *Cost efficiency is enhanced.* The nature of the psychoeducational group's purposes permits cost savings by having a larger number of participants, fewer constraints that limit the heterogeneity of the members, and a briefer overall timetable for group completion than is the case with groups that emphasize psychotherapeutic process.

INTERVENTIONS OF PSYCHOEDUCATIONAL GROUP WORK

Each psychoeducational group's specific themes, as well as its relative weighting of content directed toward possible purposes (education, skills training, or self-knowledge), will largely be determined based on the population being served and the group's overall intended function. Nonetheless, a general set of guidelines for designing interventions in psychoeducational groups has been offered by Furr (2000), who articulates a two-phased planning process: conceptual (stating the group's purpose, identifying goals, specifying objectives) and operational (selecting content, designing exercises, evaluation).

Conceptual Planning

Furr (2000) notes that the conceptualization of a group's purpose evolves from answering several questions:

1. What is the primary content focus of the group?
2. What population would benefit from participating in this group?
3. What is the purpose of intervention (e.g., remediation, prevention, or development)?
4. What is the expected outcome of participating in the group (e.g., change in cognitions, affect, behavior, or values)?

Central to Furr's model is the importance of determining for each psychoeducational group the theoretical perspective or perspectives from which pertinent goals and objectives for the group will be derived. These theoretical perspectives address the mechanisms that presumably explain change in awareness, knowledge, insight, or behavior. She offers the example of a self-esteem psychoeducational group for college students based on a cognitive-behavioral theoretical perspective. A goal derived from that perspective, learning to reduce negative self-talk, is met through objectives such as learning to identify different types of self-talk, recognizing when one is engaging in negative self-talk, understanding the impact of negative self-talk on affect, and becoming skillful in replacing negative statements with positive statements.

Operational Planning

The content of psycheducational groups generally incorporates a combination of didactic, experiential, and process components. Didactic content is likely to be more effective if it involves a learning process in which later segments, focusing on more complex material, build on earlier learning of basic concepts, on an opportunity for interaction among group members, and on a careful timing of segments that best fits members' optimal learning styles.

Experiential content facilitates the learner's application of concepts to real-life situations. When discussing didactic and experiential content, Furr (2000) calls for a continued linkage of group planning to underlying theoretical perspective(s) and offers contrasting examples of how experiential components concerning time management might differ depending on theoretical underpinnings. From a behavioral viewpoint, enhancing the individual's management of time might involve the identification and rehearsal of reinforcing antecedent behaviors. From a Gestalt perspective, the experiential activities might involve an exploration of distractions arising from unfinished business that obstruct attention to and engagement in the present.

It is important that group exercises are derived from theory and appropriate in terms of the age and experience level of group members. Activities ought to be included that prompt participant self-assessment. They can thus facilitate awareness of one's initial proficiency, as well as one's eventual progress toward change. Psychoeducational groups often incorporate exercises involving role play, imagery, and cognitive restructuring. Commonly, homework assignments are made in order to stimulate greater self-awareness, as well as the practicing of new skills.

Processing, the third of Furr's (2000) content emphases, has the goal of helping participants synthesize the experiential and didactic components. The leader's attentiveness to the choice and timing of prompts to facilitate processing is of considerable importance to its effectiveness. Midgroup process evaluation focuses on identifying possible needs for adjustments in the group's operation. In contrast, outcome evaluation contributes to the evolving knowledge base in the field by determining the extent to which a specified intervention is efficacious with a specific population and for a specific purpose.

THEORETICAL BASE

As a prelude to a discussion of the theoretical foundations of psychoeducational group work, it is important to acknowledge several important dimensions that vary across groups:

- *Target of change.* As noted at the beginning of this chapter, the participants in psychoeducational groups may be there for their own benefit, for the benefit of others who are close to them, or to ultimately change a larger community of which they are members.
- *Readiness for change.* Although some groups focus on supporting members, all of whom are presumed to be committed to making changes (e.g., recently divorced adults who seek a successful transition to single status), other groups serve individuals who are grappling with ambivalence or indecision about a key life decision (e.g., partners or spouses who are questioning whether to remain in a relationship with an abusive person).
- *Stage in the group's development.* The predominant work of a psychoeducational

group varies from its beginnings through the middle phase of work and ultimately to the phase in which focus is given to preparation for termination.

Foundation theoretical perspectives that inform psychoeducational groups include the paradigm of stages of readiness for change, principles of behavioral and cognitive practice, humanism, and principles pertaining to the diffusion of innovation. Each of these foundation perspectives is briefly discussed in the following section. The answer to the question "What facilitates change?" is discussed for each perspective.

Stage of Change: Change Is Facilitated When Interventions Are Matched to the Individual's Stage of Readiness

The stages of change model (Prochaska & DiClemente, 1984), initially developed to describe the process of smoking cessation, offers useful concepts in thinking about the behavior change process. The model has been most commonly utilized in developing interventions for addictive and compulsive disorders, yet it may offer considerable heuristic value in the design of psychoeducational groups for other purposes.

This model identifies a sequence of stages through which individuals may progress as they think about and initiate new behaviors. Part of its value is in offering ideas about how the client might be thinking, thus enabling the social worker to select strategies that are specific to the individual stage the client is in at any point in time.

This model begins with the assumption that the adoption and maintenance of behavioral change depends on the individual's readiness for each of these changes and that this readiness may shift and evolve. The model sensitizes us to the likelihood that individuals typically move back and forth between the stages and progress through change at different rates. Today, the client may be firmly committed to a specific course of action (e.g., taking steps to enhance marital satisfaction), but next week he or she may be very ambivalent about this goal. Over time, the client may progress through the following stages of readiness and experience the attitudes shown for each stage:

- *Precontemplation*
  - Not considering change.
  - May be unwilling to change behaviors.
  - Is not personally aware of a need for change, although others may believe that change is desirable.

- *Contemplation*
  - Perceives that there may be cause for concern and reasons to change behavior.
  - Is typically ambivalent about change.
  - May seek information and reevaluate current behavior.
  - Weighs the pros and cons of making a change.
  - Could remain in this stage for years.

- *Preparation*
  - Forms a commitment to making a change.
  - Sees the advantages of change as outweighing the benefits of not changing.
  - Thinks about his or her capability to be successful (i.e., self-efficacy).

- Continues the pre-behavior-change pattern, but with the intention of initiating change very soon.
- May have already attempted to change on his or her own.
- Begins to set goals and may tell others about his or her intentions.

- *Action*
  - Has chosen a goal for change and has begun to pursue it.
  - Is actively modifying behavior.
  - Can last a number of months following the initiation of change.

- *Maintenance*
  - Is making efforts to sustain the gains achieved during the action phase.
  - Is working to prevent erosion of change.

While working to adopt and maintain behavioral change, the individual may cycle repeatedly through these stages, sometimes regressing to an earlier stage. The social worker therefore needs to periodically assess the client's motivation level in order to select interventions that best fit that stage.

Behavioral Approaches: Change Is Facilitated by Enhancing Behavioral Skills

Although it is common for some practitioners to describe themselves as cognitive-behaviorists, that is, drawing from both cognitive and behavioral perspectives, each is discussed independently here for clarity. Behavioral practice had its origins in the first half of the 20th century and is based on (1) classical conditioning (the hungry dog salivates when shown food and subsequently learns to salivate to a tone after that tone has repeatedly been paired with food); (2) operant conditioning (changing behavior through positive reinforcement and negative reinforcement); and (3) modeling (behavior change following exposure to the behavior being performed by others). Behavioral practice emphasizes neither delving into unconscious process nor achieving insight about the past. Rather, it is assumed that individuals have learned current behaviors and that, through the application of behavioral principles, they can learn new behaviors, including new emotional and attitudinal patterns.

The stages of a behavioral approach commonly include: (1) establishing a strong relationship and clarifying the general goals of treatment; (2) defining the need for change (e.g., collecting baseline data on frequency, duration, and intensity of behaviors) and setting specific and measurable goals; (3) choosing techniques (e.g., modeling communication skills, introducing positive reinforcement such as self-praise when a behavior has been modified, relaxation training, systematic desensitization); (4) collecting data in order to measure progress in achieving desired outcomes; and (5) preparing for termination (e.g., discussing the possible resurgence of the targeted behavior following termination).

Cognitive Approaches: Change Is Facilitated through Identifying and Correcting Illogical Cognitions

Cognitive approaches to practice emerged in the 1960s and focus on the individual's way of viewing the world; in other words, his or her meaning-making system. Counseling based on this perspective seeks to understand this system and to find ways of intervening so as to change the client's cognitions about meaning. The premise is that irrational thinking contributes to negative emotional consequences.

Although others have offered various iterations of cognitive practice principles, Albert Ellis's (Ellis & Harper, 1961) pioneering work illustrates key steps in working with clients: (1) the worker helps the client understand that aspects of his or her thinking are irrational, (2) the manner in which the client maintains this irrational thinking is illuminated, (3) the client learns how to challenge illogical cognitions, (4) the worker educates the client about generalized irrational beliefs that may have been internalized by the client (e.g., the idea that it is a dire necessity for an adult to be loved or approved of by virtually every significant person in the community), and (5) the client practices challenging illogical cognitions.

Humanism: Change Is Facilitated through Important Qualities of the Helping Professional

Similar to the domain of interest in cognitive treatment, a key focus in practice based on humanism is seeking to understand how people construct meaning in their lives. A central tenet of humanism is that people have both free will and an inborn tendency for self-actualization. That is, when in an environment that is conducive to growth, individuals will strive to fulfill their potential. Carl Rogers operationalized the notion of an environment conducive to growth by characterizing important qualities in the effective helping professional: genuineness, empathy, and unconditional positive regard for the client (Rogers, 1951).

Rogers believed that these qualities in the counselor would facilitate the client's exploration and understanding of historical pain that resulted from conditional relationships in his or her life. That understanding was seen as laying the foundation for the client to change behaviors and move from a "false self" to a "real self." Neukrug (1999) described this evolution of growth as including an increased openness to experience, more objective and realistic perceptions, improved psychological adjustment, increased congruence, increase in self-regard, movement from an external to an internal locus of control, more acceptance of others, better problem solving, and a more accurate perception of others.

Diffusion of Innovation: Change Is Facilitated in a Larger Social System When Innovations Are Communicated by Members of That System

Everett Rogers (1995) conceptualized a process referred to as "diffusion," through which innovations (e.g., an idea, practice, or object that is perceived as new) are communicated over time among members of a social system. The rate of adoption, according to Rogers, is influenced by five characteristics of an innovation: (1) relative advantage (the degree to which the innovation is perceived as better than the idea it supersedes); (2) compatability (the degree to which the innovation is perceived as consistent with existing values and needs of the potential adopters); (3) complexity (the perception of the degree of difficulty in understanding and using the innovation); (4) trialability (the degree to which the innovation lends itself to experimental implementation); and (5) observability (the degree to which the results of the innovation are visible to others; Rogers, 2002). Within a social system, changes in the attitudes toward a new idea held by individuals are likely to be facilitated by interpersonal channels, that is, the subjective evaluations of peers who have already adopted the innovation.

In essence, Rogers was writing about change as a function of opinion leaders talking to other people. He offered an example by citing a randomized controlled trial of two strategies for changing physicians' behaviors vis-à-vis decreasing risks associated with cesarean delivery (Lomas et al., 1991). Superior outcomes resulted from the condition in which physicians were encouraged by opinion leaders, as compared with the condition in which physicians' charts were audited and feedback was given.

Rogers identifies five strategies for the diffusion of preventative innovations: (1) stress the innovation's relative advantage, (2) utilize opinion leaders to promote the new ideas, (3) promote peer support for norm change among members of the social system, (4) embed innovative preventative ideas in entertainment messages, and (5) encourage peer communication about the innovation (Rogers, 2002).

EXAMPLES

Thus far, we have made several observations:

1. Psychoeducational groups might be developed for the purpose of serving three potential targets of change (the individual, the individual's network, or the individual's community).
2. The group member might be at various points along a continuum of readiness for change (precontemplation, contemplation, preparation, action, or maintenance).
3. Several theoretical frameworks (the stages of change model, behaviorism, cognitive principles, humanism, and the concept of the diffusion of innovation) offer ways of understanding factors that facilitate change.

Before turning to examples of psychoeducational groups, a heuristic typology based on the dimensions presented thus far may be useful. In Figure 9.1, the three potential *targets of change*, the five potential *stages of readiness for change*, and three *stages of a group's development* (beginning, middle, and ending) make up a 45-cell matrix. Within each cell, effective interventions may be based on varying theoretical foundations (e.g., cognitive, behavioral, humanist, and diffusion of innovation principles) depending on the group's purpose and developmental stage.

At present, there are no published examples of psychoeducational groups to illustrate every cell of the matrix. Therefore, in addition to examples of groups that fit selected parts of the matrix, I present several ideas for possible future studies for the remaining cells. Finally, the concept of stages in a group's process (beginning, middle, and ending) is not extensively discussed.

Target/Stage: The Individual at an Early Stage of Readiness for Change (Cells 1–2)

Brekke (1989) developed and evaluated a psychoeducational group intervention for men who batter women. He noted that members of this population are difficult to reach, enter treatment involuntarily for the most part, take little or no responsibility for the interpersonal violence, minimize its severity, and exhibit distrust of helping professionals. For these reasons, a pretreatment intervention that was termed an "orientation group" was designed to prepare individuals for subsequent treatment that would be 14 weeks long, highly structured, and based on cognitive-behavioral principles.

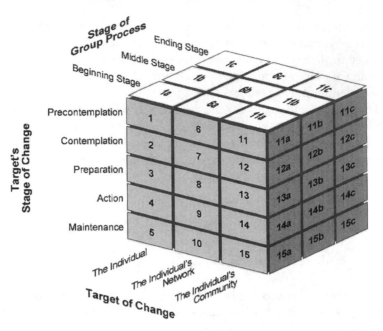

FIGURE 9.1. A stage-sensitive psychoeducational group typology.

The orientation group, meeting for five 2-hour sessions, was intended to serve several purposes:

1. *Preparation for group participation.* Clients were educated about wife abuse, aggression, and anger control and were also introduced to the skills they would be taught in treatment.
2. A *"holding tank" for individuals on the waiting list.* The group offered regular contact with the clinic in order to limit pretreatment dropout while they were waiting for treatment to begin.
3. *Selecting out.* Based on their behavior during the pretreatment group, clients who would have been inappropriate for treatment were identified and selected out.

With reference to the purpose of preparing people for treatment, the group sought to build cohesion among participants, teach the "time out" technique, provide a nonjudgmental setting in which individuals could vent their feelings about the violence and being in the group, begin educating and confronting individuals about rationalizations to justify abusive behavior, and introduce members to the model used in the treatment they were about to enter.

This pretreatment model was evaluated with a single group posttest design. Results from self-report, a measure of member cohesion, and data pertaining to attrition from the 14-week intervention suggested that the orientation group was succeeding in achieving its purposes.

Comment

Brekke's work offers an example of a psychoeducational group intervention for individuals who are already identified as clients and on a waiting list for treatment. Its focus on what

Brekke (1989) terms "attitudinal preparation" highlights the fact that it is tailored for individuals at an early stage of readiness for change.

In the near future, it is likely that more attention will be given to developing and evaluating psychoeducational group interventions for individuals who are not yet committed to change and not already "in the pipeline" awaiting treatment. The concept of a "check-up" intervention (i.e., a brief opportunity for taking stock, with no pressure to commit to change) has been reported with drinkers (Miller, Sovereign, & Krege, 1988), adult marijuana users (Stephens et al., 2000), and gay men engaging in high-risk sexual behaviors (Picciano, Roffman, Kalichman, Rutledge, & Berghuis, 2001). A style of intervening termed "motivational interviewing" is central to this work and borrows substantially from the humanist counseling principles discussed previously.

Although these and other motivational enhancement interventions designed to reach non-treatment-seekers have primarily been delivered in one-to-one formats, researchers are exploring their potential vis-à-vis group delivery (Walters, Ogle, & Martin, 2002). As this work evolves, one key issue will be how such groups are marketed. That is, what messages, images, and themes in the marketing will effectively convey the group as "a chance to take stock" versus "treatment"? A second issue pertains to the ultimate goals this type of group is intended to achieve. Will it be designed to facilitate an engagement in a candid and in-depth self-appraisal for the purpose of resolving ambivalence and making personal decisions about the future? Or will its purpose be to facilitate durable behavior change by all participants? To date, studies of check-up interventions suggest that for some participants, the brief taking-stock experience is sufficient to prompt durable behavior change. For others, participation in a subsequent intervention may be necessary to effect change.

Target/Stage: The Individual at a Later Stage of Readiness for Change (Cells 3–5)

Roffman and his colleagues developed and evaluated a telephone-delivered psychoeducational group intervention that was designed to be delivered over a 14-week period (1½ hours per week) to gay and bisexual males who sought support in reducing their HIV transmission risk (Roffman et al., 1997). Participants made use of a toll-free number to join their groups each week. In order to further reduce barriers to participation, callers were offered the choice of confidential or anonymous enrollment.

A workbook composed of 14 units accompanied these sessions and included text, illustrative case examples of specific concepts or themes, recommended exercises, and work sheets. Following an introduction that provided an overview of treatment, the next three sessions dealt with getting ready to change. The leaders talked about the difference between risk elimination and risk reduction, and the clients were assisted both in rating the relative level of risk associated with specific sexual behaviors and in setting their own personal goals for risk reduction. Accurate information concerning HIV and its transmission and details concerning the proper use of condoms were provided. An exercise concerning motivational ambivalence facilitated the goal-setting process. Clients were asked to maintain an ongoing log of their sexual activities.

In the next four sessions, clients learned to identify the specific kinds of high-risk situations in which they were most likely to slip. Considerable attention was given to coping strategies that may help avert a return to unsafe behavior, with clients being guided through role plays to practice new skills. The rights and prerogatives of each partner in a relationship were discussed, as were commonly held fears and self-defeating beliefs that may lead an individual to forgo being assertive about safety with a sexual partner. Case examples and exercises highlighted the ways in which negative self-talk can be challenged, how conflict with a partner can be understood and addressed, and how imagery can assist the client in successfully getting through a difficult situation. A part of each session was devoted to clients' debriefing of recent experiences, associated triggers, and coping strategies that were or might have been employed.

The following five sessions focused on maintenance. A concept termed the "goal violation effect" was introduced, with clients being encouraged to view a slip as an indication of need for further practice with coping skills rather than as a sign of personal weakness or failure. Group members were aided in evaluating the degree to which their friends offered support for and/or obstruction of safer sexual behavior, and strategies for expanding one's friendships were identified.

Finally, attention was given to the degree to which clients were experiencing a balanced lifestyle, that is, one in which priority is given both to meeting one's obligations and to making room for desired activities. Clients were encouraged to make lifestyle modifications that would achieve greater balance so as to facilitate the maintenance of safer sexual behaviors.

The study findings suggested the following: (1) permitting men to access HIV risk-reduction counseling via the telephone, and to enroll without divulging their identities, appeared to lower barriers to participation among less gay-identified individuals; (2) delivering cognitive-behavioral group counseling by telephone was both feasible and efficacious in reducing high-risk sexual behaviors and promoting condom use; and (3) reductions in risk behaviors, with the exception of condom utilization, appeared to be largely maintained through 12 months of posttreatment follow-up.

Comment

Although some content in this intervention focused on early stage of change issues (that is, resolving ambivalence and considering alternate goals), its primary emphasis was on skill development and behavior change maintenance. Telephone delivery and the option of remaining anonymous may be useful ways in which enhanced access for difficult-to-serve populations can be facilitated in psychoeducational groups (Roffman, Picciano, Wickizer, Bolan, & Ryan, 1998).

Target/Stage: The Individual's Network at an Early Stage of Readiness for Change (Cells 6–7)

As noted in the preceding characterization of the precontemplation stage of readiness for change, the family members, friends, and associates of individuals who are demonstrating behavior with adverse consequences may be more cognizant of the need for change than the individual whose actions have elicited concern. It is common for workers in the field of alcoholism and substance abuse to be approached by network members who seek advice about how to motivate someone to accept treatment. The issue of concern could also be affective disorders, intimate partner violence, compulsive gambling, nonadherence to medical regimens, and many other problem behaviors.

Although psychoeducational group protocols have been developed for social network members who have made the decision to seek support, ambivalent attitudes may hinder participation by the concerned person. As will be seen in the section concerning cells 11 and 12, a "pregroup" opportunity to explore the benefits and costs associated with joining a psychoeducational group may enhance eventual enrollment and engagement. To overcome apprehension about being pressured to commit, however, the design, marketing, and implementation of this psychoeducational intervention would need to be well matched to the needs of the individual in an early stage of readiness.

Target/Stage: The Individual's Network at a Later Stage of Readiness for Change (Cells 8–10)

Fristad, Arnett, and Gavazzi (1998) developed and evaluated a 90-minute psychoeducational workshop for parents of children and adolescents hospitalized for mood disorders. Earlier research with children with mood disorders had demonstrated that high levels of expressed emotion (i.e., a family climate of criticism and emotional overinvolvement) was predictive of poorer posthospitalization outcomes (Asarnow, Goldstein, Thompson, & Guthrie, 1993). Workshop topics included symptoms of major depression, dysthymia, and mania; etiology, course, and prognosis; treatment; and family factors that affect outcome. The intervention was evaluated in a single-group, pretest–posttest design involving reassessments both immediately following the workshop and 4 months later.

The outcomes in this trial reflected improved parental understanding of mood disorders, increased levels of positive expressed emotion, and decreased levels of negative expressed emotion. It appeared that fathers and mothers differed somewhat in the manner in which the psychoeducation group experience enhanced their behaviors.

Comment

There is a substantial literature describing psychoeducational groups for network members. Examples include foster parents of sexually abused children (Barth et al., 1994), families of people with mental illness (Lundwall, 1996), and children whose parents have cancer (Taylor-Brown et al., 1993).

Target/Stage: The Individual's Community at an Early Stage of Readiness for Change (Cells 11–12)

By definition, interventions in these cells of the matrix would be designed for individuals who are not yet committed to but are willing to consider participating in a psychoeducational group to prepare them for working toward change in a social system that is larger than their own social network. As such, these pregroup interventions would likely offer the opportunity to learn about what participation in a subsequent group might involve without pressure to commit, be publicized with a reinforcing message concerning the personal and community benefits to be achieved, emphasize the power of opinion leaders in changing the norms in a social system, and require minimal burden in terms of time and effort.

A hypothetical example would be a church-sponsored event, scheduled at a time that is convenient for potential participants, at which a future group would be described whose purpose would be to train a cadre of church members to work on improving dispute resolution among member families. The group session would highlight the influence of opinion leaders in changing community norms, describe the training to be provided, note the benefits to be sought, emphasize the supports that group members would receive, and present prompts for the purpose of stimulating discussion. Another example would be a school event in which students learn of the opportunity for training as opinion leaders working toward enhancing the school's spirit of inclusiveness.

Comment

As noted in the next section, psychoeducational groups can be developed to train individuals to effect change in a social system. Recognizing that potential participants in such groups might be considerably ambivalent about investing themselves in such an effort, an "orientation group" experience might be offered with the express purpose of facilitating awareness and enhancing decision making.

Target/Stage: The Individual's Community at a Later Stage of Readiness for Change (Cells 13–15)

Kelly and colleagues (1997) developed a psychoeducational group intervention for the purpose of promoting HIV risk reduction among members of a social system. Noting epidemiological reports that gay and bisexual males who lived in rural areas and small cities were behaviorally at high risk of HIV transmission, Kelly designed his intervention based on Rogers' (1995) diffusion of innovation model with the objective of effecting community-level change.

Communities with at least one gay bar were selected for the trial. Bartenders identified popular opinion leaders among bar patrons, and these individuals were invited to join a group that met for 2 hours per week for 5 weeks. The invitation was couched in an acknowledgment that AIDS was a devastating threat to gay men and that their having been identified as opinion leaders meant that they had the potential for influencing peers in important ways.

Among the foci for the group sessions were knowledge about HIV and AIDS, as well as modeling and role-play exercises to teach participants to deliver messages about behavior change (i.e., the importance of carrying condoms at all times, discussing risk reduction with partners before sex, avoiding sex when intoxicated, and refusing unwanted sexual coercion). Group leaders also taught participants to communicate the benefits of risk reduction, to correct misconceptions about risk, and to endorse safer sex practices as socially acceptable norms.

Between group sessions, participants were asked to initiate conversations with 4 to 10 peers and then debrief these experiences with other group members at the next session. Following the training, opinion leaders reported on the number of conversations they had had with peers over 3 weeks.

The outcomes of this intervention were assessed within the context of a randomized controlled trial involving eight cities. The opinion-leader intervention was implemented in four cities; the intervention in the other cities involved posting HIV-prevention educational materials in bars. Prior to the initiation of the interventions, bar patrons in all cities were asked to complete brief anonymous questionnaires concerning their sexual behaviors, beliefs, and attitudes. One year following the interventions, this data collection procedure was repeated. Kelly reported that at follow-up, the rates of high-risk sexual behaviors among bar patrons in the "opinion leader" communities were significantly lower than in the control communities. The researchers concluded that "popular and well-liked members of a community who systematically endorse and recommend risk reduction behavior can influence the sexual-risk practices of others in their social networks" (Kelly et al., 1997). Subsequent community-level HIV-prevention interventions with psychoeducational groups for women (Sikkema et al., 2000) and adolescents (Sikkema et al., 2002) residing in urban public housing developments have reported similar outcomes.

Comment

Although the opinion leaders in these studies were recruited to effect change in their social systems, it was clear from the findings that their participation contributed as well to their own knowledge, decision making, and behavior change. Rogers' conceptualization of how innovative ideas are diffused in a social system may ultimately give rise to a wide array of opinion-leader psychoeducational group interventions (e.g., dispute resolution among students in schools, social engagement among nursing home residents, medication adherence by patients, police officer behaviors to protect citizens' civil rights, infusion of diversity content in course syllabi by university professors). The leaders of groups with this purpose would need to stress the potential held by opinion leaders in influencing others, the value to the community of their using this potential, the skills in effectively communicating with others, and the manner in which such efforts can be reinforced and sustained following the group's termination.

FUTURE DIRECTIONS

Historically, psychoeducational groups have effectively supported knowledge and skill development in a wide variety of client populations with reference to a broad array of target themes. However, numerous barriers have likely prevented their optimal utilization. One barrier discussed in this chapter is mismatching a group's content vis-à-vis a prospective participant's stage of readiness for change. A second barrier is requiring in-person attendance in face-to-face sessions. Examples of psychoeducational group innovations designed to address each of these barriers have been presented in this chapter.

The brevity, cost effectiveness, and efficacy of psychoeducational groups are likely to fuel their continued growth and empirical testing in social work. Dissemination of best-practices guidelines and psychoeducational group protocols through the Internet will improve their availability to practitioners. Moreover, the delivery of psychoeducational groups via the Internet is also rapidly emerging (see Chapter 28, this volume), again indicating promise for greatly enhanced access to potential participants.

As noted in this chapter, the notion that services can be most efficacious if they are tailored to the individual's level of readiness for change will likely influence developers of future interventions. Both the challenges and opportunities presented by ambivalent individuals will likely stimulate the development of innovative models to overcome barriers to reaching and enrolling potential participants. With promising advances in the technologies of group delivery, greater awareness of the necessary processes in enhancing motivation for change of specific behaviors by specific populations, and the growing support for empirically based practice in social work, it is very likely that many more psychoeducational group protocols will be developed and evaluated in the coming years.

REFERENCES

Asarnow, J. R., Goldstein, M. J., Thompson, M., & Guthrie, D. (1993). One-year outcomes of depressive disorders in child psychiatric inpatients: Evaluation of the prognostic power of a brief measure of expressed emotion. *Journal of Child Psychology and Psychiatry, 34*, 129–137.

Barth, R., Yeaton, J., & Winterfelt, N. (1994). Psychoeducational groups with foster parents of sexually abused children. *Child and Adolescent Social Work Journal, 11*, 405–424.

Bauer, M., & McBride, L. (1996). *Structured group psychotherapy for bipolar disorder: The life goals program*. New York: Springer.

Brekke, J. S. (1989). The use of orientation groups to engage hard-to-reach clients: Model, method and evaluation. *Social Work with Groups, 12*, 75–88.

Brown, L. (1991). Types of groups. In L. Brown (Ed.), *Groups for growth and change* (pp. 47–62). New York: Longman.

Brown, N. W. (1998). *Psychoeducational groups*. Philadelphia: Accelerated Development.

Durana, C. (1996). A longitudinal evaluation of the pairs psychoeducational program for couples. *Family Therapy, 23*, 11–36.

Ellis, A., & Harper, R. A. (1961). *A guide to rational living*. Hollywood, CA: Wilshire.

Fristad, M. A., Arnett, M. M., & Gavazzi, S. M. (1998). The impact of psychoeducational workshops on families of mood-disordered children. *Family Therapy, 25*, 151–159.

Furr, S. R. (2000). Structuring the group experience: A format for designing educational groups. *Journal for Specialists in Group Work, 25*, 29–49.

Garvin, C. D. (1997). *Contemporary group work* (3rd ed.). Boston: Allyn & Bacon.

Heckman, T. G., Kalichman, S. C., Roffman, R. A., Sikkema, K. J., Heckman, B. D., Somlai, A. M., & Walker, J. (1999). A telephone-delivered coping improvement intervention for persons living with HIV/AIDS in rural areas. *Social Work with Groups, 21*, 49–61.

Kelly, J. A., Murphy, D. A., Sikkema, K. J., McAuliffe, T. L., Roffman, R. A., Solomon, L. J., et al. (1997). Randomized, controlled, community-level HIV prevention intervention for sexual risk behavior among homosexual men in U.S. cities. *Lancet, 350*, 1500–1505.

Lomas, J., Enkin, M., Anderson, G. M., Hannah, W. J., Vayda, E., & Singer, J. (1991). Opinion leaders vs. audit and feedback to implement practice guidelines. *Journal of the American Medical Association, 265*, 2202–2207.

Lundwall, R. A. (1996). How psychoeducational support groups can provide multidiscipline services to families of people with mental illness. *Psychiatric Rehabilitation Journal, 20*, 64–71.

McWhirter, J. (1995). Emotional education for university students. *Journal of College Student Psychotherapy, 10*, 27–38.

Miller, W. R., Sovereign, R. G., & Krege, B. (1988). Motivational interviewing with problem drinkers: 2. The Drinker's Check-Up as a preventive intervention. *Behavioural Psychotherapy, 16*, 251–268.

Neukrug, E. (1999). *The world of the counselor: An introduction to the counseling profession*. Pacific Grove, CA: Brooks/Cole.

Niemann, S. H. (2002). Guidance/psychoeducational groups. In D. Capuzzi & D. R. Gross (Eds.), *Introduction to group counseling* (3rd ed.). Denver: Love.

Palmer, S. E., Brown, R. A., & Barrera, M. E. (1992). Group treatment program for abusive husbands: Long term evaluation. *American Journal of Orthopsychiatry, 62*, 276–283.

Picciano, J. F., Roffman, R. A., Kalichman, S. C., Rutledge, S. E., & Berghuis, J. P. (2001). A telephone-based brief intervention using motivational enhancement to facilitate HIV risk reduction among MSM: A pilot study. *AIDS and Behavior, 5*, 251–262.

Prochaska, J. O., & DiClemente, C. C. (1984). *The transtheoretical approach: Crossing the traditional boundaries of therapy*. Malabar, FL: Krieger.

Roffman, R. A., Beadnell, B., Ryan, R., & Downey, L. (1995). Telephone group counseling in reducing AIDS risk in gay and bisexual males. *Journal of Gay and Lesbian Social Services, 2*, 145–157.

Roffman, R. A., Picciano, J. F., Ryan, R., Beadnell, B., Fisher, D., Downey, L., & Kalichman, S. C. (1997). HIV prevention group counseling delivered by telephone: An efficacy trial with gay and bisexual men. *AIDS and Behavior, 1*, 137–154.

Roffman, R. A., Picciano, J., Wickizer, L., Bolan, M., & Ryan, R. (1998). Anonymous enrollment in

AIDS prevention group counseling: Facilitating the participation of gay and bisexual men in intervention and research. *Journal of Social Service Research, 23,* 5–22.

Rogers, C. (1951). *Client-centered therapy.* Boston: Houghton Mifflin.

Rogers, E. M. (1995). *Diffusion of innovations* (4th ed.). New York: Free Press.

Rogers, E. M. (2002). Diffusion of preventive innovations. *Addictive Behaviors, 27,* 989–993.

Sikkema, K. J., Hoffman, R. G., Brondino, M. J., Anderson, E. S., Felton, C. G., Roffman, R. A., et al. (2002, July). *Outcomes of a community-level intervention among adolescents in inner-city housing developments.* Paper presented at the International AIDS Conference, Barcelona, Spain.

Sikkema, K. J., Kelly, J. A., Winett, R. A., Solomon, L. J., Cargill, V. A., Roffman, R. A., et al. (2000). Outcomes of a randomized community-level HIV prevention intervention for women living in 18 low-income housing developments. *American Journal of Public Health, 90,* 57–63.

Stephens, R. S., Roffman, R. A., & Simpson, E. E. (1994). Treating adult marijuana dependence: A test of the relapse prevention model. *Journal of Consulting and Clinical Psychology, 62,* 92–99.

Stephens, R. S., Roffman, R. A., Williams, C. D., Adams, S. E., Burke, R., & Campbell, A. (2000, November). *The marijuana check-up outcomes.* Poster presented at the annual meeting of the Association for Advancement of Behavior Therapy, New Orleans.

Taylor-Brown, J., Acheson, A., & Farber, J. (1993). Kids can cope: A group intervention for children whose parents have cancer. *Journal of Psychosocial Oncology, 11,* 41–53.

Walters, S. T., Ogle, R., & Martin, J. E. (2002). Perils and possibilities of group-based motivational interviewing. In W. R. Miller & S. Rollnick (Eds.), *Motivational interviewing: Preparing people for change* (2nd ed., pp. 377–390). New York: Guilford Press.

Yalom, I. (1995). *The theory and practice of group psychotherapy* (4th ed.). New York: Basic Books.

Zimpfer, D. (1990). Groups for divorce/separation: A review. *Journal for Specialists in Group Work, 5,* 51–60.

Chapter 10

Prevention Groups

JAMES K. NASH
SUSIE E. SNYDER

The headline from a recent issue of our local paper stated, "U.S. sees a dramatic drop in incidents of food poisoning" (McClam, 2002). The article reported that rates of six types of food poisoning dropped by 15–49% from 1996 to 2001. Public health interventions, such as tougher regulation of the food production and distribution systems, increased inspections, and consumer education, were cited as causes of the drop.

As this example illustrates, it is possible to prevent a health problem. When prevention is successful, individuals who might have become ill do not experience symptoms. Families do not have to provide care for a stricken member. Treatment—which may be unpleasant, expensive, and differentially effective—does not have to occur. In short, successful prevention produces benefits for individuals, families, and society. Consequently, prevention is at the heart of public health efforts to reduce rates of health problems in a population.

In recent years, increased attention has been given to applying prevention concepts to a wide range of problems. In the areas of mental health and psychosocial functioning, social work groups are well suited to preventing problems by providing members with opportunities to learn skills, receive and give support, and develop interpersonal networks. This chapter draws from public health to present a prevention framework and describes its use as a guide to social work group-based interventions.

PREVENTION IN PUBLIC HEALTH

A Public Health Framework

The National Institute of Mental Health (NIMH, 1998) outlined a prevention framework for mental health aimed at reducing rates of mental disorders in the U.S. population. The framework delineated three challenges for researchers and practitioners interested in prevention:

1. Gaining greater understanding of the origins of problems and disorders.
2. Identifying risk and protective factors and related risk and protective processes that are associated with problems and disorders.
3. Translating knowledge about the origins of problems and disorders and about risk and protective processes into interventions that can be evaluated and, if effective, disseminated.

These challenges highlight the links between research and practice that are central to a prevention framework (Fraser, Randolph, & Bennett, 2000; Mrazek & Haggerty, 1994). Four key ideas emerge from this framework.

Defining the Target

First, the target of prevention must be clearly defined. The "target" refers to the particular problem or disorder of interest, as well as to the population or population subgroup at risk. Social work prevention groups target a variety of problems in diverse population subgroups, for example, preventing conduct problems in children (Fraser, Nash, Galinsky, & Darwin, 2000); preventing sexually transmitted diseases in adolescents (Richey, Gillmore, Balassone, Gutiérrez, & Hartway, 1997); and preventing depression in low-income, inner-city pregnant women (Cunningham & Zayas, 2002). Although a prevention framework requires focusing on a problem, it need not be at odds with a strengths-based approach to practice. As we describe later, strengths-based and empowerment-oriented strategies are features of many prevention groups.

Understanding Risk and Protection

Second, research-based knowledge of the correlates and causes of a problem is necessary for effective prevention. In a prevention framework, factors associated with positive outcomes are known as *protective factors*, whereas factors associated with negative outcomes are known as *risk factors*. Population-based studies are required to demonstrate that an association exists between a risk or protective factor and an outcome. However, status as a risk or protective factor does not imply that a causal relationship exists between the factor and the outcome. Some risk and protective factors simply indicate increased prevalence of an outcome for one subgroup relative to others.

For example, research indicates that students from certain ethnic groups have a higher rate of school dropout relative to the overall population of students (Richman & Bowen, 1997). Ethnicity does not, however, cause dropout. Knowledge of a risk factor identifies a potential need for prevention aimed at specific subgroups. But it does not necessarily indicate how prevention should proceed. Moreover, research results from a population-based study do not automatically apply to a particular locality (Fraser, Randolph, & Bennett, 2000). Thus a school social worker might use population-based information about risk of dropout to guide further inquiry into the prevalence of dropout in her own community (e.g., by reviewing local data or surveying consumers). Suppose this inquiry identified Latina girls as a subgroup at increased risk of dropout. This knowledge, by itself, would not be sufficient to plan an effective prevention group.

To distinguish a risk indicator, such as ethnicity, from risk and protective factors that play a causal role, researchers must conduct theoretically driven longitudinal studies (Fraser, Randolph, & Bennett, 2000; Rutter, 2001). This kind of study yields knowledge about risk and protective *processes*, that is, how risk and protective factors interact over time to influence outcomes. Such knowledge informs prevention programs that aim to interrupt a risk process or promote a protective process. Consistent with an ecological–developmental perspective, a prevention framework directs attention to factors at multiple system levels, to the interaction of person and environment, and to variability across the lifespan (Farmer & Farmer, 2001).

Suppose the school social worker interested in dropout prevention for Latina girls reviews theoretical and research literature to discover what is known about a risk process for dropout. She can use tools such as focus groups with adolescents and their parents to verify whether the risk process operates in her community. She can also use this information to plan prevention. Information about a local risk process might indicate a need to focus on culturally based themes to prevent dropout instead of focusing solely on academic skills (Peeks, 1999). Similarly, this information might indicate a group format over individual counseling.

For example, Peeks (1999) described a group for middle school girls who evidenced acting-out behavior at school and low academic motivation (risk factors for dropout). Drawing on theory and prior research, Peeks identified cultural themes (e.g., family, respect, sex role expectations) that reflect key values in many Latino communities and that provide many Latina adolescents with a foundation for a strong identity. However, such values may interact with values of the dominant culture in ways that increase risk for some Latina adolescents. Latina adolescents may struggle to balance competing values (e.g., a desire for greater independence and individualism fueled by exposure to the dominant culture versus a wish to respect the family and adhere to traditional sex roles). Using information about this potential risk process as a starting point, Peeks described gathering information to verify its relevance for a particular group of girls. Peeks also noted that a group format was better suited than individual counseling to help girls negotiate competing values, because it permitted them to "discuss (common) cross-cultural conflicts ... and develop better decision-making skills" (1999, p. 141).

Research on risk and protective processes is available for many outcomes of interest to social workers (Fraser, 1997; Mrazek & Haggerty, 1994). To be sure, the amount and quality of evidence vary across populations and functional domains. Especially lacking is knowledge about risk and protection for vulnerable groups (e.g., females, people of color, older adults) and subgroups (e.g., Latina girls of Mexican origin versus Latina girls of Nicaraguan origin). When research-based knowledge of risk and protection for a particular subgroup is available, it should guide the development of prevention programs. For example, results of one study suggested that macro-level factors related to gender, race, ethnicity, and class interacted in distinct ways for African American versus European American young women to influence condom use (Gutiérrez, Oh, & Gillmore, 2000). The authors argued that prevention aimed at these subgroups must take such differences into account. As researchers and practitioners develop and implement prevention groups, they should also keep in mind that research-based knowledge of risk and protective processes reflects what is thought to be true for a population, not necessarily what will be true for a particular individual or family.

Interrupting Risk and Building Protection

Third, researchers and practitioners, often in collaboration with consumers, develop interventions designed to interrupt risk processes or promote protective processes. For example, research reveals a link between a harsh parenting style (risk factor) and child aggression (outcome). Multiple individual, family, and contextual factors contribute to the risk process. A key element involves parental modeling and reinforcement of a harsh approach to solving problems, which increases the likelihood that a child will fail to learn alternative, nonaggressive strategies for solving problems and will display a higher level of aggression relative to peers. A large body of research suggests that harsh parenting plays a pivotal role in a risk process that can lead to conduct disorder, academic failure, and delinquency. Based on this research, practitioners and researchers have developed and tested prevention efforts that emphasize building parenting skills to interrupt this risk process (Kazdin & Weisz, 1998). Many of these rely on, or include, a group component. As we describe later, a group format is ideal for helping members learn with and from each other to develop specific knowledge and skills.

Assessing the Effectiveness of Prevention

Fourth, and consistent with an evidence-based approach to social work practice (Gambrill, 1999; Rosen & Proctor, 2003), a prevention framework emphasizes a need to assess the intended effects of interventions. For example, parenting-skills training groups have been shown in multiple rigorous research studies to result in more competent parenting (short-term effect) and sustained lower levels of child aggression (long-term effect; Kazdin & Weisz, 1998). Assessing intervention effects should also include attention to differential effects across diverse population subgroups defined by factors such as age, gender, or cultural background, as well as unintended effects and iatrogenic effects (NIMH, 1998). As an example, researchers from the Metropolitan Area Child Study Research Group (MACSRG, 2002) found that the effects of a school-based violence prevention program differed across communities. The program was delivered in schools serving low-income, inner-city neighborhoods and in schools serving neighborhoods that were poor but that had relatively more resources for families and children. Participants in the latter group of schools displayed lower levels of aggression at posttest, whereas participants from low-income inner-city neighborhoods displayed higher levels of aggression at posttest.

An Example of a Social Work Prevention Group

The work of Richey and colleagues (1997), who developed a group-based intervention aimed at preventing HIV infection in adolescents, exemplifies many of these ideas. The authors reviewed research on the prevalence and correlates of HIV/AIDS to identify youth in detention facilities as a subgroup at high risk of infection. Research also highlighted risk and protective factors to target, including accurate information about HIV, attitudes about perceived vulnerability to HIV, and "beliefs about the short-term consequences of condom use, such as how easy or uncomfortable they are to use" (p. 75). Knowledge of adolescent development and of social learning and social cognitive theories suggested that a group format was especially suitable for teaching relevant knowledge and skills. Group sessions provided opportunities for adolescents to learn about and practice four skill steps to increase their ability to negotiate condom use with partners. The first step, "think it up," (Richey et al., 1997, pp. 75–76) included thinking about the goal of condom use relative to a particular situation, formulating ways to bring up the topic with a partner, and anticipating potential partner objections. In the "bring it up" step (p. 76), teens developed and practiced alternative ways (i.e., "opening lines") to initiate a discussion about condom use. Richey and colleagues also incorporated content and process features into the program to improve generalization of skills beyond the group, for example, using the power of natural consequences.

Levels of Prevention

Public health distinguishes three levels of prevention: *universal*, *selective*, and *indicated* (NIMH, 1998). Universal prevention is aimed at an entire population or population subgroup (e.g., all school-age children, all new mothers). Selective prevention targets individuals who have been identified as being at heightened risk of developing a problem or disorder. Indicated prevention efforts are aimed at "high-risk" individuals who may display symptoms of a disorder but who do not display full-blown problems—for example, symptomatic individuals who do not meet diagnostic criteria for a mental disorder. Indicated prevention may also be aimed at individuals with a diagnosis, with the aim of preventing comorbidity (NIMH, 1998).

Our focus in this chapter is on universal and, especially, selective prevention. Indicated prevention is often considered to be synonymous with *treatment*, and other chapters of this volume describe treatment groups. Although our focus is not on treatment, groups aimed at the amelioration of existing problems may also serve a prevention function and prevent future problems because they interrupt a risk process (NIMH, 1998). We believe practitioners will be more effective if they keep a prevention framework in mind as they plan and implement treatment groups.

Universal Prevention

All members of a population are eligible to participate in a universal prevention group. Membership is not based on increased risk. Universal prevention groups frequently aim to build knowledge and skills in members or to instill members with values, attitudes, or beliefs (e.g., Weisz & Black, 2001). Examples of group-based approaches to universal prevention for children include providing tobacco education or sex education content in health classes. To be effective, universal prevention groups should be tied to a risk or protective process that is grounded in theory and research. Evaluating effectiveness is critical. Universal prevention targets especially serious problems and, because all population members participate, universal prevention can be expensive. If ineffective, universal prevention wastes resources, and serious problems are not addressed. For example, Drug Awareness and Resistance Education programs have been widely used for many years to prevent youth substance use despite lack of evidence of their effectiveness (U. S. Public Health Service, 2001).

At the direct practice level, social workers are often involved in planning and facilitating universal prevention groups. Often, they work with existing groups that continue to function after the prevention program is completed. This type of group contrasts with many social work groups that come together for a specific purpose. Good examples of prevention with an existing group are violence prevention programs, such as problem-solving skills-training programs, delivered to all students in a classroom (McGinnis & Goldstein, 1997; Nash, Fraser, Galinsky, & Kupper, 2003). This approach to universal prevention has several advantages. Typically, in an existing classroom, group norms (e.g., classroom rules) are in place, roles are well defined, and cohesion is high. Beyond introducing him- or herself and describing the purpose of the group, a school social worker may need to devote little time to group-building activities. Thus a classroom-based skills-training program can begin with a presentation on a particular problem-solving skill (e.g., self-talk, accurate interpretation of others' intentions, brainstorming responses for reaching goals). The class can watch a demonstration of the skill or of problems that arise when a skill is lacking (e.g., the consequences of interpreting another person's actions as hostile when they were actually benign). Activities such as role plays allow students to learn and practice skills in the setting in which they will need to use them. Generalization is increased because fellow students are familiar with targeted skills and vocabulary (Hansen, Nangle, & Meyer, 1998).

Moving beyond direct practice, social workers can advocate for an increase in the availability of empirically based universal prevention groups and can improve access to such groups. For example, a social worker might testify before a school board and use research results to demonstrate a need for sex education groups in high schools. Advocacy by social workers can increase attention to the cultural competence and gender sensitivity of group-based universal prevention programs to insure that the content and process fit the needs and strengths of diverse subgroups (Bernal & Scharrón-Del-Río, 2001; Spencer, Lewis, & Gutiérrez, 2000).

Selective Prevention

Selective prevention programs are aimed at individuals who, relative to the population at large, are at heightened risk of developing a problem. The goal is to interrupt an emerging risk process by reducing risk factors or building protective factors. A benefit of selective prevention is the decreased cost of providing an intervention to a carefully selected subgroup instead of providing it to all population members. Additionally, selective prevention can be tailored to fit a particular group of individuals (Fraser, Randolph, & Bennett, 2000). Examples of selective prevention groups include parenting classes for pregnant adolescents (Workman & Brewer, 2002), groups for Latina adolescents aimed at building self-identity (Peeks, 1999), and groups designed to prevent depression in pregnant low-income inner-city women (Cunningham & Zayas, 2002).

Skill-building groups were one element of a selective violence-prevention program that targeted risk factors at multiple system levels (MACSRG, 2002). All students in a sample of schools serving low-income neighborhoods in Chicago and Aurora, Illinois, received a classroom-based (universal) prevention program aimed at teaching problem solving. In addition, subgroups of students at each school were selected to receive enhanced skills training in a small-group format. Small groups focused on changing beliefs about aggression and on building prosocial peer interaction skills. Students were chosen for the selective prevention groups based on scores on peer and teacher ratings of aggressive behavior.

A challenge in effective selective prevention is to identify accurately participants who are at heightened risk (i.e., screening). Heightened risk may not be due to individual and family factors alone. Societal factors, such as poverty and oppression, increase risk for specific subgroups in the United States, for example, African Americans, Latinos and Latinas, and other persons of color, girls and women, persons with disabilities, and sexual minorities. Selective prevention groups with individuals from these subgroups are likely to be more effective if contextual, as well as individual, factors are targeted (Cunningham & Zayas, 2002; Gutiérrez et al., 2000).

USING SOCIAL WORK GROUPS FOR SELECTIVE PREVENTION

Group work is well suited for selective prevention with individuals who are at heightened risk of developing problems. Certain group phenomena lend themselves naturally to prevention because they promote protective processes. For example, a well-planned and well-facilitated group creates an experience of belonging, shared meaning, and community for members (Malekoff, 2001). The group setting permits experiential, interactional, and vicarious learning, along with opportunities to apply knowledge and practice skills (Rose, 1998). It provides a chance to receive support, feedback, and confrontation from peers. Equally, it offers a chance to give support, feedback, and confrontation to peers. The group creates a normalizing experience (e.g., for participants from a marginalized population) to avoid and counter effects of stigma, oppression, and discrimination (Peeks, 1999). Many of these opportunities and experiences are difficult, if not impossible, to provide in individual-focused interventions.

Social workers can increase the effectiveness of selective prevention groups by intentionally incorporating a prevention framework into practice. As a starting point, social workers can recognize that an ecological-developmental perspective, which guides much of social work practice, also informs a prevention framework. This perspective highlights three practice principles that are especially pertinent for selective prevention groups. First, improving person–environment fit is a promising strategy for preventing mental health and psychosocial problems. Second, selective prevention groups should reflect awareness of the variability of human experience across the lifespan. Third, a prevention framework notes that mental health and psychosocial outcomes differ across cultures with respect to conceptualization, etiology, and course (Mrazek & Haggerty, 1994; NIMH, 1998). Thus attention to culturally competent practice is key in effective prevention.

Person–Environment Fit

Theoretical understanding of a phenomenon such as person–environment fit precedes effective interventions aimed at influencing the phenomenon (Kazdin, 2000). For example, many selective prevention groups use a cognitive-behavioral approach to improve person–environment fit (e.g., Cunningham & Zayas, 2002; Franklin & Corcoran, 2000; Fraser, Nash, et al., 2000; Richey et al., 1997). These groups help members to recognize their own cognitive-behavioral styles—that is, how they perceive, interpret, and respond to information from the environment—and to understand how one's style influences one's actions (Crick & Dodge, 1994). A goal of such groups is to build the capacity of members to understand, negotiate, and change their environments and to promote individual-level change in members. For example, the group model described by Richey and colleagues (1997) focused on changing adolescents' beliefs about condom use (individual change) and on equipping adolescents to negotiate condom use with a partner (environment change). The goal was to increase use of condoms and reduce risk of STDs.

Group work is often ideal for such an approach to selective prevention. The group milieu, if carefully planned, approximates the social ecologies of members. Activities such as role plays permit members to learn concepts (e.g., how beliefs influence behavior) and to practice skills for influencing the environment (Hansen et al., 1998). In addition, members can practice newly learned skills outside the group and review their success at subsequent meetings.

Human Development

Research-based knowledge of human development should guide the timing, content, and procedures of selective prevention groups (Fraser, Randolph, & Bennett, 2000; Farmer &

Farmer, 2001; MACSRG, 2002). For example, a problem-solving skills-training group may prevent conduct problems for children who are socially rejected by peers (Fraser, Nash, et al., 2000). Research on cognitive development in children and on the age at which social problem-solving skill deficits become a critical risk factor suggests that this strategy is especially important for third- through sixth-grade students. Knowledge of specific skill deficits that increase risk for children at this age indicates that the group should include content on hostile attribution bias and beliefs that legitimize aggression (Crick & Dodge, 1994). Research on possible iatrogenic effects of groups composed solely of at-risk children (especially young adolescents) suggests that the group should also include socially competent students (Dishion & Andrews, 1995; MACSRG, 2002).

Knowledge of predictable developmental transitions (e.g., puberty, retirement) also guides the development of selective prevention groups. Transitions can be "points of vulnerability" but also points of "growth and opportunity" (NIMH, 1998, chap. 2). As an example, a school social worker might provide a group for fifth-grade girls to promote a successful transition to middle school.

Culturally Competent Practice

Similar to all social work practice, cultural competence is key to effective prevention, whether universal, selective, or indicated. In recent years, a multicultural framework has emerged to guide culturally competent social work practice (e.g., Spencer et al., 2000) and research (e.g., Uehara et al., 1996). It is beyond the scope of this chapter to describe this framework in detail. Instead, we mention three features of a multicultural framework that are especially relevant to prevention groups.

First, a multicultural framework emphasizes a need for practice "to be flexible in addressing the dynamic changes and processes of the future" (Spencer et al., 2000, p. 143). From the broad macro level to the local level, change is ongoing in the systems (e.g., social, political, demographic, and economic) that make up the environment of consumers, practitioners, and researchers. For example, the events of September 11, 2001 altered the political, social, and economic landscape of the United States. Individuals and families in the areas directly affected by the attacks, especially New York City, experienced physical and psychological trauma that may have lasting effects. Collectively, such effects may alter the local psychosocial environment. Across the country, individuals, families, and communities of perceived Middle Eastern background may be more likely to experience discrimination in housing, employment, and immigration. They may also be at greater risk of being victims of violence. On a broader scale, an apparently open-ended war on terrorism may alter day-to-day life for many. It is also likely to divert resources from human services and limit the availability of supports for vulnerable groups. The economic recession that began in 2001 also contributed to increased vulnerability for many individuals, families, and communities. To the extent that selective prevention groups aim to help members understand and effectively influence the environment, it is key that practitioners and researchers remain attentive to environmental change and flexible in developing and applying knowledge about risk and protection.

A second element of a multicultural framework highlights "the importance of language used in instruments of assessment and intervention" (Spencer et al., 2000, p. 145). As described later, screening potential members is a defining feature of selective prevention. Screening lacks relevance and produces results that include an increased amount of error if procedures and instruments are not understandable or fail to reflect concepts that are culturally meaningful to consumers. For instance, Land and Hudson (1997) described a need to reconceptualize and develop new measures of *depression*, *distress*, and *coping* in a study of Latina AIDS caregivers. Existing measures reflected mainstream conceptualizations of these variables. They did not capture dimensions that were meaningful to the study's participants, even when measures were carefully translated. As an example, Land and Hudson identified strategies that were common in many Latino subcultures, such as "using herbal remedies or visiting an indigenous healer" (p. 240), that existing measures of coping failed to tap. Similar to the language used in screening and assessment, a prevention group is likely to be more effective if language used during the group sessions reflects the culture and background of members.

Finally, a multicultural framework emphasizes a need to include "the community's perspective in assessing problems and resources" (Spencer et al., 2000, p. 144). *Risk, protection*, and *problems* are abstract concepts whose conceptualization and meaning may vary across cultures, by gender, and from individual to individual. Collaboration with community members is necessary to gain understanding of cultural differences and of shared meaning. This should occur at all phases of prevention, beginning with research on risk and protection to program design and testing through implementation and evaluation of a prevention group (Land & Hudson, 1997; Uehara et al., 1996).

PLANNING SELECTIVE PREVENTION GROUPS

All groups are thought to progress through distinct phases of development, and an understanding of group development increases the effectiveness of a facilitator (Galinsky & Schopler, 1989; Northen & Kurland, 2001; Toseland & Rivas, 2001; Tuckman & Jensen, 1977). Although all phases of group development are important, our focus is on the earliest phase: planning. We believe that careful and informed planning is central to the success of a selective prevention group. Moreover, planning a selective prevention group involves a set of steps that may not occur during the planning process of other types of social work groups.

Identifying the Target of Prevention

A key step in planning a selective prevention group is to identify the target population subgroup, based on risk status, and to define key desired outcome(s). Population-based research, practice experience, and knowledge of local conditions should guide this process (Fraser, Randolph, & Bennett, 2000; Farmer & Farmer, 2001; MACSRG, 2002). There is a wealth of research-based information that practitioners can use to identify subgroups likely to be at heightened risk of a particular problem. Examples include information on risk for (1) problems affecting youth, including child maltreatment, violence, substance use, high-risk sexual behaviors, suicide, and school dropout (Fraser, 1997; McWhirter, McWhirter, McWhirter, & McWhirter, 1998; for youth violence, see also Loeber, Farrington, Stouthamer-Loeber, & Van Kammen, 1998; U.S. Public Health Service, 2001); (2) mental disorders across the lifespan (NIMH, 1998); and (3) domestic violence (Meuer, Seymour, & Wallace, 2001). Information about the prevalence of a problem and the nature and severity of its impact on individuals, families, and society is particularly relevant in planning a selective prevention group (Mrazek & Haggerty, 1994).

Collaborating with consumers to define problems and desired outcomes is likely to increase consumer engagement and participation, cultural competence, and effectiveness

(Spencer et al., 2000). Mental health and psychosocial outcomes are typically conceptualized and measured from a European American, middle-class perspective (Bernal & Scharrón-Del-Río, 2001). Selective prevention is unlikely to be effective unless practitioners understand how members think about concepts that represent targeted outcomes or risk and protective factors. For example, Peeks (1999) described a group aimed at helping bilingual Latina adolescents develop a positive sense of self-identity (a protective factor). During an early group meeting, the bilingual group leader elicited a member's understanding of a particular concept:

> [A] teen used the word "confianza" (which depending on the context, can mean trust or self-confidence) to describe her expectations about the group. To elicit clarification, the therapist asked in Spanish: "What does confianza mean to you and can you provide an example?" (p. 145)

This strategy helped the group leader to understand how this adolescent viewed a concept that was central to self-identity, using the adolescent's first language.

Identifying a Risk Process and Strategies to Interrupt Risk or Build Protection

Planning a selective prevention group involves review and synthesis of research on presumed risk factors and processes. By articulating a risk process, a researcher identifies how a combination of risk factors operates to produce a problem. Thus strategies can be designed to interrupt the risk process and prevent the problem. For example, Cunningham and Zayas (2002) postulated that individual cognitive-behavioral attributes, social network characteristics, and level of knowledge of child development interact to increase risk of depression for new ethnic-minority mothers from low-income inner city neighborhoods. Based on this framework, the authors described a multimodal program that aimed to prevent depression by teaching cognitive-behavioral skills, developing social networks (e.g., through case management and teaching self-advocacy), and providing psychoeducational information on child development.

Often, information on understanding and interrupting a risk process is presented in a manualized format to guide a prevention group (Fraser, Nash, et al., 2000; Greenberg, 1996; Grossman et al., 1997). There is debate about the advantages of using manuals in group work (Kazdin, 2000; Malekoff, 2001). Some writers argue that manuals are necessary to specify key content and procedures. Others believe that manuals remove the spontaneity and power from group work that account for its effectiveness. It is important to note that some manuals seek a balance by presenting core content and procedures while delineating how practitioners can adapt the content and procedures to meet local conditions and characteristics of a particular group (Fraser, Nash, et al., 2000).

Many empirically based and manualized prevention programs that utilize a group modality were tested on samples composed of mainly European American, often male, participants (Bernal & Scharrón-Del-Río, 2001). Fortunately, this methodology is changing, and studies increasingly include diverse samples (e.g., MACRSG, 2002). Practitioners face a dilemma when planning a selective prevention group for a population subgroup whose members have not been included in research. Some researchers argue that using an empirically based approach to prevention (e.g., in manual format) is always preferable, even for members of a subgroup who were not represented in effectiveness research. Others disagree and argue that there is an urgent need for collaborative research with diverse populations to create knowledge that will guide empirically based and culturally competent prevention (Bernal & Scharrón-Del-Río, 2001).

Screening Potential Members

Identifying individuals at heightened risk of developing a problem is a distinguishing feature of selective prevention (NIMH, 1998). Selective prevention wastes resources if it is provided to individuals who are not at heightened risk, and such individuals do not need the service. On the other hand, individuals who already evidence a problem are unlikely to benefit from a selective prevention group, and their presence may undermine the success of others. In general, selective prevention groups should include only individuals who have been identified as being at heightened risk. However, there are important exceptions to this principle. For example, there is evidence that homogeneous groups of adolescents who display increased levels of aggression relative to peers, or who simply believe in the value and efficacy of aggression to solve problems, can result in increased problem behavior for members (Dishion & Andrews, 1995; MACSRG, 2002). Thus selective prevention groups that target chronic aggression and related problems should include socially competent members, for example, members who value and routinely use nonviolent problem-solving strategies (Fraser, Nash, et al., 2000). Researchers and practitioners who adopt such an approach have an ethical responsibility to insure that (1) socially competent adolescents will not experience harmful effects from participating in the group and (2) there is a reasonable likelihood that socially competent adolescents will experience tangible benefits from participating (e.g., increased problem-solving skills).

Screening begins as a practitioner becomes aware that certain individuals appear to be at heightened risk of developing a particular problem. In practice settings, potential candidates for a selective prevention group might come to the attention of a practitioner via observation, expression of consumer interest, and referrals from professionals or family members. For example, suppose a social worker in a health clinic for seniors is approached by a consumer with concerns of feeling isolated. Suppose, further, that the social worker has observed other seniors who seem to be experiencing similar feelings. The result would be a pool of seniors for whom a group aimed at preventing depression might be indicated. Instead of simply offering a group to, say, the first eight seniors who appear to be at risk, a prevention framework highlights the importance of using additional screening procedures to identify those seniors who are at heightened risk of depression (but not in need of immediate treatment) and who are most likely to benefit from a prevention group.

Screening works best when practitioners use reliable and valid assessment procedures and instruments (Mrazek & Haggerty, 1994; NIMH, 1998). A growing number of tools are available to social workers for assessing risk and protective factors at multiple system levels (e.g., individual, family, neighborhood) related to a range of problems (see, e.g., Blythe & Reithoffer, 2000; Corcoran & Fisher, 1999; Fraser 1997). However, there is a continuing need to develop culturally sensitive, reliable, and valid measures of risk and protection. In addition to formal measures, practitioners can use information from other sources, such as interviews with consumers and family members, to assess risk level. Attention to culture when using a particular assessment tool or procedure is key (Land & Hudson, 1997; Spencer et al., 2000). Similar to other research, research on developing measures has often depended heavily on samples of European American middle-class males. The validity of such measures when used with other groups is questionable (Bernal & Scharrón-Del-Río, 2001).

Planning an Evaluation

Evaluating the short- and long-term effects of intervention is fundamental to a prevention framework (Mrazek & Haggerty, 1994; NIMH, 1998). Thus planning a selective prevention group should include identifying procedures for assessing the impact of the group. Evaluation follows from screening, because the same factors that operate in a presumed risk process should change as a result of participating in the prevention group. For example, participants in a selective group aimed at preventing child aggression by building parenting skills should be screened into the group due to a risk factor, such as harsh parenting practices. If the group is effective, parenting practices will change over the course of the group. A strategy for assessing whether this occurs is to develop a single-case study for each group participant (Abell & Hudson, 2000). This provides information on whether parenting practices change from baseline and is an example of assessing the short-term (proximal) impact of the group. The ultimate goal of the group, to prevent child aggression, implies a need to use measures of behavior (e.g., parent, child, and teacher reports) during and beyond the life of the group.

Collaboration is important if the evaluation is to be meaningful to group members (Spencer et al., 2000). Practitioners who use an existing assessment tool for initial screening may wish to discuss its content and format with participants with the aim of adapting it for use as a measure of the outcomes of a prevention group. For example, a measure of parenting practices might be changed, perhaps by adding items that reflect a parent's view of what needs to change about his or her parenting practices (e.g., tone or volume of voice) or of what he or she does well. Group members might also develop novel procedures for assessment, for example, putting a coin in a piggy bank every time a parent–child interaction goes well. Evaluation should always include meaningful indicators of members' perceptions of the group itself (e.g., relevance of material, comfort level with format and process, overall satisfaction).

USING RECREATION AND SOCIAL GROUPS FOR SELECTIVE AND UNIVERSAL PREVENTION

Kazdin (2000) noted that everyday social and recreational activities often have therapeutic effects, and as such, practitioners and researchers need to broaden their view of what is an intervention. In this spirit, it may be useful for social workers to assess the potential preventative effects of social and recreational groups. Examples of such groups include sports teams, scouting, church groups, theatre groups—the list is virtually endless. These groups may fall outside the realm of group work as traditionally conceptualized (Toseland & Rivas, 2001). But they serve a preventative function whenever members engage in activities that build protective factors or reduce risk. For example, adolescent girls may gain protective factors (e.g., peer interaction skills, internal locus of control) by playing on a soccer team (Kazdin, 2000). Recreational and social groups may foster members' interpersonal networks, from which they obtain and give instrumental and affective support. For children and adolescents, such groups may serve a preventative function by decreasing the amount of unsupervised time available for engaging in deviant activities, although this protective effect depends on group norms about deviant behavior (Hawkins, Catalano, & Miller, 1992). Social and recreational groups often provide youths with opportunities to develop a positive relationship with a caring adult, and such a relationship can serve as a protective factor for a child or adolescent (Werner, 1992).

Social workers can incorporate recreational and social groups into prevention-oriented practice by linking participants to groups, identifying and removing barriers to participation, and advocating for increased availability of such groups. To increase the likelihood that group membership will lead to desired outcomes for a particular individual, knowledge of research and assessment of a particular person–environment situation should guide such an approach. Most important, membership in a group should reflect the interests of the consumer.

FUTURE DIRECTIONS

A prevention framework serves as a promising guide for social workers interested in developing, implementing, and evaluating group-based interventions aimed at improving the mental health and psychosocial functioning of children, adolescents, and adults. A substantial body of research-based knowledge already exists to guide prevention-oriented group work. This includes knowledge of the nature and origins of problems, disorders, and desired outcomes, as well as knowledge of risk and protective processes thought to affect outcomes. It also includes research results on effective prevention programs that use a group format.

To fulfill the future promise of prevention, social workers will need to become more familiar with and use this knowledge base as they plan, implement, and evaluate the effects of prevention groups. Peer-reviewed journals in social work and other fields make up the primary repository of this knowledge base. However, selected Internet websites also provide high-quality information on issues such as risk and protection in selected populations, screening, and empirically supported group-based interventions. Examples include the sites of the American College of Preventive Medicine (ACPM, n.d.), the Office of Juvenile Justice and Delinquency Prevention (2001), and the Prevention Institute (*http://preventioninstitute.org*).

Greater use of the prevention knowledge base can lead to more effective social work groups. For instance, the ACPM website includes information on reliable and valid tools for assessing risk status for problems such as depression and family violence. Such information can help social workers screen into a selective prevention group members most likely to benefit from it and screen out those who do not need the intervention and those who need more intensive treatment.

A key challenge is for social workers to participate more fully in the building of a prevention knowledge base. Currently, a great deal of prevention science occurs in disciplines other than social work, for example, medicine, psychology, and criminology. Social workers should continue to use knowledge from these and other fields to guide prevention groups. However, social work researchers and practitioners can make important contributions to the prevention knowledge base. This is especially true for approaches to prevention that rely on a group format. Culturally relevant research on risk and protection that highlights strengths and empowerment—in addition to problems and disorders—may yield better knowledge about risk and protective processes that affect outcomes. It can also increase understanding of how participating in a group interrupts risk, builds protection, and leads to better outcomes for group members. In short, prevention-oriented research in social work can increase our ability to demonstrate and replicate the healing power of groups.

REFERENCES

Abell, N., & Hudson, W. W. (2000). Pragmatic applications of single-case and groups designs in social work practice evaluation and research. In P. Allen-Meares & C. Garvin (Eds.), *The handbook of social work direct practice* (pp. 535–550). Thousand Oaks, CA: Sage.

American College of Preventive Medicine. (n.d.). *Evidence-based recommendations for preventive services*. Retrieved September 30, 2003 from: *http://www.acpm.org*.

Bernal, G., & Scharrón-Del-Río, M. R. (2001). Are empirically supported treatments valid for ethnic minorities? Toward an alternative approach for treatment research. *Cultural Diversity and Ethnic Minority*, 7, 328–342.

Blythe, B., & Reithoffer, A. (2000). Assessment and measurement issues in direct practice in social work. In P. Allen-Meares & C. Garvin (Eds.), *The handbook of social work direct practice* (pp. 551–564). Thousand Oaks, CA: Sage.

Corcoran, K., & Fisher, J. (1999). *Measures for clinical practice: A sourcebook* (3rd ed.). New York: Free Press.

Crick, N. R., & Dodge, K. A. (1994). A review and reformulation of social-information processing mechanisms in children's social adjustment. *Psychological Bulletin*, 115, 74–101.

Cunningham, M., & Zayas, L. H. (2002). Reducing depression in pregnancy: Designing multimodal interventions. *Social Work Research*, 47, 114–123.

Dishion, T. J., & Andrews, D. W. (1995). Preventing escalation in problem behaviors with high-risk young adolescents: Immediate and 1-year outcomes. *Journal of Clinical and Consulting Psychology*, 63, 538–548.

Farmer, T. W., & Farmer, E. M. Z. (2001). Developmental science, systems of care, and prevention of emotional and behavioral problems in youth. *American Journal of Orthopsychiatry*, 71, 171–181.

Franklin, C., & Corcoran, J. (2000). Preventing adolescent pregnancy: A review of programs and practices. *Social Work*, 45, 40–52.

Fraser, M. W. (1997). *Risk and resilience in childhood: An ecological perspective*. Washington, DC: NASW Press.

Fraser, M. W., Nash, J. K., Galinsky, M. J., & Darwin, K. M. (2000). *Making choices: Social problem-solving skills for children*. Washington, DC: NASW Press.

Fraser, M. W., Randolph, K. A., & Bennett, M. D. (2000). Prevention: A risk and resilience perspective. In P. Allen-Meares, & C. Garvin (Eds.), *The handbook of social work direct practice* (pp. 89–111). Thousand Oaks, CA: Sage.

Galinsky, M. J., & Schopler, J. H. (1989). Developmental patterns in open-ended groups. *Social Work with Groups*, 12, 99–114.

Gambrill, E. (1999). Evidence-based practice: An alternative to authority-based practice. *Families in Society: The Journal of Contemporary Human Services*, 80, 341–350.

Greenberg, M. T. (1996). *The PATHS project: Preventive intervention for children*. Seattle, WA: University of Washington, Department of Psychology.

Grossman, D., Neckerman, H., Koepsell, T., Liu, P., Asher, K., Beland, K., et al. (1997). Effectiveness of a violence prevention curriculum among children in elementary school: A randomized controlled trial. *Journal of the American Medical Association*, 277, 1605–1611.

Gutiérrez, L., Oh, H. J., & Gillmore, M. R. (2000). Toward an understanding of (em)power(ment) for HIV/AIDS prevention with adolescent women. *Sex Roles*, 42, 581–611.

Hansen, D. J., Nangle, D. W., & Meyer, K. A. (1998). Enhancing the effectiveness of social skills interventions with adolescents. *Education and Treatment of Children*, 21, 489–513.

Hawkins, J. D., Catalano, R. F., & Miller, J. Y. (1992). Risk and protective factors for alcohol and other drug problems in adolescence and early adulthood: Implications for substance abuse prevention. *Psychological Bulletin*, 112, 64–105.

Kazdin, A. E. (2000). *Psychotherapy for children and adolescents: Directions for research and practice.* New York: Oxford University Press.

Kazdin, A. E., & Weisz, J. R. (1998). Identifying and developing empirically supported child and adolescent treatments. *Journal of Consulting and Clinical Psychology, 66,* 19–36.

Land, H., & Hudson, S. (1997). Methodological considerations in surveying Latina AIDS caregivers: Issues in sampling and measurement. *Social Work Research, 21,* 233– 246.

Loeber, R., Farrington, D. P., Stouthamer-Loeber, M., & Van Kammen, W. B. (1998). *Antisocial behavior and mental health problems: Explanatory factors in childhood and adolescence.* Mahwah, NJ: Erlbaum.

Malekoff, A. (2001). The power of group work with kids: A practitioner's reflection on strengths-based practice. *Families in Society: The Journal of Contemporary Human Services, 82,* 243–249.

McClam, E. (2002, April 19). US sees a dramatic drop in incidents of food poisoning. *The Oregonian,* p. A3.

McGinnis, E., & Goldstein, A. P. (1997). *Skillstreaming the elementary schoolchild: New strategies and perspectives for teaching social skills* (rev. ed.). Champaign, IL: Research Press.

McWhirter, J. J., McWhirter, B. T., McWhirter, A. M., & McWhirter, E. H. (1998*). At-risk youth: A comprehensive response* (2nd ed.). Pacific Grove, CA: Brooks/Cole.

Metropolitan Area Child Study Research Group. (2002). A cognitive-ecological approach to preventing aggression in urban settings: Initial outcomes for high-risk children. *Journal of Consulting and Clinical Psychology, 70,* 179–194.

Meuer, T., Seymour, A., & Wallace, H. (2001). Domestic violence. In A. Seymour, M. Murray, J. Sigmon, M. Hook, C. Edmunds, M. Gaboury, & G. Coleman (Eds.), *National victim assistance academy textbook* (chap. 9). Retrieved September 30, 2003 from Department of Justice Office of Victims of Crime website: *http://www.ojp.usdoj.gov/ovc/ assist/nvaa2002/chapter9.html.*

Mrazek, P. J., & Haggerty, R. J. (1994). *Reducing risks for mental disorders: Frontiers for preventive intervention research.* Washington, DC: National Academy Press.

Nash, J. K., Fraser, M. W., Galinsky, M., & Kupper, L. (2003). Early development and pilot-testing of a problem-solving skills-training program for children. *Research on Social Work Practice, 13,* 432–450.

National Institute of Mental Health. (1998). *Priorities for prevention research at NIMH.* Retrieved September 30, 2003 from: *http://www.nimh.nih.gov/research/priorrpt/index.htm.*

Northen, H., & Kurland, R. (2001). *Social work with groups* (3rd ed.). New York: Columbia University Press.

Office of Juvenile Justice and Delinquency Prevention. (2001). Blueprints for violence prevention. *Juvenile Justice Bulletin.* Retrieved September 30, 2003 from: *http://www.ncjrs.org/pdffiles1/ojjdp/ 187079.pdf*

Peeks, A. L. (1999). Conducting a social skills group with Latina adolescents. *Journal of Child and Adolescent Group Therapy, 9,* 139–153.

Richey, C. A., Gillmore, M. R., Balassone, M. L., Gutiérrez, L., & Hartway, M. (1997). Developing and implementing a group skill training intervention to reduce AIDS risk among sexually active adolescents in detention. *Journal of HIV/AIDS Prevention and Education for Adolescents and Children, 1,* 71–103.

Richman, J. M., & Bowen, G. L. (1997). School failure: An ecological-interactional-developmental perspective. In M. W. Fraser (Ed.), *Risk and resilience in childhood: An ecological perspective* (pp. 95–116.). Washington, DC: NASW Press.

Rose, S. D. (1998). *Group therapy with troubled youth: A cognitive-behavioral interactive approach.* Thousand Oaks, CA: Sage.

Rosen, A., & Proctor, E. K. (Eds.). (2003). *Developing practice guidelines for social work interventions: Issues, methods, and research agenda.* New York: Columbia University Press.

Rutter, M. (2001). Psychosocial adversity: Risk, resilience and recovery. In J. M. Richman & M. W. Fraser (Eds.), *The context of youth violence: Resilience, risk, and protection* (pp. 13–41). Westport, CT: Praeger.

Spencer, M., Lewis, E., & Gutiérrez, L. (2000). Multicultural perspectives on direct practice in social work. In P. Allen-Meares, & C. Garvin (Eds.), *The handbook of social work direct practice* (pp. 131–149). Thousand Oaks, CA: Sage.

Toseland, R. W., & Rivas, R. F. (2001). *An introduction to group work practice* (4th ed.). Boston: Allyn & Bacon.

Tuckman, B. W., & Jensen, M. A. (1977). Stages of small group development revisited. *Group and Organization Studies, 2,* 419– 427.

U. S. Public Health Service. (2001). *Youth violence: A report of the U.S. Surgeon General.* Retrieved September 30, 2003 from: *http://www.surgeongeneral.gov/library/youthviolence/youvioreport.htm.*

Uehara, E., Sohng, S. L., Bending, R. L., Seyfried, S., Richey, C. A., Keenan, L., et al. (1996). Towards a values-based approach to multicultural social work research. *Social Work, 41,* 613–623.

Weisz, A. N., & Black, B. M. (2001). Evaluating a sexual assault and dating violence prevention program for urban youths. *Social Work Research, 25,* 89–100.

Werner, E. E. (1992). The children of Kauai: Resiliency and recovery in adolescence and adulthood. *Journal of Adolescent Health, 13,* 262–268.

Workman, S., & Brewer, A. (2002, May). *Teen parents: Collaborative programs that work.* Paper presented at the Building on Family Strengths Conference, Research and Training Center, Portland State University, Portland, OR.

Part IV

Group Work Approaches Related to Setting

As we stated in the introduction to this book, groups are offered in all of the kinds of agencies in which social workers are employed to directly help people having personal difficulties. Although some ways of working may be used with all groups, other ways are idiosyncratic to the kinds of problems addressed. Some models of practice may also be more effective with one type of problem than another. We have chosen for this section a set of fields of practice that we believe represents a broad array of types of practice and includes those that are most often written about and included in group work curricula.

In this section, therefore, we have asked writers who are experts in the use of group methods with particular populations to discuss the methods and models most appropriate for use with those populations. Some of these populations are defined by age of members and some by a type of problem. In addition, some categories, such as "involuntary groups," demonstrate how to work with several types of problems such as those experienced by inmates of prisons or by perpetrators of family violence.

The first chapter in this section (Chapter 11) focuses on groups for persons dealing with either mental or physical illness or both, as we believe that many mental illnesses relate to physical conditions and many physical conditions create emotional problems. In addition, there are some commonalities in ways of helping people who suffer from a disability, whether this disability is defined as "mental" or "physical."

Chapter 12 presents ways of working with involuntary group members. This is especially important for social workers who often serve group members who are "forced" to come to the group by the criminal justice system, the family, or an institution such as the school or workplace.

We have included two chapters that focus on service to children. Chapter 13 presents the ways that a highly creative practitioner and writer works with children who come to the group for such problems as recovering from trauma, functioning poorly in school, or lacking the skills to form peer relationships. Chapter 14 considers the creation of groups in the child welfare field to help children with such problems as child abuse or the breakup of their families.

Chapter 15 discusses the many approaches that have been created to help people overcome addiction to substances. Groups are the major form of service for substance abuse, and they are offered in many ways. Practice principles need to be further developed in this large field so that practitioners can choose the most effective modality for the type of substance problem experienced by individuals.

Similarly, most programs that serve older adults offer groups to meet many kinds of needs, and Chapter 16 presents this array of services. The last chapter in this section, Chapter 17, seeks to turn the attention of group workers to a topic that was important in the early history of group work, especially in community settings. This was the use of groups to help people who were involved in intergroup conflicts due to their ethnicity, national origins, race, religion, social class, or other attributes that can separate people. These kinds of conflicts occur throughout the world today and lead to a vast amount of human suffering. It is not an accident that the author of this chapter has been involved in helping Palestinian and Jewish youth in Israel to deal with conflict in nonviolent ways.

Chapter 11

Groups in Physical and Mental Health

GEORGE S. GETZEL

$\mathbf{A}$t the beginning of a new century, it is quite appropriate for the domain of this chapter to show disregard of the Cartesian mind–body dichotomy by simultaneously addressing health and mental health as a focus for social work with groups. The aforementioned historic separation reflected long-standing conceptual and proprietary issues that have been decisively challenged by biological research that has focused on the human brain and its complex biological-chemical-physical processes linked not only to gross motor and autonomic functions but also to the complex emotional and cognitive functioning long thought outside the range of vigorous scientific inquiry and applications (Haken, 1996).

Psychiatrists have begun to pay homage to the mental health consequences of physical illnesses, as evidenced by the new diagnostic category, described globally as "Psychological Factors Affecting Medical Conditions," found in the *Diagnostic and Statistical Manual of Mental Disorders* (American Psychiatric Association, 1994, p. 675). Psychological factors may worsen a medical condition and/or significantly influence the course of its treatment. Medical illnesses and their treatments may create emotional reactions and physiological stresses. Persons with preexisting psychiatric conditions may experience exacerbations of symptoms related to either medical or psychiatric conditions.

This chapter presents historical perspectives on perennial conceptual issues in social work practice with groups in health settings. The nature of contemporary group work practice is examined. A specific conceptual framework for social work practice within health care setting is delineated, emphasizing the concepts (1) uncertain conditions, (2) crisis situations, (3) identity concerns, and (4) redistributional justice. Extensive case illustrations are presented in support of the framework.

HISTORICAL PERSPECTIVES

Bartlett (1961), in her magisterial overview of social work in health care, forecasts the emerging importance of group work for medical social workers. The use of group work in health care, which was at first cautiously approached, gained momentum in hospitals and community-based health care settings in the 1960s. Similarly, group treatment has become a core modality in the treatment of severe mental illness, alcoholism, and behavioral disorders.

After Bartlett's opening to the group work method, Frey (1966) undertook the first comprehensive examination of the value and utility of group work in health care settings. Frey suggested that the nature and function of groups used by social workers arise out of the particular goals of hospitals and organizations under whose auspices the groups fall. Group workers need to develop a deeper understanding of the organizational processes of the settings that affect the well-being of patients (the older term used for consumers) and of the goals pursued by the health care systems that reflect the concerns of persons seeking assistance. The organizational context, referred to as the "outer group" by Homans (1950), becomes a crucial point of consideration and intervention in forming and developing the small group or the "inner group" led by a group worker in a health care setting.

The establishment of group work services in complex health care organizations entails coordinated activities identified by Schwartz (1961) as *parallel processes* to the ongoing activities of the members and the group as a whole. Staff and administrators (members of an outer group) are usually wary, if not suspicious, of consumers coming together to express their needs. The inner group's expression of need may be seen as unwanted criticism or annoying complaints by ill-tempered or ignorant consumers. The "buy in" by staff and relevant administrators is important to the eventual success of a group launched on a terrain of competing professional statuses and complicated bureaucratic rules and structures.

Despite the difficulties, the last four decades of the 20th century witnessed the increased use of group work, documented first by Rosenberg and Neil (1982). They noted, in their review of group work in health care settings between 1964 and 1978, an acceleration in the number of articles describing groups that serve people with specific disease entities, groups frequently co-led with a physician or nurse in hospital settings. Rosenberg and Neil excluded articles about group work in psychiatric or mental health settings, following the division noted earlier.

EMERGING PATTERNS OF GROUP WORK IN HEALTH SETTINGS

Getzel (1986), reviewing subsequent articles through the early 1980s, reaffirmed an increase of articles on groups in health care settings, despite the reticence of mainstream overviews of social work to acknowledge the presence of group work in health settings. In addition to traditional disease-focused groups co-led by social workers and other health care professionals, Getzel noted the emergence of groups that emphasized the reciprocal engagement of the health care systems to make them more responsive to consumers' needs and the creation of emotional support groups of ill persons and their caregivers.

Lonergan (1990) stated that group work in health care settings had a combination of purposes, including assisting participants with managing physical care, emotional difficulties, and social relations affected by medical conditions. Teamwork was an integral aspect of the successful use of groups in health care's interdisciplinary culture. Consumers benefited from group participation, as it supported members by buttressing their self-esteem and high-lighting health care providers' obligations to respond humanely to individual consumers.

Schopler and Galinsky (1990) saw groups as humanizing health care and giving a more holistic perspective to consumers' care, especially because health care had grown more tech-nologically and organizationally complex, often overwhelming consumers and providers alike. Contemporary health care was fragmented with a good deal of impersonality, which may in many instances be a sign of scientific objectivity and organizational efficiency. Health care in most instances is delivered by one specialist at a time to one patient; group process seldom is considered as an option or adjunct to the one-to-one service delivery. Schopler and Galinsky (1990) argued that group work allows for mutual aid and support and is a cost-efficient means of disseminating information to health care consumers and their loved ones.

MENTAL HEALTH GROUP WORK IN ISOLATION

Group work in psychiatric settings was viewed as fertile ground in the 1950s (Konopka, 1990; Levine, 1990). Education for group workers in graduate schools typically emphasized developmental enhancement and citizen participation consonant with students' presence in settlement houses, community centers, and other community-based agencies. Historically, psychiatric settings were the domain and specialization of casework. Psychiatric work had an great appeal engendered by social work theorists' infatuations with Freud and Rank. The few early group workers in psychiatric settings had to contend with caseworkers and other professionals who were doing group work despite not having been trained in it. This devel-opment created ideological and turf-based schisms between group work and group psycho-therapy.

The challenge for group work theory in the 1960s was to define method in such a man-ner that it encompassed practice in mental health settings. Vinter (1985) presciently articu-lated that group work must use concepts from the social sciences and psychology to address social problems such as juvenile delinquency, substance abuse, and domestic violence. He saw dysfunctional behaviors embedded in social relations that become targets for change through the power and scope of carefully constructed small-group experience and extra-group interventions. Vinter and his associates at the University of Michigan began the simul-taneous tasks of theory building and experimentation (Sundel, Glasser, Sarri, & Vinter, 1985). Their approach followed a vigorous design that entailed careful intake, a thorough assessment of individual members and of the identified target behaviors to be changed, and a sequencing of interventions using the specific characteristics of group processes, such as cohesion, norms, decision making, and activities to change behaviors, as contracted early with members.

This framework was variously called the Michigan School approach, the remedial ap-proach, and the rehabilitative and prevention approach. It remains a very useful perspective for its broad applications and the specificity of its concepts and practice prescriptions. Eval-uation research is an integral aspect of its philosophy. Cognitive-behavioral approaches fit easily into the framework. It can be readily applied to problems of health and mental health (Rose, 1990b). The reciprocal, or interactionist, approach was conceptualized by William Schwartz (1961, 1994), and its more generalized character presaged the issues of health and groups in terms now associated with holistic health concepts and environmental medicine. Schwartz (1994) argued that all human beings, in interaction with all living creatures, seek symbiotic union for their immediate survival and well-being and, on a grander scale, that a species' survival over time is dependent on its ecological fit with other living things. The group itself is a means and context for participants to find health, belongingness, and growth. Schwartz's ideas continue to influence a range of practitioners, theorists, and teachers (Gitterman & Shulman, 1994).

A REVIEW OF GROUP WORK PRACTICE AND HEALTH

Because there has been so much innovation and turbulence in health care, abetted by rapid changes in medical technology and in the organization of health care delivery and its funding, it is useful to look at the group work literature in health care to note emphases and trends. From even a selective examination of the growing professional literature, it is clear that considerable evidence shows the creative of use of groups in addressing medical conditions and mental illness. The majority of articles examined came from journals specific to social work and group work.

Disease-specific groups continued to be a focus of the literature on group work in health care. For example, sickle-cell disease groups for adults (Butler & Beltran, 1993) were strongly recommended for persons with this as yet incurable, painful, life-threatening condition, even though more attention has been given traditionally to support and psychoeducational groups for children, adolescents, and family caregivers. The group foci were patient education, support, and task-oriented activities. The themes in the group included death anxiety, social isolation, questions of dependency on drugs, and problems with family and health care providers. Sickle-cell groups were a growing phenomenon (Kramer & Nash, 1995). Adolescents with sickle-cell disease may come to groups to learn about the disease, but long-time attenders tend to use groups to work on personal problems and learn to skills and strategies to deal with difficult life experiences (Telfair & Gardner, 2000).

Cwikel and Behar (1999), in their review of outcome studies of psychosocial intervention with cancer patients, found individual and group interventions equally helpful, more so during the treatment phase than at terminal stage, as did Glajchen & Magen (1995) on the outcomes of community cancer support groups. Duhatschek-Krause (1989) discussed a support-group-work model for patients with life-threatening illnesses. Group members focused on strategies of coping with existential concerns, similar to analyses of groups of persons with end-stage AIDS/HIV symptoms and disease (Getzel, 1991; Getzel & Mahony, 1991).

Folzer (2001) saw the importance of group work with mildly brain-injured patients to learn psycho-social skills that could be practiced in the group. The safety of the peer environment allowed for greater candor about symptoms and functional disabilities. Avery (1998) advocated on behalf of groups composed of women with severe mental illness to introduce a feminist perspective to counter the deleterious effects of the medical model and the isolation and oppression of women. Special groups for young women with early onset Parkinson's disease have been started (Posen et al., 2000).

Bond and De Graaf-Kaser (1990) reviewed the relative merit of groups in the rehabilitation and treatment of persons with profound mental illness on a fourfold matrix of natural versus artificial/sheltered environments and experiential versus structured group formats. They stated that systematic research on traditional group therapy, education groups, self-help groups, and skill-building groups is rare.

Camblin, Stone, Merritt, and De Graaf-Kaser (1990) wrote that group work with persons living with chronic mental illness should focus on socialization, problem solving, and controlling emotional expressions in verbal exchanges in the group. Garvin (1992) argued that deinstitutionalization of persons with chronic illness lent itself to testing a task-centered group work approach. There is significant research support for the use of groups that have structured interventions and a time-limited format with this population. The classical task-centered model emphasizes on goal formulation and attainment and behaviorally specific outcomes.

Moore and Starkes (1992) saw the use of group work with mentally ill individuals who were in institutions for short stays as beneficial in that it maximized their use of available services in the setting. Group work was identified as an antidote for the toxic effects of a total institutional environment in a similar way to that recommended by Glassman (1991). Groups simultaneously provide a therapeutic milieu for solving extant psychosocial problems and serve as points of contact for patients to address problems they are experiencing in the institutional environment. The skills of environmental competence and upward and outward influence learned by group members better prepares them for reentry into the community.

Roberts and Smith (1994) felt that groups created a sense of community in the psychiatric ward and prepared patients better for adaptation to the external community. Lee and Gaucher (2000) described a comprehensive program using intensive group work interventions with adolescents dually diagnosed as developmentally disabled and mentally ill; an evaluation indicated significant improvements in social skills.

Armstrong (1990) wrote of the benefit of groups that focused on future plans, practical concerns, and available resources in assisting the discharge of patients in acute psychiatric inpatient units; this method differs from that of discharge groups with chronically impaired patients that heavily focus on feelings of separation and loss. Miller and Mason (1998) described the sensitive use of group work with clients who experience their first episodes of schizophrenia. Grillo-Di Demenico (1990) advocated for educational groups to assist chronically mentally ill persons with occupational issues.

The use of cognitive approaches in groups has been a major theme over the past 10 years. Albert (1994) strongly recommended, for chronically mentally ill older adults, the use of cognitive therapy groups that used techniques that challenged members' self-degrading images of themselves as mentally ill. Agencies were seen as reinforcing negative self-concepts by suppressing the discussion of mental illness and its stigma. Cognitive techniques were judged as consonant with support and socialization in the group (Rose, 1990a).

Rose (1990b) persuasively argued for the integration of careful exposure experiences to high-anxiety situations into the group as a whole and for group discussion using cognitive interventions for the treatment of agoraphobia. Strong empirical validation for the approach was noted. Fisher (1995) stated that cognitive-behavioral approaches optimized results in an outpatient setting and that a combination of disease-recovery and cognitive-behavioral approaches was more effective in an inpatient setting. Rittner and Smyth (1999) developed cognitive-behavioral groups for suicidal adolescents that focused on contracting, identifying triggers for depressive/suicidal ideations, engaging in writing exercises (postcards to the group), and group decision making and activities. Rhodes (1995) recommended an educational group format for young children in addictive families who are often overlooked and are at multiple risk for emotional problems and substance abuse. Cognitive-behavioral techniques have become the primary tools used in AIDS/HIV prevention groups with different populations at risk of infection or reinfection (Hackl, Somlai, Kelly, & Kalichman, 1997; Pomeroy, Rubin, Van Laningham, & Walker, 1997; Roffman et al., 1997).

Earnshaw(1991) recommended cognitive-behavioral groups for adults on probation in England who volunteered to participate in a community center program focused on skill building and resocialization. The initial emphasis of the program and the groups was self-image, which has been replaced by the here-and-now addressing of lapses in thinking and reasoning as adults that place the group members at risk for recidivism. This corresponds to the experience of the use of group work in a probation program for young, violence-prone male offenders in New York City (Goodman, Getzel, & Ford, 1996).

The AIDS movement continued to make varied use of groups: groups that use a narrative approach (Dean, 1995); groups for persons who are HIV positive (Greene, McVinney, & Addams, 1993); telephone support groups (Heckman et al., 1999); groups in a homeless shelter (Mancoske & Lindhorst, 1991) and in a pediatric clinic (Mayers & Spiegel, 1992); and groups for women (Edell, 1998).

Specific strategies in groups with regressed populations were noted in the literature. Ryan and Doubleday (1995) described the difficulties in providing mental health services to isolated, depressed elderly and recommended the establishment of support groups with a socialization function and a topical psychoeducational emphasis. With time and determined professional guidance, such groups can take on a therapeutic character. Group members empower themselves and make demands on the worker to address more long-term emotional and personal concerns.

Lynn and Nisivoccia (1995) wrote that little emphasis was placed on the use of program activities with persons with chronic mental illness and suggested that group activities are useful because they can be built into time-limited groups that avoid insight techniques. Simple group activities enhance socialization skills and positive feedback. Schnekenburger (1995) reviewed her work with a poetry writing group that was successfully launched in a residence for persons with chronic mental illness, noting its benefits for members and the general community.

Walsh, Richardson, and Cardey (1991) recommended the use of structured fantasy approaches in working with emotionally disturbed children who had severe cognitive and social impairments; they made use of creative drama, videotaping, and playback discussions. Craig (1990) demonstrated the value of group work with children who survived sexual abuse and who moved from a sense of being victims to seeing themselves as survivors. Tutty and Wagar (1994) developed a structured group work approach for children who have witnessed family violence that used storybooks that addressed themes such as divorce, fighting, and anger, as well as creative drama with video-feedback discussion. Schamess (1990) saw the importance of integrating family treatment and group work intervention in working with children at risk; he started a group for children who were reacting to their parents' divorces and/or separations, using their genograms and a mother–child group for single teenagers and their infants to challenge dysfunctional interactions.

Finzi and Stange (1997) developed an innovative short-term group intervention for children with adjustment problems related to having parents with mental illness.

Group work in special settings continued to be a focus of the literature. Wolozin and Dalton (1990) developed a group for men who were separated from their families in a maximum security prison. Richman (1990) emphasized the importance of group support for staff and volunteers in hospice settings who face the serial deaths of consumers. In addition, groups are central in enhancing teamwork, volunteer training, and coordinating multidisciplinary practitioners in their demanding work. He suggested the value of bringing in an outside consultant to lead staff support groups in a hospice in order to provide comfort and safety in discussing personally identified issues and concerns. Forte, Barrett, and Campbell (1996) evaluated a bereavement group for staff members as positively helping participants reconnect to their social networks and lowering their incidents of grief. Similar recommendations were made for staff and volunteers in AIDS programs (Cushman, Evans, & Namerow, 1995; Garside, 1993; Grossman & Silverstein, 1993)

Another area of growing interest was groups for caregivers. McCallion and Toseland (1995) researched the effects of groups for caregivers of the frail elderly. Morris and Woods (1992) analyzed the research on the benefits of both educational and problem-solving groups for caregivers of persons with Alzheimer's disease and related dementias. Support groups for partners of adult survivors of sexual abuse (Reid, Mathews, & Liss, 1995) were organized out of the recognition that partners were themselves secondary victims who provided caregiving to primary victims. Parker, Hutchinson, and Berry (1995) developed a support group for family members of personnel in the Persian Gulf War in 1991.

There have been many reports of groups for couples, other family members, and caregivers of persons living with and affected by HIV/AIDS (Ball, 1998; Edell, 1998; Hayes, McConnell, Nardozzi, & Mullican, 1998; Livingston, 1996; Moore, 1998) Support groups for caregivers of persons with AIDS, connected through telephone conference calls, were successfully conducted with members spread throughout urban and rural areas of North Carolina (Meier, Galinsky, & Rounds, 1995) and elsewhere (Weiner, 1998; Weiner, Spencer, Davidson, & Fair, 1993).

From this review of the most recent literature, it is clear that group work has moved to the center of practice attention in a number of areas of health care. Practice skills with groups have become an absolute requisite for work with people in health settings. Societal interest in conditions that affect subpopulations, such as HIV/AIDS, breast and ovarian cancers, and sickle-cell disease, has made these conditions major foci, which may reflect social workers' commitment to oppressed and underserved populations. It would be important in the future to point out conceptual and practical bridges between disease-specific group work efforts.

Group workers must follow changes in health technologies that have profound effects on the well-being of people. Whether it be new medications, testing procedures for biological abnormalities, surgical techniques, or treatment protocols, the use of group work to assist persons to understand technologies and to make informed choices becomes critical. Consumers' sense of well-being can be enhanced by peer groups that identify decision-making options and the consequences of actions. Such groups blend education and advocacy objectives.

Paradoxically, as more complicated health-related technologies develop, so also do the self-care and mutual aid requirements for consumers and related kin in home health care. Groups that reinforce self-care as part of aftercare and that support family caregivers will continue to grow in importance as the duration of stays in health care facilities decrease.

The centrality of group work in treatment programs for the persistently mentally ill and persons with histories of substance abuse is clearly established. The emergence of group work in community-based programs for these populations must grow in sophistication through enhanced professionalization of service providers and the design of group services. Social workers with groups can play a significant role in training staff members who work with consumers during acute episodes and in aftercare-recovery programs.

The health care consequences of trauma and the use of groups have been clearly established over the past 20 years; unfortunately, violence in communities and in the world will call for even wider use of group support strategies. Finally, the worldwide phenomenon of aging populations in developed countries presents special challenges for group workers to enhance the psychosocial well-being of elders living into their 80s and beyond who are coping with multiple disabling conditions and chronic illnesses.

UNIFIED APPROACH TO GROUP WORK FOR HEALTH CARE

A unified approach to group work consists of a formulation with common concepts to assist the practitioner in working fluidly with group members on problems that historically have been defined as either medical or psychiatric. A unified approach should address those cross-cutting situations, such as emotional reactions to physical illness. A useful conceptual formulation should encompass the characteristics of a variety of illnesses and disabling conditions encountered in institutional environments and community-based settings. Finally, an effective unified approach should address the complexities of medical technologies and their consequences to consumers, kinship systems, and communities.

I argue that there are specific variables that merit attention in considering the membership of groups in health care. The interpenetrated variables of (1) uncertain conditions, (2) crisis situations, (3) identity concerns, and (4) redistributional justice options are proposed as vital in thinking about and forming groups. People typically are drawn to each other as they face conditions of uncertainty and search for cognitive, instrumental, and emotional guidance. When uncertainty reaches overwhelming proportions, it becomes a crisis. Typically, a crisis entails the breakdown in predictable patterns of adaptation to the inner and external environments. Behavioral responses and available environmental resources are not available, and people become vulnerable to crisis reactions. A diagnosis of cancer, the onset of major depression, or posttraumatic stress reactions to a terrorist attack are events that incur crisis responses, which typically involve strong shifts in emotions, thoughts, and behaviors.

The emergence of identity questions, simply described as confusions about a person's sense of self, are confounded by health-related crises and alterations in how persons are now treated by kin, friends, neighbors, health providers, and others. Identity questions may be short term or transitory in the case of acute illness (a child hospitalized for dehydration from a respiratory infection) or more serious in cases of chronic illness (a young adult diagnosed with schizophrenia and hospitalized three times for suicide attempts).

Identity concerns are evident in cases of profound shifts of experience to what Viktor Frankl (1984) has called the "existential triad" of illness, dying, and meaninglessness. The encounter with highly charged life-threatening experiences transports the person irrevocably to another psychic place; life will never be the same. The security and predictability of everyday life vanishes or is greatly diminished. It is as if one is forcibly expelled from one country into a strange new one. Being placed on a hemodialysis machine after kidney failure or losing an adult child in the collapse of the World Trade Center are examples of life-altering existential encounters.

In summary, when persons share crisis events that create identity concerns and point to underlying boundary conditions, the use of groups is vital and has special allure and utility for consumers and providers in health care settings and contexts. The need for groups is seeded and grown in the rich soil of uncertainty; groups positively thrive with gentle doses of conflict, controversy, and contradiction. If you grow anxious about uncertain conditions, you will reach out to others for data and for emotional support. For example, if your immune system is compromised by HIV or diabetes, and you are told that you are ineligible for smallpox injections in anticipation of biological attack by terrorists, what do you do? What are your options? Will your needs be addressed? Will your voice be heard? Boundary changes also raise important questions about the goodness of environments in which group members live and how fairly people are treated by organizations, governments, and others in society. Group members may find common cause in inequities and choose to empower themselves by seeking options for redistributional justice.

IMPLICATIONS FOR THE FORMATION
OF GROUPS IN HEALTH CARE

Pregroup planning for groups has been amply discussed over the past 20 years (Kurland, 1978), and its relevance for health care groups is no less significant. According to Kurland, group work practitioners should give special attention to group purpose, shared needs, agency context, structure, content, and salient composition factors.

Uncertainty or a health crisis can bring together diverse people who have shared concerns. Such groups may be short term or of longer duration and often allow for heterogeneity because stressors may mitigate segregating factors such as age, race, class, and ethnicity. Cognitive groups can provide health information and can focus more on content than group process. Short-term groups are often the only practical format in complex health settings that emphasize shorter stays. Community support groups may be long term, with stability of membership over time. The need to overcome attendant fears of illness or disability was vividly exemplified by groups of persons who saw the growing HIV/AIDS pandemic in large urban centers more than 20 years ago or of postal workers who saw colleagues become ill from an anthrax attack spread through the mail system in Washington, D.C.

Groups that provide education, abet the prevention of illness, provide support for the ill and their families, and incur social action in behalf of consumers naturally come to mind. The technology for treating and preventing illness and disease is a key consideration in the design of group work services in health care. Consumers must develop the skills and the understanding to use and benefit from the diagnostic and treatment potential of complex medical technologies. Compliance and benefits from drugs for mental illness, chemotherapies for cancers, or antiviral treatments for HIV of necessity entail the engagement of consumers and providers in a variety of formal and informal group interactions. Groups can support the mutually beneficial collaboration of providers and consumers together or in separate and coordinated efforts. Groups to educate consumers about disease prevention and treatment brings providers and consumers closer together.

Consumers in their own groups can learn how to support each other and more effectively deal with health providers. Providers in their own groups can seek out support in handling the stresses of dealing with the vicarious trauma of serving very ill and dying patients. Family members who take on critical caregiving roles need group education about illness and treatment, as well as peer support, in caring for a demented older spouse or a child with a life-threatening blood disorder. Variation of group composition and membership must be related to group purpose and members' special needs. Health settings also lend themselves to short-duration groups (Ebenstein, 1998; Gladstone & Reynolds, 1997), as well ones of longer duration. The problems in health care require a variety of groups with coordinated functions in institutional, as well as community-based agencies and contexts. The content of groups flows from need and purpose and may involve discussion, activities, audiovisual material, telephone links, and computer-assisted group and group-like experiences.

EXAMPLES FROM THE WORLD OF PRACTICE

The following cases illustrate the central characteristics of group work in health care in contemporary practice context in what have previously been called medical and mental health settings. Although these characteristics of group work in health care may appear at any time in the life of a group, the examples to follow approximate the phases of beginnings, middles, and endings. Practice challenges and skill demands are noted.

Uncertain Conditions

Uncertainty typically is expressed during the beginning phase of a group, but it may occur at any time in group development. Group members during this phase express deep ambivalence about being in a group and about what they may learn about themselves and from each other and the worker. Rather than confront uncertainty in their lives, they may wish to protect themselves against anxiety through simple denial. The group worker should encourage the explorations of group conflicts as problems for the members to solve together, thus avoiding the tendency to become the professional expert and mentor (unwitting savior of a seemingly floundering group). The group members may want the group worker's expertise and then angrily reject it.

In the following case of a group of adults with chronic mental illness, the group worker assists members with uncertain conditions that create conflict in the group itself and some anger directed at him in an unexpected way.

The incident occurred after Paul returned to the group after a hospitalization for a suicide attempt. Members of the group seemed to avoid mention of Paul's absence and instead engaged in an intense discussion about whether medication works well for people with depression. Paul asked, in a light, casual way, if the discussion was boring to the social worker. Other group members stopped and stared at the worker, who became self-conscious and sweaty. Looking at Paul and the other group members, the worker said, "The group seems to be reacting to Paul's important question to me."

In defense of the social worker, another member, Mary, said that one did not need to be mentally ill or hospitalized to lead the group. The worker indicated that this might be so but wondered if Paul and other group members might feel differently. An intense discussion ensued in which Paul talked about his anger at himself for trying to kill himself and his distrust of anyone who had not suffered severe depression. Some members, while defending the worker, acknowledged their jealousy toward others who were not troubled or who showed no sympathy for people living with mental illness. A little while later in the process, the worker helped members discuss their feelings about Paul's recent hospitalization and their fears of the same.

During the next session, the worker found the opportunity to say that, on reflecting on the previous session, he wondered if it was all right for the group to be angry or distrusting of the worker for not being a patient with a history of serious mental illness. Larry, a fairly outspoken member, said that the worker should not give himself so much credit; that maybe the group would drive the worker insane. Amid good-natured laughter, Linda said that the group would have to decide whether the worker was crazy enough to join them. More laughter ensued.

Crisis Situations

The social worker must see the group members as capable of accepting crisis situations that arise among the membership, avoiding an overprotective stance. To the extent that the social worker encourages members to discuss how they have handled similar situations, group-as-a-whole mutual aid will be encouraged instead of flight behavior, taking the form of facile advice-giving on a one-to-one basis. Mutual interaction is more apt to occur and to be effectively addressed after a group has passed through the issues of formation and beginning. It is important to point out themes that reflect emotions and ideas shared by the members and to assist the group in identifying the universality of their plight. A crisis presented by one member is understood by others in the group in a more profound way. A crisis may belie existential issues too painful to address fully at that particular time but that are apt to be raised at future sessions. The group displays several gestures of mutual aid.

A crisis situation was revealed in a group of women living with AIDS when Mary, in a tearful, agitated manner, told the other members that she had been diagnosed with cervical cancer and would be hospitalized the next day. Mary told the group that she did not care whether she lived or died and felt shame for what would happen to her two young children. Shaking convulsively, Mary wept, saying that she had not planned for guardianship after her husband died 6 months previously.

Joan held Mary, and the group began telling Mary that they were very worried about her. Tanya said that she used a lawyer from the agency when she panicked during a recent hospitalization. The group worker told the group that it seemed very hard to make a will and guardian provisions. Joan said that people just don't want to think about dying but that one has to be realistic, concluding, "Better late than never." The group then began a discussion about how, after being diagnosed, they have grown more responsible in thinking about their children.

Identity Concerns

The theme of identity shifts emerges in groups that consist of people who have serious illness or have encountered profound trauma. Identity concerns tied to health conditions or a stigmatized status in society occur routinely in support and treatment groups of consumers. Groups are powerful vehicles for learning from other members how you are perceived by others (interpersonal learning input) and how to behave differently (interpersonal learning output); Yalom (1995) had identified these as therapeutic factors deemed most important by group members in treatment groups. Groups that have developed strong cohesion and patterns of mutual aid can more openly address identity questions.

In a mental health program for isolated adolescents, identity concerns are normative and especially overwhelming for a transgendered young man who simultaneously must cope with questions of gender and sexual orientation. A group of gay and lesbian youths becomes a safe context in which to begin the tentative exploration of these issues and the attendant emotions of confusion, alienation, anger, and sadness when identity is not supported by others.

Malcolm came to the group looking very depressed and unkempt, a significant change from his usual appearance. The group members disregarded him for the first 15 minutes of the session. The group took on a somber tone when the group worker noted that Malcolm was uncharacteristically quiet. In defense of him, Meg angrily told the worker that Malcolm would talk when and if he wished. Leonardo broke through the group's silence by attacking Meg for protecting Malcolm. Leonardo said, "Other guys will continue to attack Malcolm if he does not stand up for himself and quit acting like a fag. You look for trouble wearing eye makeup."

Malcolm said that he regretted bothering the group but cryptically indicated that no one should worry because he intended to quit high school or "do something else." Several members became quite concerned and asked him what he meant. The social worker intervened, saying that he, too, was concerned not only with what Malcolm was saying but with how he was saying it. Malcolm cried. Other members took hold of his hands after he wiped tears and mascara off his cheeks.

The worker, directing himself to the group as a whole, asked what was going on with members after Malcolm shared his pain. This started a discussion about a magnet school for gay and lesbian youths who cannot make it in regular high school. It was not clear whether Malcolm was listening, as he sat quietly in his chair.

Redistributional Justice Options

The application of the principles of social justice for a group begins when they have sufficient group solidarity and problem-solving capacity, allowing thinking that extends outside the boundary of the group to the external environment. The group members demonstrate an interest in and capacity for acting in behalf of their collective interests with social entities seen as affecting them as individuals and as a collectivity. A growing sense of injustice arises from the operation of other social systems. Group members make choices based on their evolving concept of social justice. Their choice as a group might be to support an aggrieved member or for the group as a whole to join a coalition advocating a common cause. Any action by the group would inevitably involve the group worker with the politics of his or her social agency (Getzel, 2003).

An example of a support group developing a social action focus occurred in a group of parents of children who had been victims of homicide. The mothers asked for a separate group to address their specific concerns as oppressed survivors of this horrific tragedy. Over time, they identified with the powerful image within the group. They later were moved to engage government representatives about their concerns.

The group frequently discussed how their children's bodies looked after the murders. Some mothers suffered because they were unable to have their children in open caskets.

This central group image of mothers of murdered children gave courage to the women to offer testimony before the state legislature. They succeeded in getting the legislature to pass an appropriation subsidizing mental health services to family survivors of homicide. The mothers argued that this was reparation for the government's failure to protect their children.

FUTURE DIRECTIONS

Rapid changes in health care technology and the organization of health service delivery now and in the future will determine the shape of group work services and programs. Advances in biological research will make ever-changing requirements on consumers for knowledge and cooperation to reap the benefits of new treatments, which in turn will affect the quantity and quality of the lives of beneficiaries and their loved ones. Groups for education and the engagement of consumers are likely to multiply, with interdisciplinary leadership in both institutional and community-based health environments. For economic and technological reasons, treatment will continue to grow in outpatient settings and in consumers' homes. Family caregiving will be an integral aspect of this trend; thus the need for support for kin and kith assisting in the care of others.

Genetic testing can anticipate hereditary diseases such as Huntington's disease, forms of breast cancer, and other serious disabling and life-threatening illnesses. Advances in genetic testing will pose profound choices for couples contemplating having children; once again, groups will be needed for education, support, and psychologically sound decision making.

Although medical advances can relieve human pain and suffering, they also can do the reverse by keeping persons alive who are in pain with no hope of recovery. Groups have a great deal of potential to help consumers with the overwhelming emotional task of writing advance directives (medical proxies, living wills, powers of attorney, etc.). Family members with decision-making authority for a relative or friend who is no longer competent to make medical decisions on his or her own may need individual and group support.

The growing proportion of persons living into late life will require a blending of social supports and health care in assisted living environments and in private residences. Group work programs for the frail elderly in day programs and institutions is an important growing area of activity. The cultural diversity of the aging population will require group workers to be sensitive to ethnic, gender, and lifestyle differences of members of groups. Workers will need to provide group support in settings such as nursing homes and hospices or during events of large-scale death (natural disasters, wars, or terrorist attacks).

Community-based programs for persons with physical and psychological disabilities present daunting challenges to the group worker for outreach and engagement. The obstacles to overcome are overwhelming: scarce health and human resources and the additional social problems of homelessness, substance abuse, domestic violence, and HIV/AIDS. There is a strong need for innovative, low-threshold individual and group services to engage people who fall below the safety net of entitlements and traditional services. Useful technologies via computer links hold the promise of opening group ties and enhanced communication for the homebound and the disabled in the community.

Group workers must begin to see the recovery movement (Alcoholics Anonymous and sister fellowships) as a resource in their work with persons with a variety of addictions and find ways to integrate recovery groups and their principles into their practice as appropriate. Groups with a spiritual/religious emphasis should be considered as a form of complementary care. Group workers would be wise to renew an emphasis on nonverbal activities to reach verbally inaccessible and ego-impoverished consumers.

Finally, the potential of group work in health care to address social justice issues is of great importance at a time when the federal government has eviscerated health and human resources and state and local governments are desperate to balance budgets at the expense of the poor and sick. In the years ahead, the practice of group work in health care must be synonymous with a concept of social justice. Without broad participation in the quest for social justice, personal healing and human solidarity withers and dies. No greater challenge confronts social workers with groups today.

REFERENCES

Albert, J. (1994). Rethinking difference: A cognitive therapy group for chronic mental patients. *Social Work with Groups, 17,* 105–121.

American Psychiatric Association. (1994). *Diagnostic and statistical manual of mental disorders* (4th ed.). Washington, DC: Author.

Armstrong, K. (1990). The discharge issues group: A model for acute psychiatric inpatient units. *Social Work with Groups, 13,* 93–103.

Avery, L. (1998). A feminist perspective on group work with severely mentally ill women. *Women and Therapy, 21,* 1–14.

Ball, S. (1998). A time-limited group model for HIV-negative gay men. *Journal of Gay and Lesbian Social Services, 8,* 23–42.

Bartlett, H. M. (1961). *Social work practice in health care.* New York: National Association of Social Workers.

Bond, G. R., & De Graaf-Kaser, R. (1990). Group approaches for persons with severe mental illness: A typology. *Social Work with Groups, 13,* 21–35.

Butler, D. J., & Beltran, L. R. (1993). Functions of an adult sickle cell group: Education, task orientation, and support. *Health and Social Work, 18,* 49–56.

Camblin, L. M., Stone, W. N., Merritt, L., & De Graaf-Kaser, R. (1990). An adaptive approach to group therapy for the chronic patient. *Social Work with Groups, 13,* 21–36.

Craig, E. (1990). Starting the journey: Enhancing the therapeutic elements of groupwork for adolescent female child sexual abuse victims. *Groupwork, 3,* 103–117.

Cushman, L. F., Evans, P., & Namerow, P. B. (1995). Occupational stress among AIDS social service providers, *Social Work in Health Care, 21,* 115–131.

Cwikel, J. G., & Behar, L. C. (1999). Social work with adult cancer patients: A vote-count review of intervention research. *Social Work in Health Care, 29,* 39–67.

Dean, R. G. (1995). Stories of AIDS: The use of narrative as an approach to understanding in an AIDS support group. *Clinical Social Work Journal, 23,* 287–304.

Duhatschek-Krause, A. L. (1989). A support group for patients and families facing life-threatening illness: Finding a solution to non-being. *Social Work with Groups, 12,* 55–69.

Earnshaw, J. (1991). Evolution and accountability: Ten years of groups in a day centre for offenders. *Groupwork, 4,* 231–239.

Ebenstein, H. (1998). Single-session groups: Issues for social workers. *Social Work with Groups, 21,* 49–60.

Edell, M. (1998). Replacing community: Establishing linkages for women living with HIV/AIDS: A group work approach. *Social Work with Groups, 21,* 49–62.

Finzi, R., & Stange, D. (1997). Short term group intervention as a means of improving the adjustment of children of mentally ill parents. *Social Work with Groups, 20,* 69–80.

Fisher, M. S. (1995). Group therapy protocols for persons with personality disorders who abuse substances: Effective treatment alternatives. *Social Work with Groups, 18,* 71–89.

Folzer, S. M. (2001). Group psychotherapy with "mild" brain-injured adults. *American Journal of Orthopsychiatry, 71,* 245–251.

Forte, J. A., Barrett, A. V., & Campbell, M. H. (1996). Patterns of social connectedness and shared grief work: A symbolic interactionist perspective, *Social Work with Groups, 19,* 29–51.

Frankl, V. E. (1984). *Man's search for meaning: An introduction to logotherapy* (3rd ed.). New York: Simon & Schuster.

Frey, L. A. (1966). *Uses of groups in the health field.* New York: National Association of Social Workers.

Garside, B. (1993). Physicians mutual aid group: A response to AIDS-related burnout. *Health and Social Work, 18,* 259–267.

Garvin, C. (1992). A task centered group approach to work with the chronically mentally ill. *Social Work with Groups, 15,* 67–81.

Getzel, G. S. (1986). Social work groups in health care setting: Four emerging approaches. *Social Work in Health Care, 12,* 23–38.

Getzel, G. S. (1991). Survival modes of people with AIDS in groups. *Social Work, 36*, 7–11.

Getzel, G. S. (2003). Group work and social justice: Rhetoric or action. In N. E. Sullivan, E. S. Mesbur, N. C. Lang, D. Goodman, & L. Mitchell (Eds.), *Social work with groups: Social justice through personal, community and social change* (pp. 53–64). New York: Haworth Press.

Getzel, G. S., & Mahony, K. (1991). Confronting human finitude: Group work with people with AIDS. *Journal of Gay and Lesbian Psychotherapy, 1*, 105–120.

Gitterman, A., & Shulman, L. (1994). *Mutual aid groups: Vulnerable populations and the life cycle.* New York: Columbia University Press.

Gladstone, J., & Reynolds, T. (1997). Single session group work intervention in response to employee stress during workforce transition. *Social Work with Groups, 20*, 33–51.

Glajchen, M., & Magen, R. (1995). Evaluating process, outcome and satisfaction in community-based cancer support groups. *Social Work with Groups, 18*, 27–40.

Glassman, U. (1991). The social work group and its distinct healing qualities in the health care setting. *Health and Social Work, 16*, 203–212.

Goodman, H. G., Getzel, G. S., & Ford, W. (1996). Group work with high-risk urban youths on probation. *Social Work, 41*, 337–432.

Greene, D. C., McVinney, L. D., & Addams, S. (1993). Strengths in transition: Professionally facilitated HIV support groups and the development of client symptomatology. *Social Work with Groups, 16*, 41–54.

Grillo-DiDemenico. (1990). An educational occupational issues group for the chronic psychiatric patient. *Social Work with Groups, 13*, 113–127.

Grossman, A. H., & Silverstein, C. (1993). Facilitating support groups for professionals working with people with AIDS. *Social Work, 38*, 144–151.

Hackl, K. L., Somlai, A. M., Kelly, J. A., & Kalichman, S. C. (1997). Women living with HIV/AIDS: The dual challenge of being a patient and a caregiver. *Health and Social Work, 22*, 53–62.

Haken, H. (1996). *Principles of brain functioning: A synergetic approach to brain activity, behavior and cognition.* New York: Springer.

Hayes, M. A., McConnell, S. C., Nardozzi, J. A., & Mullican, R. J. (1998). Family and friends of people with HIV/AIDS support group. *Social Work with Groups, 21*, 35–47.

Heckman, T. G., Kalichman, S. C., Roffman, R. R., Sikkema, K. J., Heckman, B. D., & Somali, A. M. (1999). A telephone-delivered coping improvement intervention for persons living with HIV/AIDS in rural areas. *Social Work with Groups, 21*, 49–61.

Homans, G. C. (1950). *The human group.* New York: Harcourt Brace.

Konopka, G. (1990) Thirty-five years of group work in psychiatric settings (Part 2). *Social Work with Groups, 13*, 13–15.

Kramer, K. D., & Nash, K. B. (1995). The unique social ecology of groups: Findings from groups for African Americans affected by sickle cell disease. *Social Work with Groups, 18*, 55–65.

Kurland, R. (1978). Planning: A neglected component of group development. *Social work with Groups, 1*, 173–178.

Lee, M. Y., & Gaucher, R. (2000). Group treatment for dually diagnosed adolescents: An empowerment-based approach. *Social Work with Groups, 23*, 55–79.

Levine, B. (1990). Thirty-five years of group work in psychiatric settings (Part 1). *Social Work with Groups, 13*, 1–11.

Livingston, D. (1996). A systems approach to AIDS counseling for gay couples. *Journal of Gay and Lesbian Social Services, 4*, 83–93.

Lonergan, E. C. (1990). *Group intervention: How to maintain groups in medical and psychiatric settings.* New York: Aronson.

Lynn, M., & Nisivoccia, D. (1995). Activity-oriented group work with the mentally ill: Enhancing socialization. *Social Work with Groups, 18*, 95–107.

Mancoske, F. J., & Lindhorst, T. (1991). Mutual assistance groups in a shelter for persons with AIDS. *Social Work with Groups, 14*, 75–86.

Mayers, A., & Spiegel, L. (1992). A parental support group in a pediatric AIDS clinic: Its usefulness and limitations. *Health and Social Work, 17*, 183–193.

McCallion, P., & Toseland, R. W. (1995). Supportive group intervention with caregivers of frail older adults. *Social Work with Groups, 18,* 11–15.

Meier, A., Galinsky, M. J., & Rounds, K. A. (1995). Telephone support groups for caregivers of persons with AIDS. *Social Work with Groups, 18,* 99–108.

Miller, R., & Mason, S. E. (1998). Group work with first episode schizophrenia clients. *Social Work with Groups, 21,* 19–33.

Moore, E. E., & Starkes, A. J. (1992). The group-in-institution as the unit of attention: Recapturing and refining a social work tradition. *Social Work with Groups, 17,* 171–193.

Moore, P. J. (1998). AIDS bereavement supports in an African American church: A model for facilitator training. *Illness, Crisis and Loss, 7,* 390–401.

Morris, R. G., & Woods, R. T. (1992). The use of a coping strategy focused support group for carers of dementia sufferers. *Counseling Psychology Quarterly, 5,* 337–349.

Parker, S., Hutchinson, D., & Berry, S. (1995). A support group for families of armed services personnel in the Persian Gulf War. *Social Work with Groups, 18,* 89–97.

Pomeroy, E. C., Rubin, A., Van Laningham, L., & Walker, R. J. (1997). "Straight Talk": The effectiveness of a psychoeducational group intervention for heterosexuals with HIV/AIDS. *Research on Social Work Practice, 7,* 149–163.

Posen, J., Moore, O., Tassa, D. S., Ginzburg, K., Drory, M., & Giladi, N. (2000). Young women with PD: A group work experience. *Social Work in Health Care, 32,* 77–91.

Reid, K., Mathews, G., & Liss, P. S. (1995). My partner is hurting: Group work with male partners of adult survivors of sexual abuse. *Social Work with Groups, 18,* 81–87.

Rhodes, R. (1995). A group intervention for young children in addictive families. *Social Work with Groups, 18,* 123–133.

Richman, J. M. (1990). Group work in a hospice setting. *Social Work with Groups, 12,* 171–184.

Rittner, B., & Smyth, N. J. (1999). Time-limited cognitive-behavioral group interventions with suicidal adolescents. *Social Work with Groups, 22,* 55–75.

Roberts, J., & Smith, J. (1994). From hospital community to the wider community: Developing a therapeutic environment on a rehabilitation ward. *Journal of Mental Health, 3,* 69–79.

Roffman, R. A., Downey, L., Beadnell, B., Gordon, J. R., Craver, J. N., & Stephens, R. S. (1997). Cognitive-behavioral group counseling to prevent HIV transmission in gay and bisexual men: Factors contributing to successful risk reduction. *Research on Social Work Practice, 7,* 165–186.

Rose, S. D. (1990a). Group exposure: A method of treating agoraphobia. *Social Work with Groups, 13,* 37–51.

Rose, S. D. (1990b). Putting the group into cognitive-behavioral treatment. *Social Work with Groups, 13,* 71–83.

Rosenberg, G., & Neil, G. (1982). Group services and medical illness: A review of literature between 1964–1978. In A. Lurie, G. Rosenberg, & S. Pinsky (Eds.), *Social work with groups in health care* (pp. 30–53). New York: Prodist.

Ryan, D., & Doubleday, E. (1995). Group work: A lifeline for isolated elderly. *Social Work with Groups, 18,* 65–78.

Schamess, G. (1990). New directions in children's group therapy: Integrating family and group perspectives in the treatment of at risk children and families. *Social Work with Groups, 13,* 67–92.

Schopler, J. H., & Galinsky, M. J. (1990). Introduction. Social group work: Promoting a more holistic approach to health care. *Social Work with Groups, 12,* 1–6.

Schnekenburger, E. (1995). Waking the heart up: A writing group's story. *Social Work with Groups, 18,* 19–40.

Schwartz, W. (1961). The social worker in the group. In *New perspectives on services to groups: Theory, organization, and practice* (pp. 7–34). New York: National Association of Social Workers.

Schwartz, W. (1994) Between client and system: The mediating function. In T. Berman-Rossi (Ed.), *Social work: The collected writings of William Schwartz* (pp. 324–346). Itasca, IL: Peacock Press.

Sundel, M., Glasser, P., & Sarri, R., & Vinter, R. (1985) *Individual change through small groups* (2nd ed.). New York: Free Press.

Telfair, J., & Gardner, M. M. (2000). Adolescents with sickle cell disease: Determinants of support group attendance and satisfaction. *Health and Social Work, 25,* 43–49.

Tutty, L. M., & Wagar, J. (1994). The evolution of a group for young children who have witnessed family violence. *Social Work with Groups, 17,* 89–104.

Vinter, R. (1985). An approach to group work practice. In M. Sundel, P. Glasser, R. Sarri, & R. Vinter (Eds.), *Individual change through small groups* (2nd ed., pp. 5–10). New York: Free Press.

Walsh, R. T., Richardson, M. A., & Cardey, R. M. (1991). Structured fantasy approaches to children's group therapy. *Social Work with Groups, 14,* 57–73.

Wiener, L. S. (1998). Telephone support groups for HIV-positive mothers whose children have died of AIDS. *Social Work, 43,* 279–285.

Wiener, L. S., Spencer, E. D., Davidson, R., & Fair, C. (1993). National telephone support groups: A new avenue toward psychosocial support HIV-infected children and their families. *Social Work with Groups, 16,* 55–71.

Wolozin, D., & Dalton, E. (1990). Short-term group psychotherapy with the "family-absent father" in a maximum security psychiatric hospital. *Social Work with Groups, 13,* 103–111.

Yalom, I. D. (1995). *The theory and practice of group psychotherapy* (4nd ed.). New York: Basic Books.

Chapter 12

Involuntary Groups

RONALD ROONEY
MICHAEL CHOVANEC

In this chapter, we define involuntary groups, describe the purpose of social work with involuntary clients in groups, delineate appropriate interventions and their theoretical and empirical bases, and suggest guidelines for use of the interventions, with examples. We present an integration of individual and group stages of change and, finally, consider future directions for such work.

DEFINITION OF SOCIAL WORK PRACTICE WITH INVOLUNTARY CLIENTS IN GROUPS

Social workers often practice with involuntary clients in mandated groups and also in groups that are otherwise voluntary. Involuntary clients are persons who experience legal or nonlegal pressure to accept social services (Rooney, 1992). Some groups are composed of members who are either coerced or in other ways pressured to participate (Behroozi, 1992). *Mandated involuntary groups* are those in which coercion occurs through external, legal pressure (Rooney, 1992). For example, groups in corrections and with domestic violence perpetrators include legal mandates. In other cases, social workers encounter involuntary clients in otherwise voluntary groups. For example, some members may not freely choose to participate in a voluntary parenting group. The reason may be that they were referred by a child welfare worker who would monitor their participation as a factor in influencing a recommendation about child custody.

PURPOSE OF SOCIAL WORK PRACTICE WITH INVOLUNTARY CLIENTS IN GROUPS

Social workers who practice with involuntary clients in groups perform dual roles of supporting social control and promoting individual growth potential. They perform a social control purpose of community protection and client resocialization to roles that clients might not choose for themselves (Garvin, 1981). The profession has an extensive history of work with clients who are involuntary without using that term to describe them (Konopka, 1950; Pray, 1945; Roberts & Brownell, 1999). In the past 10 years, more attention has been devoted to such clients, using the term "involuntary" (Ivanoff, Blythe, & Tripodi, 1994; Rooney, 1992; Trotter, 1999). Applications to social group work with involuntary clients in corrections have also been reported (Goodman, 1997; Goodman, Getzel, & Ford, 1996).

Social workers employ a variety of strategies to promote individual growth potential. One major strategy is the principle of mutual aid designed to enhance individual growth potential (Behroozi, 1992; Goodman, 1997). For example, in addition to working toward protecting society from further crime, it has been possible to work with offenders to develop voluntary goals such as pursuing educational and employment opportunities (Goodman, 1997; Goodman et al., 1996).

INTERVENTIONS AND THEIR
THEORETICAL AND EMPIRICAL BASES

Five sources of interventions and their theoretical and empirical bases are reviewed. First, reactance theory provides a conceptual and theoretical basis for understanding opposition to change and ways to reduce that opposition. Second, the stages of change model provides a useful framework for assessing motivation for change among involuntary clients. Third, motivational interviewing adds specific intervention guidelines directed to particular stages of change. Fourth, we review stages of change in groups for involuntary clients. And finally, we review a series of techniques that are useful in enhancing participation by involuntary group members. Based on these interventions, a matrix for conceptualizing involuntary groups and involuntary clients in otherwise voluntary groups is presented.

Reactance Theory

Reactance theory provides a useful framework for understanding clients who perceive themselves as being coerced into treatment. The theory assumes that people have a variety of behaviors that they are free to exercise at any time. When some of those presumed free behaviors are threatened or eliminated, a person experiences *reactance*, or a motivational drive to restore those free behaviors (Brehm & Brehm, 1981). For example, the "free behavior" of not attending treatment is threatened or eliminated when a person is mandated to attend a treatment program. The theory suggests that persons who are feeling pressured or coerced will behave in a variety of predictable ways, such as expressing anger toward the group leader, passive group participation, or withdrawal from treatment. The Therapeutic Reactance Scale (TRS) measures level of reactance within individuals (Dowd, Milne, & Wise, 1991; Dowd & Wallbrown, 1993). The TRS, in combination with clinical indicators such as refusal to complete homework assignments or previous poor treatment response, can be used to assess levels of reactance early in treatment (Beutler & Berren, 1995; Beutler, Kim, Davidson, Karno, & Fisher, 1996; Groth-Marnat, 1997; Prochaska, Norcross, & DiClemente, 1994).

Reactance theory suggests a variety of strategies to either increase or decrease opposition to change. For example, efforts to reduce reactance can include providing choices or clarifying what is and is not mandated (Rooney, 1992). One might wish to increase reactance if a client appeared to be unaware of the consequences of critical decisions he or she might make. To increase reactance, one would emphasize the consequences of failure to follow through with mandated changes for the involuntary client's future freedoms. Providing emotional support and reflection are recommended for highly reactant clients. Structure through contracting or use of contingencies is recommended with low-reactant clients. Early attention to reactance allows practitioners to engage the client more quickly and to increase the chances for a more successful outcome.

Stages of Change Model

The stages of change model evolved from research examining how people overcome addictive behaviors such as smoking, drinking, and excessive weight loss (Norcross, Beutler, & Clarkin, 1998; Prochaska et al., 1995). A series of five stages are identified related to changing of addictive behavior. In the *precontemplation stage*, clients do not recognize problems, but others in their environment perceive them as having problems. In the *contemplation stage*, clients identify problems but are not ready to act on those problems. In the *preparation stage*, clients are ready to begin preliminary efforts toward change. Those preliminary efforts become consistent in the *action stage*. Finally, in the *maintenance stage*, clients attempt to maintain changed behaviors.

The stages of change model has been applied to both chemical dependency groups (Yu & Watkins, 1996) and domestic abuse groups (Daniels & Murphy, 1997). The stages of Change Scale (SOCS) has been developed for assessing client motivation (McConnaughy, DiClemente, Prochaska, & Velicer, 1989). Application of this instrument has helped to build growing evidence that precontemplators are common among those clients seeking mental health treatment.

Motivational Interviewing

Motivational interviewing suggests specific interventions designed to assist individuals in progressing along the stages of change. It was developed for work with clients with chemical dependency concerns, particularly those who were opposed to entering treatment (Miller & Rollnick, 1991). In this approach, however, resistance is reframed as ambivalence, and strategies are offered to address it. Motivational interviewing group facilitators are proactive in engaging individual clients at any point on the continuum of motivation for change. In addition, client self-motivating statements toward change are identified and supported. For example, the group leader will take the lead in exploring ambivalence and eliciting self-motivating statements among clients in the precontemplation stage (Miller & Rollnick, 1991). This model has been used in combination with the stages of change model with work in groups of men who batter (Daniels & Murphy, 1997; Murphy & Baxter, 1997).

Stages of Group Change for Involuntary Groups

In addition to models of individual change in motivation over time, social workers have long found it useful to conceive of stages of change as applied to groups. Such stages were originally posed as applying relatively universally to most kinds of groups (Bennis & Shepard, 1956; Garland, Jones, & Kolodny, 1965). More recently, those stages have been adapted for specific populations such as women (Schiller, 1995, 1997) and groups of older institutionalized persons (Berman-Rossi & Kelly, 1998). Unfortunately, the applications to date assume that all clients are voluntary, and hence they do not address the coercive forces that affect the group process for involuntary clients. In addition, a pregroup or preliminary stage of group development is not included in the aforementioned models. This stage is significant for involuntary groups, as potential group members make critical decisions about whether and how to engage in the group process prior to the first session. Most of the interventions articulated in this chapter focus on engaging the client and enhancing more voluntary participation in the group process. In this chapter, the Kurland and Salmon (1998) model of group development, which includes a preliminary stage, will be integrated with the individual stage of change approach to help examine the change process for involuntary clients within the group setting and suggest appropriate interventions.

Involuntary groups include a *pregroup planning phase*, in which potential leaders and organizations decide whether and how to form groups. Because involuntary groups are likely to stimulate reactance and to bring together persons many of whom are not eager to change, the first decision to be made is whether to form the group and, if so, how. Involuntary groups can provide an opportunity for *in vivo* learning in which members can learn from others, including peer modeling; can learn how to help others; and can provide a source of support for risk taking and making efforts to change. They can also be a source of effective confrontation or persuasion to stimulate dissonance (Rooney, 1992, p. 281). On the other hand, fellow members of involuntary groups can serve as role models for antisocial, as well as prosocial, behavior, and some potential members do not learn well in groups and hence may make the experience less positive for others (Rooney, 1992, p. 284; Trotter, 1999). In this regard, it is useful to consider what kinds of choices are possible for group members and in what ways they can perceive personal benefit from group participation (Rooney, 1992).

Having decided to offer an involuntary group, the next step is pregroup contact (Kurland & Salmon, 1998). Potential group members are secured for the group and oriented to group participation. Such orientation includes discussing the voluntarism issue and eliciting the potential group member's thoughts and feelings about it. In this step with involuntary groups, leader efforts are made to enhance choices, however constrained, and to stimulate self-motivation for participation rather than relying exclusively on threats of punishment or promises of reward. Changes that are motivated by a perception that an individual will be benefited, hence self-attributed, are more likely to be long lasting than changes that occur as a result of either threats or rewards (Rooney, 1992). In this step, potential members are familiarized with rules, nonnegotiable policies, and choices available in the group. Such use of orientation for group members entering a program has been supported as a way of reducing group attrition in domestic violence programs (Brekke, 1989; Tolman & Bhosley, 1987).

In the *beginning stage* of group development, Kurland and Salmon (1998) indicate that members are anxious about the unknown, so themes of trust and distrust are prominent. Also members present both approach and avoidance behaviors, as they want acceptance and want to change yet fear being hurt or made vulnerable. The major tasks in the beginning stage include orientation to the group, clarification of group purpose and norms, and finding commonalities between group members to build cohesion.

In the beginning stage of involuntary groups, members often do not detect a strong connection between their difficulties and those faced by others and hence have doubts about the likelihood of being helped by the group (Berman-Rossi & Kelly, 2000). Thus avoidance behaviors are more likely to be emphasized by group members. For example, in domestic abuse groups, men often present themselves in a wary, noncommittal fashion. Providing an opening statement that anticipates and addresses some of the initial concerns that men typically present is useful in reducing these avoidant behaviors and engaging men in the group process. In addition, it is important when clarifying norms that group leaders make explicit which norms are negotiable and which are not as a way of reducing reactance. Similar to those in voluntary groups, worker tasks at this stage include attempting to link individual motivations into a shared stake in the outcome of the group. In addition, group members often present themselves through anger and frustration early on in the development of involuntary groups. Reactance theory suggests that those who feel coerced into joining the group are more likely to express their frustration and anger toward the group leader. Group leaders are tested early and need to respond to the men's complaints in an empathic and respectful way without condoning their problem behaviors. Articulating group members' anger and frustration early on reduces opposition or avoids its being driven underground by threats of retribution. The group leader who responds to anger in a respectful way rather than cutting off or avoiding the issue models a way of dealing with anger without putting others down. For example, responding respectfully to anger in domestic abuse groups and not avoiding it provides an alternative to the use of anger for power and control that many of the men in the group have experienced.

In the *middle stage* of group development, Kurland and Salmon (1998) suggest that the group leader's role is less central, with support provided for increased leadership and mutual aid between group members. They suggest that group members are likely to be more comfortable with the group process and with examining their similarities to and differences from other members. Members test the group leader to see to what extent they can express their feelings and bring problems to the group without being rejected or punished.

Depending on the extent to which conflict is identified and responded to in a respectful and empathic way, the middle stage is very similar to that in traditional or voluntary groups. Group leadership is tapped and support is provided for the exchange of mutual aid between members. For example, veteran members can be encouraged to explain ground rules or assist in providing guidance for new members in completing required tasks. The group leader in involuntary groups continues to have a power to reward and punish that does not disappear. The leader can, however, specify that recommendations will not be made capriciously based on likes and dislikes but rather based on accomplishment of tasks. How well the initial anger and frustration that group members present is responded to determines whether the group becomes a safe place to support individual change or never reaches the level of cohesion and trust needed to fully experience this middle stage.

In the *ending* stage, Kurland and Salmon (1998) suggest that the group leader's role is to guide the differentiation process, assisting group members to articulate the changes they have made and supporting their efforts to reconnect with resources outside the group.

Similar to the middle stages of involuntary groups, the ending stages are strongly dependent on how well initial contacts with group members are made. If the initial anger and frustration is addressed directly and in a respectful way, endings appear similar to those in voluntary groups. A key factor is whether the group is closed or open ended. In open-ended groups, the ending process is less intense as members are leaving at different times. Also there are typically completion requirements that determine when a group member ends that add more structure to the ending process. In addition, the levels of changes made by individuals vary widely. Changes made by group members need to be articulated and validated by the group member, the leader, and others in the group.

Techniques for Engaging Involuntary Clients in the Group Process

Thomas and Caplan (1999) propose 56 useful techniques for enhancing participation of involuntary clients in groups and place those techniques into three major categories of enhancing *process, inclusion,* and *linking.* The group facilitator uses *process* interventions to identify the emotional message behind the client's statement and reflects the client's worldview. *Linking* interventions are used to connect clients' individual issues with those of others in the group and to allow the group leader to make generalized statements about the group itself. *Inclusion* interventions encourage uninvolved group members to join the group discussion and include didactic and projective exercises that allow group members to voice their opinions without being singled out.

Techniques for Examining Faulty Beliefs

How can group members be helped to address critical issues without feeling singled out and blamed? For example, in the corrections field, leaders who utilize a cognitive restructuring framework consider that some of the difficulties experienced by law violators emerge from faulty thinking patterns. Some group members, for instance, may believe that "money will solve all my problems." Such beliefs are not socially acceptable, and members might not readily attest to belief in them. Using the *sophistry* method, group members who have committed crimes are asked to debate the pros and cons of such beliefs without immediately acknowledging their own views about these beliefs. For example, some group members would argue in favor of the position that "if I have been treated unfairly, I have a right to treat others unfairly," whereas others would be asked to dispute that position (Evans & Kane, 1996, p. 114). Such examination can then engage members in assessing whether those beliefs may play a part in their legal difficulties.

Techniques for Appropriately Confronting Clients

More forceful addressing of critical issues occurs when members are confronted about harmful thoughts and behavior. Confrontational approaches were introduced into the chemical dependency field in the 1970s and 1980s (Thomas & Yoshioka, 1989). In the domestic abuse field, confrontation has been used to address men's rationalizations about abusive behavior and as a way of discussing gender, power, and control issues (Pence & Paymar, 1993). Motivational change approaches based on the stages of change conception and reactance theory provide alternatives to these traditional confrontational approaches. Murphy and Baxter (1997) describe the negative consequences of using a highly confrontational approach with domestic abuse perpetrators that might increase their defensiveness and reinforce their belief that relationships are based on coercion. That is, if members believe that group leaders can impose their will and beliefs on abuse perpetrators because they possess the power to coerce, then their belief that power in a relationship is based on ability to coerce is not being challenged.

There is also evidence that highly confrontational approaches lead to poor client outcomes (Yalom & Leiberman, 1971) and that clients with low self-esteem and poor self-concepts are more likely to deteriorate within the group setting (Lambert & Bergin, 1994). A confrontation–denial cycle has been described as occurring in many groups, whereby intensive confrontations by leaders stimulate a round of denials by clients, setting off another wave of confrontations and denials (Murphy & Baxter, 1997). Interventions that do not insist that clients label themselves as deviant but rather focus on those actions that are likely to help them achieve their goals are less likely to provoke this confrontation–denial cycle (Murphy & Baxter, 1997). In this approach, the group leader attempts to understand the world from the client's viewpoint and supports the client's ownership of responsibility for change (Kear-Colwell & Pollock, 1997). Emphasis is placed on understanding pathways that have led to undesirable outcomes.

GUIDELINES AND EXAMPLES FOR SOCIAL WORKERS WITH INVOLUNTARY GROUPS THROUGHOUT STAGES OF DEVELOPMENT

Based on the preceding perspectives, the following seven guidelines are suggested for work with involuntary client groups and individuals in otherwise voluntary groups. As we present the guidelines for intervention, we integrate them with the expected stage of group development and individual motivation for change (see Table 12.1).

1. *Make an appropriate organizational decision about whether a group needs to be involuntary.* Because involuntary groups contain both opportunities and challenges, the first question to be answered is whether the group needs to be involuntary, and, if so, what are these requirements? Hence the first step is to identify those non-negotiable parts of the group's mission from the organization. For example, patients on an inpatient psychiatric unit might be expected to participate in group treatment as determined in their treatment plans. Similarly, a group for domestic violence perpetrators must explore alternatives to violent resolution to disputes. The more freedoms that are threatened, the more likely that reactance will be stimulated. Hence, in addition to non-negotiable requirements, it is important to explore what portions of the purpose and methods of a group can either be negotiable or include choices to be made by members. Hence, if members of groups on psychiatric units can have some say in the topics to be discussed or some choice regarding which groups they participate in, reactance could be expected to be reduced. For example, men in a domestic violence program must complete at least 12 of 15 group sessions in order to graduate; they can, however, choose which sessions, if any, they will not attend. Choices can be increased for those potential members who complain about the length or cost of the program by providing the phone numbers of surrounding programs to increase their range of selection.

2. *Conduct pregroup orientation.* Pregroup orientation is useful for members of voluntary groups as well, but particular advantages accrue for involuntary groups. By assessing the potential client's current motivation on the cycle of change, the leader can present interventions that fit the motivation of members. Similarly, reactance may be reduced by clarifying expectations, including negotiable options and choices. These sessions can also raise the opportunity for contracting concerning other, more voluntary problems acknowledged by potential members, such as securing further education.

Similar guidelines can be followed to enhance voluntarism of members who experience pressure to participate in an otherwise voluntary group. For example, with the parent who is referred to a parenting group, the group leader can first identify and empathize with the pressure felt by the potential member. The leader can then clarify that the potential member can in fact choose *not* to be a member of this group and take the consequences from the re-

TABLE 12.1. Interventions, Group Stages of Change, and Stages of Individual Development

Interventions	Stage of change	Anticipated level of individual development
1. Make organizational decision about use of involuntary group.	Pregroup planning	Precontemplation

2. Pregroup orientation.
  a. Initial orientation of group.
  b. Reframe from resistance to ambivalence.
  c. Clarify choices.		

3. Emphasize joining and inclusion.
  a. Clarify non-negotiables.
  b. Support positive choices made to date.
  c. Provide emotional support.
  d. Identify self-motivating statements.
  e. Provide opening statement addressing client initial concerns/fears.
  f. Link to process.
  g. Support inclusion.
  h. Link members to each other.
  i. Stimulate nonthreatening attention to issues.
  j. Continue reframing resistance as ambivalence.
	Beginning	Precontemplation

4. Decide to make a change.
  a. Assist in assessing costs and benefits of change.
  b. Provide information about choices.
	Middle	Contemplation

5. Support in planning actions.		Action
6. Emphasize responsibility for choices rather than confrontation.		
7. Utilize clear criteria for group completion. a. Plan for maintenance; address relapse.	Ending	Maintenance

ferring worker or solicit a different referral. In this way, the leader can begin to emphasize choice in participating in this group. If the potential member then *chooses* to be a member, he or she can also decide to pursue personal goals, as well as to carry out the mandated participation. For example, he or she might choose to seek support for circumstances as a single parent and choose to focus on parenting supports and strategies for single parents.

3. *Emphasize methods to assist in joining and inclusion in early sessions.* Special efforts have to be made in involuntary groups to assist members to join the group in the *beginning phase* and feel included. The leader can assume that most members of an involuntary group are initially at the *precontemplation* stage of individual motivation for change, in which they do not now recognize a need for change. Interventions that engage members in taking in new information about the costs and benefits of behaviors without forcing them to accept those attitudes and beliefs are appropriate for this stage. This phase also contains explicit contracting that includes both required group goals and problems and those selected more voluntarily by individuals.

A prepared opening statement by the group facilitator can be an important part of an orientation session. This opening statement allows the facilitator to join with the potential group members by anticipating some of the major questions and concerns members are expected to bring with them as they enter a program. For example, the following is an opening statement one could use with men entering a domestic abuse program. Techniques utilized and their purposes are indicated in *italics*.

> "Welcome to the program. I know many of you may feel as if you have been forced to come here. Many men who are in similar situations never make it this far to come to the first meeting. I support your choice in attending the program [*emphasizing choices already made*]. You may think that we will try to force you to change. The reality is that no one can make you change [*emphasizing choice to reduce reactance*]. All we ask is that you listen to what is said and take the bits and pieces of the program that make sense to you and that can help you avoid future problems and contact with the court system [*limited, clear requirements to reduce reactance*].
>
> "You may also fear that you will be judged as guilty or shamed for the incident that brought you here. Many of you have already gone through the court system. We are not here to judge you as guilty or innocent for the charges you bring with you [*clarifying role and avoiding emphasis on blaming*]. Our focus is on helping you to learn from whatever incident brings you in. Our task is to create a safe environment for men to examine their actions and learn from their mistakes [*positive, future-oriented focus*].
>
> "The group has some rules. Physical or verbal abuse is not tolerated in our group sessions. If you cause it, you will be asked to leave the group session. What we say here is confidential and should not be shared outside the group [*clarifying non-negotiable requirements*]. I cannot force group members to do this but expect you will keep confidence in respect for others in the group. I have to break confidentiality if you tell me that you are in danger of hurting yourself or others, since legally I must report that information to other professionals or the authorities [*clarifying rights and limitations*".]

The preceding statement emphasizes choices and avoids blaming statements in an effort to reduce reactance. Nonnegotiable rules are shared, as well as their rationale. After this introduction, members are asked to share information about the circumstances of their referral and the goals they are setting for themselves for group participation.

In the circumstance of the involuntary member in an otherwise voluntary group, efforts at this stage can similarly reinforce choices about participation and freedom to choose not to participate actively but to learn by observing persons who are further along in the change process. So, for example, the reluctant participant in the parenting group could choose to be an observer until he or she feels more comfortable about group participation.

4. *As group members progress into the contemplation phase, emphasis is placed on deciding to make a change.* While some members are progressing into the *contemplation* phase of individual motivation for change, the group as a whole may be in the middle phase. As noted, as many as a third or a quarter of involuntary clients may be at the *contemplation* phase of individual motivation at the beginning of the group. Leader efforts at this stage are focused on helping clients to examine the costs and benefits of change and to make a decision to change or not to change. Individual ambivalence is explored, and particular themes in each member's struggle to change are identified and then linked to the other group members. This intervention provides an opportunity for all group members to contribute (inclusion) and builds group cohesion.

For example, a client in the domestic violence group, Jack, reports in the fourth session: "I have decided that I will not try to contact my ex-partner anymore. My ex-partner should have a group like this, but I know I did shove her. I am realizing that I was a jerk at times.

Things just started building up and when she got in my face and told me she didn't love me anymore I couldn't handle it."

LEADER: It takes a lot of courage to look at oneself and take responsibility [*rewarding acknowledging responsibility*]. What helped you do this? (*after hearing Jack's response*) It sounds as if you wanted to make sure this type of incident doesn't happen again. Certainly staying sober is a good first step in figuring out what to do differently. How is not drinking working for you [*supporting and reinforcing choices*]?

After Jack responds to this question asking him about a choice and a strength, the leader turns to the group: "Has anyone else decided not to use alcohol or drugs as a result of the incident that brought them in to the program?" The leader reinforces Jack's self-motivating statement about maintaining sobriety and tries to link Jack's process in staying sober with others in the group. In the process, other men may identify self-care strategies that might be useful for Jack.

JACK: I just decided it was time to quit using because I have had nothing but trouble when I start drinking. I am getting tired of it. Sure, I get urges to use every day, but I just think about being in jail and decide I'm not going there.

LEADER: So, Jack, you think about the consequences and make a decision that drinking is not working for you; it can be a trigger to violence. What kinds of triggers have the rest of you noticed that often come before a violent episode?

The leader is linking Jack's concerns with those of other group members, attempting to stimulate inclusion in the group as others relate to precipitants toward violence. The leader expresses empathy, articulates the ambivalence, and focuses on the positive side toward change. He identifies what the client takes responsibility for, supports positive changes already made, and draws on other members for support.

5. *Members are assisted in the action phase to plan specific actions to address the problem.* Examining alternatives is most relevant in the action phase of individual motivation for change. For example, men in groups for domestic violence perpetrators often have to complete a role-play task demonstrating that they have a plan for dealing with a potential conflict with someone in their current lives. In this potential future encounter, they are asked to identify the various cues they anticipate in interactions with this person and how they will address anger and keep themselves calm during the exchange.

In the parenting group, the initially reluctant member, along with other participants, would be asked to make a plan based on skills learned so far for addressing a potential parenting conflict that they are concerned about. For example, the reluctant member might be concerned with getting her child to go to bed on time. This issue may or may not be considered significant by the referring worker, but it is a voluntary issue to the parent. By emphasizing choice about what situation to select and which strategies to employ, the leader can emphasize self-attribution and support choices.

6. *Emphasis on taking responsibility for choices rather than confrontation.* If the leader emphasizes taking responsibility for choices, reactance should be reduced, and influence efforts can be focused productively around areas of motivation. For example, Roger, another member of the domestic violence group, reports the following in a middle session: "My wife and kids won't talk to me. I call them and they hang up. She's got this restraining

order so I can't even talk to her and the kids. That's not right. I should be able to talk to my own family. I am tired of all this. I am going to go over there and handle it."

When the leader clarifies that by handling it, Roger means going over to his wife's home and talking to her, thereby violating the restraining order, he turns to others in the group to ask: "What do you think of Roger's plan? Do you think that is going to help him get out of this group successfully and get back with his wife and kids [*articulating Roger's personal goals for the program*]?" Group members point out to Roger that this is the kind of decision that got him into the group in the first place and that his situation will only get worse. The leader points out to Roger that, if he chooses to violate the restraining order and potentially endanger his wife, the leader will have to warn her, and Roger will not be able to continue in the group. This fact is presented not as a humiliating confrontation but as a statement of consequences. He then goes on to ask Roger and other group members: "Can you think of other ways Roger might be able to initiate contact with his wife and kids without violating the restraining order or acting against their will [*alternative means to reach the same goal*]?" This move to problem solving leads the group to recommend that Roger write a letter to his wife and children telling them how much he cares for them and how he is working in the group to get control of his anger.

7. *Utilize clear criteria for group completion.* Reactance is likely to be reduced by having clear behavioral goals rather than vague, amorphous ones. Consequently, if the criteria for group completion clearly spell out what a member is to do, reactance should be reduced. For example, in the domestic violence group, a commitment to carrying out specific tasks designed to implement nonviolent solutions is easy to assess regarding group completion. The group for domestic violence perpetrators contains the requirement of attending 15 group sessions and completing eight tasks. A tracking sheet is shared with men in orientation that identifies the topics covered over the 15 weeks and lists the tasks they are required to complete. This tracking sheet is then given to the probation officer once the men have completed the program, with program participation measured by sessions attended and tasks completed. Expectations and instructions for completing each task are available for review before they begin to work on them.

Similarly, in the parenting group, all group members—but especially those who are initially reluctant—will benefit from a clear delineation of the expectations for successful completion of the group. For example, each member is expected to attend regularly, to listen to presentations on different topics, and to choose an area most applicable to him or her in which to focus planning for improvement. Focusing attention on a self-selected area, such as interaction around bedtime, is likely to increase voluntarism.

SUMMARY AND CONCLUSIONS

We have explored how social workers can perform dual roles in work with involuntary clients in groups pursuing social control and fostering individual growth. This dual pursuit suggests two areas for continued development: the systems context for work with involuntary clients and evaluation of intervention.

The Systems Context for Work with Involuntary Clients

Social workers operate within a systems perspective that examines the conditions under which illegal behavior or behavior labeled as deviant occurs. In this regard, social workers are mindful of overrepresentation of members of oppressed groups and persons of color among involuntary clients (Diorio, 1992; Horejsi, Heavy Runner-Craig, & Pablo, 1992; Longres, 1991; Rooney & Bibus, 1995). Hence, social workers are aware of over-representation of persons of color among more restrictive treatments across many populations and problems. For example, persons of color are more likely to be in prison and to receive more restrictive options for mental health problems and are more likely to have their children in out-of-home care (Dewberry Rooney, 2001; Morton, 2001).

Social workers note that restricted access to resources, as well as living in unsafe neighborhoods with inadequate schools, plays a part in determining which members of society are likely to become involuntary clients. Many treatment approaches for work with offenders emphasize examination of personal choices and taking responsibility for behavior. Social workers support that emphasis to a degree. Looking at individual pathways that have led into particular choices and behavior can be constructive. Instead of ineffectual or harmful raging against persons and systems considered unfair, the group can be an arena for learning safe, effective methods of negotiating systems. Anger can be channeled into empowering, rather than abusive, actions. Clients such as Roger can be taught to work with an attorney to assure regular, consistent, safe visitation with their children rather than threatening their spouses.

Social workers employ an empowering perspective to look beyond individual pathways and examine group pathways and access to resources. Hence, social workers examine those social conditions that made that involuntary contact more likely. For example, Roger may link with others in the group who are having difficulty making contact with their children and develop strategies for working with probation and law enforcement to increase opportunities to demonstrate the changes they are making and improve access to their children. Similarly, an empowerment perspective would suggest exploring messages about violence in the media and providing opportunities to learn alternatives to violence in schools. An empowerment perspective also suggests exploring organizational factors and attitudes that contribute to disproportionate racial representation among clients in fields such as child welfare (Dewberry Rooney, 2001).

The Importance of Evaluation

Much of the work with involuntary clients in groups appears untested and/or ineffective. In the area of domestic violence, between 40% and 60% of the men who enter a treatment program have been reported to drop out within the first three sessions (Gondolf, 1997), with one study examining the attrition rate from inquiry to treatment completion and finding that less than 1% completed the 8-month program (Gondolf & Foster, 1991). Failure to complete a treatment program can have a significant impact on men's partners, as well. Gondolf (1988) found that when men reported to their partners that they were attending treatment, those partners were more likely to return to them. Hence high attrition rates in domestic abuse treatment put women at risk for future abuse.

In addition, group leaders of involuntary groups are in explicit positions of power, influencing program participants and determining who graduates. Many involuntary clients have experience with authority figures who have used abusive power over them. Ongoing group evaluation that assesses program interventions and outcomes helps insure that programs do not replicate the abusive background that many clients entering involuntary groups have experienced.

Evaluation of involuntary groups needs to address the achievement of both social control and individual growth goals. That is, evaluation needs to address whether, for instance, violence is reduced and whether repeated offenses decline. But evaluation should also explore whether members set and reach personal growth goals. Process studies are needed that show whether members learn new skills and whether engagement methods such as those described in this chapter enhance attendance and group completion.

Finally, social workers who lead involuntary groups have an ethical responsibility to evaluate their practice and base their interventions on best practices such as those suggested herein. If social workers are to achieve success in pursuing both social control and individual growth with members of involuntary groups, they will need to employ effective skills in engaging participants in the group process and to evaluate the success of those methods and groups. Only through this regular examination of the involuntary process found in a variety of groups will clients, their families, and the community be better served.

REFERENCES

Berman-Rossi, T., & Kelly, T. (2000, March). *Teaching students to understand and utilize the changing paradigm of stages of group development theory.* Paper presented at the annual program meeting of the Council on Social Work Education, New York, NY.

Behroozi, C. S. (1992). A model for social work with involuntary applicants in groups. *Social Work with Groups, 15*(2/3), 223–238.

Bennis, W., & Shepard, H. (1956). A theory of group development. *Human Relations, 9,* 415–437.

Berman-Rossi, T., & Kelly, T. B. (1998, March). *Advancing stages of group development theory.* Paper presented at the annual program meeting of the Council on Social Work Education, Orlando, FL.

Brehm, S., & Brehm, J. (1981). *Psychological reactance: A theory of freedom and control.* New York: Academic Press.

Brekke, J. (1989). The use of orientation groups for hard-to-reach clients: Model, method and evaluation. *Social Work with Groups, 12*(2), 75–88.

Beutler, L. E., & Berren, M. (Eds.). (1995). *Integrative assessment of adult personality.* New York: Guilford Press.

Beutler, L. E., Kim, E. J., Davidson, E., Karno, M., & Fisher, D. (1996). Research contributions to improving managed health care outcomes. *Psychotherapy, 33,* 197–206.

Daniels, J. W., & Murphy, C. M. (1997). Stages and processes of change in batterers' treatment, *Cognitive and Behavioral Practice, 4*(1), 123–145.

Dewberry Rooney, G. (2001). History and significance. In *Breaking the silence: A candid discussion on the disproportionality of African American children in out-of-home placement.* Retrieved October 2003 from University of Minnesota, Center for Advanced Studies in Child Welfare website: *http://ssw.che.umn.edu/cascw/pdf/2001%20PROCEEDINGS.pdf*

Diorio, W. (1992). Parenting perceptions of the authority of public caseworkers. *Families in Society, 73*(4), 222–235.

Dowd, T., Milne, C. R., & Wise, S. L. (1991). The Therapeutic Reactance Scale: A measure of psychological reactance. *Journal of Family Issues, 6,* 229–247.

Dowd, T., & Wallbrown, F. (1993). Motivational components of client reactance. *Journal of Counseling and Development, 71,* 533–538.

Evans, T. D., & Kane, D. P. (1996). Sophistry: A promising group technique for the involuntary client. *Journal for Specialists in Group Work, 21*(2), 110–117.

Garland, J. A., Jones, H. E., & Kolodny, R. L. (1965). A model for stages of development in social work groups. In S. Bernstein (Ed.), *Explorations in social group work.* Boston: Boston University, School of Social Work.

Gondolf, E. W. (1988). The effects of batterer counseling on shelter outcome. *Journal of Interpersonal Violence, 3*(3), 275–289.

Gondolf, E. W. (1997). Batterer programs: What we know and need to know. *Journal of Interpersonal Violence, 12*(1), 83–98.

Gondolf, E. W., & Foster, B. (1991). Preprogram attrition in batterer programs. *Journal of Family Violence, 6,* 337–349.

Goodman, H. (1997). Social group work in community corrections. *Social Work with Groups, 20*(1), 51–64.

Goodman, H., Getzel, G. S., & Ford, W. (1996). Group work with high-risk urban youths on probation. *Social Work, 41*(4), 375–381.

Groth-Marnat, G. (1997). *Handbook of psychological assessment* (3rd ed.). New York: Wiley.

Horejsi, C., Heavy Runner-Craig, B., & Pablo, J. (1992). Reactions by Native American parents to child protection agencies. *Child Welfare, 71,* 329–342.

Ivanoff, A., Blythe, B., & Tripodi, T. (1994). *Involuntary clients in social work practice: A research-based approach.* New York: Aldine de Gruyter.

Kear-Colwell, J., & Pollock, P. (1997). Motivation or confrontation: Which approach to the child sex offender? *Criminal Justice and Behavior, 24*(1), 20–33.

Konopka, G. (1950). The social group work method: its use in the correctional field. *Federal Probation, 14,* 25–30.

Kurland, R., & Salmon, R. (1998). *Teaching a methods course in social work with groups.* Alexandria, VA: Council on Social Work Education.

Lambert, M. J., & Bergin, A. E. (1994). The effectiveness of psychotherapy. In A. E. Bergin & S. I. Garfield (Eds.), *Handbook of psychotherapy and behavior change* (4th ed., pp. 143–189). New York: Wiley.

Longres, J. F. (1991). Toward a status model of ethnic sensitive practice. *Journal of Multicultural Social Work, 1*(1), 41–56.

McConnaughy, E. A., DiClemente, C. C., Prochaska, J. O., & Velicer, W. F. (1989). Stages of change in psychotherapy: A follow-up report. *Psychotherapy, 26,* 494–503.

Miller, W. R., & Rollnick, S. (1991). *Motivational interviewing: Preparing people to change addictive behavior.* New York: Guilford Press.

Morton, T. (2001). Where does it begin? In *Breaking the silence: A candid discussion on the disproportionality of African American children in out-of-home placement.* Retrieved October 2003 from the University of Minnesota, Center for Advanced Studies in Child Welfare, website: *http://ssw.che.umn.edu/casw/pdf/2001%20PROCEEDINGS.pdf.*

Murphy, C. M., & Baxter, V. A. (1997). Motivating batterers to change in the treatment context. *Journal of Interpersonal Violence, 12*(4), 607–619.

Norcross, J. C., Beutler, L. E., & Clarkin, J. F. (1998). Prescriptive eclectic psychotherapy. In R. A. Dorfman (Ed.), *Paradigms of clinical social work* (Vol. 2). New York: Brunner/Mazel.

Pence, E., & Paymar, M. (1993). *Education groups for men who batter: The Duluth model.* New York: Springer.

Pray, K. L. (1945). The place of social casework in the treatment of delinquency. *Social Service Review, 19*(2), 235–248.

Prochaska, J., Norcross, J., & DiClemente, C. (1995). *Changing for good.* New York: Avon Books.

Roberts, A. R., & Brownell, P. (1999). A century of forensic social work: Bridging the past to the present. *Social Work, 44*(4), 359–369.

Rooney, R., & Bibus, A. (1995). Multiple lenses: ethnically sensitive practice with involuntary clients who are having difficulties with drugs or alcohol. *Journal of MultiCultural Social Work, 4*(2), 59–73.

Rooney, R. H. (1992). *Strategies for work with involuntary clients.* New York: Columbia University Press.

Schiller, L. Y. (1995). Stages of development in women's groups: A relational model. In R. L. Karland & R. Salmon (Eds.), *Group work practice in a troubled society: Problems and opportunities* (pp. 117–138). New York: Haworth Press.

Schiller, L. Y. (1997). Rethinking stages of group development in women's groups: Implications for practice. *Social Work with Groups, 20*(3), 3–19.

Thomas, E. J., & Yoshioka, M. R. (1989). Spouse interventive confrontations in unilateral family therapy for alcohol abuse. *Social Casework: The Journal of Contemporary Social Work, 70,* 340–347.

Thomas, H., & Caplan, T. (1999). Spinning the group process wheel: Effective facilitation techniques for motivating involuntary client groups. *Social Work with Groups, 2*(4), 3–21.

Tolman, R. M., & Bhosley, G. (1987, May). A comparison of two types of pregroup preparation for men who batter. Paper presented at the Symposium for the Empirical Foundations of Group Work, Chicago, IL.

Trotter, C. (1999). *Working with involuntary clients.* London: Sage.

Yalom, I. D., & Lieberman, M. A. (1971). A study of encounter group casualties. *Archives of General Psychiatry, 25,* 16–30.

Yu, M. M., & Watkins, T. (1996). Group counseling with DUI offenders: A model using client anger to enhance group cohesion and movement. *Alcoholism Treatment Quarterly, 14*(3), 47–57.

Chapter 13

Strengths-Based Group Work with Children and Adolescents

ANDREW MALEKOFF

This chapter introduces a framework for strengths-based group work practice with children and adolescents. At the heart of the presentation are seven practice principles that are described and illustrated:

1. Form groups based on members' felt needs and wants, not diagnoses.
2. Structure groups to welcome the whole person, not just the troubled parts.
3. Integrate verbal and nonverbal activities.
4. Decentralize authority and turn control over to group members.
5. Develop alliances with relevant other people in group members' lives.
6. Maintain a dual focus on individual change and social reform.
7. Understand and respect group development as a kcy to promoting change.

To set the stage, I present an original poem—"My Kind of Group Work"—which exemplifies strengths-based group work. The themes echoed by the poem are explored throughout the chapter. Following the poem is a summary of research on strengths-based social work, an introduction to youth assets, and reflections on the relationship between cognitive-behavioral approaches and strengths-based group work. Practice applications for strengths-based group work follow.

The settings in which the illustrations take place include an outpatient mental health clinic, a community center, public schools, a youth drop-in center/coffeehouse, a therapeutic summer camp, and a school-based mental health/day treatment facility. References in the text and footnotes are made to settings (e.g., inpatient, residential) that are not specifically illustrated. The strengths-based practice described has universal application across settings and populations served.

MY KIND OF GROUP WORK (GW)

It's the GW with ragged edges that belie its genius
It's the GW that can be messy and noisy and chaotic and profound, all at once
It's the GW where children and youth are group members, not clients or patients
It's the GW where the group worker does with the group, not for or to the group
It's the GW where learning by doing is as important as insight by talking
It's the GW that is not ashamed to laugh and have fun
It's the GW that makes use of everyday life and not only canned curricula
It's the GW where worker and group members share responsibility
It's the GW that threatens grown-ups who are uptight
It's the GW that welcomes parents, and doesn't avoid them
It's the GW that invites the rational and spontaneous
It's the GW that lets difficult, painful, and taboo subjects see the light of day
It's the GW that begins with felt need, not a label and diagnosis
It's the GW that respects pathology, but never worships it
It's the GW that embraces strengths, not deficits
It's the GW that welcomes the whole person, not just the troubled parts
It's the GW that has a social conscience and social consciousness
It is the GW with a dual focus of individual change and social reform
It's the GW that is a rare gem in the human services, yet faces extinction
It's the GW that is the hidden treasure in youth development
It's the GW that needs workers to stay the course
   administrators to support the way
    and missionaries to spread the word

—MALEKOFF (2002b)

STRENGTHS-BASED SOCIAL WORK:
TAPPING IN TO WHAT ONE HAS TO OFFER

Knowing something about the history and tradition of group work is a good first step to understanding their relationship to strengths-based practice. Social group work's origins are a melding of three early 20th-century social movements: the settlement movement, the progressive education movement, and the recreation movement (Alissi, 2001; Breton, 1990). What all three have in common is the conviction that people have much to offer to each other to improve the quality of their lives. Each movement realized this by organizing neighbors to challenge and change unacceptable social conditions in the community, by enabling students to practice democracy and learn citizenship in the classroom, and by providing people of all ages opportunities to experience the profound joy of participation in a creative group.

The practice of drawing on what people have to offer is another way of saying that strengths matter. Helping people to discover the resources to improve their situations is not an option for social workers but an obligation (Weick & Saleebey, 1995). It is our duty to understand what people know, what they can do, and what they and their environments have to offer. To do this we must be willing to look beyond labels, categories, and diagnoses (Kemp, Whittaker, & Tracy, 1997; Powell, 2001). We need to assume a "stance of uncertainty" (Pozatek, 1994), a commitment to developing relationships with children, adolescents, and parents that transcends the traditional paradigm of practitioner as knowledgeable expert and client as naïve initiate, relationships that capture the joy of human collaboration (Malekoff, 1997). Establishing a strengths perspective is a good starting point.

RESEARCH ON STRENGTHS-BASED PRACTICE

The effectiveness of the strengths-based framework presented herein has not been formally evaluated. Instead, I present literature on core influences on this framework: strengths-based social work and youth development.

Some of the "converging lines of research and practice" that support the strengths perspective are in the areas of developmental resilience, health and wellness, story and narrative, and solution-focused approaches (Saleebey, 1996, 2001, 2002). A recent example is a study that points to the effectiveness of strengths-based practice for case management with people suffering from serious emotional disturbances (Rapp, 1998).

Developmental resilience studies provide a valuable perspective on the growth-enhancing impact of protective factors and the strength-based variables that mitigate against risk. Extensive studies (Rutter, 1995; Werner, 2000; Werner & Smith, 2001; Werner, Smith, & Garmezy, 1998) found that stimulating and supportive environments are a significant counterforce to constitutional vulnerabilities in children and youths. There are young people who, despite an exposure to multiple risk factors, do not succumb to serious health and behavior problems (e.g., substance abuse, violence, teen pregnancy, school dropout, and delinquency). As Hawkins (1995, p. 14) states, "Protective factors are conditions that buffer young people from the negative consequences of exposure to risk by either reducing the impact of the risk or changing the way a person responds to risk." In the assessment arena, a series of measures and protocols have been designed to help practitioners recognize and work with strengths in children and families (Early, 2001; Gilgun, 1999; Gilgun, Keskinen, Marti, & Jones, 1999; Graybeal, 2001; Malekoff, 1997).

Another fertile area for building strengths among children and adolescents is in the classroom group. A recent national study of 90,000 seventh to twelfth graders across the United States concluded that school connectedness is a critical variable for students' success in school (Blum, McNeely, & Rinehart, 2002). Those who feel connected are less likely to engage in high-risk behaviors. The study concluded that well-managed classrooms are essential to insuring school connectedness. Classroom management can be improved, the study suggests, by providing teachers with strategies for engaging and disciplining students. Knowledge and skill about group work will be an invaluable aid in helping teachers to develop the skills necessary to carry out such strategies in the classroom-group context.

An important arena for strengths-based research is in the youth development field (Catalano, Berglund, Ryan, Lonczak, & Hawkins, 1998). At the core of youth development research is the identification of personal and social assets (i.e., strengths) that facilitate positive youth development (Benson, 1997; Eccles & Gootman, 2002).

STRENGTHS-BASED BUILDING BLOCKS

The Search Institute developed a framework of assets that are signposts of positive child and adolescent development. A review of more than 800 studies provided a scientific foundation for the 40 developmental assets identified by the Search Institute (Scales & Leffert, 1999).

As both a theoretical and research framework, the assets are divided into external (e.g., factors in the environment that promote health and strengths) and internal (e.g., factors in the individual, such as competencies and prosocial values, that represent strengths).

External assets are divided into four subgroups (support, empowerment, boundaries and expectations, and constructive use of time). Examples of specific assets in these subgroups are:

- *Caring neighborhood and school climate*—the young person experiences a caring neighborhood and caring school climate.
- *Safety*—the young person feels safe at home and in the community.
- *Youth as resources*—the community provides young people with useful roles.
- *High expectations*—parents and teachers have high expectations for youths.

Internal assets are also divided into four subgroups (commitment to learning, positive values, social competencies, positive identity). Examples of specific assets in these subgroups are:

- *Achievement motivation*—the young person is motivated to do well in school.
- *Caring*—the young person values helping other people.
- *Planning and decision making*—the young person knows how to plan ahead and make choices.
- *Sense of purpose*—the young person reports, "my life has a purpose."

Group work and youth development are not new. Both have existed since the early part of the 20th century. In fact, group work was the bedrock of early youth development, and group workers the driving force in community centers, neighborhood clubs, and camps and on playgrounds and street corners (Malekoff, 1998, 2002b). The assets have relevance to group workers working with children and adolescents from a strengths-based perspective. They offer group workers some direction for identifying needs and setting group goals, establishing alliances with parents and relevant others, stimulating creative activities, and developing leadership skills.

COGNITIVE-BEHAVIORAL APPROACHES, STRENGTHS-BASED GROUP WORK, AND BEYOND

At the beginning of the 21st century, decreasing dollars for human services, the privatization of mental health care, and the advent of managed care have led to greater attention to short-term, "solution focused" interventions for troubled youth. As a result, the cognitive-behavioral approach has gained great visibility. This approach is based on the principle that behavior, emotions, and cognitions are learned and therefore can be changed by new learning. The emphasis is on addressing problematic behavior as a target for modification, rather than as a symptom of an underlying condition or situation.

A leading proponent of the sociobehavioral approach in the field of group work with children and youth is Sheldon Rose. He developed the cognitive-behavioral interactional approach of group therapy (1998). In this model, the small group is the context for social reinforcement of prosocial behavior, a concept most significant for group work with children and adolescents. As the child begins to step beyond the family unit in adolescence, he or she forms a growing attachment to the peer group. Included among the various behavioral methods of teaching coping skills to children and adolescents are problem solving and sociorecreational methods,[1] both derivatives of the progressive education and recreation movements.

In changing times, different theoretical approaches gain favor as an accommodation to the social, political, and economic realities of the day. Group workers who decide to adapt various approaches can integrate them with the strengths-based principles described herein. For example, using a cognitive-behavioral approach in group work with adolescents does not preclude fostering mutual aid, using the group to promote competence and autonomy, actively engaging parents, or understanding the role of group process as a powerful change dynamic. The challenge for group workers subscribing to strengths-based principles is to create avenues for integration across disciplines and models.

A FRAMEWORK FOR STRENGTHS-BASED GROUP WORK WITH CHILDREN AND ADOLESCENTS

The following seven-principle framework for strengths-based group work with children and adolescents evolved from my group work practice experience over the past three decades (Malekoff, 2001, 2002d). Readers should take special note of Saleebey's (2002) principles of the strengths perspective:

> Every individual, group, family, and community has its strengths; trauma and abuse, illness and struggle may be injurious but they may also be sources of challenge and opportunity; assume that you do not know the upper limits of the capacity to grow and change and take individual, group, and community aspirations seriously; we best serve clients by collaborating with them; every environment is full of resources; and caring, care taking, and context count. (pp. 13–18)

The seven principles are described and then illustrated to bring to life their practical application. The illustrations are a combination of practice summaries, brief vignettes, and longer narratives. Readers should note that, although examples are chosen to illustrate specific principles, the principles are overlapping and interrelated.

Principle 1: Form Groups Based on Members' Felt Needs and Wants, Not Diagnoses

Groups must not be formed on the basis of a diagnosis or a label. Groups should be formed on the basis of felt needs and wants. Felt needs are different from ascribed labels. Understanding members' felt needs is where we begin in group work. Such a simple concept, yet so foreign to so many.[2]

Failed groups may be blamed on unmotivated and resistant children and adolescents or uncooperative and sabotaging parents when, all too often, the real culprit is poor planning. One example of a creative rationale for several failed groups came from a beleaguered practitioner in an inpatient psychiatric setting.

He confidently asserted, "the literature states that groups don't work for ADD kids" (ADD and ADHD are shorthand labels for people diagnosed with attention-deficit disorder and attention-deficit/hyperactivity disorder). Sweeping generalizations and global statements are rarely helpful. Without agreement among group members and between the worker and members about what needs and wants a group will attempt to meet, without clarity in regard to group purpose and individual goals, the effectiveness of a group cannot begin to be measured or evaluated.

Felt needs refers to individual wants, desires, and areas of concern that are both *unique* to individuals in the target population and *universal* to individuals in the target population (i.e., normative adolescent issues, developmental tasks, the need to negotiate difficult environments).

A group for juvenile offenders is offered as an illustration of blending unique and universal needs. The group was formed around the activity of boxing (Wright, 2002). The purposes of the group, to learn the art and science of boxing, to prevent violence, and to enhance personal and social growth, represent the two levels of felt need. Learning the skill of boxing represents a unique need, a desire of the boys who were recruited for this particular group. In today's world, violence prevention could be viewed as a universal need or for this group, a unique need, given their juvenile offender status and the dangerous context of their lives. The need to enhance personal and social growth is universal. Learning boxing helps the group members to reach several physical goals (e.g., boxing, rope skipping, calisthenics). It also helps them to address social and personal growth in the areas of identity, defense, impulse control, patience, focus, commitment, respect (for self, others, and referee), stress relief, and peer support.

Understanding felt needs is a prerequisite to establishing group purpose, deciding on group composition, setting individual and group goals and objectives, and determining what content or means a children's or adolescents' group will use to reach its ends (Malekoff, 1997, pp. 53–80). Knowledge and use of the often-neglected planning process is a prerequisite for workers with all sound groups (Northen & Kurland, 2001).

The following discussion utilizes an illustration of a child who has been labeled with attention-deficit/hyperactivity disorder.

Principle 2: Structure Groups to Welcome the Whole Person, Not Just the Troubled Parts

Group workers must learn to structure groups to welcome the whole person and not just the troubled, hurt, or broken parts (Breton, 1990). There is so much talk these days about strengths and wellness. This is hardly a new and revolutionary concept. But it has been neglected for too long. Good group work practice has been paying attention to people's strengths and assets since the days of the original settlement houses over 100 years ago, mostly without any fanfare (Malekoff, 2002b).

A children's group is a great place for young people to come face-to-face with various levels of difference, to confront the impulse to isolate and objectify the unfamiliar, and to reach for strength amid diversity.[3] In an early meeting of the "changing-family group," in a child guidance center (Malekoff & Laser, 1999), the themes of difference and inclusion came to the fore. Each of the seven 9- and 10-year-old group members had experienced upheaval in his or her families. The parents had divorced, separated, or died. The purpose of the group was to reduce isolation, to explore feelings of loss, and to help members learn how to cope with these changes.

Near the end of the third meeting of the group, the group worker gave a homework assignment: "Over the next week think of something that is important to you, something that you really value, and bring it in to the next group meeting to share with the group." Allie, a 9-year-old whose father had died just months before, said, "I know what I'd like to bring . . . but I'd have to dig him up." Time seemed to stand still as the group worker silently awaited a response from the group.

And then unexpectedly Jimmy, the most physically active and distractible member of the group, who was by then all over the room and into the toys and games on the shelves, stopped what he was doing. He bounded over to Allie and got about as physically close to her as he could without making physical contact. Without asking her what she had meant by her statement, Jimmy said softly, "You could bring a picture."

After another pause in the action, Allie reached into her pink plastic purse and removed a tattered photograph. Her action spurred the others to form a semicircle around her so that each could get a good look at the snapshot she held of her smiling father.

What the group learned weeks later was that Jimmy knew the feeling that comes with being an annoyance to almost everyone. When asked for his own impressions of what his teachers thought of him, he hesitated and shrugged. But after a moment or two his cheeks reddened, and, with his mouth forming an ironic smile, he said, "They all hate me."

In this example, the principle of welcoming the whole person and valuing members as helpers is stimulated as the group worker steps aside, tacitly inviting full participation, and enabling the group to respond to Allie's lament, "I know what I'd like to bring . . . but I'd have to dig him up." As a result, Jimmy stepped forward with a touching sensitivity, typically hidden from the view of others in his day-to-day interactions.

Principle 3: Integrate Verbal and Nonverbal Activities

Competent group work requires the use of verbal and nonverbal activities. Group work practitioners must, for once and for all, learn to relax and to abandon the strange and bizarre belief that the only successful group is one that consists of people who sit still and speak politely and insightfully (Malekoff, 1997, pp. 146–165).

Activity is more than "tool," more than programmed content, more than "canned" exercises, and more than a mechanistic means to an end. Middleman (1985) aptly described the "toolness of program more as putty than a hammer, that is, as a tool that also changes as it is used" (p. 4). In addition to a wealth of structured resource material available (e.g., games, exercises, and curricula), there are activities that grow spontaneously out of the living together that the group members do. These are the creative applications, the member- and worker-initiated innovations that can be cultivated and brought to life in the group, contributing to a growing sense of groupness and rich history of experience together (Malekoff, 1997, p. 148). A simple homework assignment in the changing-family group, illustrated in the previous section, led to a profound moment and empathic connection for Allie, Jimmy, and their fellow group members who had lost so much in their young lives.

The following two vignettes offer additional angles on the use of activity by illustrating (1) how the use of art and action research were used to combat homophobia and (2) how the decision of a group of children to wear their glasses to group meetings opened a pathway to greater intimacy. These illustrations reflect work in two kinds of settings: a drop-in center and coffeehouse for lesbian and gay youths and a residential therapeutic camp for school-age children.[4]

Isolation or Inclusion: Creating Safe Spaces for Lesbian and Gay Youths

A recent action research project was launched with the aim of improving the lives of lesbian and gay youths by raising awareness of school-based homophobia (Peters, 2001, 2003). The action research process (Malekoff, 1994) involved surveying more than 1,000 high school students and then presenting the results for discussion by youths and adults in an all-day conference. The purpose was to raise consciousness, stimulate interaction, and motivate change. The settings for this illustration involved a collaborative effort by a coffeehouse for lesbian, gay, bisexual, transgender, and questioning youths; a community mental health center; several public high schools; a community center; and several advocacy groups.

The project began with groups of youths and adults brainstorming to create questionnaires to probe student and faculty attitudes and experiences with homophobia in local high schools. The process enabled the participants to sharpen their thinking in an attempt to gather data that would strengthen their roles as advocates. This group process also illustrates Principle 6, *maintain a dual focus on individual change and social reform*.

Beyond developing questionnaires, a group of older adolescent boys formed a creative art group that arrived at the idea to create almost-true-to-life school lockers defaced with anti-gay slurs (e.g., faggot) as a means of raising consciousness on a more visceral level. According to one of the student group leaders (Zaleznick, 2001) in the creative art group, "Every day gay, lesbian, bisexual, and transgender teens are 'gay bashed' in school and many have nowhere to turn. The art group . . . created model lockers to represent the homophobia that exists in schools." Ultimately the lockers, realistic and shocking, became a traveling exhibit used to encourage the development of GSA's (gay–straight alliances) in schools.

In the following example, a younger group participating in a therapeutic camp found another way to shed some light on a troubling matter.

Shedding Some Light

Ivan, who lived in a foster family, was a member of a therapeutic summer camp group for children with serious emotional disturbances. He lived with a foster family with a history of alcoholism. He had extremely poor vision and was too embarrassed to wear his thick-lensed, and broken glasses, held together at the bridge of his nose with white adhesive tape. He was afraid that he would be teased by the group and called names, such as "four-eyes." This was the treatment he had grown accustomed to in the school and neighborhood.

He shared his fears in the group, and the members agreed to be kind and not tease him. To support Ivan, everyone in the group who wore glasses decided to wear theirs if Ivan would wear his. This act, a simple nonverbal activity that emerged directly from the life of the group, spoke volumes.

After some hesitation, unsure about whether he could trust the others and the situation, he finally agreed to wear his glasses. The first day after the agreement, he wore his glasses for an hour. No one made fun of him, and all were pleased that he could see better and perform better while playing board games.

The next day he came to the group with a pair of new glasses and solicited the worker's and group's opinions of the style of frames he had chosen. The group was approving, validating his choice, which made him smile. He willingly wore the glasses and, some weeks later, asked the others if they wished to know why his vision was so poor, requiring corrective lenses. The group became quiet as he told his story of living in an eastern European orphanage until the age of 4. He revealed that he was strapped down to a bed in the evenings and that, whenever he cried or refused to go to sleep, nurses shined a flashlight in his eyes.

Ivan seemed relieved after sharing his story. The others remained pensive as they grappled with this information that he hoped would help them to understand him better.

The young men's art group and the summer camp group also illustrate Principle 4, *decentralize authority and turn control over to group members*. The group members' initiative is demonstrated in both examples. In the first, the use of art provided both a reflection of group members' painful life experiences and a tool for social action. In the second, the simple act of deciding to wear eyeglasses in solidarity with a fellow member opened an unexpected door of understanding and intimacy. In the following illustration, turning control over to group members takes a different "twist."

Principle 4: Decentralize Authority and Turn Control Over to Group Members

Group workers need to understand that losing control is not what you want to get away from; it's what you want to get to. What this means is that when control is turned over to the group, and when the group worker gives up his or her centrality in the group, then mutual aid can follow, and members can then find expression for what they have to offer. Encouraging "what they have to offer" is the kind of group work we need to practice; it is what real empowerment is all about.

In the following example, a variation on Fritz Redl's "life-space interviewing" (1966) demonstrates its application with a group in a day treatment/therapeutic school setting.

Groups-on-the-Go: Mutual Aid in the Moment

This illustration presents *groups-on-the-go* (Jagendorf & Malekoff, 2000), spontaneously formed, mutual aid groups for children and adolescents. "Spontaneously formed groups" refers to groups that are formed in response to a pressing need. They are composed of individuals known to one another who voluntarily agree to participate. These groups are offered in an agency that provides sanction and support (and of course adequate space) for the activity.

Groups-on-the-go is an extension of life-space interviewing (Redl, 1966, pp. 35–67), the purpose of which is to address problems in adolescents' direct here-and-now life experience.[5] Group workers must be problem focused, clear about goals, and active in the pursuit of their aims. However, they must also be prepared for emergent problems that occur in the life of the group, to expect the unexpected, and to be ready for "group work on the go" (Malekoff, 1997, viii).

The two major tasks of life-space interviewing are clinical exploitation of life events and emotional first aid on the spot. These terms refer to "interviewing (that) is closely built around the child's direct life experience in connection with issues that become the interview focus" (Redl, 1966, p. 41). Groups-on-the-go adds a third feature, mutual aid in the moment, by which peers are purposefully introduced into the helping mix.

Pregroup planning is critical for effective group work; however, spontaneous interventions are frequently necessary.[6] For example, when a number of students in a school are unaccounted for at the same time, the reaction can range from a "here we go again" shrug of the shoulders to general alarm about their whereabouts. Group workers must pay attention to administrative details, such as obtaining passes for permission for students to leave class.

They must also be prepared to describe the value of the intervention and to demystify the process for the gatekeepers in the organization who might otherwise squash such efforts. With these caveats in mind, readers are introduced to *the dance group*.

In this illustration, the group worker is a team member in a school-based mental health program. She represents a community mental health center that formed a partnership with the school to provide services on site in the school for children and adolescents who have been identified as having serious emotional disturbances. The dance group begins with an individual meeting between the social worker and Jay.

> Jay sat in session upset, dirty blonde hair over his eyes, with no expression on his face. Jay loves music and plays the keyboard. He often spoke about the music he listened to. He likes grunge rock groups that sing about depressing, painful themes. Jay said that he was invited to Maria's sweet-sixteen party this Friday and that all his friends from school were going. Jay said, "But I'm not going. And if I go, I'll stay outside and smoke cigarettes or sit in the corner like I did at the prom last year. I'll just sit like this all night." He proceeded to cross his arms, slump down in his chair and look depressed.
>
> We talked for a while about why Jay didn't want to go to Maria's sweet sixteen. Jay finally blurted out, "I can't dance." "No? You've never danced at a party or a concert?" I asked. "Well, I jump into the mosh pit. Don't get me wrong, that's fun: banging heads and pulling at people's clothes. But I don't think they'll have that at the sweet sixteen."
>
> There was a knock on the door, and Jerold bounced in. Jerold has great energy and poise. And he is a wonderful dancer. "Jerold, perfect timing. Jay, can I tell Jerold about your dilemma?" Jay seemed to shrug his response, "Sure, tell him."
>
> "You're going to Maria's sweet sixteen, right, Jerold," I asked.
>
> "Oh, yeah," he said.
>
> "Well, Jay doesn't want to go."
>
> Jerold turned to Jay. "No way, how come?"
>
> "'Cause I don't know how to dance."
>
> "You can dance, Jay," Jerold said.
>
> "No, I don't know how. If I go I'm just going to sit in the corner or stay outside until it's over. I'll wear my torn pants and a tie-dyed shirt. Maybe they won't even let me in."
>
> "Jerold, you're a great dancer," I said. "Do you think you could teach Jay to dance?"
>
> "Yeah, I could teach you, give you some moves. You could do it."
>
> "What do you say, Jay? You both could come to my office, I'll lock the door, and we could have a dance lesson." (In time two girls joined this group-on-the-go. Ultimately, Jay attended the sweet-sixteen party . . . and danced.)

Far from coming into conflict with the culture of the host setting, groups-on-the-go can positively influence organizational culture. The worker's faith in mutual aid and in what young group members have to offer, willingness to take the risk of forming a group-on-the-go, and readiness to navigate obstacles and manage logistics can favorably influence the environment. By emphasizing members' strengths, maintaining an optimistic outlook that problems can be solved, and never losing sight of the normative experiences of young people who are most often identified by deficits, a group-on-the-go can go a long way to adding spirit and character to a school (or other setting inhabited by children and teens) and instilling a sense of hope in both the youth and adults who inhabit such a space together.

With the dance group, the worker paid careful attention to including school personnel in the mix. In the illustration of Principle 5, this is taken a step further, as indicated, by detailing a careful negotiation with elementary school teachers to gain sanction for a group idea that was at first greeted with ambivalent feelings.

Principle 5: Develop Alliances with Relevant Other People in Group Members' Lives

Group workers involved with children and youths must understand that anxious and angry parents, teachers, and school administrators are not our enemies and that we must collaborate with them and form stable alliances with them if we are to be successful with their children. We must learn to embrace their frustration and anxiety, rather than becoming defensive and rejecting. Alliances are needed with relevant others who are deeply invested in the plight of our group members.

The example to follow also illustrates Principle 3, *integrating verbal and nonverbal activities*, in groups and shows how members with different skill and competency levels can work together if program content is carefully chosen. The setting for this illustration is a therapeutic elementary school program.[7]

A Poetry Club for Kids

A group work service for a classroom group in a special education school setting presents group workers with a unique set of challenges. One group worker knew that he needed to contract with the classroom teachers, integrate group purpose with academic and behavioral goals, and support the prosocial values promoted daily in the classroom. He thought that a poetry club (Malekoff, 2002a) could build spirit, tap students' creativity, provide an alternative and fun means of expression, and cultivate an appreciation for poetry that could extend beyond the life of the group itself.

The classroom composition in the program was six students, one teacher, and one aide, they are referred to as "6-1-1 classes." At the time, three students were in each of two classes, one older and one younger class. The worker asked them to think about the concept of "poetry in motion" and explained that all poetry didn't have to be regimented pencil-to-paper work and that together they could help the students discover means for finding poetic expression verbally, musically, and physically, as well. For example, one of the group activities involved photography, with members taking turns to arrange the group into their own unique poetic tableau to be preserved photographically.

The group worker presented the idea of mutual aid as a core principle. Older students could help the younger ones, and younger ones could encourage the efforts of the older ones. The staff could easily relate to the prosocial value of promoting mutual aid.

The teachers provided a list of academic goals representing the grade level of students in their classes. Samples of the stated goals are: *students will learn to comprehend a story; students will learn to listen to and enjoy stories; students will recall important facts and ideas; students will learn to read orally with phrasing and expression, pacing, and volume; students will express personal opinions about readings*. It is important to work collaboratively with teachers and to respect the goals they wish to accomplish and to standards they aim to maintain if one expects to be a welcomed guest in their classrooms. In reviews with the teachers, it became clear that academic goals were compatible with group purposes and goals.

The purpose and goals of the group were conceived as follows:

The Poetry Club is a weekly group that is about learning to work together, share, have fun, and build confidence through the self-expression of poetry. The goals of Poetry Club are related to academic goals, including following directions, participating in discussions, and reading aloud fluently and accurately. The Poetry Club members will learn to help one another, applaud one another, and appreciate one another.

The Poetry Club met once a week over 10 weeks for about 40 minutes each session.

The group meetings began with a reading of a "guess what" poem: poetry that described something for them to discover together. Key words were left out of the poems to create mystery. The group's assignment was to guess what the poem described. After the poem was read, the group was instructed to huddle up, as a football team might, and discuss what they thought the poem was about. Finally, when the members thought they had arrived at the correct answer, they would say so. The first poem was about a giraffe. An added bonus was that the poem itself was shaped like a giraffe.

    A longer term project was guided poetry. The members were given open-ended sentences to complete about themselves and their fellow group members that probed their thoughts, interests, experiences, and strengths. The raw material was drafted as a "poem under construction," and each week the members would work toward the goal of refining their poem into a finished product to be included in a group-ending Poetry Club journal that would record all of their work.

Allowing adequate time for a good ending is essential. In a short-term group such as the Poetry Club, members should be reminded of how many group meetings are remaining from the very beginning and along the way. This can be done verbally or on a calendar for those members who are more inclined to integrate information visually. By providing reminders in a thoughtful manner, the end of the group does not come unexpectedly to the members, and planning for a meaningful separation is made possible.

The last three ending-phase meetings were bittersweet, with the members enjoying readings from the Poetry Club journal, chronicling their good work. The younger boys, in particular, loved gift-wrapping extra journals that they would bring home to their families. Free access to scissors and Scotch tape was heaven for the 5-, 6-, and 7-year-olds. The boys openly wished that Poetry Club could continue and questioned why it had to end. Transition. Separation. Loss. Not an easy subject for this group.

Along the lines of advocating for a group service in a school or other system, group workers practicing strengths-based group work need to maintain a dual focus of individual change and social reform. This principle has been illustrated in the creative arts group that aimed to raise consciousness about homophobia in high schools. The next two examples provide further illustrations.

Principle 6: Maintain a Dual Focus on Individual Change and Social Reform

Group workers must stay tuned in to the "near things of individual need and the far things of social reform" (Schwartz, 1986). This dual vision was first conceptualized by one of the earliest group work researchers, Wilbur Newstetter (1935). Group workers must help group members to become active participants in community affairs, so that they might make a difference, might change the world one day whereas others have failed. A good group can be a great start for this kind of consciousness development and action.

Understanding the dual focus is especially critical for youths today, when so many world-shattering and traumatic events influence lives. The illustrations that follow describe group work responses to the Columbine High School tragedy in 1999 and the terrorist attack on America on September 11, 2001.

Beyond shattering one's sense that the world is a safe place, traumatic events undermine basic attachments of family, friends, and community (Herman, 1997; van der Kolk, 1987). As a result, trauma survivors feel abandoned and isolated. One of the goals of recovery is to restore "the connection between survivors and community" (Herman, 1997, p. 50). If trauma isolates, group work connects.

In the Aftermath of Columbine: An Intergenerational Collaboration

The Columbine massacre, although it took place in Colorado, affected young people, parents, and school officials all across the United States. Schools redoubled efforts to insure security, emergency rooms and outpatient clinic emergency visits spiked, and a general sense of anxiety filled schools across the United States.

Two weeks after the massacre in Columbine, in one northeastern suburb a group of 12 teenagers and 8 adults was formed for a one-session group to videotape a program for broadcast. Following is the group worker's account of this group (Malekoff, 1999):

> The meeting started with a pre-group warm up in which the members got acquainted with one another and the purpose of the group. They were all group members from various other settings including a high school, a mental health center, drop-in center for lesbian and gay youth, an outreach program for Latino youth, a chemical dependency program, and a street outreach program. The purpose of the one-session group, which was to be video taped for educational purposes, was *to explore, identify, and emphasize what youth need in the aftermath of Columbine*. The participants understood this opportunity as one that would enable them to debrief and give voice to their impressions and concerns to a wider audience.
>
> As the 90-minute group meeting unfolded the eyes of the adult participants and observers widened. They were caught by surprise as they listened to the young people who ranged in age from 13 to 18. After some discussion about school safety and what some described as "fascist" measures taken by school administrators (e.g., requiring transparent book bags, administering random locker checks, searches and pat downs) they talked about, as one 16-year-old girl stated, "What do we really need."
>
> To everyone's surprise they said that what they really needed and wanted was closer relationships with adults in home and at school. The group worker remarked to the teens, "You seem to be starving for someone to simply listen to you."
>
> Intergenerational groups have the benefit of providing both generations an opportunity to "practice" communication with both adults and youth, other than those with whom they have daily contact at home or in school. In this group, participation in a recorded intergenerational exchange in the aftermath of Columbine was the participants' way of spreading the message of their experiences and perceptions to others who might also be struggling. It was their way of making a difference. (p. 1)

A Gift from the Children of Oklahoma to the Children of New York Following 9/11/2001

Among the services offered by a mental health agency in the metropolitan New York area in the aftermath of September 11, 2001, are bereavement groups for children who lost parents in the World Trade Center (Malekoff, 2002c; Morse, 2002). One group worker in a Project Liberty agency (the Federal Emergency Management Agency [FEMA]-funded post-9/11 crisis counseling program) made contact with an Oklahoma City organization to exchange information and experiences in order to prepare for the work ahead. One day a large box arrived in the mail. It was addressed to the children in the New York bereavement groups. It came from a group of elementary school children in Oklahoma City.

Inside the box were 55 teddy bears. A laminated card bordered by American flags was hanging from a string around each teddy bear's neck. Each card contained a message written by an Oklahoma City child to a child from New York. One of the cards said,

> Dear New York,
>
> I am very sorry about the plane crash. And I am very sorry if someone special to you died in it.

In both of these examples, young people responded in the aftermath of horrific events. Group workers need not feel that all groups should take some form of dramatic social action to qualify as strengths-based group work. More to the point is that group workers maintain awareness of appropriate opportunities to take social action and to be flexible enough to help the group to see possibilities for action.

Participating in a change effort that includes identifying a problem, exploring it in some depth, seeking solutions, and implementing and evaluating them is an important learning experience for young group members trying to make sense of the world and a good practical lesson about the problem-solving process (Malekoff, 1997, pp. 119–145).

Principle 7: Understand and Respect Group Development as a Key to Promoting Change

Each good group has a life of its own, each one with a unique personality—what group workers refer to as a culture. All those who work with groups must learn to value the developmental life of a group. A greater understanding of and respect for group development, amidst the noise and movement and excitement of a typical kids' group, can lead to a feeling of greater confidence in the group worker, confidence that he or she will move ahead and hang in there and not bail out, as too many an adult already has.

A vital tenet of group work practice is that "the worker must actively understand, value, and respect the group process itself as the powerful change dynamic that it is" over time and in each meeting (Middleman & Wood, 1990, p. 11). This tenet demands that the practitioner have a good knowledge base, reinforced by practice experience, of group developmental theory. Group developmental theory refers to group dynamics and tasks that are unique to progressive stages (or phases) from the first to last moments of a group's time together. Group development reflects a group's path toward closeness, interrelatedness, and, ultimately, separation. Group development is not always a neat and orderly process. A group is subject to regression when it confronts obstacles and crises.

Two distinguished developmental models, Schwartz's interactional model (Berman-Rossi, 1994; Gitterman & Shulman, 1985/1986) and the Boston model (Garland, Jones, & Kolodny, 1973), are good starting points. Some group leaders have an intuitive sense of group development, as illustrated by a Little League coach who understood his team's need for a good ending as the season came to a close.

> One Little League coach instituted an annual ritual of a postseason combination barbecue and parent–child softball game. As the end of the season approached, the players (boys and girls), their siblings, parents and grandparents started buzzing about the barbecue, making plans from

the sidelines. Compare the feeling in this leave-taking scenario to that of the team whose ending would come and go as swiftly as the final pitch of the final game of the season. (Malekoff, 1997, p. 176)

CONCLUSION AND FUTURE DIRECTIONS

This chapter presents a strengths-based framework for group work with children and adolescents. Seven principles were offered to serve as a foundation to inform practice so that it can be flexibly and purposefully practiced regardless of chosen model, approach, or curriculum.

Group workers who rely on curricula, agendas, and exercises require accompanying knowledge and skill necessary to promote interaction, mutual aid, and spontaneity among group members. Otherwise, rather than curriculum-guided tools, these activities then become curriculum-driven procedures. Without a good practice foundation, packaged approaches risk controlling children and youths by inhibiting creative expression.

The strengths-based principles are overlapping and interrelated. They call for group workers to consider the felt needs of group members, to recognize and activate what group members have to offer, to use a variety of activities and media to engage and challenge children and youth in groups, to reach out to parents and relevant others in group members' lives, to recognize opportunities for group members to practice social action and citizenship, and to become familiar with the developmental path of groups.

The future of group work with young people rests with practitioners who are well grounded in the foundations and traditions of group work. In addition, today's practitioners need to develop special knowledge and skill in working with violence, trauma and loss, and intercultural issues.

Although the September 11, 2001, attack on America is the most horrific public event in recent memory, it only underscores the increasing violence that children and youths are exposed to in public arenas (e.g., gang violence, the Columbine shootings, the Oklahoma City bombing, the Beltway sniper) and in private settings (e.g., child abuse, domestic violence, witnessing violence). It is clear that we need a public health approach to violence prevention, an approach that offers a continuum of services from prevention to treatment (Prothrow-Stith, 1993, 2002). Among its many roles, group work can promote intercultural relations, teach peaceable conflict resolution, and build supportive groups for survivors of violence.

Research on the impact of violence on children and adolescents and on the role of group work in prevention and treatment will be critical in the future (Glodich & Allen, 1998). Of equal importance is developing and evaluating approaches for intercultural relations that reduce prejudice, foster understanding, promote peace, and provide youths with the skills to become active participants in community affairs (Malekoff, 1997).

The future of group work with children and adolescents relies on educators and practitioners who advocate for integrating group work values, knowledge, and skill into youth development programs and the classroom. As the studies referred to earlier suggest, connectedness—attachment to peers, teachers, and relevant other adults—is a good educational and public health strategy that promotes strengths in young people.

Regardless of the problem to be addressed or the theoretical approach, group workers should be mindful that children and adolescents want to be taken as whole people with something to offer, not broken objects to be fixed. Tuning in to and grounding oneself in the seven principles of strengths-based group work is a good starting point.

NOTES

1. For recent examples of the efficacy of cognitive-behavioral group therapy for children and adolescents with serious emotional disorders see Thienemann, Martin, and Cregger (2001) and Mendlowitz, Manassis, and Bradley (1999), who present studies on groups for adolescents with obsessive–compulsive disorders and children with anxiety disorders. Mendlowitz et al. (1999) highlight the role of parental involvement.

2. Beyond identifying need, good group work practice with children and adolescents requires a planning process that includes gaining sanction and support from agency administration, developing a clear purpose, selecting and screening members carefully, attending to the structural details (i.e., time and space) of the effort, and identifying appropriate content and materials for the group to meet its goals (Malekoff, 1997, pp. 53–80).

3. Engaging the whole person requires paying attention to intercultural issues. Addressing diversity in the group can help to promote prejudice reduction, intergroup relations, and group identity. Later in this chapter an illustration of a group project to fight homophobia in high schools is presented. For a comprehensive discussion of intercultural issues and group work with youth see Malekoff (1997, pp. 189–214).

4. Passi (1998) offers a rich assortment of suggestions for creative group programming in psychiatric day hospitals and residential centers. Her ideas are well suited for an older adolescent population and, in some instances, can be easily adapted for group work with children and younger adolescents.

5. The group work described by Fritz Redl and David Wineman has been referred to as "programming for ego support" and was forged from their direct experiences in a residential setting (Pioneer House) for preadolescents. Their landmark books, *Controls from Within* (1952) and *Children Who Hate* (1951), are essential resources for all group workers.

6. This also holds true for residential and other settings (i.e., day treatment, camp, day care) in which children and youths spend all or the better part of their days.

7. Regarding group work with youth in inpatient settings, Stein and Kymissis (1989) highlight the importance of a good interrelationship among team members and between team members, parents, and children. This is essential in insuring that dysfunctional patterns of communication are not replicated in the treatment setting.

REFERENCES

Alissi, A. (2001). *The social group work traditions: Toward social justice in a free society.* Weatogue, CT: The Social Group Work Foundation.

Benson, P. (1997). *All kids are our kids: What communities must do to raise caring and responsible children and adolescents.* San Francisco, CA: Jossey-Bass.

Berman-Rossi, T. (Ed.). (1994). *Social work: The collected writings of William Schwartz.* Itasca, IL: Peacock.

Blum, R., McNeely, C., & Rinehart, P. (2002). *Improving the odds: The untapped power of schools to improve the health of teens.* University of Minnesota, Center for Adolescent Health and Development.

Breton, M. (1990). Learning from social group work traditions. *Social Work with Groups, 13*(3), 21–24.

Catalano, R., Berglund, M., Ryan, J., Lonczak, H., & Hawkins, D. (1998). *Positive youth development in the United States: Research findings on evaluations of positive youth development programs.* Seattle, WA: University of Washington, Social Development Research Group.

Early, T. (2001). Measures for practice with families from a strengths Perspective. Families in Society, *82*(3), 225–232.

Eccles, J., & Gootman, J. (Eds.). (2002). *Community programs to promote Youth development.* Washington, DC: National Academy Press.

Garland, J., Jones, H., & Kolodny, R. (1973). A model for stages of development in social work with groups. In S. Bernstein (Ed.), *Explorations in group work* (pp. 17–71). Boston: Milford House.

Gilgun, J. (1999). CASPARS: New tools for assessing client risks and strengths. *Families in Society*, 80(5), 450–459.

Gilgun, J., Keskinen, S., Marti, D., & Jones, D. (1999). Clinical applications of the CASPARS instruments: Boys who act out sexually. *Families in Society*, 80(6), 629–641.

Gitterman, A., & Shulman, L. (Eds.). (1985/1986). The legacy of William Schwartz: Group practice as shared interaction [Special issue]. *Social Work with Groups*, 8(4).

Glodich, A., & Allen, J. (1998). Adolescents exposed to violence and abuse: A review of the group therapy literature with an emphasis on preventing trauma reenactment. *Journal of Child and Adolescent Group Therapy*, 8(3), 135–154.

Graybeal, C. (2001). Strengths-based social work assessment: Transforming the dominant paradigm. *Families in Society*, 82(3), 233–242.

Hawkins, D. (1995). Controlling crime before it happens: Risk focused prevention. *National Institute of Justice Journal*, 229, 10–18.

Herman, J. (1997). *Trauma and recovery*. New York: Basic Books.

Kemp, S., Whittaker, J., & Tracy, E. (1997). *Person–environment practice: The social ecology of interpersonal helping*. Hawthorne, NY: Aldine de Gruyter.

Jagendorf, J., & Malekoff, A. (2000). Groups-on-the-go: Spontaneously formed mutual aid groups for adolescents in distress. *Social Work with Groups*, 22(4), 15–32.

Malekoff, A. (1994). Action research: An approach to preventing substance abuse and promoting social competency. *Health and Social Work*, 19(1), 46–53.

Malekoff, A. (1997). *Group work with adolescents: Principles and practice*. New York: Guilford Press.

Malekoff, A. (1998). Keys to integrating family support and youth development through group work. *Family Resource Coalition of America Report*, 17(1), 9–10.

Malekoff, A. (1999). From the editor. *HUH?!?: A Newsletter about Working with Children and Youth in Groups*, 4(4), p. 1.

Malekoff, A. (2001). The power of group work with kids: A practitioner's reflection on strengths-based practice. *Families in Society*, 82(3), 243–249.

Malekoff, A. (2002a). "What could happen and what couldn't happen": A poetry club for kids. *Families in Society*, 83(1), 29–34.

Malekoff, A. (2002b, March). *Group work: The hidden treasure in youth development*. Paper presented at the biannual conference of the Long Island Institute for Group Work with Children and Youth of the North Shore Child and Family Guidance Center, Melville, NY.

Malekoff, A. (2002c). The longest day. In A. Gitterman & A. Malekoff (Eds.), *Reflections: Narratives of professional helping, September 11 memorial issue*, 8(3), 28–35.

Malekoff, A. (2002d). The power of group work with kids: Lessons learned. In R. Kurland & A. Malekoff (Eds.), *Stories celebrating group work: It's not always easy to sit on your mouth* (pp. 73–86). Binghamton, NY: Haworth Press.

Malekoff, A., & Laser, M. (1999). Addressing difference in group work with children and young adolescents. *Social Work with Groups*, 21(4), 23–34.

Mendlowitz, S., Manassis, K., & Bradley, S. (1999). Cognitive-behavioral group treatments in childhood anxiety disorders: The role of parental involvement. *Journal of the American Academy of Child and Adolescent Psychiatry*, 38(10), 1223–1229.

Middleman, R. (1985, March 22). *Integrating the arts and activities in clinical group work practice*. Paper presented at the Center for Group Work Studies, Barry University School of Social Work, Miami Shores, FL.

Middleman, R., & Wood, G. (1990). From social group work to social work with groups. *Social Work with Groups*, 13(3), 3–20.

Morse, K. (2002). A lump in my throat and a gift from a far away place. In A. Gitterman & A. Malekoff (Eds.), *Reflections: Narratives of professional helping, September 11 memorial issue*, 8(3), 63–65.

Newstetter, W. (1935). What is social group work? In *Proceedings of the National Conference of Social Work* (pp. 291–299). Chicago: University of Chicago Press.

Northen, H., & Kurland, R. (2001). *Social work with groups*. New York: Columbia University Press.

Passi, L. (1998). *A guide to creative group programming in the psychiatric day hospital*. Binghamton, NY: Haworth Press.

Peters, A. (2001). From the guest editor. *HUH?!?: A Newsletter about Working with Children and Youth in Groups, 6*(3), 1.

Peters, A. (2003). Isolation or inclusion: Creating safe spaces for lesbian and gay youth. *Families in Society, 84*(3), 331–337.

Powell, W. (2001). The eye of the beholder. *Families in Society, 82*(3), 219–220.

Pozatek, E. (1994). The problem of certainty: Clinical social work in the postmodern era. *Social Work, 39*(4), 396–404.

Prothrow-Stith, D. (1993). *Deadly consequences: How violence is destroying our teenage population and a plan to begin solving the problem.* New York: Harper Collins.

Prothrow-Stith, D. (2002) Youth violence prevention: The intersection between public health and justice. *Contemporary Justice Review, 5*(2), 121–131.

Rapp, C. (1998). *The strengths model: Case management with people suffering from severe and persistent mental illness.* New York: Oxford University Press.

Redl, F. (1966). The life space interview: Strategies and techniques. In F. Redl (Ed.), *When we deal with children* (pp. 35–67). New York: Free Press.

Redl, F., & Wineman, D. (1951). *Children who hate.* New York: Macmillan.

Redl, F., & Wineman, D. (1952). *Controls from within: Techniques for the treatment of the aggressive child.* New York: Macmillan.

Rose, S. (1998). *Group therapy with troubled youth: A cognitive-behavioral interactive approach.* Thousand Oaks, CA: Sage.

Rutter, M. (Ed.). (1995). *Psychosocial disturbances in young people: Challenges for prevention.* New York: Cambridge University Press.

Saleebey, D. (1996). The strengths perspective in practice: Extensions and cautions. *Social Work, 41*(3), 296–305.

Saleebey, D. (2001). Practicing the strengths perspective: Everyday tools and resources. *Families in Society, 82*(3), 221–222.

Saleebey, D. (2002). *The strenghts perspective in social work practice.* Boston, MA: Allyn & Bacon.

Scales, P., & Leffert, N. (1999). *Developmental assets: A synthesis of the scientific research on adolescent development.* Minneapolis, MN: Search Institute.

Schwartz, W. (1986). The group work tradition and social work practice. *Social Work with Groups, 8*(4), 7–28.

Stein, M., & Kymissis, P. (1989). Adolescent inpatient group psychotherapy. In F. Cramer & L. Richmond (Eds.), *Adolescent group psychotherapy* (pp. 69–84). Madison, WI: International Universities Press.

Thienemann, M., Martin, J., & Cregger, B. (2001). Manual-driven group cognitive-behavioral therapy for adolescents with obsessive-compulsive disorder: A pilot study. *Journal of the American Academy of Child and Adolescent Psychiatry, 40*(11), 1254–1260.

van der Kolk, B. (1987). The role of the group in the origin and resolution of trauma response. In B. van der Kolk (Ed.), *Psychological trauma* (pp. 153–171). Washington, DC: American Psychiatric Press.

Weick, A., & Saleebey, D. (1995). *A postmodern approach to social work practice.* The 1995 Richard Lodge Memorial Lecture, Adelphi University School of Social Work, New York.

Werner, E. (2000). Protective factors and individual resilience. In S. Meisels & J. Shonkoff (Eds.), *Handbook of early childhood intervention* (pp. 115–134). New York: Cambridge University Press.

Werner, E., & Smith, R. S. (2001). *Journeys from childhood to midlife: Risk, resiliency and recovery.* Ithaca, NY: Cornell University Press.

Werner, E., Smith, R. S., & Garmezy, N. (1998). *Vulnerable but invincible: A longitudinal study of resilient children and youth.* New York: Adams, Bannaster, Cox.

Wright, W. (2002, October). *Keep it in the ring: A violence prevention boxing program for juvenile offenders.* Paper presented at the annual symposium of the Association for the Advancement of Social Work with Groups, New York, New York.

Zaleznick, A. (2001). The Locker Room Project. *HUH?!?: A Newsletter about Working with Children and Youth in Groups, 6*(3), 4.

Chapter 14

Group Work in Child Welfare

BARBARA RITTNER

The function of child welfare is to ensure that workers evaluate incidents of potential maltreatment, supervise children deemed at risk for ongoing abuse and neglect, develop effective services to reduce reoccurrence of maltreatment, and discharge those children believed to be safe (Rittner, 2002). Almost everything that happens in child welfare settings happens in groups of one sort or another. Child welfare organizations are composed of groups of administrators, supervisors, workers, and support staff. Child welfare personnel often interact with a variety of service vendors, court personnel, and treatment professionals. These interactions regularly occur in groups as well.

Many of the children who come under supervision are temporarily placed in group shelter settings in which many children reside. They may move in with foster families, where groups of foster and other children also live. Some are placed in small group homes or larger residential facilities. In large part, foster families are trained in groups, as are adoptive families. The training of agency intake workers, foster care workers, shelter staff, and supervisors generally occurs in groups. Many child welfare workers participate in interdisciplinary team meetings to assess and develop interventions for at-risk children and their families.

It is not uncommon for child welfare clients to be treated in traditional remedial groups, many of which are open ended (Galinsky & Schopler, 1989); some of these are dedicated exclusively to treating abusive family members. Caretakers with problems that affect their ability to provide for the care and safety of their children are mandated to enter groups that treat drug addiction, sexual assault, anger management problems, or mental illness. These groups are generally open ended and foster the development of mutual aid to change behaviors or ameliorate the impact of abuse and neglect (Shulman, 1984).

Despite the ubiquity of groups and group processes in child welfare settings, little has been written about how group dynamics in these settings facilitate the reduction of reoccurrences of maltreatment and how failure to attend to group dynamics may create barriers to effective interventions. Much of what we need to know about these groups can be derived from other sources—that is, from the literature about task and remedial groups.

Clearly, then, much of what happens at administrative levels and in service units relies on the dynamics inherent in task group processes (Ephross & Vassil, 1988). Nonetheless, group dynamics as a central component of training success is absent from many of the protocols used to train professionals or caretakers. Although those engaged in treatment groups are aware of the power of group interventions for people with abuse and neglect histories, few child welfare workers use group interventions in child welfare settings. This chapter discusses the role of task, remedial, and training groups within the context of child welfare settings. I address the group practice skills needed by administrators, unit supervisors, child welfare workers, mental health social workers, and trainers to be effective in child welfare settings or with child welfare populations.

AGENCY-BASED TASK GROUPS

Lohmann and Lohmann (2002) observed that administrators, in general, are responsible for providing leadership and oversight, for making decisions, and for building an organization. Middle and upper-level managers in child welfare agencies are responsible for program planning and development, work flow, coordination of services, and evaluation of performance in concert with federal and state policies and procedures (Austin, 1981; Harris & Warner, 1988; Lewis, Lewis, & Souflée, 1991). Continuous changes in policy and shrinking economic support frequently bring various levels of administrators together to assess how they can provide needed services within the constraints of available resources. Inherent in the process is complex decision making that may be subject to the scrutiny of the press and the community (Rittner, 1995).

As Toseland and Rivas (1984) observed, organizational groups have two primary functions—meeting the needs of the agency and meeting the needs of the clients. Administrators frequently convene and conduct meetings to address the performance of an agency without necessarily fully attending to group process. The ability of child welfare organizations to meet the complex needs requisite to protecting children largely depends on how well various task group members work together toward common goals and how well they can engage in problem solving as they confront constant shifts in service demands. Further complicating the situation is the fact that these administrative groups often have changing memberships that reflect the high turnover rates in child welfare agencies. As people are promoted or hired, they join others in the context of hierarchical associations within tables of organization as members of "administrative teams."

Direct service units and middle managers, like their higher level administrative counterparts, also regularly meet in groups. There is evidence that when these groups are employed for more than simple information dissemination, they can foster an environmental culture that protects workers from burnout. Burnout is common in human service agencies and is associated with high levels of turnover, large caseloads, and stressful jobs (Leiter & Maslach, 1988). There is no question that working in child welfare is stressful. Direct service workers are exposed to a constant barrage of abhorrent abusive behaviors and abject neglect perpetrated against children. They face unrelenting demands to dislocate and relocate children from one setting to another. At times they deal with hostile parents and demanding legal systems that may hold them responsible for predicting the behavior of others. In addition, many workers labor under large caseloads in constant states of crises, with very little respect from the community for the difficult job they perform. They are generally poorly paid for their efforts, and many only stay for a few years. These dynamics make them especially vulnerable to burnout (Miller, Ellis, Zook, & Lyles, 1990; Rittner, 1995).

AGENCY GROUP PROCESS AND SKILLS

The more workers and line supervisors see the environment as supportive, the less likely they are to experience burnout and the more likely they are to provide higher levels of service (Leiter & Maslach, 1988; Maslach & Jackson, 1981; Miller et al., 1990). If administrators and supervisors have fundamental authoritarian and supportive functions (Miller et al., 1990), then it becomes self-evident that how they convene groups and facilitate group process can determine how well members manage the demands made on them. There are three key elements to effective agency-based groups: membership androles, purpose, and process. Each of these will be addressed in turn.

Membership

The first challenge that conveners of working groups in child welfare face is deciding on membership. Ironically, this is a decision that is rarely made proactively. Most often the membership of administrative and supervisory groups is directly related to position or rank on tables of organization. It is not uncommon for child welfare administrators to meet with those who report directly to them in groups. Likewise, unit supervisors regularly meet with their immediate supervisor, unit workers with their supervisors, and so on. In large part, this is because most of these groups reflect the ongoing business of the agency—that is, administrative, staff, and unit meetings. In these cases, membership is directly related to function and span of control. Further, these groups rarely need to consider expanding or changing their memberships except on an ad hoc basis. They rely more on how well the group is functioning than on who should be attending.

In some cases, however, membership in the group should be carefully considered. Ephross and Vassil (1988) suggest that membership should be based on two principles: what the member will contribute and what benefits the member will derive from attending. This is particularly true when ad hoc groups are formed to address specific problems or issues or when groups are charged with strategic planning, goal setting, policy and procedure implementation, or program evaluations. Once the purpose of the group shifts from "business as usual" to planning or evaluative functions, then membership needs to be expanded to help the organization adapt to changes in funding, roles, structure, and procedures or to evaluate how well the agency or units have met their goals. Determining which potential members possess critical knowledge, have key skills, or will benefit from participating will enhance the outcomes of the group process and the products of the group (Ephross & Vassil, 1988).

Often the inclusion of representative members in these groups insures that constituents feel that they have had a role in the process and increases their sense of investment in the outcomes. In child welfare, representative members may include the major stakeholders: administrators, unit supervisors, direct service workers, consumers, and vendors (Lohmann & Lohmann, 2002). The more those who are or will be doing the job are included in planning, decision making, and evaluation processes, the greater the probability that the goals set and procedures developed will be congruent with organizational mission, resource availability, worker capabilities, and knowledge. Equally important, barriers to successful implementation are more likely to be identified and corrected early if membership is broadly based. Finally, inclusive membership reduces the potential for duplication of services either within the agency or across service providers (Austin, 1981; Harris & Warner, 1988; Lewis et al., 1991). It is not always possible to include broad representation from large child welfare organizations or from very rural ones. Some child welfare agencies in major cities have hundreds of workers providing services to thousands of families, making the selection process difficult; whereas smaller, rural organizations have limited numbers of workers scattered over large geographical areas, making availability difficult.

Despite the logic of representative membership with shared power, agency-based groups are historically top-heavy and tend to embody autocratic leadership. As a result, they are often perceived by line workers as nothing more than gatherings to inform workers about new policies and procedures or as potentially punitive sessions in which unit supervisors and workers are castigated for perceived failures with little appreciation of the real nature of the work they do. As Glisson and James (2002) observed in their comparative study of human service delivery teams, cultures within organizations shape the perceptions of participants based on their function and ranks within the agency. Their findings are consistent with other literature on organizational cultures that suggests that there are important differences in the lenses through which administrators and line workers view systems and functions and, more important, that those lenses shape the attitudes, perceptions, and decisions made by each level. This approach can avoid the "us versus them" attitudes that prevent effective group dynamics from emerging (Hopkins & Hyde, 2002).

Recently, institutionalized group planning activities have occurred with the development of strategic mapping and quality assurance groups (Joyner, 2002; Tausch & Harter, 2001). These models of decision making and quality assurance depend on an inclusionary process, with representatives from complementary functions involved in goal setting and tracking successes. The literature on these models clearly supports the importance of broad representation in both goal setting and goal attainment evaluation. The consensus-building strategy inherent in these models encourages evaluating effectiveness of service delivery beyond case reporting (Marshall, Solomon, & Steber, 2001).

Group Leadership Roles

Regardless of the type of agency-based group, the next major decision that many groups face is designating or selecting a leader (Cohen, 1994). In reality, the more hierarchical the agency is, the more difficult it is for leadership to be flexible. The assumption often is that the person with the highest rank is the leader, even though at times that person may not be the best person to lead. In child welfare hierarchies, rank has implicit and explicit power attached to it. It is difficult in those settings for a leader to fully empower the members in a group if he or she holds a higher rank. This is particularly true for working groups that fall outside the scope of the "business as usual" group meeting.

Ideally, leadership can be a "distributive function" (Ephross & Vassil, 1988, p. 100) that adapts to the emerging needs or demands of a group. In that case, the leadership role can be selected by the members based on either the knowledge or the leadership skills that a member brings to facilitating group process or consensus building. It may also be that leadership shifts as demands on groups change. If distributive leadership is impractical—and there are likely to be times at which it is—then how administrators and managers use the leadership role is important. Effective administrative and supervisory leaders recognize the limitations of shared power and authority in naturally occurring groups, including those in child welfare agencies. They use their leadership position to develop strategies that can facilitate open communication and planning, and they tolerate productive conflict within the group. In this way, the organization can utilize broad group representation without expecting to realize unattainable presumptions of equality.

Real-Life Example from a Child Welfare Agency Experience

Ample real life examples exist of how unit supervisors can effectively engage group process in their units by strengthening the dynamics inherent in unit meetings. One such unit supervisor where I worked began having Friday morning coffee with her unit of nine workers. Generally lasting $1\frac{1}{2}$ hours, the time was spent drinking coffee, eating food that the members brought in, and reviewing the week in a fashion that closely resembled Duffy's (1994) recommended "check-in." The discussions might focus on problem cases, interagency frustrations, changes in court procedures, or interventions and resources that were effective. Over time, the unit began talking extensively about the problems that adolescents in care were creating. Eventually, other workers and supervisors were invited to join the discussion to insure a fuller understanding of the problems these adolescents faced and the demands they were putting on the units. The units documented the problems that existed and talked about a variety of possible solutions, culminating in a proposal for the formation of an adolescent unit that was brought to the larger administrative group by the unit supervisors. The plan was quickly adopted by the administrators, and the unit was implemented and populated with workers who enjoyed working with that population.

INTERDISCIPLINARY GROUPS

The four major issues that emerge in child welfare interdisciplinary groups are membership, roles, client selection, and reimbursement. Once these issues are resolved, group meetings are more likely to focus on the types of services that can be provided. It is critical that the planning stage of interdisciplinary groups include representative membership and shared leadership so that the goals established incorporate the best interests of clients in coherence with the best interests of service providers. The absence of clear expectations about what agencies want and need from each other can create a tendency for agencies to attempt to "cherry pick" the best clients and refer the most difficult clients to each other. This is especially true if the basis for continuation of contracts is measured solely by success rates.

One of the most common forms of interdisciplinary groups is that in which service providers meet to discuss intervention options for child welfare families. In some cases, the services are provided to address a particular type of abuse (Lyon & Kouloumpos-Lenares, 1987), whereas in other instances a variety of service vendors are present to explore referral options (Wagner, 1987). Toseland, Ivanoff, and Rose (1987) examined child welfare treatment conferences, a form of interdisciplinary group. The membership included representatives from child welfare, mental health settings, residential care facilities, public health, the courts, and "others." The group members' educational levels reflected those that are typically found in interdisciplinary groups—ranging from those with undergraduate degrees to those with doctoral level degrees (including MDs and PhDs). Their findings are encouragingly positive about the benefits of these groups. Besides documenting greater treatment successes, they found that the conferences kept staff informed about client progress, reduced redundancies in services, and avoided contradictory recommendations. Further, team conferences tended to provide a venue for staff to learn from each other in supportive ways.

One of the most robust new treatment modalities in child welfare services is family group conferencing (Macgowan & Pennell, 2001; Sieppert, Hudson, & Unrau, 2000). This model is not only interdisciplinary in nature but also brings family and nonfamily groups together to plan for the safety and well-being of at-risk children. Also referred to as family mediation, it is a resource-intensive model of intervention in which the family as a group is brought together with service providers (often as a group), with the expectation that the various groups will work together to develop services that will delimit future maltreatment. The group leader is often the child protective services worker who has as his or her primary goal the brokering of services across constituencies. Undoubtedly a group model, it brings together all stakeholders in child welfare to negotiate care and safety plans.

Interdisciplinary groups do have some drawbacks and known failures (Byles, 1985; West & Poulton, 1997). Byles (1985) describes difficulties encountered in simply making some interdisciplinary programs or services operational because of mismatched agendas, differing desired outcomes, or unresolved power differentials. Ephross and Vassil (1988) would argue that success is dependent on a supportive structure that includes predictable patterns within the group. These patterns might well include consistency in meeting place, agenda items, and leadership. Toseland et al. (1987) raised concerns about the complex problems that emerge in selecting and providing leadership in these groups because the skills with which leadership roles are executed can have a major impact on their success. In many ways, the degree to which all of the stakeholders feel that their issues, concerns, and desires are being met may have a great deal to do with how successful these groups are. Therefore, the degree to which the group leaders are trained as skilled group workers is an essential element that may not be adequately addressed by the sponsoring agencies.

All interdisciplinary team programs struggle with concerns about possible levels of consumer participation. In child welfare, there are additional issues. Among them is the question of who is the consumer—the child(ren), the biological parents, the foster parents, or the adoptive parents. Further, there may be very tense relationships among child welfare consumers—that is, among foster or adoptive parents and biological parents. In some cases, the roles that families can assume in these teams may be uncertain. Child welfare clients are never voluntary service recipients, even if they are not adjudicated and are cooperative. Often the people in these teams have the power to remove or return children or to determine the type of services or placement that the parents or children will have. Finally, in some cases because of potential litigation, consumers may be excluded from participation in a particular team even if generally they are included.

In summary, child welfare workers and administrators would do well to develop skills as task group leaders. The power of these groups to augment the quality of services to children and their families is often overlooked, suggesting that training components that focus on task group leadership skills should be on the agenda of human resources departments.

DIRECT SERVICES TO CHILD WELFARE CLIENTS

Group services are provided to abusing and neglecting parents, to children and adolescents under supervision, and to adult survivors of abuse and neglect in a variety of venues. This section addresses the role of group work as a means of direct remedial intervention with children and biological parents. Again, little has been specifically written about best practices for child welfare clients, but there is an abundance of research about groups addresses problems shared by child welfare clients.

Group Work with Children under Child Welfare Supervision

Children who come into child welfare services often have experienced multiple levels of abuse and neglect. Their experiences predispose them to social and emotional problems. Current research demonstrates that the earlier maltreatment occurs, the more likely the child is to develop associated behavioral and emotional problems that may well persist into adulthood (Heffernan & Cloitre, 2000; Zanarini et al., 2002).

Children in foster care are rarely treated together in groups unless they are in a residential setting with a high number of adjudicated children. Even then, not all the other members have histories of abuse and neglect that brought them under child welfare supervision. Rather they are referred to groups because of problems that emerge as a result of the abuse and neglect they experience—emotional or behavioral problems, as well as adjustment problems. Among the earliest reported children's groups were those developed to help children cope with parental divorce (Titkin & Cobb, 1983), paralleling circumstances faced by foster children who may have experienced domestic violence, loss of contact with parents, and repeated changes in residences and caretakers (Rittner, 1995). Likewise, Knittle and Tuana (1980) were among the earliest clinicians to report using group work to treat girls who were victims of interfamilial sexual abuse, a trauma that is often seen in foster children.

Most empirically supported groups with children focus on adolescents rather than on children of latency and prelatency ages. In recent years, the emphasis has been on group treatment with a cognitive-behavioral therapy (CBT) orientation, which appears to be as effective as individual treatment in reducing symptoms of depression and anxiety, posttraumatic stress disorder, school problems, substance abuse problems, and poor peer relations (Manassis et al., 2002). Generalizing from studies with nonabused adolescents, it becomes apparent that CBT groups could be effective in treating children with abuse and neglect histories (Kaminer, Burleson, & Goldberger, 2002; Manassis et al., 2002). For example, Manassis et al. (2002) found that children with high levels of social phobia did better in individual therapy than those with more generalized anxiety and hyperactivity, who were treated effectively in CBT-oriented groups. Both anxiety and hyperactivity are common presenting problems in children with abuse and neglect histories.

Abused and neglected adolescents, like their nonabused counterparts, develop problems with depression and substance abuse, as well as problems associated with eventual development of personality disorders (borderline and antisocial personality disorders; Heffernan & Cloitre, 2000; Kaminer et al., 2002; Zanarini et al., 2002). Kaminer et al. (2002) noted that adolescent participants in a CBT group manifested marked decreases of depression and anxiety symptoms, reduction of substance abuse, and improved family and peer relationships. In addition, the members sustained gains in a variety of associated areas over a 9-month period after leaving treatment.

Real-Life Example: An Adolescent Foster Care Group

Once the adolescent unit previously discussed was developed, I volunteered to be a part of it. One day, as I drove one of my repeat runaway foster children from juvenile detention to a temporary shelter, I asked her why she ran away from every placement. She complained about her new school (she had been in four or five schools in the previous 1½ years because of her constant changes in placements), her foster parents, and her lack of friends. At the time, I also had three other runaways in the shelter. I sat down with all four of them and asked why it was so hard for them to stay put. As they talked, I realized that they needed to be meeting in a group exclusively for adolescents in foster care. With the approval of both agencies (child welfare and the shelter), I started a group that met every other day at the shelter. After a tentative start, the youths started talking about what it was like to be in foster care. By the third meeting, they wanted to know if other "kids in the system" could join. We expanded the group to 10 adolescents, spanning ages 11 to 17. It became apparent to me that I did not understand what it felt like to be a foster child at the mercy of a system that rarely consulted them about their needs and wants. They talked about what it was like to be around peers complaining about their parents. Most of them had very complicated relationships with their parents and foster parents. Some didn't know who their parents were, others couldn't live with their parents, and a few didn't know where their parents lived anymore. They talked about running from their parents almost as often as they ran to their parents. Every day they felt that they were the "only ones," the ones without parents.

Over time the group became a place where these adolescents belonged, where others also understood exactly what it was like to be a foster child. They taught each other survival skills in foster care—how to live, if necessary, like a boarder in a foster home and how to use school activities to avoid having to go "home." They talked about their experiences when other adolescents in their schools found out they were in foster care. They talked about depression and ways to manage it; they talked about the trauma and abuse they had experienced in the system and outside of the system; they talked about how painful it was to lose siblings into the child welfare system and not be able to find them anymore; they talked about their uncertain futures; they talked about using drugs to dull the pain; and they talked about living and barely surviving on the streets. They came to group every week and, remarkably, stayed put, in part so they could attend the group.

Group Work with Biological Parents

In fact, the very things that brought these children into the system and into the group are the very things that also bring many adults into groups. Many practitioners treat the survivors of abuse and neglect in mental health settings. Sometimes they come because of the consequences of their childhood experiences, and at other times they are mandated into treatment by the courts.

Most child protective service workers develop agreements with abusive and neglecting parents about needed services that are expected to reduce the risk of future maltreatment. Employing casework strategies, they monitor compliance with case plans through visitations that evaluate the ongoing safety of supervised children. Compliance with those plans is then used as a basis to decide whether to continue supervision (Rittner & Dozier, 2000).

The literature supports a triadic connection between trauma, alcohol and other drug (AOD) problems, and abuse and neglect of children (Blackson, Tarter, Loeber, Ammerman, & Windle, 1996; Chaffin, Kelleher, & Hollenberg, 1996; Cohen et al., 2002; Miller, Smyth, & Mudar, 1999; Rittner & Dozier, 2000; Sagatun-Edwards, Saylor, & Shifflett, 1995). Miller et al. (1999) found that women with higher levels of punitiveness toward their children were more likely to be in domestically violent relationships, to have AOD problems, and to have childhood histories of abuse. This is consistent with the work of others, who report high levels of co-occurring mental health and substance-related problems (Sacks,

2000). It is possible that the lack of adequate trauma assessment of parents under child welfare supervision may partly explain why substance abuse treatment dropouts and failures are so common in that population (Murphy et al., 1991; Rittner & Dozier, 2000).

One of the dilemmas that workers face is how to make the kinds of referrals that can delimit future abuse events. A number of established comprehensive models of group treatment have proven effective with abusive parents. The most common are multiple family treatment models, self-help groups, and groups that address the major underlying problems that those parents have that potentially compromise their ability to care for their children.

From its inception, treating groups of abusing parents together in what has been known as multiple family treatment (MFT) has been shown to be effective (Benningfield, 1978; Shorkey, 1979). When used in conjunction with regularly scheduled home interventions, MFT has been associated with a reduction in subsequent reports of maltreatment, better parenting skills, and creation of supportive networks (McKay, Gonzalez, Stone, Ryland, & Kohner, 1995). MFT often employs a curriculum-driven group model designed to enhance a parent's understanding of developmental issues, challenge and modify dysfunctional parenting behaviors, enhance anger management, create resource and support networks, and reinforce effective parenting skills (Constantino et al., 2001). In addition to parenting skills, some models of MFT focus on reestablishing mutual attachments between the child and parents (McKay et al., 1995). Despite findings that suggest that the group dynamics help families to work together to resolve multiple and complex problems, MFT is underused (OShea & Phelps, 1985).

Abusing and neglecting parents have been referred to a variety of self-help groups, including Parents Anonymous (PA; Bly, 1988). PA group membership includes peer role models and professionally trained leaders as facilitators who rely on a structured group curriculum to help parents learn how to effect changes in their disciplinary behaviors (Garvin, 1987). These groups are among the few groups specifically developed to serve parents who are referred, or likely to be referred, to child welfare services. Like all self-help groups, these groups have a strong identity with mutual aid group dynamics and processes, as members connect through shared understanding of the problems they face and derive support and help from each other in solving those problems.

Many parents are mandated into substance abuse treatment or anger management groups on the assumption that abuse and neglect is a consequence of AOD use (Rittner & Dozier, 2000). Unfortunately, in child welfare, this may be an overly simplistic understanding of the dynamics of abuse and neglect in parenting behaviors. This statement is particularly true for mothers who abuse and/or neglect their children (Miller et al., 1999).

The assessment and treatment of trauma in caretakers who abuse may be an important step in delimiting future abuse events. Once the assessment has been made, a referral to an adult survivor group may be indicated. These groups are important resources for those with histories of childhood sexual abuse, as well as other types of abuse (Morgan & Cummings, 1999; Nesbit Wallis, 2002). Survivors commonly experience higher levels of depression, various symptoms of posttraumatic stress disorder, interpersonal relationship and social adjustment problems, and anger management problems (Morgan & Cummings, 1999). Importantly, these consequences are just as likely to be present whether the victims experienced one or multiple events of sexual abuse (Hazzard, 1993; Heffernan & Cloitre, 2000; Zanarina et al., 2002). Survivor groups provide a safe environment in which to process traumatic events with other victims with similar experiences.

The current research suggests that CBT is effective in treating survivors. Some study findings, however, suggest that the best outcomes are associated with many exposures to group and individual treatments over time rather than with a single group experience of a specific type. This finding may reflect the fact that trauma survivors are slow to trust and share their life experiences with others. Follette, Alexander, and Follette (1991) and others (Morgan & Cummings, 1999) found that when sexually abused women had prior exposure to group treatments, they derived more symptom relief. It would appear that a normalizing process occurs in these groups when trauma survivors realize that they have developed coping strategies that mirror those used by other survivors. Over time, survivors become more open to the influence of other members and begin to see them as powerful allies in shaping new self-images and coping strategies.

Finally, many parents charged with abuse and neglect are referred to substance abuse treatment groups. The reason is that, when abuse and neglect are found to be present, workers often presume substance abuse is also present (Chaffin, Kelleher, & Hollenberg, 1996; Rittner & Dozier, 2000; Wolock & Magura, 1996). It is imperative that the evaluation of substance-related problems be comprehensive enough to determine whether it is the major factor that is contributing to abuse and neglect of children (Rittner & Dozier, 2000). This is especially true if the treatment focus is primarily on establishing abstinence. Once it is determined that substance-related disorders are the primary problem affecting parenting behavior, then substance-abuse treatment should be pursued (see Fisher, Chapter 15, this volume).

TRAINING: GROUP-BASED LEARNING

Child welfare training for staff members and caretakers generally occurs in group settings. It is obviously more efficient to do so. Employees are usually trained in groups before entering units, and adoptive parents, as well as foster parents, receive preservice training in groups. This section focuses on foster and adoptive parent group training models.

Foster and adoptive parents need training to enhance their knowledge about the various systems they will encounter. It is important that foster parents, especially those who might adopt placed children, understand the potential losses they will experience with possible reunification of the children with their birth parents. These parents require many skills in dealing with children with severe attachment disorders, trauma histories, and acting-out behaviors. Because of these unique parenting demands, there is growing evidence that group training enhances the attitudes and skills necessary to become effective and satisfied foster or adoptive parents (Burry, 1999; Gillis-Arnold, Crase, Stockdale, & Shelley, 1998).

Formal group training for foster and adoptive parents grew out of what was previously the "certification" of them (that is, making sure they and their homes met standards). Initially, it was assumed that people wanting to be foster parents were already knowledgeable about being parents. Over time, it became evident that being a "parent" to foster or adopted children was very different from raising biological or even stepchildren. The failure to fully prepare parents for what they would face in fostering and adopting abused and neglected children led to high levels of aborted placements, especially in foster care (Runyan & Fullerton, 1981).

Only a few studies have evaluated foster or adoptive parent training. Hampson and Tavormina (1980) published one of the earliest studies, which compared foster parents trained to use behavioral modification programs with those trained in more self-reflective, psychoeducationally oriented support groups. They concluded that the best training incorporated elements of both, because neither one was found to be independently effective. This study was followed by a study that compared foster parents trained in groups with those trained individually in their homes (Hampson, Schulte, & Ricks, 1983). Both of these studies support the understanding that foster parents who are assigned to group trainings tend to have better attendance and tend to rate children's behaviors more positively.

Since the 1980s, adoptive and foster parent training has primarily occurred in groups, with most states adopting the Model Approach to Partnership in Parenting Program (MAPP, 1987). Even though the focus and content of this training tends to vary from program to program and from state to state (Lee & Holland, 1991), most generally use a 30-hour group training format to help prospective parents decide if adopting or foster parenting is for them (Baum, Crase, & Crase, 2001). Those parents who go through the entire training obtain skills and attitudes believed to be associated with successful adoptive or foster parenting, particularly in skill acquisition (Burry, 1999).

The MAPP model uses lectures, role playing, and group discussions to facilitate learning. In addition, participants are provided with "homework" assignments that are intended to help prospective parents develop insights into their potential success as foster parents. Although studies have examined the impact of MAPP training on parenting attitudes (Lee & Holland, 1991), few have evaluated possible group-process benefits. MAPP is a curriculum-driven training that relies on a prescriptive, formatted curriculum. Group activities are built into each module primarily in the form of role plays and group discussions. Unfortunately, although the parents meet in groups and are trained in a group-based model, it is questionable whether the model in fact uses group skills specifically to reinforce the potential long-range mutual aid that these parents need. Hampson and Tavormina's (1980) early study should serve as a reminder to trainers that foster parents trained in groups can benefit from the elements of mutual aid in group dynamics and processes that are incorporated into the sessions.

Real-Life Example: Group Home versus Foster Family

Once the previously cited adolescent unit was developed, it became apparent in the group that one of the problems these youths faced was directly connected to being in foster homes. Many of the adolescents in the group admitted that they preferred living on the streets or in shelters to living with foster families. A number of factors drove those feelings. For some, the challenges of being part of a family were overwhelming. They had been in the system long enough or had come from such severely dysfunctional families that the intimacy and closeness of foster family life substantially increased their feelings of anxiety and depression. Others found that foster parents did not necessarily understand the degree to which they relied on their own autonomy for survival, autonomy that the foster parents resented. Others admitted that feeling dependent was threatening to them. As this area of discussion continued, it became clear that we needed to advocate with caseworkers for different kinds of placements for some of the youths in the group. That conclusion eventually led to a meeting with a local service provider to expand nontherapeutic residential care to older adolescents in the system. This action may have accounted for the fact that this community was one of the earliest to adopt an "independent living" unit for adolescents aging out of the foster care system.

CONCLUSION

Foster care is a complex service delivery system that often relies on groups to provide a range of services to at-risk children. All of these groups have as their goal to keep children safe. The achievement of this goal may well depend on the degree to which members of naturally occurring and remedial groups collaborate with each other to achieve the goal of reducing the risk of subsequent maltreatment. It is critical that researchers develop effective means of studying and analyzing child welfare–based group dynamics and processes so that administrators and service providers can better understand what factors in these groups contribute to meeting that essential goal—keeping our children safe.

Finally, there is a movement in child welfare to develop more empirically based practice models. People working in groups will continue to frame much of what is planned, developed, and implemented to better serve at-risk children and their families. Too often those plans do not adequately examine the role of group dynamics as central to the group's success (Bronstein, 2003). It would be helpful if research on planning and implementing groups looked at which kinds of groups are most effective. Inasmuch as the role of group-based decisions is likely to continue to be central to child welfare, research on how those groups contribute to the successes, as well as the failures, is key to the development of better programs to serve this population.

REFERENCES

Austin, M. J. (1981). *Supervisory management for human services*. Englewood Cliffs, NJ: Prentice-Hall.

Baum, A. C., Crase, S. J., & Crase, K. L. (2001). Influences on the decision to become or not become a foster parent. *Families in Society, 82*(2), 202–213.

Benningfield, A. B. (1978). Multiple family therapy systems. *Journal of Marriage and Family Counseling, 4*(2), 25–34.

Blackson, T. C., Tarter, R. E., Loeber, R., Ammerman, R. T., & Windle, M. (1996). The influence of parental substance abuse and difficult temperament in fathers and sons on sons' disengagement from family to deviant peers. *Journal of Youth and Adolescents, 25*, 389–411.

Bly, L. N. (1988). Self-help and child abuse: Victims, victimizers, and the development of self-control. *Contemporary Family Therapy, 10*(4), 243–255.

Bronstein, L. R. (2003). A model for interdisciplinary collaboration. *Social Work, 48*(3), 297–306.

Burry, C. L. (1999). Evaluation of a training program for foster parents of infants with prenatal substance effects. *Child Welfare, 78*(1), 197–214.

Byles, J. A. (1985). Problems in interagency collaboration: Lessons from a project that failed. *Child Abuse and Neglect, 9*(4), 549–554.

Chaffin, M., Kelleher, K., & Hollenberg, J. (1996). Onset of physical abuse and neglect: Psychiatric, substance abuse, and social risk factors from prospective community data. *Child Abuse and Neglect, 20*(3), 191–203.

Cohen, L. J., McGeogh, P. G., Sniezyna, W., Nikiforov, K., Cullen, K., & Galynker, I. I. (2002). Childhood sexual history of 20 male pedophiles vs. 24 male healthy control subjects. *Journal of Nervous and Mental Disease, 190*(11), 757–766.

Cohen, M. B. (1994). Who wants to chair the meeting? Group development and leadership patterns in a community action group of homeless people. *Social Work with Groups, 17*(1–2), 71–87.

Constantino, J. N., Hashemi, N., Solis, E., Alon, T., Haley, S., McClure, S., et al. (2001). Supplementation of urban home visitation with a series of group meetings for parents and infants: Results of a "real world" randomized controlled trail. *Child Abuse and Neglect, 25*(12), 1571–1581.

Duffy, T. (1994). The check-in and other go-rounds in group work: Guidelines for use. *Social Work with Groups, 17*(1–2), 163–175.

Ephross, P. H., & Vassil, T. V. (1988). *Groups that work*. New York: Columbia University Press.

Follette, V. M., Alexander, P. C., & Follette, W. C. (1991). Individual predictors of outcomes in group treatment for incest survivors. *Journal of Consulting and Clinical Psychology, 59*(1), 150–155.

Galinsky, M., & Schopler, J. (1989). Developmental patterns in open-ended groups. *Social Work with Groups, 12*(2), 99–114.

Garvin, C. (1987). *Contemporary group work* (2nd ed.). Englewood Cliffs, NJ: Prentice-Hall.

Gillis-Arnold, R., Crase, S. J., Stockdale, D. F., & Shelley, M. C. (1998). Parenting attitudes, foster parenting attitudes, and motivations of adoptive and non-adoptive foster parent trainees. *Children and Youth Services Review, 20*(8), 715–732.

Glisson, C., & James, L. R. (2002). The cross-level effects of culture and climate in human service teams. *Journal of Organizational Behavior, 23*(6), 767–794.

Hampson, R. B., Schulte, M. A., & Ricks, C. C. (1983). Individual vs. group training for foster parents: Efficiency/effectiveness evaluations. *Family Relations, 32*, 191–201.

Hampson, R. B., & Tavormina, J. B. (1980). Relative effectiveness of behavioral and reflective group training with foster mothers. *Journal of Consulting and Clinical Psychology, 48*, 294–295.

Harris, N., & Warner, T. W. (1988, Summer). Turning CPS philosophy into action. *Public Welfare,* 11–17.

Hazzard, A. (1993). Trauma-related beliefs as mediators of sexual abuse impact in adult women survivors: A pilot study. *Journal of Child Sexual Abuse, 2*(3), 55–69.

Heffernan, K., & Cloitre, M. (2000). A comparison of posttraumatic stress disorder with and without borderline personality disorder among women with a history of childhood sexual abuse: Etiological and clinical characteristics. *Journal of Nervous and Mental Disease, 188*(9), 589–595.

Hopkins, K. M., & Hyde, C. (2002). The human service managerial dilemma: New expectations, chronic challenges and old solutions. *Administration in Social Work, 26*(3), 1–15.

Joyner, J. (2002, March 1). Strategic goals map future for IT department: Concepts include quality, service, commitment to employees, new venture strategy. *Computing Canada, 28*(5), 19.

Kaminer, Y., Burleson, J. A., & Goldberger, R. (2002). Cognitive-behavioral coping skills and psychoeducation therapies for adolescent substance abuse. *Journal of Nervous and Mental Disease, 190*(11), 737–745.

Knittle, B. J., & Tuana, S. J. (1980). Group therapy as primary treatment for adolescent victims of intrafamilial sexual abuse. *Clinical Social Work Journal, 8*(4), 236–242.

Lee, J. H., & Holland, T. P. (1991). Evaluating the effectiveness of foster parent training. *Research on Social Work Practice, 1*(2), 162–174.

Leiter, M. P., & Maslach, C. (1988). The impact of interpersonal environment on burnout and organizational commitment. *Journal of Organizational Behavior, 9*, 297–308.

Lewis, J. A., Lewis, M. D., & Souflée, F. (1991). *Management of human services programs.* Belmont, CA: Brooks/Cole.

Lohmann, R. A., & Lohmann, N. (2002). *Social administration.* New York: Columbia University Press.

Lyons, E., & Kouloumpos-Lenares, K. (1987). Clinician and state children's services worker collaborate in treating sexual abuse. *Child Welfare, 6*(6), 517–527.

Macgowan, M. J., & Pennell, J. (2001). Building social responsibility through family group conferencing. *Social Work with Groups, 24*(3–4), 67–87.

Manassis, K., Mendlowitz, S. L., Scapillato, D., Avery, D., Fiksenbaum, L., Freire, M., et al. (2002). Group and individual cognitive-behavioral therapy for childhood anxiety disorders: A randomized trail. *Child and Adolescent Psychiatry, 41*(12), 1423–1430.

Marshall, T., Solomon, P., & Steber, S.-A. (2001). Implementing best practice models by using consensus-building process. *Administration and Policy in Mental Health, 29*(2), 105–116.

Maslach, C., & Jackson, S. E. (1981). The measurement of experienced burnout. *Journal of Occupational Behavior, 2*, 99–113.

McKay, M. M., Gonzalez, J. J., Stone, S., Ryland, D., & Kohner, K. (1995). Multiple family therapy groups: A responsive intervention model for inner city families. *Social Work with Groups, 18*(4), 41–56.

Miller, B. A., Smyth, N. J., & Mudar, P. J. (1999). Mothers' alcohol and other drug problems and their punitiveness toward their children. *Journal of Studies on Alcohol, 60*(5), 632–642.

Miller, K. I., Ellis, B. H., Zook, E. G., & Lyles, J. S. (1990). An integrated model of communication, stress, and burnout in the workplace. *Communication Research, 17*(3), 300–326.

Model approach to partnerships in parenting: Group preparation and selection of foster and/or adoptive families. (1987). Atlanta, GA: Child Welfare Institute.

Morgan, T., & Cummings, A. L. (1999). Change experienced during group therapy by female survivors of childhood sexual abuse. *Journal of Consulting and Clinical Psychology, 67*(1), 28–36.

Murphy, J. M., Jellinek, M., Quinn, D., Smith, G., Poitrast, F. G., & Goshko, M. (1991). Substance abuse and serious child mistreatment: Prevalence, risk, and outcome in a court sample. *Child Abuse and Neglect, 15,* 197–211.

Nesbit Wallis, D. A. (2002). Reduction of trauma symptoms following group therapy. *Australian and New Zealand Journal of Psychiatry, 36*(1), 67–74.

OShea, M. D., & Phelps, R. (1985). Multiple family therapy: Current status and critical appraisal. *Family Process, 24*(4), 555–582.

Rittner, B. (1995). Children on the move: Placement patterns of children under children's protective services. *Families in Society, 76*(8), 469–477.

Rittner, B. (2002). The use of risk assessment instruments in child protective services case planning and closures. *Children and Youth Services Review, 24*(3), 189–207.

Rittner, B., & Dozier, C. D. (2000).Effects of court-ordered substance abuse treatment in child protective services cases. *Social Work, 45*(2), 131–140.

Runyan, A., & Fullerton, S. (1981). Foster care provider training: A preventative program. *Children and Youth Services Review, 3,* 127–141.

Sacks, S. (2000). Co-occurring mental health and substance use disorders: Promising approaches and research issues. *Substance Use and Misuse, 35*(12–14), 2061–2093.

Sagatun-Edwards, I. J., Saylor, C., & Shifflett, B. (1995). Drug exposed infants in social welfare system and juvenile court. *Child Abuse and Neglect, 19*(1), 83–91.

Shorkey, C. T. (1979). A review of methods used in the treatment of abusing parents. *Social Casework, 690*(6), 360–367.

Shulman, L. (1984). *Skills of helping individuals and groups* (2nd ed.). Itasca, IL: Peacock.

Sieppert, J. D., Hudson, J., & Unrau, Y. (2000). Family group conferencing in child welfare: Lessons form a demonstration project. *Families in Society, 81,* 382–391

Tausch, B. D., & Harter, M. C. (2001). Perceived effectiveness of diagnostic and therapeutic guidelines in primary care quality circles. *International Journal for Quality in Health Care, 13*(3), 239–246.

Titkin, E. A., & Cobb, C. (1983). Treating post-divorce adjustment in latency age children: A focused group paradigm. *Social Work with Groups, 6*(2), 53–66.

Toseland, R. W., Ivanoff, A., & Rose, S. R. (1987). Treatment conferences: Task groups in action. *Social Work with Groups, 10*(2), 79–94.

Toseland, R. W., & Rivas, R. (1984). *An introduction to group work practice.* New York: Macmillan.

Wagner, W. G. (1987). Child sexual abuse: A multidisciplinary approach. *Journal of Counseling and Development, 65*(8), 435–439.

West, M. A., & Poulton, B. C. (1997). A failure of function: Teamwork in primary health care. *Journal of Interprofessional Care, 11*(2), 205–216.

Wolock, I., & Magura, S. (1996). Parental substance abuse as a predictor of child maltreatment re-reports. *Child Abuse and Neglect, 20*(12), 1183–1193.

Zanarini, M. C., Yong, L., Frankenburg, F. R., Hennen, J., Reich, B., Marino, M. F., & Vujanovic, A. A. (2002). Severity of reported childhood sexual abuse and its relationship to severity of borderline psychopathology and psychosocial impairment among borderline inpatients. *Journal of Nervous and Mental Disease, 190*(6), 381–387.

Chapter 15

Groups for Substance
Abuse Treatment

MAURICE S. FISHER

Group work approaches are a mainstay of inpatient programs and treatment and are the cornerstone of most outpatient programs for substance abusers. Although group work is not a panacea, this method continues to be the most commonly applied modality for the treatment of alcoholism and other substances (Fisher, 1995; Golden, Khantzian, & McAuliffe, 1994; Rotgers, Keller, & Morgenstern, 2003). Many consider group work to be the treatment of choice for addicted persons (Cooper, 1987; Fisher & Bentley, 1996; Matano & Yalom, 1991).

This use of groups is widespread because group members can help one another examine what has, as well as what has not, worked and under what conditions. Group work using cognitive-behavioral techniques may be particularly helpful with self-regulation and personal management of deficits. Additionally, professionally led groups, like self-help groups such as Alcoholics Anonymous (AA), Cocaine Anonymous (CA), and Narcotics Anonymous (NA), have the benefit of a common history among the membership in terms of their alcohol and other drug use experiences.

The purpose of this chapter is to describe and provide an analysis of four group work models currently in common use. Two of the models, the disease-and-recovery model and the cognitive-behavioral model, have been specifically suggested for persons dually diagnosed with mental health and substance use disorders.

RATIONALE FOR USING GROUP WORK MODELS
WITH SUBSTANCE-ABUSING CLIENTS

For clients who have a substance use disorder, recovery can be aided by improving their social skills and the quality of their interpersonal relationships. Because group work focuses explicitly on these issues, it is an important component of substance abuse treatment. Group authorities in the chemical addiction field (i.e., Fisher, 1995; Flores, 1997) advocate for groups for the following reasons:

1. Groups reduce the sense of isolation often experienced by persons with substance use disorders, who may experience a sense of relief to discover that other people are struggling with similar problems.
2. Groups help instill hope in persons with substance use disorders such that they can experience recovery; this generally occurs when they observe other members of the group who are recovering from chemical addictions.
3. Groups provide an opportunity for the members to learn how to cope with chemical addictions, as well as other psychosocial problems, by observing how others with similar sorts of situations cope with them.
4. Groups can provide a good deal of new information to members through material presented by the group work leader or via guest facilitators, instructors, and other members.
5. Groups help members to develop enhanced self-concepts (e.g., self-worth and self-image) or to modify distorted self-concepts because of the feedback members receive from other members as to their worth, skills, and abilities.
6. Groups provide reparative family experiences as the group members offer each member support and nurturance that may be lacking in their own families. Group interactions may also help members to experiment with alternative ways to create improved interactions in their families.
7. Groups provide emotional and affective support when members undertake anxiety-provoking or difficult tasks in their life situations outside the group. This may take the form of encouragement, reinforcement, or coaching.
8. Groups help members to acquire the social skills that they need to cope with life situations instead of using substances to overcome feelings of inadequacy in these situations. Groups offer many opportunities to learn social skills through observing others and being coached by other members. Members can then try the skills out in a safe and supportive environment.
9. Group members may confront each other in very powerful ways regarding chemical (licit and illicit) use or any other dysfunctional behaviors. The effectiveness of confrontation within the social work group context lies in the potency of receiving the same feedback from several people, especially people who come from similar situations and have similar problems. (The use of confrontation is frequently found in groups of substance abusers because of the use of the defense mechanisms of denial. The appropriate uses of confrontation must be carefully assessed in terms of the needs and capacities of the members being confronted.)
10. In view of the large numbers of people who require substance use treatment, group services may create some economic advantages in the use of professional personnel because of the ability of groups to help a number of people concurrently.
11. The effects of the group treatment may extend beyond the boundaries of the group context or individual meeting by encouraging members to provide support to one another outside the group session.

Persons experiencing substance abuse problems frequently enter treatment with distorted views of the world in which they live owing to years of drug use that impaired their perceptual capacities. Drug use also tends to be highly associated with social skill deficits, feelings of isolation, and a general distrust of others. This is especially true of persons who have lost or destroyed any healthy or pseudohealthy relationships they may have had through the use of drugs and the lifestyle they have adopted.

Additionally, obvious difficulties are inherent in treating clients who still use their drug(s) of choice in the same group with persons who have abstinence as their goal. There is concern that the "users" will monopolize the group process and that members with alternative goals (e.g., quitting or, in the case of alcohol, moderation) will tend to assume responsibility for the ones still uncommitted or unmotivated to modify their drug usage. Based on the client's stage of change seeking, my recommendation is to assign active substance users to groups that focus on motivational modalities prior to active group therapy in more change-oriented groups (see Prochaska, Norcross, & DiClemente, 1994).

DIFFERENCES BETWEEN SUPPORT GROUPS
AND GROUP WORK MODELS

It is necessary to differentiate group therapy from self-help groups such as AA, CA, and NA. Social group work is defined here as:

> an orientation and method of social work intervention in which small numbers of people who share similar interests or common problems convene regularly and engage in activities designed to achieve their common goals. In contrast to group psychotherapy, the goals of group work are not necessarily the treatment of emotional problems. The objectives also include exchanging information, developing social and manual skills, changing value orientations, and diverting antisocial behaviors into productive channels. Interventive techniques include, but are not limited to, controlled therapeutic discussions . . . education, and tutoring. (Barker, 1999, p. 449)

Social group work models of substance abuse treatment stress the difficulties members have in integrating and modulating their affective lives. In contrast to self-help groups, group work is conducted by a practitioner who uses a psychosocial model of substance abuse on which to base decisions about group composition, interventive strategies, and therapeutic goals. Other group experiences, especially AA, CA, and NA, may provide crucial support to members who experience periods of painful uncovering in group work. Hence it is possible to see other groups complementing the efforts of group work (Fisher, 1994; Mack, 1981). Yet it is important to note that support groups are not treatment per se; they are ancillary and collateral to treatment efforts and prove helpful for a person who lacks a supportive interpersonal network.

DESCRIPTIONS OF SOCIAL WORK GROUPS
AND THEIR RELATIVE EFFECTIVENESS

The question regarding the effectiveness of group work for persons with substance-abuse and dependence is critical. Part of the rationale for using group work methods lies within the typical defensive nature and style of the persons with abuse or dependence. According to Flores (1997) this characteristic style involves a defensive posture commonly referred to as denial. Moreover, people with substance abuse and dependence usually present with a complexity of myriad defenses and character pathologies, and the workers need to have a concise understanding of the individual member's defensive process and character dynamics if they intend to help each member benefit from treatment. Also, each person who has a substance use disorder has a unique history of biological, psychological, and social causes that led to the problem of abuse and/or dependency.

This section discusses four major group work approaches for people who abuse substances. For each approach I describe the theoretical underpinnings utilized by the approach, the outcomes sought, the general length of treatment, the structure of sessions, the typical techniques employed, and the evidence of relative effectiveness.

Interactional Group Psychotherapy

Theoretical Foundation

This approach is based on the following assumptions: (1) Interpersonal relationships play a critical role in the development of the individual; (2) maladaptive patterns result in psychiatric symptomatology; (3) the interactive group process focuses on the dynamic interplay of individuals within the "here and now" of the group meeting; (4) interpersonal learning— insight that results from the examination of this dynamic—is considered a primary vehicle of therapeutic change (Matano, Yalom, & Schwartz, 1997, p. 303).

Matano et al. (1997, p. 303) propose that "the effective use of the here and now occurs in two stages":

First, the group must plunge into its own interaction. Second, the group has to step outside itself and begin to understand what has just transpired. An interactive approach assumes that clients within the group context will eventually tend to display the same maladaptive thoughts and behaviors they exhibit outside therapy. Additionally, through the reactions and feedback of other group members, clients become acutely aware of their maladaptive behaviors and alternative approaches within the safe confines of the therapy group.

Although the preceding represents the basic heuristic of writers such as Yalom who have done the most to advance and develop interactional group approaches, other writers on this approach also integrate a great deal of psychodynamic theory into their work. As Flores (1997) states with reference to the work of Louis Ormont, a more explicitly psychoanalytic theorist:

> Ormont, like most modern psychoanalysts and self-psychologists, sees pathology as the result of self-defeating defenses or resistances that are erected against transference wishes, shame, guilt, and fears of oedipal and pre-oedipal retaliations. He views these defenses as necessary, though maladaptive, attempts at self-preservation that are the consequences of unmet developmental needs. (p. 144)

Desired Outcomes

The posture of writers who take an interactional perspective contrasts with many others. An interactional approach "stresses the role of the interpersonal relationships in the genesis and perpetuation of addiction" (Matano et al., 1997, p. 305). Therefore, the idea that addiction is to be viewed primarily as a disease is not a central one in this model, although Matano et al. state that both models have validity and that the challenge is to integrate models (i.e., disease and recovery and the interactional approaches) and to know when to emphasize which one. Important outcomes stressed by these authors are a priority on recovery, identification as an "alcoholic" or "addict," modulation of anxiety levels, a therapeutic approach to responsibility, and incorporation into the language and belief systems of AA (p. 305). These outcomes are not antithetical to the goals of AA, and Matano and colleagues indicate their respect for AA and the need for an integration of support groups and group therapy approaches.

Length of Treatment

Treatment of people with substance use disorders is viewed as a long-term process with individual variations depending on the characteristics of the group members and their stage of recovery. Flores (1997) states: "The therapist may find that in some cases the entire first year of treatment may be spent on 'just' maintaining sobriety, with little or no active encouragement of personality modification" (p. 173). Such periods of growth take place over time periods ranging from 2 to 5 years of abstinence (p. 175).

Recruitment of Members

Flores (1997) sees it as inevitable that persons who are determined to be chemically dependent and in need of treatment should and will be referred to psychotherapy groups. Nevertheless, he asserts that these clients may not affiliate with these groups because they are poorly prepared for groups by professionals who underestimate the initial anxiety clients feel about such referrals as well as the fact that they may be in an acute state of withdrawal and toxicity. Flores (1997, p. 71), based on the work of Rutan and Stone (1984), indicates that such preparation must accomplish the following:

1. Establish a preliminary alliance between client and therapist.
2. Gain a clear consensus about the client's therapeutic hopes.
3. Offer information and instruction about group psychotherapy.
4. Deal with the initial anxiety about joining a group.
5. Present and gain acceptance of a contract.

Structure of Sessions

Flores (1997, pp. 164–165) presents the following protocol for group psychotherapy treatment with addicted populations:

> The early stages of therapy should be patterned after Cummings' description of "exclusion therapy" (1979). Essentially this approach requires that the issue of drug usage be approached first and the client excluded from therapy unless he or she agrees to the goals of abstinence. Alcohol, or other drug, addiction should therefore be the primary focus during the early stages of treatment.
>
> During the first two months of treatment, much of the group's time would be spent on education of the disease concept of alcoholism/addiction and the development of what Yalom describes as group cohesiveness (1985). The group at this point would provide support and structure as Wallace recommends (1978). Gradually the shift should be initiated to move the group from a support model to an interactional model as described by Yalom (1974). During this time, directive and active leadership required at this early stage (Wallace, 1975) should shift to allow the group to take a more active and responsible role in the group process.

...

Much of the time throughout treatment should be spent on confronting the addicted person's denial system (Cummings, 1979; Wallace, 1975). A heavy focus should be directed toward getting the addicted person to make a gradual recognition of their buried feelings. Usually, feelings of extreme guilt would be best dealt with by providing an overall simplistic cognitive structure of their illness (Wallace, 1975).

Techniques Utilized

The following are some of the major techniques employed by practitioners of this approach. These are not listed in any particular order but are provided with reference to the actual group situation at the time:

1. *Confrontation.* This consists of realistic feedback about the member's behavior as seen by the practitioner. According to Flores (1997), this must be offered with empathy, concern, and caring, especially concern about the member's dangerous, self-defeating behaviors.

2. *Promote optimal level of anxiety.* The worker must assess whether the amount of anxiety elicited by the group experience will be disabling or will foster change. As Matano and Yalom (1991) note:

> A number of therapeutic techniques can help reduce the [client's] anxiety. Generally speaking, the more structure and support provided, the lower the anxiety. This can best be accomplished if the therapist is active, supportive, and explicitly teaches about the process of group therapy and addiction. If here-and-now interactions become emotionally charged, then the therapist can titrate the level of anxiety by steering the group into a stage of objective reflection about the interaction.
>
> Thus, the therapist does not aim to eradicate anxiety from the group but to manage it carefully according to the [client's] tolerance levels. By successfully navigating anxiety-producing situations, a [client] can develop confidence about performing adequately in similar interactions outside the group and may also learn that such negative emotional states can be tolerated without recourse to drugs or alcohol. (pp. 276–277)

3. *Promote a here-and-now, process-oriented focus.* This is especially important in the later stages of treatment, when the members are ready to examine their interactions in the group, experiment with new interpersonal behaviors, and receive and offer feedback from others about their behavior in the group (Levine & Gallogly, 1985).

4. *Confront group obstacles.* Group conditions, especially those related to safety, honesty, openness, and authenticity, that impede the therapeutic work must be challenged (Levine & Gallogly, 1985).

5. *Work to prevent relapse or to handle it when it occurs.* This involves confronting denial or refusal to do work in the group, making the principles on which the group operate (e.g., "one day at a time") simple, and maintaining the members' humility in the face of reverses that occur within the group context.

Evidence of Effectiveness

Most of the materials on which this discussion of interactional group psychotherapy has been based provide anecdotal evidence as to the effectiveness of this approach but do not present data from experimental designs. One exception to this type of evaluation is an article by Sandahl, Herlitz, Ahlin, and Roennberg (1998). These authors engaged in a project in Sweden in which they compared psychodynamically oriented time-limited group psycho-therapy with a cognitive-behavioral treatment of a homogeneous group of male and female clients who were moderately alcohol dependent. Members were randomly assigned to the two treatment groups. At 15-month follow-up, clients from both groups had improved. Those in the psychodynamic group, however, seemed to have been able to maintain a more positive drinking pattern during the whole follow-up period compared to the clients in the cognitive-behavioral treatment who seemed gradually to deteriorate.

Social Skills Training

Theoretical Foundations

The basic premise of this approach is that "through a variety of learning techniques (e.g., behavioral rehearsal, modeling, cognitive restructuring, didactic instruction), people and their social networks can be taught to use alternative methods of coping with the demands of living without using maladaptive addictive substances such as alcohol" (Monti, Abrams, Kadden, Cooney, & Ned, 1989, p. 1). Such addictive behaviors are understood to be mal-adaptive, or irresponsible, ways of managing both small and large stressors in daily life (Baer, Kivlahan, & Marlatt, 1995).

Desired Outcomes

The group members are helped to acquire skills to cope with the stresses that elicit or main-tain the use of substances. These skills include social skills, assertiveness, refusal skills, main-taining close relationships, enhancing social support, problem solving, relaxation, anger management, and managing emergencies.

Length of Treatment

Social skills training is typically short term. Hester (1995) suggests that length of treatment involvement is correlated with the individualized goals (e.g., sobriety vs. moderation man-agement) of the client. Hence each client would utilize group treatment (i.e., contracting for specific numbers of sessions) based on an individualized plan of recovery.

Recruitment of Members

Full social skills training is introduced to members when they have made a commitment to change. Nevertheless, the processes of skill and motivational enhancement (Miller & Rollnick, 1991) are not seen as separate but complementary, with attention to both present at all times in the group context.

Structure of Sessions

Once an assessment has identified the kinds of skill deficits group members must work to overcome, sessions are devoted to specific tasks, homework assignments, and practice opportunities to develop such skills. Psychoeducational approaches may also be used to instruct clients in the essential components of the skills. Anxiety and stress management, as well as community reinforcement and behavioral self-control procedures, are introduced as needed. The group context is a good one for these activities because of the opportunities the group offers for modeling and practice of skills with peers.

Techniques Utilized

The following are techniques that are frequently used for skills training:

1. Assessment of skill deficits. An example of an instrument for this is the Alcohol-Specific Role Play Test (Monti et al., 1989).
2. Modification of maladaptive cognitions. The practitioner helps members to identify cognitions that prevent their acquiring the skills and to replace these with appropriate cognitions.
3. Teaching of coping behaviors through instruction, modeling, directed practice, and feedback. The practitioner may make use of written handouts, presentation of information, short lectures, and role plays. In the role plays, either the practitioners or other members offer themselves as models of the appropriate behaviors. Short film clips may be utilized for the same purpose.
4. The teaching of problem-solving strategies. The practitioner instructs the members in how to specify problems, generate alternative solutions, evaluate each solution, choose the best, most responsible solution, and implement the solution.
5. The use of self-reward systems. The client is helped to select and administer self-rewards after utilizing the skill. Examples of these self-rewards are treating ones self to a good meal, going out to a movie with a significant other, or relaxing in a hot tub. The practitioner ascertains the kinds of rewards that are most gratifying to the client but that are not related to the use of drugs or to destructive outcomes.

Evidence of Effectiveness

The social skills approach has been proposed as an alternative to confrontation, to hostile, controlling, and blaming approaches (Miller & Rollnick, 1991). The former approach demonstrates that empathy and supportive measures are important (Baer, Kivlahan, & Marlatt, 1995; Najavits, Weiss, Shaw, & Muenz, 1998). The evidence shows that through social skills approaches, coping skills are elicited and natural coping resources are developed (Baer, Kivlahan, & Marlatt, 1995).

Cognitive-Behavioral Groups

Theoretical Foundations

A behavioral approach contends that all behavior is a product of *antecedent* events that elicit the behavior and the *consequences* of the behavior that maintain it and make it more likely to reoccur (e.g., reinforcements and punishments). A cognitive-behavioral approach is based on the idea that these antecedents and consequent events are not limited to acts that people perform but also include the thoughts (cognitions) and feelings of the individual, as well as others. For example, a drug user might experience the antecedent events of (1) a belief that an environmental stress will be overwhelming and (2) an offer of drugs. In this instance, the consequences might be an immediate feeling of pleasure and a set of beliefs that all problems will now be solved. A cognitive-behavioral intervention will seek to help the individual modify the antecedents or consequences or both. In groups, other members may suggest alternative ways of modifying these forces and support the member in doing so.

Additionally, many advocate treatment that uses a cognitive-behavioral approach for the client with a dual diagnosis (mental illness and substance abuse). For instance, Osher and Kofoed (1989) describe an integrated perspective based on a cognitive-behavioral approach (i.e., self-medication model) of addiction. Cooper (1987) argues that a cognitive-behavioral approach portrays substance use disorders as being related to efforts to self-medicate for particularly painful affective states. Beck, Wright, Newman, and Liese (1993) argue that "cognitive therapy is ideally suited for these individuals, since it has been developed and tested on patients with depression, anxiety, and personality disorders" (p. 10). In fact, Beck et al. (1993) note that cognitive therapy treatment for clients with dual diagnoses is based on an integrated perspective. That is, they strongly suggest that, when a co-occurring psychiatric syndrome is found to exist in a client with alcohol or other drug use, the therapist should focus simultaneously on substance abuse and the symptoms of the mental disorder, as well as on any other factors of interaction, such as social problems. So as to gain necessary pretreatment data, Beck and colleagues (1993) suggest the use of a "case conceptualization" (Persons, 1989) defined as the evaluation and integration of historical information, psychiatric diagnosis, cognitive profile, and other aspects of functioning.

Desired Outcomes

Cognitive-behavioral groups seek to help members prevent lapse (i.e., a deviation in rational judgment) and relapse (i.e., resuming a pattern of substance misuse) by reducing the average number of drinks or other drugs taken on a daily basis, as well as the total number of substance-using days. Intermediate outcomes sought include regular attendance in the group, completion of homework assignments, and staying in the group treatment until completion. Lifelong abstinence with involvement in support groups is encouraged.

Length of Treatment

A well-documented study of cognitive-behavioral treatment (Graham, Annis, Brett, & Venesoen, 1996) indicated that the inpatient treatment component consisted of 12 weekly sessions that lasted for 60–90 minutes. Participants in an evening outpatient program attended groups twice weekly for the 12 weeks, and abstinence was required during the 12 months that clients were in the full program.

Recruitment of Members

In the Graham et al. study (1996), members were participants in a 12-step, 26-day residential program or an evening group counseling program. Clients in the residential program tended to have moderate to severe alcohol problems, with the majority having both alcohol and other drug problems. These participants received a variety of services, including group discussion, rational self-counseling, anger management, and goal setting. Clients in the evening program were mild to moderate substance abusers. In another study reported by Washington (1999), participants had a primary diagnosis of substance abuse, were addicted to at least one chemical substance, and were nonpsychotic.

Structure of Sessions

In the Graham et al. (1996) study, the groups were highly structured. Clients were asked to complete a weekly homework assignment in which they prepared for and experienced a high-risk event. They also completed weekly reports of cravings for and use of alcohol and other drugs. Graham et al. (1996) reported: "Each session generally included: group or individual discussion of desires to use or actual use during the previous week; discussion of common high-risk situations; anticipating individual high-risk situations likely to occur in the coming week; and planning for how these situations could be handled without relapse" (p. 1131).

Techniques Utilized

In the first session in the Graham et al. (1996) project, clients discussed their responses to a standardized measure of high-risk situations (Inventory of Drinking Situations; Annis, Graham, & Davis, 1987; Inventory of Drug-Taking Situations; Annis & Martin, 1985). Session 2 initiated the process of helping clients "identify upcoming high-risk situations, evaluate their own desires to use and identify strategies, in advance that would help them to avoid use" (p. 1131).

The authors described subsequent sessions as follows:

> Sessions 3–10 continued the process and also included discussion of general types of high-risk situations that tend to be common for many people, such as negative emotions and conflict with others. Sessions 11 and 12 attempted to bring the client's focus to the most likely relapse circumstances and involved discussion of strategies for avoiding relapse, even this "worse case scenario." The homework assignments for each session provided a structure for clients to focus on practicing both cognitive and behavioral rehearsal of strategies for avoiding relapse in real life high-risk situations. In so far as real-life situations allowed, the counselors guided the clients . . . through successful mastery of the "less risky" high-risk situations, avoiding the riskiest situations until the client was ready. (p. 1131)

Evidence of Effectiveness

Graham et al.'s (1996) study compared persons receiving group versus individual cognitive-behavioral training. Washington's (1999) study compared individuals receiving cognitive versus experiential group therapy. In the former study, both individual and group formats were well received by clients. Clients in both conditions completed homework assignments and completed the program to about the same degree. There was, however, a greater tendency for the group residential clients to stay with the program until the final stages (82.6% for the group compared with 61.9% for the individual treatment). The same was true for the evening group clients (74% for group and 64.7% for individual). There were no other significant differences in substance use between group and individual treatments. The same lack of difference appeared at 12-month follow-up. In summarizing the implications of these findings, Graham and her colleagues (1996) state:

> The present study tested a group approach that was closely comparable with the individual method developed by Annis. The findings suggest that this group approach is as successful as the individual approach. Based on this finding, research focusing on enhancing group approaches would be desirable. The present study has shown the viability of using individual identification of

and planning for high-risk situations in a format that incorporates the advantages of group support and feedback. Research is needed to further develop this model to obtain greater increases in rates of maintaining gains from treatment. (p. 1137)

Washington's (1999) study compared cognitive group therapy with experiential group therapy. The participants were all women with chemical dependence. Women in the cognitive group had higher scores on the outcome measures that examined self-efficacy. As the author states: "The general pattern of positive change demonstrated by the cognitive group on social self-efficacy is meaningful considering the loneliness and isolation that are characteristic of chemically dependent women" (p. 193). A similar pattern was found with reference to general self-actualization. A major limitation of this study was the absence of random assignment to the groups.

Disease-and-Recovery Group Therapy

Theoretical Foundations

This approach is anchored in the 12-step principles and traditions of Alcoholics Anonymous. The core aspects of this model are: (1) accepting that people are not always responsible for their thoughts, behaviors, and emotions; (2) accepting that people arc limited in what they are able to control and at times are at the mercy of their biopsychosocial makeup; (3) accepting an "alcoholic" or "addict" identity; and (4) accepting abstinence as the treatment goal.

Group members should recognize that they have arrived at a crisis in their lives, are powerless over alcohol or other drugs, and must surrender to a "higher power" in order to recover from the disease of addiction. Also, members should strive for total abstinence from all illicit drugs; this is attained through an effort to abstain "one day at a time." Additionally, members should acknowledge their personality defects and wrongdoings and make amends to people whom they have abused. From this perspective, members should understand that people with alcohol or other drug use problems have an underlying biological vulnerability characterized by a loss of control over the substance.

Minkoff (1989), Daley, Moss, and Campbell (1987), and Evans and Sullivan (1990) describe the disease-and-recovery model as holistic in its approach to the treatment of both mental health and substance abuse issues. Each of these authors argues that the disease-and-recovery approach has many similarities to and is comparable to those approaches utilized in mental health treatment. For example, they claim that both mental health and substance abuse problems share the same concepts of illness (Minkoff, 1989), the general goal of recovery (Evans & Sullivan, 1990), and complementary interventions, such as group therapy and peer support (Daley et al., 1987). In this treatment approach, the consumer is seen as powerless over the reality of having comorbidity and powerless to cure it, powerless to consistently control the symptoms of each disease, and ultimately powerless to consistently prevent harmful consequences of the symptoms. Each disorder is viewed as having a complex, multifactorial etiology in which a hereditary or congenital biological predisposition interacts with psychosocial stressors to result in the emergence of symptoms (Lamb, 1982). Profound denial is seen as a prominent characteristic of comorbidity, and overcoming denial by way of a recovery process is viewed as the first major treatment task. Analogous recovery processes have been described for both substance use and mental disorders (Alcoholics Anonymous, 1975; Harding, Brooks, & Ashikaga, 1987).

Desired Outcomes

Disease-and-recovery group therapy seeks to prevent relapse by achieving the proximal outcomes of development of an "alcoholic" or "addict" identity, acknowledgement of a loss of control, acceptance of abstinence as the main treatment goal, and participation in ongoing support group activities (e.g., getting a sponsor, attending AA, CA, and/or NA meetings). Reliance on external control (i.e., a higher power) limits individual responsibility (Fisher, 1994). Acceptance by the members that their "disease" is chronic, progressive, and eventually fatal is considered by Fisher and Bentley (1996) as a paramount client internalization.

Length of Treatment

In a 1996 quasi-experimental group comparative study across inpatient and outpatient domains, Fisher and Bentley (1996) found that by using an intensive program of 45-minute groups held three times weekly (with a total of 12 group sessions), a disease-and-recovery group had about the same positive outcomes in decreasing substance abuse severity as did a cognitive-behavioral group design. However, in the same study, the disease-and-recovery group was shown as less effective than a cognitive-behavioral group for outpatient clients.

Recruitment of Members

In the Fisher and Bentley (1996) study, members were referred by mental health and substance abuse professionals who utilized specific inclusion criteria provided to them. The inclusion criteria was that each member meet the current DSM criteria for substance use disorder (type unspecified) and for an Axis II personality disorder (type unspecified). This study was aimed at clients who were not psychotic (i.e., actively hallucinating) to increase the chances of facilitating group interaction among membership.

Structure of Sessions

The Fisher and Bentley (1996) study utilized a strict 12-session protocol. Each session generally included discussion of the concepts of "disease" and of "powerlessness." Didactic materials from AA, CA, and NA were used, as well as homework assignments. Additionally, clients were requested during each session to assess potential triggers for relapse, their individual motivation to manage the "disease," and potential obstacles for their continued recovery.

Techniques Utilized

In the disease-and-recovery group designed for Fisher and Bentley's (1996) study, the 12 sessions were divided into three traditional phases, beginning, middle, and end. The authors indicated that in the beginning phase (three sessions) the acceptance of the "disease" concept is begun. Heavy emphasis is placed on helping the group members understand the 12 steps and how to therapeutically use them. Additionally, emphasis is placed on core concepts such as "surrender," as in surrendering one's reluctance to begin treatment, "powerlessness" (over the disease alone), as well as understanding the concept of "one day at a time" (relative to staying present oriented).

The second phase of treatment, the middle six sessions, shifts focus to increasing clients' sense of responsibility in for using and abusing behaviors. Errors in not taking responsibility for substance using and abusing (i.e., blaming, minimizing, and justifying), as well as other unmanageable behaviors, are stressed by all members. Heavy emphasis is placed on promoting the notion and use of a "higher power," on which ultimate responsibility for recovery is placed. Emphasis is also placed on "letting go" of resentments that may serve as a catalyst to relapse. During the last three sessions, the termination phase, Fisher (1995) notes that heavy reinforcements are given for honesty and thoroughness of understanding oneself through confrontation. Detailed attention is paid to the "sick" and "bad" behaviors as part of the "disease of addiction." Throughout all 12 sessions, Fisher (1995) supports members' attendance at support groups (AA, CA, and/or NA) in order to maintain the individual member's recovery plans.

Evidence of Effectiveness

As mentioned, Fisher and Bentley (1996) reported on pre- and posttest evaluations using the Addiction Severity Index (ASI; McLellan, Luborsky, O'Brien, & Woody, 1980). Results showed improved interpersonal relationships with families and a lessening of overall alcohol and drug use. Among outpatients, the disease-and-recovery group showed less promise in overall reduction of alcohol and drug use severity than did a group using the cognitive-behavioral model (Fisher & Bentley, 1996).

PRACTICAL GUIDELINES FOR IMPLEMENTATION OF SOCIAL GROUP MODELS

Group therapy is useful for persons who have dual diagnoses, particularly those with personality disorders, who can learn to identify errors in their own thinking and in the thinking of others (Center for Substance Abuse Treatment [CSAT], 1994). Specifically, group work, as proposed in cognitive-behavioral and disease-and-recovery models, helps members identify erroneous thinking about alcohol, other drug use, and relapse. For example, when a group member glamorizes stories of alcohol and/or drug use or criminal behaviors and acting-out behaviors, these group models are useful in limiting their views.

The following guidelines help maximize membership participation within the context of all of the four models. These guidelines are primarily derived from my clinical practice experience in conducting groups from this population (Fisher & Bentley, 1996).

First, these models are not suggested for persons who are actively psychotic or who have poor reality testing abilities. The rationale here is that the disease-and-recovery model centers much of its focus on appealing to "higher powers," which may exacerbate some clients' delusional systems. The cognitive-behavioral model requires that one be able to understand the use of what is sometimes a rather abstract concept for the purpose of predicting potential relapse situations. Initial screening should also assess the existence of a personality disorder, along with substance abuse, but should also screen for psychopathology. An instrument that has been found useful to this end is the Structured Clinical Interview for DSM-IV Personality Disorders (SCID II; American Psychiatric Association, 1997).

Second, at the start of the initial session, therapists should make individual contracts with each member to encourage prosocial behaviors and to avoid attempts to dominate, control, or compete for attention with other group members (CSAT, 1994). Also, such contracting gives members an opportunity to begin development of aftercare treatment designed to enhance relapse prevention.

Third, group workers should avoid creating groups that consist entirely of clients dually diagnosed with one type of personality disorder to enhance mutual learning from diverse personality characteristics. The group models as proposed are best conducted with a mix of consumers who suffer from a range of personality disorders. As noted earlier, contemporary substance abuse involves multiple substances (Wallen & Weiner, 1989); thus having a mix of persons using a variety of substances seems inevitable. In this way, it is believed that the heterogeneity of the group composition will increase the potential for ego integration and sharing of ego strengths (Fisher, 1994).

A fourth and final guideline is related to having understandable and specific group rules. The cognitive-behavioral model and the disease-and-recovery model are best conducted in an inpatient setting in which the group therapists have control over the environment. This allows the group members to develop a degree of security and comfort so that they can more fully share and take potential risks as group cohesion increases. In a similar manner, groups require rules so as to maintain motivation for treatment.

The outcomes of substance abuse groups have been poorly studied (Fisher & Bentley, 1996). There is a need to develop a more comprehensive understanding of the role that the group worker should play to enhance the outcome of treatment effects among members. Finally, there should be additional studies comparing models such as the disease-and-recovery model and the cognitive-behavioral model among different populations and settings so as to establish the best fit for consumers.

REFERENCES

Alcoholics Anonymous. (1975). *Living sober.* New York: Alcoholics Anonymous World Services.

American Psychiatric Association. (1997). *SCID: Structured Clinical Interview for DSM-IV.* Washington, DC: American Psychiatric Press.

Annis, H., Graham, J., & Davis, C. (1987). *Inventory of drinking situations (IDS): Users guide.* Toronto, Ontario, Canada: Addiction Research Foundation.

Annis, H., & Martin, G. (1985). *Inventory of drug taking situations (IDTS).* Toronto, Ontario, Canada: Addiction Research Foundation.

Baer, J., Kivlahan, D., & Marlatt, G. (1995). High-risk drinking across the transition from high school to college. *Alcoholism: Clinical and Experimental Research, 19*(1), 54–61.

Barker, R. (1999). *The social work dictionary* (4th ed.). Silver Spring, MD: NASW Press.

Beck, A. T., Wright, F. D., Newman, C. F., & Liese, B. S. (1993). *Cognitive therapy of substance abuse.* New York: Guilford Press.

Center for Substance Abuse Treatment. (1994). *Assessment and treatment of patients with coexisting mental illness and alcohol and other drug abuse.* (DHHS Publication No. 94-2078). Rockville, MD: Substance Abuse and Mental Health Services Administration.

Cooper, D. (1987). The role of group psychotherapy in the treatment of substance abusers. *American Journal of Psychotherapy, 12,* 55–67.

Cummings, N. (1979) Turning bread into stones. *American Psychologist, 34*(12), 1119–1129.

Daley, D., Moss, H., & Campbell, F. (1987). *Dual disorders: Counseling clients with chemical dependency and mental illness.* Center City, MN: Hazelden Education Materials.

Evans, K., & Sullivan, J. M. (1990). *Dual diagnosis: Counseling the mentally ill substance abuser.* New York: Guilford Press.

Fisher, M. (1994). *Effectiveness study of two group models with substance abusing mentally ill (multi-

challenged) consumers. Unpublished doctoral dissertation, Virginia Commonwealth University School of Social Work, Richmond.

Fisher, M. (1995). Group therapy protocols for persons with personality disorders who abuse substances: Effective treatment alternatives. *Social Work with Groups, 18*(4), 71–89.

Fisher, M. S., & Bentley, K. J. (1996). Effectiveness study of two group therapy models with dually diagnosed consumers. *Psychiatric Services, 47*(11), 1244–1250.

Flores, P. (1997). *Group psychotherapy with addicted populations*. New York: Haworth Press.

Golden, S. J., Khantzian, E. J., & McAuliffe, W. E. (1994). Group therapy. In M. Galanter (Ed.), *Substance abuse treatment* (pp. 303–315). New York: American Psychiatric Press.

Graham, K., Annis, H., Brett, P., & Venesoen, P. (1996). A controlled field trail of group versus individual cognitive-behavioral training for relapse prevention. *Addictions, 91*(8), 1127–1139.

Harding, C., Brooks, G., & Ashikaga, T. (1987). The Vermont longitudinal study of persons with severe mental illness: 2. Long-term outcome of subjects who retrospectively met DSM-III criteria for schizophrenia. *American Journal of Psychiatry, 144*, 727–735.

Hester, R. (1995). Behavior self-control training. In R. Hester & W. Miller (Eds.), *Handbook of alcoholism treatment approaches: Effective alternatives* (pp. 148–159). Boston: Allyn & Bacon.

Lamb, H. (1982). *Treating the long-term mentally ill*. San Francisco: Jossey-Bass.

Levine, B., & Gallogly, V. (1985). *Group therapy with alcoholics: Outpatient and inpatient approaches*. Beverly Hills, CA: Sage.

Mack, J. E. (1981). Alcoholism, A.A., and the governance of the self. In M. H. Bean & N. E. Zimberg (Eds.), *Dynamic approaches to the understanding and treatment of alcoholism* (pp. 128–162). New York: Free Press.

Matano, R. A., & Yalom, I. D. (1991). Approaches to chemical dependency: Chemical dependency and interactive group therapy: A synthesis. *International Journal of Group Psychotherapy, 41*, 269–293.

Matano, R. A., Yalom, I. D., & Schwartz, K. (1997). Interactive group therapy for substance abusers. In J. L. Spira (Ed.), *Group therapy for medically ill patients* (pp. 296–325). New York: Guilford Press.

McLellan, A. T., Luborsky, L., O'Brien, C. P., & Woody, G. E. (1980). An improved evaluation instrument for substance abuse patients: The addiction severity index. *Journal of Nervous and Mental Disorders, 168*, 26–33.

Miller, W., & Rollnick, S. (1991). *Motivational interviewing: Preparing people to change addictive behaviors*. New York: Guilford Press.

Minkoff, K. (1989). An integrated treatment model for dual diagnosis of psychosis and addiction. *Hospital and Community Psychiatry, 40*, 1031–1036.

Monti, P., Abrams, D., Kadden, R., Cooney, N., & Ned, L. (1989). *Treating alcohol dependence: A coping skills training guide*. New York: Basic Books.

Najavits, L., Weiss, R., Shaw, S., & Muenz, L. (1998). Seeking safety: Outcomes of a new cognitive-behavioral psychotherapy for women with posttraumatic stress disorder and substance dependence. *Journal of Traumatic Stress, 11*(3), 437–456.

Osher, F., & Kofoed, L. (1989). Treatment of patients with psychiatric and psychoactive substance abuse disorders. *Hospital and Community Psychiatry, 40*, 1025–1030.

Persons, J. (1989). *Cognitive therapy in practice: A case formulation approach*. New York: Norton.

Prochaska, J., Norcross, J., & DiClemente, C. (1994). *Changing for good: The revolutionary program that explains the six stages of change and teaches you how to free yourself from bad habits*. New York: Morrow.

Rotgers, F., Morgenstern, J., & Walters, S. T. (Eds.). (2003). *Treating substance abuse: Theory and technique* (2nd ed.). New York: Guilford Press.

Rutan, J., & Stone, W. (1984). *Psychodynamic group psychotherapy*. Lexington, MA: Collamore Press.

Sandahl, C., Herlitz, K., Ahlin, G., & Roennberg, S. (1998). Time limited group psychotherapy for moderately alcohol dependent patients: A randomized controlled clinical trial. *Psychotherapy Research, 8*(4), 361–378.

Wallace, J. (1975). *Tactical and strategic use of the preferred defense structure of the recovering alcoholic*. New York: National Council on Alcoholism.

Wallen, M., & Weiner, H. (1989). Impediments to effective treatment of the dually diagnosed patient. *Journal of Psychoactive Drugs, 21*(2), 161–168.

Washington, O. (1999). Effects of cognitive and experiential group therapy on self-efficacy and perceptions of employability of chemically dependent women. *Issues in Mental Health Nursing, 20*, 181–198.

Yalom, I. D. (1974). Group therapy and alcoholism. *Annals of the New York Academy of Sciences, 233*, 85–103.

Yalom, I. D. (1985). *The theory and practice of group psychotherapy* (3rd ed.). New York: Basic Books.

Chapter 16

Groups for Older Adults

RUTH CAMPBELL

In recent years, groups held with and by older adults have increased considerably as research has identified the multiple losses and deficits of aging, as well as the strengths and potential of this later stage of life. The settings in which groups are held have also expanded with the development of new geriatrics programs at medical facilities, adult day centers for people with memory loss, an increase in assisted living residences, lifelong learning programs such as Elderhostels, and other community-based programs.

Two widely recognized facts about the older adult population are (1) that the percentage of Americans over age 65 is rapidly increasing and that within that population the largest increase will be in the percentage over age 85 (Administration on Aging, 2002) and (2) that the group we label as "old" represents a very heterogeneous group, spanning at least two generations, with a wide range of health status, racial and ethnic background, education, income, and experience. This diversity is reflected in the many different kinds of groups involving older adults, including those that are purely educational or psychoeducational, support and self-help groups, recreational and creative activities, groups for those with a specific illness such as depression or Alzheimer's disease, and political and community action groups.

Group work with the elderly, according to Toseland (1995), developed over the early part of the 20th century in three distinct settings: settlement houses and community centers, homes for the aged, and state mental institutions. Maurice Linden (1953), a psychiatrist, was one of the early leaders, co-leading a group therapy program for elderly regressed women in a state mental institution in Pennsylvania (Burnside & Schmidt, 1994). Kubie and Landau (1953) described their experience in developing a senior center program for low-income elderly in New York. Group work in homes for the aged and nursing homes (Konopka, 1954; Shore, 1952) focused on helping residents adjust to the nursing home, remain socially active, and enhance their physical and cognitive functioning.

The two most comprehensive books in the field, by Toseland (1995) and by Burnside and Schmidt (1994), document how group work can be utilized by healthy, active elderly people, by those with chronic conditions, and by the frail elderly with physical and cognitive impairments. Toseland (1995) notes that there are three categories of contraindications for group participation. These are (1) practical barriers such as transportation, frailty, or lack of enough people in a setting to support a group; (2) people's particular therapeutic needs, such as acute crisis situations or material too personal to disclose in a group; (3) people with certain personality or mental health problems. However, it is often possible to target groups especially for certain populations or to start with individual counseling and gradually move to a group.

Interest is increasing in the geropsychiatric literature as models used with younger populations, such as cognitive-behavioral therapy, dialectical behavior therapy, and interpersonal therapy group methods, are adapted and evaluated for use with an older population. Research has demonstrated the effectiveness of these therapies, as well as provided some evidence that these psychosocial interventions offer broader effects and greater stability of response than seen with medications alone (Hollon, 2002). Practitioners are also drawing on existing gerontological research to explore new group options for the elderly. A cognitive therapy group for the elderly, an intergenerational reminiscence group, a "meaning of life" group, and writing groups are examples of groups that grew from practitioners' recognition of the special needs of their clients (Ingersoll-Dayton & Campbell, 2001).

Groups are viewed as especially powerful agents of change for the elderly, uniquely suited to the challenges of the aging process: coping with loss, shrinking support networks, societal change, and chronic illness. Although recreational groups are certainly important, this chapter focuses on some of the newer interventions in psychotherapy: reminiscence, caregiver, and other support groups and groups using creative methods. Most of these have generated empirical evidence supporting outcomes and also point the way to future development of the field.

THE PURPOSE OF GROUP WORK WITH THE ELDERLY

The purpose of group work, regardless of the intervention and the physical and cognitive level of the participants, is to enable the older adult to function at the highest level possible and to push the boundaries of what the individual, family, or society at large expects from a certain person in a certain situation. Groups provide a cushion, a way to safely explore one's own identity and to forge new connections with others. For the elderly, groups may often represent a surrogate family, a new network of friends, and a way to explore areas in their lives that they never had the time or opportunity to do earlier. For the leader, groups with the elderly are a particular challenge, a balancing act between asserting leadership, providing counseling and support, and stepping back to allow the group to take over. The purpose of the group will often depend largely on how the group defines it. The significant role of the group worker is to develop groups that are sensitive to the changing needs of this population and to the wide diversity of roles, abilities, and as yet unfulfilled desires of adults in the later stages of life.

Several theoretical approaches provide the framework for group work practice with the elderly. Rowe and Kahn (1987, 1997), in their concept of successful aging, pointed out that many characteristics of aging, such as decreased mobility and physical and cognitive decline, that are thought to be normal stages of the aging process are actually due to lifestyle and other factors that can potentially be modified through exercise, nutrition, cognitive training, or active participation in life. The concept of selective optimization with compensation, developed by Baltes and Baltes (1990), emphasizes the variability among individuals as they age and affirms that the self does remain resilient in later life.

These concepts confront the idea that used to be prevalent, even in the professional community, that older people cannot change: "If he never joined a group before, why would he now? What can be gained from working with people with memory loss?" Groups themselves, as Yalom (1985) wrote, instill hope. The purpose of being in a group is to make some change that will enhance one's life, reinforce one's ability to cope, and build on existing strengths.

Social support is also a significant element of successful aging. Studies have shown that older people who maintain meaningful ties with others are likely to be in better physical and mental health than those who do not (Krause, 2001). As people age, they are more likely to be living alone; for example, about half of women over the age of 75 lived alone in 2000 (Administration on Aging, 2002). Even elderly couples may find themselves isolated due to chronic illness, caregiving demands, distance from family members, and changes in their social networks. Groups offer a more structured opportunity to gradually and safely make new friendships and replenish support networks.

Aging is often depicted as a time of loss. Spouses, friends, and significant family members die, become ill, or move. Retirement may bring a loss of role, status, and income. Chronic illness, which affects about 80% of people over age 65, imposes limitations that affect mobility, transportation, enjoyment of familiar activities, and daily functioning. Sensory losses in vision and hearing, in particular, require major life adjustments, and declining memory, even in the earliest stages, challenges an individual's sense of self and identity. The proliferation of support groups to address these specific needs (groups concerned with losses of hearing and vision, diabetes, cancer, etc.) has been an important development in helping older adults learn new coping patterns and flexibility. The ability to give as well as to receive assistance is an important characteristic of social support (Ingersoll-Dayton, 2001), which is, in itself, a powerful argument for group participation.

An important perspective in dealing with these losses is recognizing and reinforcing strengths relevant to later life. Wisdom, according to Baltes, Smith, Staudinger, and Sowarka (1990), includes a deep understanding of human nature, knowledge about social relationships, and a recognition of life's uncertainties (Ingersoll-Dayton, 2001). Another strength of older adults is resilience, the ability to cope with setbacks and recover. Resilience also implies the ability to reframe cognitively what has happened, changing the meaning of the event (Pearlin & Skaff, 1995) in order to deal with unbearable losses.

Yalom's (1975) classic description of the curative factors of group therapy has been adapted to apply to the aging by Toseland (1990), Ronch and Crispi (1997), Burnside and Schmidt (1994), Erwin (1996), and others. The following are especially important for group leaders working with the elderly to strive to achieve: instillation of hope; universality (learning that others have had similar experiences); a sense of belonging and affiliation; the opportunity to learn and assume new and meaningful roles; receiving and sharing information and skills in problem solving; consensual validation and affirmation; offering a safe place for ventilation and integrating diverse experiences; and encouragement to explore creativity both in the arts and through new ways of thinking about life.

INTERVENTIONS

Group interventions in the following categories are discussed: psychotherapy, reminiscence and life review, caregiver groups, support and self-help groups, community action, and educational and arts groups.

Psychotherapy

Although the prevalence of major depression among the elderly is lower than in adults at midlife and younger, the potential adverse effects of depression, such as suicide, neglect of health, and stress on physical and social functioning, make it a significant issue faced by professionals working with the elderly. It is estimated that about 2% of community elderly suffer a major or clinical depression; another 2%, dysthymia; and an additional 4–8% suffer depressive symptoms secondary to bereavement, adjustment to physical illness, and other life changes. Among residents of long-term care institutions and the medically ill, clinical depression is found in about 12–16% of the population, and depressive symptoms affect an additional 20–30% (Blazer, 1998). Other emotional problems seen in practice include anxiety, suspiciousness and agitation, sleeping problems, long-standing mental health problems such as schizophrenia, and alcohol and drug abuse.

The specific characteristics of these problems and the attributes of group therapy are well matched. Leszcz (1997) writes, "An overarching concept is that of the unique capacity of group psychotherapy to offer a self-esteem enhancing, relational matrix to its participants" (p. 93). Multiple medications make it difficult to manage these conditions with medications alone. Cognitive impairment, loss of supportive relationships, and physical disability present other challenges to treatment (Hollon, 2003). Group therapy is less expensive than individual therapy, and being part of a group may also reduce the stigma attached to therapy that prevents some older adults from seeking treatment. Only about one-fourth of depressed older adults actually are treated for depression. Low-income and minority elderly people are even less likely to receive treatment. Hollon (2003) notes that researchers have found a greater stability of response with psychosocial methods than with medications alone.

Standardized Therapies

Standardized therapies consisting of structured, manual-based interventions that involve cognitive and behavioral strategies have been effectively used with younger adults and also have the most empirical support with the elderly. Brief standardized psychotherapies focus on the stressors and losses common in late life, with the goal of reducing psychopathology and increasing quality of life (Klausner & Alexopoulos, 1999). Treatment focuses on changing patterns of thinking, learning new skills, and improving problem-solving abilities.

1. *Dialectical behavior therapy (DBT)*. Lynch, Morse, Mendelson, and Robins (2003) adapted DBT for use with depressed older adults. They found the following components of standard DBT treatment relevant in treating this population: acceptance of elements of life that cannot be changed (radical acceptance), increased awareness without judgment (mindfulness), attentional control (mindfulness), better tolerance of pain, acting contrary to depressive urges, and increased interpersonal effectiveness. By focusing on maladaptive coping styles and behaviors functionally related to depression, the researchers hoped that these behaviors and coping styles could be modified to decrease the likelihood of future depressive episodes.

Thirty-four depressed people age 60 and over living in the community were randomly assigned to either 28 weeks of standard medication management or medication management in combination with a DBT weekly skills training group plus weekly half-hour individual telephone coaching. Group sessions lasted 2 hours. Four group sessions focused on education about depression, teaching core mindfulness concepts and practices, and encouraging participants to develop daily mindfulness practices. Two sessions focused on better tolerance of pain and distress, three sessions on emotional regulation skills, and five sessions on interpersonal effectiveness skills. After this, the 14 sessions were repeated so each topic was covered twice. Besides receiving weekly 30-minute telephone contact with the therapist, members could also call their therapist between group sessions if there was a crisis. After the 28 weeks, telephone coaching that reinforced the use of these skills continued every 2 weeks and then was reduced.

Patients in the DBT group sessions showed significant improvements on self-rated depression scores and adaptive coping. They also were less concerned about being liked and hurting others' feelings, were better able to say no to requests, were less apologetic, and felt less responsible for other people's problems compared with patients receiving medication only. The DBT group members also showed nearly significant improvements in hopeless thoughts, which should reduce their vulnerability to suicide.

2. *Cognitive-behavioral therapy.* The goals of cognitive-behavioral therapy are to change thoughts, improve skills, and modify emotional states that contribute to psychopathology (Klausner & Alexopoulos, 1999). Developed in the late 1950s by Aaron Beck (1972), it has become one of the most successful and widely utilized psychotherapies for treating a wide range of problems. As Fogler and Edwards (2001) point out, the emphasis in cognitive therapy on educational methods and concrete techniques for change make it especially acceptable to older adults. Their group, "New Ways to Feel Good," appeals to older adults intimidated by the term "cognitive therapy." Two social workers conduct 10 weekly group sessions with a maximum of 10 members who have DSM-IV diagnoses of depression and/or anxiety. Each group session starts with a brief go-around question, then a short lecture presenting the basics of cognitive therapy, group discussion of problems, goal setting, and goal review and homework assignments.

Brok (1997) states, "As a general rule, the more structure there is in a group, the less the manifest anxiety" (Brok, 1997, p. 117). He stresses the importance of flexibility of method in his "life enrichment counseling approach," which aims to help older people develop ways of making meaningful use of leisure time. Group members list leisure activities on a structured form, evaluate them for enjoyment, and then participate in cognitively based, theme-oriented group discussion. For example, one member listed piano playing as a favorite activity. In group discussion, it became clear that she had not played the piano in many years. The group explored this further. One member suggested where a piano was available, and others talked about how and when the woman might play it. The group then was able to activate a long dormant interest (Brok, 1997, p. 127).

3. Leszcz (1997) proposes a model of integrated group therapy drawing on the theoretical perspectives of the various clinical strategies. Rather than selecting from a single focus on social support, interpersonal skills, coping skills, or distorted cognitions, he believes it is consistent to integrate these various methods, employing therapeutic strategies as opportunities arise in the group. Therapy interventions must always be clearly rooted in patient need and evaluated in an ongoing fashion, collaboratively with the patient (Leszcz, 1997).

This approach is integrative, not eclectic, in that all strategies proceed from overarching theoretical perspectives. The interpersonal focus gives a picture of the individual's intrapersonal world, through exploring the individual's subjective sense of self historically and currently. The group processes of cohesion, acceptance, and empathic exploration can provide feedback and add new perspectives. Reminiscence can be helpful in gaining a clearer understanding of the individual member. Developmental and self-psychological factors address the causes of guilt, demoralization, and fears of engagement, stimulating openness in members who may not have previously experienced this. As members require specific skills to acquire self-mastery, cognitive-behavioral methods can be used, cognitive distortions confronted, and homework assigned to reinforce behavioral change. Another aspect of integration involves the concurrent use of medication. Group members exchange information about medications, sharing anxieties and fears, and responding to side effects.

In all methods, effectiveness of group therapy is rooted in the individuals' engagement and interaction within the group and the feeling of success and connection they experience in the group. In all of these interventions, the therapist's attitude of respect, hopefulness, and genuine warmth and empathy is essential. The therapist working with the elderly has to be more active than is needed with a younger group to insure a nonfailure experience and to help members' integration into the group through therapist bridging, reframing, or translating patient verbalizations and behaviors (Lesczc, 1997).

Nonstandardized Therapies

Nonstandardized therapies do not rely on structured, manual-based treatment and vary from short term to longer term or ongoing groups. They focus on feelings, change over the life course, and deal with issues from the individual's past, as well as the present. Psychodynamic psychotherapy focuses on resolution of interpersonal conflicts, understanding and acceptance of achievements and disappointments in life, and adaptation to current losses and stressors. For frail elderly group members, the goal is to help members come to some acceptance of physical limitations, to grieve losses of both relationships and physical functioning, to address fears of dependency, and to repair or optimize personal interactions with others in their lives (Klausner & Alexopoulos, 1999).

A short-term therapy group with Holocaust survivors and second-generation members who were not related is an example of a supportive, psychodynamic approach. The group aimed to integrate the past by focusing on the conflicts of the Holocaust. The survivors felt the support of the second generation, who asked to hear their stories, and the second generation was supported when they could share their angry feelings and have them heard and validated (Erlich, 2002). The groups meet for 10 to 12 weekly sessions for 1½ hours. Common themes for the survivors and second-generation members included separation, mourning of loss, anger, and feelings of inadequacy. These common feelings facilitated empathy, understanding, and identification between the two generations.

Group therapy in nursing homes helps residents maintain control in their lives, recognize their fears, express feelings of loss, deal with loneliness, and provide affirmation of each other. Ronch and Crispi (1997) observe that, although task-oriented groups are valuable in nursing homes, discussion-oriented groups provide many benefits for the residents. They present a nonthreatening environment in which to discuss topics they are unable to discuss elsewhere. They can find commonality of experience and develop more meaningful relationships with other members, creating a buffer for loneliness and isolation.

The orientation of Ronch and Crispi's (1997) groups is interactive, with a here-and-now focus. Residents are referred because staff or family members recognize a maladaptive behavior syndrome or a diagnosable mental disorder. Ronch and Crispi (1997) advocate the importance of focusing on the purpose of the group, as well as their perceived problems. They ask, "Why is this resident experiencing difficulties at this time?" Domains include losses, somatic complaints, personality disorders, and issues concerning the resident's autonomy and perceptions of aging and what is expected of them in this situation. Therapists can question the validity of these expectations and clarify situations in which relations between individuals and staff members are built on inaccurate perceptions. These groups, most of all, provide a safe place to express feelings and individuality, which may not be possible in the public atmosphere of institutional living.

Written and Oral Reminiscence

Reminiscence as an intervention grew out of the seminal article by Robert Butler (1963) on life review, which he characterized as "a naturally occurring, universal mental process characterized by the progressive return to consciousness of past experiences, and, particularly the resurgence of unsolved conflict; simultaneously and normally, these reviewed experiences and conflicts can be surveyed and reintegrated" (Butler, 1963, p. 66). Recent writers have challenged the idea that life review is a natural process occurring in individuals before death (Wink & Schiff, 2002). Studies have shown that not all older adults want to review their lives or feel the need to do so.

Reminiscence groups have been widely utilized, both with healthy older adults and with those with Alzheimer's disease and other physical and cognitive problems. Burnside sees reminiscence as having a narrower focus than life review, serving a supportive, restorative function. Reminiscence groups help group members relive and appreciate events in the past that are personally significant (Burnside, 1995).

The process of reminiscing in a group can restore a sense of self, as individuals talk about events in their lives that have real meaning for them. There are big differences in how this intervention is used. The group leader has to assure that everyone has a chance to speak, that the group does not become a series of monologues, and that the talking, listening, and sharing is deepening members' engagement with each other. When painful memories surface in the group, individual sessions with the group leader may be necessary in order to fully address the emotions arising from the reminiscence session. LoGerfo (1980–1981) distinguished three types of reminiscence: (1) informative—the sharing of stories; (2) evaluative—similar to a life review process; and (3) obsessive—rumination, repetitive thoughts, obsessive mourning. Experienced leaders need to recognize the obsessive reminiscences and address the needs of the individuals involved without allowing them to dominate the group.

Many reminiscence groups are structured through themes. Burnside (1995) reports that most themes use a lifespan, chronological order, such as first pet, first job, first day of school. She recommends that leaders should be flexible about themes and change them if the group is not interested. The wording for themes should be very precise and easily understood. Gender and cultural aspects of the group need to be taken into account (see Nomura, 2001, for examples of themes used with Japanese elderly). Although a variety of professionals and staff members lead reminiscence groups, the availability of kits and other structured programs can, with an inexperienced leader, result in sterile, rote kinds of groups without significant interaction and engagement among members. Props, including those that stimulate the senses—hearing, smelling, and touching—can be effective in eliciting memories: the smell of coffee, the odor of mustard plasters used on the body, the feel of a familiar lotion smoothed on hands, the sound of music both long past and current. Sherman (1995) studied the relationship between objects and reminiscence, finding in several cases that cherished objects not only stirred memories but also triggered a process of related memories, reconstructing certain periods in people's lives. He also found that the over-80-year-old group had significantly fewer personally meaningful memorabilia and also were less likely to engage in reminiscing.

However, Erwin (1996) and others have designed specific modules for more frail elderly in day care centers and nursing homes that use reminiscence selectively and effectively. Using the topic of "favorite vacations," for example, the group leader begins by talking about her own favorite vacation. As group members identify vacation places they enjoyed, the leader puts a sticker marking each location on a large map. The leader may prompt questions for sites, smells, sounds, weather, or people who were part of the vacation. She also suggests that guided imagery can be used, if the group leader can do this, to further enhance the imaginative experience. Erwin's topics are not based on the past but incorporate the present, with topics such as lifelong learning, a family genogram, and seasons of the year.

Besides the oral reminiscence groups just described, an increasing trend is toward written reminiscence, such as the guided autobiography groups developed by James Birren (Birren & Cochran, 2001). The process of writing stimulates further recall and gives group members a chance to rehearse and edit the memories before they present them to the group. Birren and Cochran (2001) organize group sessions around themes which are more reflective than the themes discussed in oral reminiscence: the major branching points in one's life; your family; the role of money in one's life; major life work or career; health and body; sexual identity; experiences with and ideas about death, spiritual life, and values; goals and aspirations. They also suggest expanded themes for specific groups, such as war veterans, prospective retirees, and ethnic minorities. The goals of this kind of group include: (1) helping to build a sense of community; (2) developing strategies to deal with life changes; (3) helping group members understand their pasts and also explore future directions; and (4) helping members find resources to face challenges and losses.

Other, less structured writing groups combine both the practice of writing at home and reading in the group with group discussion about the writings. Chandler and Ray (2001) describe a "senior memories" group with primarily African American seniors. Members gathered to write memories of Detroit, and their writings conveyed a strong sense of place, "the dirt streets, the tired horse and wagon tumbling full of what any household could part with for the money" (Chandler & Ray, 2002, p. 79). They also reflected on their own lives, their childhoods, work, and families. Leaders did not assign topics but prompted as needed. Participants agreed that they said things in this group that they hadn't told their friends or families (a common finding in writing groups).

Such diverse groups as Hispanic elderly in a New York settlement house, retired seamen, and participants meeting at an African American library are described by the writers, social workers, and artists who facilitated these groups, which were sponsored by a writing project in New York City (Kaminsky, 1984). Written, as opposed to oral, reminiscence has the value of creating a concrete product that can be shared by many others outside the group and that exists as a legacy after the person has died. Writing also bestows a new identity, that of a "writer," to group members, which makes this process more acceptable to many seniors than group therapy or a recreational group.

Most of the writing groups described in this chapter are short term, lasting 8–10 weeks with possible follow-up sessions. The benefit of a long-term writing group continuing more than 20 years is described by Campbell (2001). Men and women from very different backgrounds, educational levels, and beliefs, through their writing, become a kind of surrogate family, sharing intimate stories, helping each other when they are ill, providing food and transportation when needed, and attending memorial services as members die. Although members do write memoirs, they also write fiction, poetry, letters to the editor, and philosophical essays. The group is loosely structured so that the members request assignments as needed from the group leader. However, frequently they respond to what is happening currently in their lives, as well as to memories stimulated by writings of other group members. In a recent group session, Mr. B began with a letter to the editor about politics in Washington; Ms. C wrote about her recent surgery and slow recovery; Ms. D began writing about an argument she had as a child with her cousin over a pet, which led to the revelation by her cousin that Ms. D had been adopted, a fact she had not known before. The readings and discussions form an intricate pattern, going back and forth among past, present, and future. Although this group is led by a social worker, another, similar group has been facilitated by a volunteer for many years. The cohesion and success of many short-term groups offer possibilities for continuation that should be explored.

Other innovative uses of reminiscence groups for the frail elderly are described by Supiano, Ozminkowski, Campbell, and Lapidos (1987). Volunteers were used to take down the oral compositions of nursing home residents. Many group participants achieved important benefits: reduced depression, improved interactions with other nursing home residents, and a restored sense of identity and achievement. Writings were displayed in several nursing homes, and a collection was published and distributed to friends and family members. The effect on the nursing home staff was also positive, as they observed residents engaged in a very different way than was usually seen on the floor.

Groups for Family Caregivers

Family members provide most of the care given to frail older persons in the community. Caregivers can find satisfaction and also stress in caregiving (Kramer, 1997). Significant levels of stress, feelings of burden, compromised physical health, and even premature mortality are reported in the caregiving literature (Sorensen, Pinquart, Habil, & Duberstein, 2002). Many of these informal caregivers, primarily spouses but also adult children, are themselves over the age of 60 and coping with their own aging issues. Because of growing concern with the needs of these caregivers, group work with family caregivers has developed into a major focus of the group work literature for the elderly. In particular, support groups for caregivers of people with Alzheimer's disease, who generally experience the highest level of stress, are widely available in the community and in hospitals and nursing facilities. Three different types of group treatment are discussed in this section: psychoeducational groups, psychotherapy groups, and support groups.

Psychoeducational Groups

Psychoeducational interventions are a recently increasing way of addressing the problems of caregiving. A general stress mediation model (Aneshensel, Pearlin, Mullan, Zarit, & Whitlatch, 1995) suggests that multidimensional mediation may be needed to improve outcomes in a stressful situation. Ostwald, Hepburn, Caron, Burns, and Mantell (1999) developed a 14-hour training program of weekly, 2-hour sessions for primary caregivers and their families based on this model. At least one additional family member other than the primary caregiver was required to accompany the caregiver and patient to the seven weekly sessions. Patients participated in a concurrent day care program, making it easier for the caregiver to attend the group. The structured content began with information about dementia; in subsequent sessions, caregivers viewed videos of the assessment of their relatives and were told their family members' functioning levels. The last two sessions focused on caregiving skills, with an emphasis on involving all family members as active learners. An interesting outcome of this program was that improvement on the burden score was not apparent until the 5-month follow-up interview. Compared with the waiting-list control group, who showed substantial increases in their burden scores during this same period of time, the treatment group on average showed a reduction in feelings of burden, and the treatment also seemed to prevent any significant increases (Ostwald et al., 1999).

In one program (Gallagher-Thompson & DeVries, 1994), wives and daughters of individuals with dementia attended "coping with frustration" classes, in which they were taught specific skills, such as relaxing in a stressful situation and learning to be appropriately assertive with their elder and other relatives. The strategy of using "classes" instead of "group therapy" reduces the stigma that many people attach to seeking help. Three models of psychoeducational intervention have been developed by Gallagher-Thompson and colleagues (1997): coping with depression, increasing problem-solving skills, and anger management. Caregivers monitored their moods and pleasant events and set step-by-step goals to increase these events. Participants showed decreases in depression and increases in morale when compared with a control group. The problem-solving class focused more on problem-solving strategies for daily life, whereas the anger management class incorporated relaxation techniques and taught participants to identify specific situations that precipitated anger, as well as the physical manifestations of anger (Gallagher-Thompson, Lovett, & Rose, 1991).

All of these classes were attended by European Americans. Gallagher-Thompson et al. (1997) adapted the program to make it specifically relevant to Hispanic caregivers of dementia patients. One change was to begin each session with a "check-in," time because the Hispanic caregivers wanted to talk to each other informally before the class began. The leaders also noted that the pace of information was too fast and the homework too complicated and that the reading material, translated into Spanish, needed to be modified to be more relevant to the Hispanic situation. A great deal of interaction and peer support arose among the caregivers as a result of the skills training component.

Hebert and colleagues (2003) developed a group program based on a transactional theory of stress and coping (Folkman et al., 1991). The purpose of the program was to improve stress management skills by teaching caregivers how to respond to difficult behaviors, thereby reducing their burden, distress, and anxiety and enhancing their well-being. The program consisted of 15 two-hour weekly sessions with two components. The first component, cognitive appraisal (four sessions), aimed to help the caregiver identify specific stressors, distinguish between the changeable and unchangeable aspects of the stressor, and choose coping strategies. The caregivers also received a home assignment to practice their ability to identify four specific stressors, the changeable and unchangeable elements, and their own emotional reactions. The second component (11 sessions) taught three specific coping strategies: problem solving, reframing, and seeking social support. In a randomized controlled study of this program, Hebert et al. (2003) found that it decreased the frequency of and reactions to behaviors, especially disruptive ones. However, there was no indirect effect on more general problems such as burden, stress, psychological distress, affect, and lack of social support. Although Hebert et al. (2003) recommend that this kind of program, which aims at targeted outcomes, should replace the more traditional support groups currently organized by the Alzheimer's Association, it is hard to see how the vast network of Alzheimer's support groups, often peer led, could support this much more intensive intervention.

Psychotherapy Groups

Shaw (1997) co-led a long-term Alzheimer's Association family support group guided by the modern analytic group principles of paying attention to the resistances brought up in the group process and the transferences to other group members or group leaders. The group had a maximum of 12 members and was culturally, socially, economically, and religiously diverse. Loneliness and loss of companionship were common themes. When one man talked about his 24-hour devotion to nursing his wife, refusing to place her in a nursing home, the leader used a bridging technique to help build emotional connections between him and other group members. The leader asked group members why the man continued in these devoted efforts while depriving himself of pleasure. The group noted his sadness, frustration, and moral conflict. He was able to share his anger and disappointments within the empathic safety of the group.

Support Groups

Support groups differ from traditional group therapies in that their goal is not to change the members' problematic behaviors. They are widespread, inexpensive to run, and can be professionally led or peer led, often organized by a local or national group such as the Alzheimer's Association. Although many reports suggest that these groups are effective at relieving caregivers' levels of stress, the majority of controlled experimental studies have not shown that they have any significant effect (Hebert et al., 2003). However, most of the groups studied have used, on the average, eight weekly 2-hour sessions, frequently using information and emotion-sharing strategies. Hebert et al. (2003) suggest that these programs need to be spread over a longer period, to have a specific theoretical framework, and to focus especially on the management of difficult behaviors and the responses they create. The University of Michigan's Turner Geriatric Clinic has two ongoing support groups, as well as a structured six-session lecture/discussion format, which is held two or three times a year. The ongoing groups, one for adult children and another for spouses ("Caring for Your Mate"), allow caregivers to attend regularly or irregularly, depending on their situation. The groups have a strong nucleus of participants who both receive and give support and information. A peer volunteer contacts members in the Caring for Your Mate group in between sessions, and members often contact each other between meetings as well. New members can join at any time; members frequently remain in the group for an extended period of time after the person they were caring for dies.

Two problems with support groups are that they reach a relatively small percentage of those who need help and that they are predominantly composed of white, middle-class, more highly educated individuals. An eight-week series for African American women caring for a parent with dementia (Sistler & Washington, 1999) used the serenity prayer as a major theme of their sessions. Caregivers discussed what factors they could not change, such as their parents having the disease and the progression of the illness. Problem-solving activities focused on difficult behaviors, on identifying feelings of both the caregiver and care receiver, on caring for oneself, and on keeping the care receiver active. Participants discussed religion, prayer, and their feelings about God. Combining problem solving with the serenity prayer helped participants improve in self-confidence, well-being, and happiness, as measured in posttests. Targeting a specific homogeneous group is effective in reaching caregivers who do not usually attend support groups.

A multicomponent model in an outpatient clinic combined the support-group approach with two individual and four family task-oriented counseling sessions. Spousal caregivers were required to attend weekly support groups, which continued indefinitely. Counselors were always available to help deal with crises and to meet changing needs. As a result, spouses in treatment groups were able to delay nursing home placement almost a year longer than the control group for patients in the early to middle stages of dementia, when placement is probably least appropriate (Mittelman, Ferris, Shulman, Steinberg, & Levin, 1996).

A meta-analysis of caregiver interventions (Sorenson et al., 2002) found that multicomponent interventions—combining group sessions with individual treatment, as in the aforementioned study—were particularly effective in reducing caregiver burden and also had positive outcomes on well-being and knowledge but were less effective than psychotherapy and psychoeducational groups in reducing caregiver depression and care-receiver symptoms. Respite and day care interventions did reduce caregiver burden and depression and increased well-being. Support groups were also effective at reducing caregiver burden and improving knowledge and skills. Sorenson et al. (2002) conclude that group interventions are more effective than individual treatment in alleviating care-receiver behaviors. This is probably due to the group setting, which promotes the exchange of experiences and allows rehearsal of specific caregiving skills.

Because individuals have a wide variety of needs and preferences, it is helpful to have a repertoire of strategies, not a "one-size-fits-all" approach. Clinicians should identify the goals of the group in order to determine which intervention to use. Interventions of seven to nine sessions are adequate to address knowledge and skills but may not provide enough time to improve depression or alleviate burden.

Groups for the Frail and Cognitively Impaired

As diagnosis of Alzheimer's disease becomes more sophisticated, early diagnosis is increasingly common. Many of the group strategies described here can be adapted for people with cognitive difficulties. Cognitive-behavioral interventions and other psychotherapeutic methods for treating depression can be of great value to people with early dementia and even middle-stage dementia (Teri & Gallagher-Thompson, 1991). Using a support group format, the "Coffee House" ("Memory Café," 2001), a group for people with early dementia, meets weekly for 5 hours, beginning with structured group discussion in which members cover such issues as the effects of the diagnosis, their memory problems, and their anger about not being able to drive and being "bossed" around by spouses or adult children. Guided by co-leaders, participants are encouraged to openly discuss the losses they are feeling and their anger, fear, and other emotions. It has also become an activist group. Members compile "tip sheets" to advise others how to communicate with someone with memory loss and to discuss how they would like to be treated. "Don't speak louder. Take your time. Give me time to answer. Don't say a lot at once." Several members also appeared on a panel at professional meetings to talk openly about their experiences and to tell professionals what they need from them.

Besides participating in the support group, members exercise, have lunch together, and work on individual projects such as guided autobiography. Some have compiled memory books or tried painting and other art projects. They attended a lecture on Alzheimer's disease that was part of a large Learning in Retirement program. The object is to find ways to maintain the participants' existing strengths and to respond to the individual's entire life history, not just their status as a person with memory loss.

Geriatric skills enhancement (GSE) was developed in institutional settings to bridge the gap between recreation and psychotherapy. The aim was to work with the skills deficits and psychosocial losses of aging persons at various levels of functioning (Erwin, 1996). Patient focus groups identified concerns such as social isolation and reduced social networks, limited mobility, declining physical strength, and a sense of powerlessness. Core group modules were developed that incorporated music, art, photography, humor, reminiscence, sensory awareness, and movement. The goals are to review how individuals became invested in the larger community and the results of their participation. Talking about school, neighborhood, church, and city affairs recognizes the desire of adults in a nursing home to still feel part of a community.

A group for cognitively impaired men was formed at a Japanese nursing home to give the men a place where they could meet together and talk about their work and their interests. In most nursing homes, men are the minority, surrounded by women. In this group, men exchanged name cards (made for them by the staff) and not to know about each other's former occupations, war experiences, and current lives (Kurokawa, 2002).

Support, Educational, and Advocacy Groups

Support groups help members work through difficult life transitions—illnesses, widowhood, retirement. Often these groups combine an educational purpose with support, as in an 11-week Pathfinders class for recently bereaved widows and widowers (Caserta, Lund, & Rice, 1999), which focuses on increasing competency in self-care skills such as meal planning, household maintenance, and managing finances. The hospice movement has made extensive use of bereavement support groups as an integral part of the grieving process. The telephone conference call offers an innovative method of reaching homebound elderly persons and caregivers who might not otherwise be able to participate in a group. Kaslyn (1999) discusses the logistics and benefits of this kind of group, emphasizing the considerable advantages of accessibility, anonymity, and convenience. On-line groups for caregivers are becoming increasingly popular for the same reasons. Each person can participate at his or her own convenience and can offer advice and encouragement, as well as receive it.

In groups for special populations, such as older gays and lesbians, Fassinger (1997) emphasizes the importance of going beyond psychological interventions to encompass advocacy, consultation, and attention to social systems. Advocacy groups and political movements, such as the AARP and the Gray Panthers, offer leadership roles to older adults and opportunities to make an impact on society. Retirees make up a substantial proportion of board members of nonprofit organizations and are a significant force in many volunteer groups aimed at social change or helping others. Resident councils in nursing homes, when working with collaborative management, can also empower nursing home residents to contribute to their environment (Lee & Carr, 1994). In volunteer groups such as peer counseling, older adults plan and implement programs to benefit their peers and provide a link between professionals and elderly clients (Bratter & Freeman, 1990; Campbell, 1995).

Other group interventions that exist outside the usual group work literature include the Elderhostel and Learning in Retirement programs, which have responded to the increasing education levels in the older population and their enthusiasm for continued learning and teaching. Classes, often taught by retirees themselves to their peers, cover an extensive range of topics and offer the stimulation of challenging ideas, along with group interaction. Their widespread popularity can be seen in the thick pages of the Elderhostel catalogue and the rapid increase of Learning in Retirement programs throughout the country.

Finally, art, music, dance, and drama groups nurture talents that may not have been evident in earlier years. Well-known folk artists such as Harry Leiberman have emerged from art classes in senior centers. Perlstein (1984) developed living history plays that were written and acted by older adults and performed to other older adults in senior centers and nursing homes. Worley and Henderson (1995) used creative drama as a means to help older adults integrate their thoughts and dramatize personal narratives. Aging can liberate individuals from earlier roles or obligations and spur those who always wanted to act or write or paint to do it now before time runs out.

FUTURE DIRECTIONS

The much anticipated baby boom generation is expected to present a new face of aging. In terms of education, income, skill with new technologies, and a greatly increased population of older Hispanics and Asian Americans, the look of future generations is bound to be different. What that will mean for group work can be seen in the success of current examples discussed herein, such as Learning in Retirement and new ways of working with the cognitively impaired. This generation will also be more accustomed to psychotherapeutic and self-help interventions than the current group of older adults. Leadership will more often be assumed by the elderly, who will have a stronger voice in directing the types of groups and level of professionalism involved.

The rapid growth of assisted living creates a new category of group living that presents opportunities for different kinds of group work and exploring new kinds of communities of the elderly. Individuals fully accustomed to and comfortable with the computer and the Internet will develop new kinds of virtual groups, which can already be seen among caregivers, people with Parkinson's disease and other chronic illnesses, and the many seniors involved in the Seniornet internet community.

As more people live to advanced old age, the profession needs to explore how to work with "individualized" group plans and evaluate which are effective with diverse populations in terms of race, ethnicity, education, and physical and cognitive ability. It is hopeful to observe that many of the interventions described here are being systematically studied, often using control groups, to determine exactly what benefits can be expected from certain interventions. The field has gone beyond mere pre- and posttests of one group.

The challenge is not only to continue intensive evaluation of group methods but also to develop new ways of collaborating with older adults in clarifying expectations for groups and developing flexible models that can change as the needs of members change. For the generation that brought new meaning to the term "commune," it will be interesting to see what new forms of groups will emerge to meet the multiplicity of experiences that are part of aging. Perhaps the most difficult challenge is to train practitioners in group work and to integrate groups more completely into senior settings. It is unsettling to look at a large number of activities programs in institutional settings and day care programs and observe such a limited range of formulaic activities, such as trivia and bingo, and few opportunities to share feelings, anxieties, and common experiences. As discussed here, many group modalities are being developed and studied. The next step is to train professionals in the field to use them effectively to enhance the quality of life for older adults and their caregivers.

REFERENCES

Administration on Aging. (2002). *A Profile of Older Americans: 2002*. Rockville, MD: U.S. Department of Health and Human Services.

Aneshensel, C. S., Pearlin, L. I., Mullan, J. T., Zarit, S. H., & Whitlatch, C. J. (1995). *Profiles in caregiving: The unexpected career*. San Diego: Academic Press.

Baltes, P. B., & Baltes, M. M. (Eds.). (1990). *Psychological perspectives on successful aging: The model of selective optimization with compensation*. New York: Cambridge University Press.

Baltes, P. B., Smith, I., Staudinger, U. M., & Sowarka, D. (1990). Wisdom: One facet of successful aging? In H. R. Moody (Ed.), *Aging concepts and controversies* (pp. 427–431). Thousand Oaks, CA: Pine Forge Press.

Beck, A. (1972). *Depression: Cause and treatment*. Philadelphia: University of Pennsylvania Press.

Birren, J. E., & Cochran, K. N. (2001). *Telling the stories of life through guided autobiography groups*. Baltimore: Johns Hopkins University Press.

Blazer, D. (1998). *Emotional problems in late life: Intervention strategies for professional caregivers* (2nd ed.). New York: Springer.

Bratter, B., & Freeman, E. (1990, Winter). The maturing of peer counseling. *Generations*, 49–52.

Brok, A. J. (1997). A modified cognitive-behavioral approach to group therapy with the elderly. *Group*, 21(2), 115–134.

Burnside, I. (1995). Themes in reminiscence groups with older women. In J. Hendricks (Ed.), *The meaning of reminiscing and life review* (pp. 159–172). Amityville, NY: Baywood.

Burnside, I., & Schmidt, M. G. (Eds.). (1994). *Working with older adults: Group process and techniques* (3rd ed.). Boston: Jones & Bartlett.

Butler, R. N. (1963). The life review: An interpretation of reminiscence in the aged. *Psychiatry, 26*, 65–76.

Campbell, R. (1995). A peer counseling program for older persons. In S. L. Hatch (Ed.), *Peer programs on the college campus*. San Jose, CA: Resource.

Campbell, R. (2001). Re-creating family through a writing group. In B. Ingersoll-Dayton & R. Campbell (Eds.), *The delicate balance: Case studies in counseling and care management for older adults* (pp. 129–148). Baltimore: Health Professions Press.

Caserta, M. S., Lund, D. A., & Rice, S. J. (1999). Pathfinders: A self-care and health education program for older widows and widowers. *Gerontologist, 39*(5), 615–620.

Chandler, S., & Ray, R. (2002). New meanings for old tales: A discourse-based study of reminiscence and development in late life. In J. D. Webster & B. K. Haight (Eds.), *Critical advances in reminiscence work: From theory to application* (pp. 76–94). New York: Springer.

Erlich, S. (2002). Short-term group therapy with Holocaust survivors and the second generation. *Group, 26*(2), 163–171.

Erwin, K. T. (1996). *Group techniques for aging adults: Putting geriatric skills enhancement into practice*. Washington, DC: Taylor & Francis.

Fassinger, R. E. (1997). Issues in group work with older lesbians. *Group, 21*(2), 191–210.

Fogler, J., & Edwards, S. (2001). The power of group cognitive therapy. In B. Ingersoll-Dayton & R. Campbell (Eds.), *The delicate balance: Case studies in counseling and care management for older adults* (pp. 99–112). Baltimore: Health Professions Press.

Folkman, S., Chesney, M., McKusick, L., Ironson, G., Johnson, D. D., & Coates, T. J. (1991). Translating coping theory into an intervention. In J. Eckenrode (Ed.), *The social context of coping* (pp. 239–260). New York: Plenum Press.

Gallagher-Thompson, D., & DeVries, H. M. (1994). "Coping with frustration" classes: Development and preliminary outcomes with women who care for relatives with dementia. *Gerontologist, 34*(4), 548–552.

Gallagher-Thompson, D., Leary, M. C., Ossinalde, C., Romero, J. J., Wald, M. J., & Fernandez-Gamarra, E. (1997). Hispanic caregivers of older adults with dementia: Cultural issues in outreach and intervention. *Group, 21*(2), 211–232.

Gallagher-Thompson, D., Lovett, A., & Rose, J. (1991). Psychotherapeutic interventions for stressed family caregivers. In W. A. Myers (Ed.), *New techniques in the psychotherapy of older patients* (pp. 61–78). Washington: DC: American Psychiatric Press.

Hebert, R., Levesque, L., Vezina, J., Lavoie, J. P., Ducharme, F., Gendron, C., et al. (2003). Efficacy of a psychoeducative group program for caregivers of demented persons living at home: A randomized controlled trial. *Journal of Gerontology: Social Sciences, 58B*(1), S58–S67.

Hollon, S. D. (2003). Psychotherapy research with older populations. *American Journal of Geriatric Psychiatry, 11*(1), 7–8.

Ingersoll-Dayton, B. (2001). Intervention issues with older adults. In B. Ingersoll-Dayton & R. Campbell (Eds.), *The delicate balance: Case studies in counseling and care management for older adults* (pp. 7–15). Baltimore: Health Professions Press.

Ingersoll-Dayton, B., & Campbell, R. (Eds.). (2001). *The delicate balance: Case studies in counseling and care management for older adults.* Baltimore: Health Professions Press.

Kaminsky, M. (Ed.). (1984). *The uses of reminiscence: New ways of working with older adults.* New York: Haworth Press.

Kaslyn, M. (1999). Telephone group work: Challenges for practice. *Social Work with Groups, 22*(1), 63–77.

Klausner, E. J., & Alexopoulos, G. S. (1999). The future of psychosocial treatments for elderly patients. *Psychiatric Services, 50*(9), 1198–2204.

Konopka, G. (1954). Social group work in institutions for the aged. In G. Konopka (Ed.), *Group work in the institution: A modern challenge* (pp. 276–285). New York: Whiteside & Morrow.

Kramer, B. J. (1997). Gain in the caregiving experience: Where are we? What next? *Gerontologist, 37*, 218–232.

Krause, N. (2001). Social support. In R. H. Binstock & L. K. George (Eds.), *Handbook of aging and the social sciences* (pp. 272–294). San Diego, CA: Academic Press.

Kubie, S. H., & Landau, G. (1953). *Group work with the aged.* New York: International Universities Press.

Kurokawa, Y. (2002, January 19). *Archipelago special. The long road now brightens—Reminiscence method: A chronicle of one year* [Television program]. Tokyo, Japan: NHK.

Lee, J., & Carr, M. B. (1994). Coming together for change: Workshops for women in the nursing home. *Gerontologist, 34*(2), 261–266.

Leszcz, M. (1997). Integrated group psychotherapy for the treatment of depression in the elderly. *Group, 21*(2), 89–113.

Linden, M. (1953). Group psychotherapy with institutionalized senile women: Study in gerontologic human relations. *International Journal of Group Psychotherapy, 3*, 150–170.

LoGerfo, M. (1980–1981). Three ways of reminiscence in theory and practice. *International Journal of Aging and Human Development, 12*, 39–48.

Lynch, T. R., Morse, J. Q., Mendelson, T., & Robins, C. J. (2003). Dialectical behavior therapy for depressed older adults: A randomized pilot study. *American Journal of Geriatric Psychiatry, 11*(1), 33–45.

Memory café. (2001, November 1). *Family Circle,* p. 18.

Mittelman, M. S., Ferris, S. H., Shulman, E., Steinberg, G., & Levin, B. (1996). A family intervention to delay nursing home placement of patients with Alzheimer's disease: A randomized controlled trial. *Journal of the American Medical Association, 276*(21), 1725–1731.

Nomura, T. (2002). Evaluative research on reminiscence groups for people with dementia. In J. D. Webster & B. K. Haight (Eds.), *Critical advances in reminiscence work: From theory to application* (pp. 289–299). New York: Springer.

Ostwald, S. K., Hepburn, K. W., Caron, W., Burns, T., & Mantell, R. (1999). Reducing caregiver burden: A randomized psychoeducational intervention for caregivers of persons with dementia. *Gerontologist, 39*(3), 299–309.

Pearlin, L. I., & Skaff, M. M. (1995). Stressors and adaptation in later life. In M. Gatz (Ed.), *Emerging issues in mental health and aging* (pp. 97–123). Washington, DC: American Psychiatric Association.

Perlstein, S. (1984). A stage for memory: Living history plays by older adults. In M. Kaminsky (Ed.), *The uses of reminiscence: New ways of working with older adults* (pp. 37–52). New York: Haworth Press.

Ronch, J. L., & Crispi, E. L. (1997). Opportunities for development via group psychotherapy in the nursing home. *Group*, *21*(2), 135–158.

Rowe, J. W., & Kahn, R. L. (1987). Human aging: Usual and successful. *Science*, *237*, 143–149.

Rowe, J. W., & Kahn, R. L. (1997). Successful aging. *Gerontologist*, *37*(4), 433–440.

Shaw, S. B. (1997). A modern psychoanalytic approach to caregiver support groups. *Group*, *21*(2), 159–174.

Sherman, E. (1995). Reminiscentia: Cherished objects as memorabilia in late-life reminiscence. In J. Hendricks (Ed.), *The meaning of reminiscence and life review* (pp. 193–204). Amityville, NY: Baywood.

Shore, H. (1952). Group work program development in homes for the aged. *Social Service Review*, *26*(2), 181–194.

Sistler, A., & Washington, K. S. (1999). Serenity for African American caregivers. *Social Work with Groups*, *22*(1), 49–62.

Sorensen, S., Pinquart, M., Habil, D., & Duberstein, P. (2002). How effective are interventions with caregivers? An updated meta-analysis. *Gerontologist*, *42*(3), 356–372.

Supiano, K. P., Ozminkowski, R. J., Campbell, R., & Lapidos, C. (1987). Effectiveness of writing groups in nursing homes. *Journal of Applied Gerontology*, *8*(3), 382–400.

Teri, L., & Gallagher-Thompson, D. (1991). Cognitive-behavioral interventions for treatment of depression in Alzheimer's patients. *Gerontologist*, *31*(3), 413–416.

Toseland, R. W. (1990). *Group work with older adults*. New York: New York University Press.

Toseland, R. W. (1995). *Group work with the elderly and family caregivers*. New York: Springer.

Wink, P., & Schiff, B. (2002). To review or not to review? The role of personality and life events in life review and adaptation to old age. In J. D. Webster & B. K. Haight (Eds.), *Critical advances in reminiscence work: From theory to application* (pp. 44–60). New York: Springer.

Worley, K., & Henderson, S. (1995). Speaking of difficult choices: The creation of a drama and dialogue group on end-of-life choices. *Gerontologist*, *35*(3), 412–414.

Yalom, I. D. (1975). *The theory and practice of group psychotherapy* (2nd ed.). New York: Basic Books.

Yalom, I. D. (1985). *The theory and practice of group psychotherapy* (3rd ed.). New York: Basic Books.

Chapter 17

Groups for Reducing Intergroup Conflicts

DAVID BARGAL

Had René Descartes, the famous philosopher, lived today, he probably would have modified his famous saying—*cogito ergo sum* (I think, therefore I exist)—to the following: "I am in conflict, therefore I exist." The current reality for people who live in Western pluralistic societies is full of conflict. In the interpersonal realm, there are conflicts in families, for example, between children and parents and husbands and wives. In workplaces, we witness conflicts among employees and between management and workers. At the community level, there are ethnic, racial, and interest group conflicts. At the international level, conflicts between states are prevalent. In retrospect, it seems that the 20th century was one of the cruelest times in human history, as regards the number of wars and conflicts and the high costs in terms of human life and material damage.

In Western democracies, which are characterized by pluralism, various racial, ethnic, and interest groups hold divergent outlooks. Each group pursues its own goals and seeks to gain influence, power, and resources from the available pool of material, social, legal, and political means. Traditionally, such conflicts have been resolved either through violence or through legal action. Although such means may offer immediate solutions to concrete issues, they cannot in themselves achieve long-range settlement of the conflict. Nor do they create a climate for ongoing dialogue between the parties in conflict. It is possible, however, to develop conflict management strategies to help the rival parties engage in more open and rational dialogue in order to achieve their goals through negotiation and mutual consent.

This chapter presents the rationale, theoretical background, and intervention principles for conducting workshops to improve relations and reduce conflict between groups. A detailed description of an intervention that I conducted illustrates an attempt to improve intergroup relations between Arab and Jewish youth in Israel and serves as the main source of data. It is argued that social work, and group work in particular, may provide appropriate settings for promoting interventions aimed at improving intergroup relations in many situations encountered by clients. In accordance with this approach, social work with groups should deal more with ethnic, cultural, racial, community, and organizational conflicts and should offer a repertoire of interventions to cope with these issues.

ARAB–JEWISH RELATIONS IN ISRAEL AND CONFLICT MANAGEMENT WORKSHOPS

The Israeli–Palestinian conflict is a protracted one and has recently even escalated to the point of frequent suicide bombings and harsh responses by the Israeli army. About 18% of the population of the State of Israel is composed of Arabs, who identify with many of their relatives residing in the Palestinian Authority. However, the Arabs residing in Israel are considered full-fledged citizens of the state and are entitled to full legal, social, educational, and welfare privileges. In practice, because of the ongoing conflict between the Arab countries and the State of Israel, its Arab citizens have been subject to discrimination, deprivation of some rights, and isolation from the Jewish population for almost 50 years.

Although behavioral sciences may not have a direct impact on the political process, which affects Israeli–Palestinian relations, it is possible to bring about change among individuals at the level of interpersonal and intergroup relations. One of the interventions that has been developed to improve relations between Arab and Jewish youth who are citizens of Israel is the conflict management workshop (CMW).

Bargal and Bar (1990a) defined the CMW as:

> organizational arrangements devised to bring together two opposing groups (on ethnic, political, or interpersonal grounds) at a relatively isolated location. Through the use of interpersonal, group, and organizational means, the two parties come to know each other's members closely. Some of the roots and manifestations of the conflict between the groups are brought out into the open, discussed and clarified, in order to enable them to get along more satisfactorily. (p. 5)

INTERGROUP RELATIONS AND INTERGROUP CONFLICTS

The study of intergroup conflict is viewed as a derivative of intergroup relations, which are an inseparable facet of the structure and composition of almost every modern pluralistic society. Tajfel (1982), a prominent contributor to this area of study, has described intergroup relations as "one of the most difficult and complex knots of problems which we confront in our times" (p. 1). Another renowned scholar in the field of intergroup conflict, Sherif (1966), defined intergroup relations as follows: "Whenever individuals belonging to one group interact, collectively or individually, with another group or its members in terms of their group identification, we have an instance of intergroup behavior" (p. 12).

On the basis of their "in-group," individuals develop stereotypes, prejudice, and discrimination toward members of other groups. Moreover, conflictual intergroup relations may escalate toward hostility, animosity, and even violence. These negative emotions and their concomitant behaviors in the forms of delegitimacy, aggression, and, in some cases, even deprivation of human rights emanate from several sources (for detailed surveys of the topic, see Brewer & Brown, 1998; Stephan, 1985; Stephan & Stephan, 1996; and Stephan & Stephan, 2001). Numerous attempts to understand intergroup conflict and discrimination have focused on the following main factors: social cognitive processes, personality development, social-cultural influences, social identity, and conditions of intergroup conflict and competition for realistic resources.

First, regarding social cognitive processes, Fiske and Taylor (1991) define social cognition as a theoretical perspective that explains how information is processed and stored. The assumption underlying the social cognition approach is that humans have limited cognitive capacity to manage the overload of daily social and interactive stimuli. Therefore, the mind categorizes information about situations, objects, and people "before engaging memory or inferential processes" (Howard, 2000, p. 368). The cognitive products of these processes are schemata, or representations regarding oneself or one's social world. Regarding the role of schemata in social interaction, Howard (2000) points out that they lead us to reduce and summarize information by its basic elements. Such categorization is a cognitive device for storing information, but important facts may be lost in the process. Moreover, categorization frequently implies the evaluation of some categories as better or worse than others. Thus social cognitive processes are not only related to perception but also actually define social relationships. In addition, they have an impact on the development of biased stereotypes (prejudice) and discriminatory behavior.

Attribution processes also manifest themselves in the service of social cognitive processes (Stephan, 1985). Attribution processes provide the "rules" used by humans to perceive and explain other people's behavior. Because very little information is available to the perceiver, who is also biased by in-group affiliation, he or she tends to attribute bad characteristics to the other group members and to blame those characteristics on their personalities rather than on circumstances or on social, political, and historical contexts. For example, whites may perceive blacks as lazy, uncivilized underachievers. Much of the blame in this instance is put on the individual black person rather than on economic, political, and cultural circumstances.

The second theoretical approach to the development of intergroup discrimination is rooted in the dynamics of personality development. According to the psychodynamic approach (Adorno, Frenkel-Brunswick, Levinson, & Sanford, 1950), manifestations of prejudice and discrimination reflect a deep personality conflict that stems mainly from an authoritarian personality makeup. The expression of prejudice serves as an outlet for hostility that is harbored as a result of harsh methods of upbringing during childhood. Although the authoritarian personality construct has been a topic of numerous studies, a direct link could not be established between socialization practices and the prejudice of one group against another (Ashmore & Delboca, 1976). More recent research (Altmeyer, 1998) established the empirical existence of a new type of authoritarian personality.

The third, sociocultural, explanation for the development of prejudice and discriminatory behavior is based on the assumption that these patterns are learned in the same way as other preferences, beliefs, and values—through interaction with one's sociocultural environment (Ashmore & Delboca, 1976). Socialization, which embodies the various mechanisms through which culture is transmitted from one generation to the next, operates through various channels. Four major channels of socialization have been distinguished: parents, peers, schools, and mass media. However, most of the research evidence on this issue is correlational, and "it is not clear exactly how cultural patterns are transformed into the prejudice of individuals and the relative importance of the various agents of socialization is not known" (Ashmore & Delboca, 1976, p. 97).

According to the fourth approach, social identity theory (Tajfel & Turner, 1986), prejudice and intergroup tension originate in the individual's affiliation with a group. The group serves as the individual's main source of social identity: The in-group is perceived in positive terms, and its members are viewed in a differentiated and personal way, whereas the out-group is perceived in a negative light, as a depersonalized collective. Intergroup discrimination is motivated by a desire for a positive social identity that can enhance self-esteem.

"Realistic group conflict theory" is the fifth approach to explaining the development of intergroup discrimination (Campbell, 1965; Sherif, 1966). According to this theory, prejudice is the product of a negative interdependence between different social groups. Such interdependence is manifested in relations between a conqueror and the conquered population or between a dominant majority and a suppressed minority. In this context, the dominant group uses its power and status to keep subordinate groups in an inferior position. Members of the dominant group tend to view their subordinates in terms of negative stereotypes and act accordingly. Ultimately, this approach is used to rationalize the attempt to maintain the inferior status of less powerful groups and even justify their exploitation. Prejudice may also be part of a psychological reaction to competition between two groups for valued, scarce, or limited resources (Sherif, 1966).

Within the conflict between Arab and Jews in the State of Israel, elements of the theories discussed here can be identified. The Jewish population may perceive their Arab counterparts as dangerous and unreliable, whereas the Jews may be perceived as domineering and discriminatory. The two national groups isolate themselves from one another, each focusing on its distinct identity, history, values, and beliefs. The Jewish group makes up 82% of Israel's population, and the Arabs make up the rest. There is little constructive interaction between them, and competition for scarce resources such as land generates negative dependence and hostility, which is manifested in prejudice and discrimination toward the Arab minority group members. It seems that the only way to alleviate this situation is through planned activities aimed at reducing tension and fostering social justice. The next section deals with the principles guiding these attempts to reduce intergroup tension.

THEORETICAL APPROACHES AND PRINCIPLES FOR REDUCING INTERGROUP CONFLICTS

Two major approaches have been employed to reduce intergroup tension and improve intergroup relations: facilitative conditions and conflict management workshops or encounters.

Facilitative Conditions

Facilitative conditions are based on Allport's (1954) contact hypothesis. This hypothesis, which was elaborated by Amir (1969), has recently been upheld and reconfirmed empirically (Pettigrew, 1998; Pettigrew & Tropp, 2000). According to this approach, the following conditions may strongly contribute toward the improvement of intergroup relations between adversarial groups (Fisher, 1990):

1. Contact in an intimate, pleasant, and rewarding organizational climate.
2. Equal status between the two groups.
3. The existence of cooperative superordinate goals (Sherif, 1958), which participants in the two groups work together to accomplish.
4. Strong institutional support for the program.

Conflict Management Workshops

The conflict management approach derives its principles of intervention from several sources:

1. The notion of reeducation (Lewin, 1945/1948), or resocialization, which suggests that individuals may undergo changes in knowledge, values and standards, emotional attachments, and conduct mainly through *interaction in small groups* (Lieberman, 1980, 1983).

2. The course of change that occurs among participants in the group is characterized by three phases: "unfreezing," "movement," and "refreezing." "Unfreezing" is the phase in which the motivation and readiness for the change are emphasized. "Movement" refers to the phase in which the participants gradually change their attitudes and reframe their cognitive beliefs toward their own group and toward out-group members. "Refreezing" refers to the institutionalization of the change in the form of new habitual attitudes or behavior to be applied within, as well as beyond, the group's meetings (Lewin, 1947/1958).

3. The facilitators of the group are the most important agents of change that help participants modify their attitudes, emotions, and behavior. The facilitators employ basic counseling skills such as positive regard, empathy, and support for the participants (Carkhuff, 1969; Egan, 1986), who may engage in a prejudiced discourse in the group sessions. In this context, the facilitators convey the message that the encounter is a safe setting in which participants can renounce biased beliefs about members of other ethnic and social groups. The facilitators also give minilectures concerning issues related to prejudice, stereotypes, group processes, and intergroup conflicts. The lectures are intended to help the participants understand and incorporate the changes, which they undergo more fully (a detailed example of the facilitator's activities is provided later in this chapter). According to Bargal and Bar (1994), the optimal encounter focuses on three main target units: the individual, the small group and its dynamics, and intergroup relations. The following is a general description of each of the three target units.

The Individual Participant's Personality

The participant's personality is at the center of the intervention. The components of the participant's personality include cognitive mechanisms for organizing his or her impression of the social world, such as stereotypes regarding members of the other group and feelings toward them. Specifically, the intervention focuses on prejudiced and discriminatory behavior manifested by participants toward each other. The principal psychological processes by which stereotypes and prejudice can be modified are: creation of a supportive climate by the facilitators; catharsis of feelings when needed; and planned confrontations regarding participants' biased perceptions of others or themselves. The facilitators are in charge of developing intimate and meaningful contacts among members of the group, in addition to encouraging discussions about beliefs and feelings and enhancing participants' insight into biased attitudes and feelings they hold toward themselves and others.

The Individual Group Member and Group Affiliations

The second target of intervention is at the group level. At the center are the participants' multiple group affiliations, which generate multiple identities. As mentioned, the participants' in-groups are perceived in positive, differentiated terms, whereas out-groups are perceived in a negative, generalized way. The group achieves its goal of molding participants to its standards and norms by exerting pressure (Tajfel & Turner, 1986). The participants are sensitized to these mechanisms as a first step toward alleviating these pressures and developing a more individualistic, independent perspective toward their group affiliations and identities.

Intergroup Relations in a Diverse, Pluralistic Society

The third target of intervention focuses on the intergroup level and on relations among ethnic, gender, and social groups in a pluralistic society. Topics dealt with in minilectures, discussions, and experiential activities focus on issues of inequality and injustice in the relations between the majority group (Jews) and the minority group (Arabs). Common behavioral manifestations of minority–majority relations, such as respect, patronage, and exploitation, are examined. Participants become aware of the need to play an active role as agents of change and point to ways in which they can mitigate social injustice. In this spirit, cooperative projects continue even beyond the duration of the workshop. The projects generally focus on educational and social activities, which are conducted in schools and surrounding communities.

Conflict management workshops have been conducted in an attempt to deal with international conflicts (Burton, 1969), including tensions in Ireland (Doob, 1970; Doob & Foltz, 1973) and in the Middle East (Cohen & Azar, 1981; Cohen, Kelman, Miller, & Smith, 1977; Kelman & Cohen, 1979, 1986). These workshops are based on principles and methods derived from small-group research, as well as from research on attitude change and counseling. Since Lewin first proposed this approach toward managing intergroup conflict (Lippitt, 1949), several modifications have been introduced. Blake, Mouton, and Sloma (1965) and Blake and Mouton (1984) offer a model that entails working with parties in conflict on their images of each other, as well as opening avenues of communication, and working together on solutions to specific problems.

CONFLICT MANAGEMENT WORKSHOPS AT THE NEVE SHALOM SCHOOL FOR PEACE

The Jewish–Arab village of Neve Shalom ("Oasis of Peace") was founded in 1970 to encourage and enhance meaningful and enduring contact between Jews and Arabs in Israel. The village is a model of Arab–Jewish cooperation based on equality and mutual trust. Residents live and work together for the attainment of mutual "superordinate" goals within a fully integrated community. Members of each national group are encouraged to maintain and take pride in their separate religious, cultural, and national identities (see Shipler, 1986).

The School for Peace at Neve Shalom is an educational entity that is located in the village but operates autonomously. The school conducts conflict management workshops aimed at promoting peaceful Arab–Jewish coexistence based on equality, mutual trust, and respect. Since its establishment, numerous workshops have been held for Arab and Jewish youths, with a total of 5,000 participants from both nationalities over the years. Although the majority of youths participated in a single workshop, some of them attended several additional meetings as well.

The workshops were held in a "cultural island" (the village of Neve Shalom), where cooperation between the two national groups is put into practice. Several aspects of the workshop have been dealt with in earlier publications (on the role problems of facilitators, see Bargal & Bar, 1990a; on preparation of participants, see Bargal & Bar, 1990b; on the application of Lewinian theory in the workshops, see Bargal & Bar, 1992).

The workshop model applied at Neve Shalom incorporates many of the structural principles of management, training, and evaluation proposed for conflict management workshops (Bargal, 1992). Details regarding the structure, process, and intervention principles that may be generalized and adapted to different cultural settings are presented next.

Components of the Conflict Management Workshops

Objectives

As suggested by Bargal and Bar (1990b), the workshops aimed to achieve the following objectives: (1) to initiate contacts and acquaintances among participants belonging to the two national (Arab and Jewish) groups; (2) to arouse awareness of the complexity of the Arab–Jewish conflict situation; (3) to change previous distorted stereotypes and prejudices that the members of the two national groups hold toward each other; (4) to help participants develop impartial behavior and attitudes toward one another; (5) to teach basic skills for conflict management; (6) to help participants develop humanistic, democratic perspectives and an orientation toward working for social justice.

The detailed description of the encounter between Palestinian and Israeli youths gives an idea of how these objectives were realized. In a subsequent part of the chapter, the process of intervention in the workshop unfolds and the intrapsychic, interpersonal, and intergroup mechanisms that operated are described and explained.

Selection of Participants

The selection of the appropriate participants for the workshops may largely determine the extent of their success. Research into group work emphasizes the importance of prior selection of candidates for group interventions in order to attain attitudinal change and symptom reduction (on social work with groups, see Glasser, Sarri, & Vinter, 1974; Toseland & Rivas, 1984; on group psychotherapy, see Melnick & Woods, 1976; Moreland, Levine, & Wingert, 1996; and Yalom, 1985).

The groups of Jewish and Arab youths who took part in the workshops were paired in terms of socioeconomic background in order to promote maximum symmetry between them (Allport, 1954; Amir 1969). Moreover, the participants in both groups resided in close geographical proximity to each other, in order to enable continued interaction between them after the workshop ended.

Based on theory, research, and professional experience, it was decided to select participants on the basis of three qualities: (1) high motivation to take part in the conflict management workshops, which is a prerequisite for many change-oriented activities (Egan, 1986; Lieberman, 1983; Yalom, 1985); (2) empathy with and sensitivity to others (the ability to enter the "other person's shoes"), a prerequisite for encounters that involve changing negative stereotypes and identifying with the other's sorrow, humiliation, and injustice (Stephan & Finlay, 2000); (3) leadership qualities, for example, "gatekeepers" (Lewin, 1947/1958) or influential members of the class or community. Influential people may disseminate the messages of the workshops to their groups and communities of origin.

Preparation of Participants

In order to enhance the impact of the workshops on the participants, preworkshop anticipatory programs were designed for each national group. In these programs, the groups met separately on their own grounds, and sessions were led by the prospective facilitator or facilitators from the same national group (for a detailed discussion of the preworkshop preparations, see Bargal & Bar, 1990b). The preliminary meetings aimed to provide the potential participants with three elements: basic information on the workshop setting, increased cognitive awareness, and emotional preparation.

The information provided at the preworkshop program included a general orientation to the schedule, activities, and accommodations at the School for Peace. At the cognitive level, the prospective participants in the preparatory phase were expected to heighten their awareness regarding the importance of tolerance toward different attitudes and values to be exercised at the workshop. An additional issue emphasized in the preparatory sessions concerned the deep cultural differences between the groups who would be meeting under very intimate conditions. Notably, Arab society—be it Christian or Muslim—was alien to the Jewish participants. For the Arab participants, who had never met with Jewish youths on close terms before, the open interpersonal relationships—especially between boys and girls—and the spontaneous expression of feelings were often strange and even threatening. The third type of knowledge focused on differential "emotional inoculation" of the two national groups. The Jewish participants had to be emotionally prepared to overcome their fear of Arabs, which is rooted in the persistent threat of annihilation by the surrounding Arab countries. The Arab participants had to be reassured that in the workshop they would be able to disclose their personal experiences of humiliation and rejection by members of the Jewish majority.

These three dimensions of preparation prior to the workshop enhanced the change processes among participants in the actual encounter.

Change Processes That Affect Participants' Attitudes, Perceptions, and Behavior

The mechanisms for effecting change during the workshop focused primarily on the emotional and cognitive dimensions, such as exposing participants to new sources of information, allowing them to reflect on the sociocultural and political contexts in which they live and interact, and enabling them to restructure their social perceptions (Babad, Birnbaum, & Benne, 1983; Lewin, 1945/1948; Lieberman, 1983). This section focuses on analysis of the processes of change that occurred during the workshop from four perspectives: participants, facilitators, workshop structure, and content topics (Bar & Bargal, 1995).

PARTICIPANTS

The main cognitive and emotional mechanisms that operated in the intervention processes were cognitive dissonance; decategorization; limiting the use of denial, splitting, and projection as defense mechanisms; and anxiety aroused as a consequence of fading illusions (Schein, 1979).

Participants in the conflict management workshops described a change in attitudes resulting from cognitive dissonance (Bargal & Bar, 1992; Maoz, 2000). This dissonance was reflected in the discrepancy between their perceptions of the other group and the actual behavior of participants in that group with whom they interacted intensively. The process of attitude change has been referred to as decategorization or destereotyping (Brewer & Brown, 1998; Lewin, 1945/1948). In this process, negative characteristics attributed to the other national group based on ascription of collective attributes and stereotypes were gradually replaced by new impressions that developed as a result of personal acquaintance with individuals in the other group.

This suggests that stereotypes may ultimately be undermined as a result of favorable personal experiences with members of the other group. However, changes in cognitive perceptions are not immediately incorporated into the psyche. Feelings of frustration may be aroused by awareness of the need to alter distorted perspectives and develop new perceptions of oneself. In addition, feelings of anxiety may be aroused by fear of restructuring cognitive and emotional frames of mind embedded in each individual, for example, perceptions of oneself as inherently bad, irrational, violent, and uncompromising. At this point, the reality personified by individuals in the other group may clash with the mechanisms of denial and splitting that participants have employed all of their lives. Notably, the anxiety and fear associated with giving up the use of these mechanisms may cause participants to express intense anger and to blame members of the other group for the political situation.

This emotionally charged and dissonant situation also provides the "building blocks" for restructuring participants' new social perceptions. The educational tools for facilitating this situation are group and intergroup dynamics created through the facilitators' interventions, as well as themes focusing on development of perceptions and skills conducive to "living with conflict" (Bar & Bargal, 1995; Bargal & Bar, 1994). Two important interpersonal processes facilitate changes in self-perceptions and perceptions of the other group: identification with participants from the other group and identification with facilitators of both nationalities.

FACILITATORS

The workshop facilitators bore most of the responsibility for effecting change. In short, during this phase of the workshop, it is very important for participants to experience group and interpersonal dynamics that facilitate change processes. These dynamics are largely affected by the facilitators' style and the nature of the intervention, which are instrumental in creating these conditions.

In the intervention process, the facilitators make it possible for participants to express some of their disappointments, frustrations, and anxieties through catharsis. The facilitators employ basic counseling principles such as positive regard, empathy, and support for participants (Carkhuff, 1969; Egan, 1986) in the encounters. In so doing, they convey the message that the encounter is safe enough to enable participants to reassess previous beliefs and express feelings and opinions that they had never dared express before. Although these principles are *a sine qua non* for efforts to change attitudes and behavior, and although provision of support and security may be effective and even vital conditions, they are not sufficient to effect change. Facilitators must focus on utilizing skills that help participants deal with contradictory views and feelings toward themselves or other group members. This is done via the use of confrontational means utilized by the facilitators (Egan, 1986). Such confrontations help participants achieve the cognitive dissonance described previously. Facilitators also provide feedback to participants who express feelings and behavior that can help counteract prejudiced and unrealistic views of their own group or members of the other group. Moreover, facilitators are in a position to provide alternatives to violence as a means of solving controversial political or ideological issues.

At this stage, facilitators also use a strategy referred to by Yalom (1985) as "instillation of hope." The intensity of the conflictual situation may encourage participants to adopt a fatalistic, pessimistic approach, which signals passiveness and withdrawal from coping with the object of their relationships. Thus facilitators aim to preserve a group climate that portrays the difficult, complex reality of the conflict between the two nations on the one hand and opens a window of hope on the other. Because people create the conflict, there is hope that people may also find a way to solve it.

Another strategy at the facilitators' disposal is cognitive reframing. Every change in self, even in the emotional sphere, is transformed into a cognitive framework of human consciousness. Words, concepts, rationales, attitudes, and values reflect various perceptual and cognitive "gestalts" that are elaborated and adopted by the self. Hence, the facilitator's function in this phase is to explain and clarify the meanings of the changes within the group from a "here and now" time perspective (Egan, 1986). This is done without ignoring their implications for the external social-political and cultural reality of the participants' lives.

Finally, the facilitator's task is to contain difficult feelings expressed by the participants, especially anger and anxiety. The facilitator clarifies that the participants' feelings at this stage reflect an imbalance in their perceptual and emotional orientation, which is a prerequisite for change. Facilitators also provide information and explanations regarding the intra- and intergroup processes experienced by participants, for example, pressure to conform to the norms of one's group and demonization of the other group. Moreover, participants gain insight into the group and intergroup dynamics that they experience in the workshops and in the real world. In addition, they become more aware of their impact on shaping behavior and attitudes (Bargal & Bar, 1994).

WORKSHOP STRUCTURE

Work in a relatively large binational group creates a paradoxical situation. On the one hand, an atmosphere of cohesiveness and solidarity is formed as a result of the intensive interpersonal relationships and close contact that develop under the conditions of an isolated "cultural island." On the other hand, the topics discussed and the constant feeling that one's own national group is right and good and that the other group is bad generate an atmosphere of anxiety and disharmony among the group members. Even under these circumstances, however, each participant can still identify with the pain, injustice, fear, and other intense personal emotions genuinely conveyed by members of the other group. This identification helps break down the "walls of hate" and counteract stereotyped categorization while enabling participants to see the other side's point of view. Concurrently, activity among homogeneous national groups, in which participants are able to share the feelings of anxiety aroused by cognitive dissonance, help them incorporate identification with the other group into themselves. In this process, participants begin to understand their need to preserve their own social and national identity, bearing in mind the emotional cost of ignoring the other group's identity.

An additional change mechanism at the disposal of participants at this stage of the workshop is identification with the facilitators. In particular, participants can identify with facilitators of the same national group as models who have managed to find a balanced way of living with the contradictory contexts of Arab and Jewish society (Bargal & Bar, 1990a).

In this connection, facilitators are viewed as individuals who have managed to adopt a complex perspective of the situation while remaining confident enough of their own social identities to be able to understand the other side's point of view. In many respects, the workshop participants aspire to achieve this state, especially when they feel somewhat confused and threatened and need a model to help them implement the desired change. Mature interpersonal relationships between Arab and Jewish facilitators, which are based on consideration and sensitivity, also serve as model for workshop participants to emulate.

CONTENT TOPICS

One of the main contributions of the facilitators was inculcation of the concept of "living with conflict" (Bar & Bargal, 1995). At this stage, the participants experienced the meaning of living with conflict in their interactions—a conflict that emanates from the respective identities of each group. In this phase, the facilitators provide information regarding majority–minority relations while portraying the asymmetry between the two groups and its implications for political processes. Minority groups are often underrepresented and deprived of privileges granted to the majority group (e.g., Jewish Israelis receive a monetary allowance after completion of compulsory army service, but Arab citizens of Israel are not entitled to this compensation because they do not serve in the army).

Facilitators point out the similarities, as well as the differences, between the two groups. They emphasize the overall need for national group identity and the importance of each group's unique history. In this connection, it is noted that both groups have suffered traumas and disasters (e.g., Jewish participants are affected by the memory of the Holocaust, and many Arab participants have relatives who were exiled following the War of Independence). These examples serve to highlight similarities in the concerns and aspirations of each national group. The dialogue that ensues among the participants also exposes different political solutions to the conflict proposed by each group. The main strategy for coping with the conflict is acknowledgement of each party's right to autonomous existence. In the case of Israeli Arabs, emphasis is placed on acknowledgement of their full rights and acceptance as equals by the Jewish majority.

At this stage, it is assumed that participants are able to integrate the new perspectives they have incorporated and to practice the new behavior or express the reframed attitudes in real-life situations (Lewin, 1947; Schein, 1979). In accordance with the afore-mentioned objectives of the workshop, at the end of the process participants are expected to better understand themselves and realize the complexity of the social-political situation (i.e., that there are no clear-cut solutions to the Arab–Israeli conflict).

Evaluation and Operational Recommendations

According to the participants' verbal reports, as well as the results of the questionnaires (Bargal, 2000; Bargal & Bar, 1992; Maoz, 2000), it seems that the participants benefited from the workshops on the whole. However, because workshops are short-term interventions, they cannot be expected to bring about significant change in all participants. It is even more presumptuous to think that at this stage most participants are able to integrate the content of the workshops and reframe their cognitive and social perceptions. In fact, some may not realize the impact of the workshop until later, and others may revert to their original attitudes toward the other national group and the Arab–Israeli conflict. In order to examine these questions, it would be worthwhile to conduct follow-up studies, which are very rare in the literature because of their complexity and the high costs involved in their implementation (Stephan & Stephan, 2001).

From our own observations, it is evident that a one-time conflict management workshop will not suffice to effect meaningful change in the participants. In the policy conclusions of earlier studies (Bar & Bargal, 1995), several workshop models are recommended. Based on the experience gained from these workshops, the most effective model is a three-phase workshop sequence. According to this model, participants meet in homogenous national groups in the first phase. These sessions focus on anticipatory socialization, that is, airing fears, conveying information about the intergroup encounter, and developing realistic expectations, emotional resilience, cognitive openness, and tolerance toward the other group. In the second phase, sessions are held in a mixed group, based on the format of the intergroup encounter described here. In the third phase of the model workshop, which takes place at some point after the intergroup encounter, participants meet again in homogenous national groups in order to reintegrate what they learned during the intergroup phase in a more secure group atmosphere.

An additional intervention with a potential long-term impact is a cooperative effort to pursue superordinate goals, such as working on mutual community development projects. The design of long-range cooperative projects devoted to issues that concern both groups may strengthen the bonds created during the workshop. Such cooperation may also help preserve the changes in the participants' cognitive beliefs and social identities that occurred during the workshop. Furthermore, the cooperative effort may insure that workshop participants selected on the basis of their ability to serve as gatekeepers will succeed in disseminating the messages of tolerance, antidiscrimination, and humaneness as they interact with classmates who did not take part in the workshop.

FUTURE DIRECTIONS

Intergroup conflicts dominate the scene in Western democratic societies. As suggested in the literature review, these conflicts emanate from personality and cognitive distortions, which breed stereotypes and prejudice (Adorno et al., 1950; Altmeyer, 1998; Brewer & Brown, 1998). They are the consequence of rigid and extreme perpetuation of ethnic and racial boundaries and may also be generated by ideological and political dissension regarding allocation of resources and feelings of injustice (Ashmore & Delboca, 1976; Campbell, 1965; Sherif, 1966).

The attainment of justice in multicultural and heterogeneous societies depends largely on the ability of ethnic, racial, gender, and interest groups to obtain resources and exercise their rights through democratic means. Notably, pluralistic societies are fraught with conflicts that must be resolved through legal means or through strategies of conflict management. Toward this end, conflict management workshops and intergroup dialogues (Schoem & Hurtado, 2001) have been used to deal with some cases of dissension between groups, such as community conflicts, intergroup conflicts in educational settings (Stephan, 1999), and even parties at war (Kelman, 1997). The groups in conflict, as shown in this presentation of a conflict management workshop for Arab and Jewish youths, have several characteristics. They consist of a small number of participants and can thus develop intimate relationships among their members. During the meetings, the focus of the discussions is on the distorted and prejudiced images each party holds regarding the other and on ways of guiding social institutions toward the pursuit of equality and justice. Individual group members are perceived as representatives of different ethnic and social groups. Therefore, the changes they experience on a personal level may project to the intergroup realm as well.

Group work as a method of intervention in social work was historically involved in education for democracy and intervening in community problems. However, it seems that the present concern of the field is confined to intragroup structures and processes and focusing on interpersonal and intrapsychic problems. A recent textbook on social work with groups (Toseland & Rivas, 1995) has no chapters dealing with intergroup relations or with intergroup conflicts. A survey of about 160 articles published in *Social Work with Groups* between 1992 and 2002 revealed only 6 articles dealing with intergroup conflicts. Two articles focused on the use of small groups to sensitize students to diversity issues in society (Miller & Donner, 2000; Rittner & Nakanishi, 1993). A similar experience, in which social work students participated in dialogue groups, is reported by Nagda et al. (1999). Abrams (2000) dealt with ethnic conflicts among group members, and Mondros, Woodrow, and Weinstein (1992) focused on the use of groups to solve interorganizational conflicts. The two remaining articles dealt with the encounter between Arab and Israeli youths (Bargal, 1992; Bargal & Bar, 1994).

The approach presented here offers an important repertoire of interventions in social work with groups that may also be applied in the American context, which is characterized by prevalent racial, ethnic, gender, and ideological conflicts (for a detailed presentation of the framework, see Bargal & Bar, 1994). Notably, the intervention principles presented here (Allport, 1954; Fisher, 1990; Pettigrew, 1998; Stephan & Stephan, 2001), as well as my own professional experience conducting workshops (Bargal & Bar, 1990a, 1990b, 1992, 1994), may provide a solid base of knowledge that can be adopted by scholars and practitioners who deal with social work in group settings.

REFERENCES

Abrams, B. (2000). Finding common ground in a conflict resolution group. *Social Work with Groups, 23*(4), 55–69.

Adorno, T. W., Frenkel-Brunswick, E., Levinson, D. J., & Sanford, R. M. (1950). *The authoritarian personality*. New York: Harper.

Allport, G. W. (1954). *The nature of prejudice*. Cambridge, MA: Addison-Wesley.

Altmeyer, B. (1998). The other authoritarian personality. In M. Zana (Ed.), *Advances in experimental social psychology* (Vol. 30, pp. 47–92). New York: Academic Press.

Amir, Y. (1969). Contact hypothesis in ethnic relations. *Psychological Bulletin, 71*, 319–342.

Ashmore, R., & Delboca, F. (1976). Psychological approaches to understanding intergroup conflict. In P. Katz (Ed.), *Toward the elimination of racism* (pp. 73–123). New York: Pergamon.

Babad, E., Birnbaum, M., & Benne, K. (1983). *The social self*. Beverly Hills: Sage.

Bar, H., & Bargal, D. (1995). *Living with the conflict*. Jerusalem, Israel: The Jerusalem Institute for the Study of Israel (Hebrew).

Bargal, D. (1992). Conflict management workshops for Palestinian and Jewish youth: A framework for planning, intervention and evaluation. *Social Work with Groups, 15*(1), 51–68.

Bargal, D. (2000, April). *Education for peace: Description, conceptualization and evaluation of a workshop for Palestinian and Jewish youth*. Paper presented at the conference on the Global Program on Youth, Ann Arbor, MI.

Bargal, D., & Bar, H. (1990a). Role problems of facilitators in an Arab-Jewish conflict management workshop. *Small Group Research, 21*(1), 5–27.

Bargal, D., & Bar, H. (1990b). Strategies for Arab-Jewish conflict management workshops. In S. Wheelan, E. Pepitone, & V. Abt (Eds.), *Advances in field theory* (pp. 210–229). Beverly Hills, CA: Sage.

Bargal, D., & Bar, H. (1992). A Lewinian approach to intergroup workshops for Arab-Palestinian and Jewish youth. *Journal of Social Issues, 48*(2), 139–154.

Bargal, D., & Bar, H. (1994). The encounter of social selves approach in conducting intergroup workshops for Arab and Jewish youth in Israel. *Social Work with Groups, 17*(3), 39–59.

Blake, R., & Mouton, J. (1984). *Solving costly organizational conflicts.* San Francisco, CA: Jossey-Bass.

Blake, R., Mouton, J., & Sloma, R. (1965). The union management intergroup laboratory: Strategy for resolving intergroup conflict. *Journal of Applied Behavioral Science, 1,* 87–114.

Brewer, M., & Brown, R. (1998). Intergroup relations. In D. Gilbert, S. Fiske, & G. Lindzey (Eds.), *The handbook of social psychology* (Vol. 2, pp. 554–593). Boston: McGraw-Hill.

Burton, J. (1969). *Conflict and communication: The use of controlled communication in international relations.* London: Macmillan.

Campbell, D. (1965). Ethnocentric and other altruistic motives. In D. Levine (Ed.), *Nebraska Symposium on Motivation* (Vol. 13, pp. 283–311). Lincoln: University of Nebraska Press.

Carkhuff, R. (1969). *Helping and human resources.* New York: Holt, Rinehart, & Winston.

Cohen, S., Kelman, H., Miller, F., & Smith, B. (1977). Evolving intergroup techniques for conflict resolution: An Israeli-Palestinian workshop. *Journal of Social Issues, 33,* 165–189.

Cohen, S. P., & Azar, E. E. (1981). From war to peace: The transition between Egypt and Israel. *Journal of Conflict Resolution, 25,* 87–114.

Doob, L. (Ed.). (1970). *Resolving conflicts in Africa.* New Haven, CT: Yale University Press.

Doob, L., & Foltz, W. (1973). The Belfast workshop: An application of group techniques to destructive conflict. *Journal of Conflict Resolution, 17,* 489–512.

Egan, G. (1986). *The skilled helper: A systematic approach to effecting helping.* Monterey, CA: Brooks/Cole.

Fisher, R. J. (1990). *The social psychology of intergroup and international conflict resolution.* New York: Springer.

Fiske, S., & Taylor, S. (1991). *Social cognition* (2nd ed.). New York: McGraw-Hill.

Glasser, P., Sarri, R., & Vinter, R. (Eds.). (1974). *Individual change through small groups.* New York: Free Press.

Howard, S. (2000). Social psychology of identities. *Annual Review of Sociology, 26,* 369–393.

Kelman, H. (1997). Group processes in the resolution of international conflicts. *American Psychologist, 52,* 212–220.

Kelman, H., & Cohen, S. (1979). Reduction of international conflict: An interactional approach. In W. G. Austin & S. Worchel (Eds.), *The social psychology of intergroup relations* (pp. 288–303). Belmont, CA: Wadsworth.

Kelman, H., & Cohen, S. (1986). Resolution of international conflict: An interactional approach. In S. Worchel & W. G. Austin (Eds.), *Psychology of intergroup relations* (pp. 323–342). Chicago: Nelson Hall.

Lewin, K. (1947). Frontiers in group dynamics (Part 2). *Human Relations, 1,* 143–153.

Lewin, K. (1948). Conduct, knowledge, and acceptance of new values. In K. Lewin (Ed.), *Resolving social conflicts* (pp. 201–218). New York: Harper & Row. (Original work published 1945)

Lewin, K. (1958). Group decision and social change. In E. Maccoby, T. Newcomb, & E. Hartley (Eds.), *Readings in social psychology* (pp. 197–211). New York: Holt. (Original work published 1947)

Lieberman, M. (1980). Group methods. In F. Kanfer & A. Goldstein (Eds.), *Helping people change* (pp. 470–536). New York: Pergamon.

Lieberman, M. (1983). Comparative analyses of change mechanisms in groups. In H. Blumberg, P. Hare, V. Kent, & M. Davies (Eds.), *Small groups and social interaction* (Vol. 2, pp. 239–252). New York: Wiley.

Lippitt, R. (1949). *Training in community relations.* New York: Harper & Row.

Maoz, I. (2000). An experiment in peace: Reconciliation aimed workshops for Jewish-Israeli and Palestinian youth. *Journal of Peace Research, 37*(6–7), 721–736.

Melnick, J., & Woods, M. (1976). Group composition research and theory for psychotherapeutic and growth oriented groups. *Journal of Applied Behavioral Science, 12*(4), 493–512.

Miller, J., & Donner, S. (2000). More than just talk: The use of racial dialogues to combat racism. *Social Work with Groups, 23*(1), 31–53.

Mondros, J., Woodrow, R., & Weinstein, L. (1992). The use of groups to manage conflict. *Social Work with Groups, 15*(4), 43–57.

Moreland, R., Levine, J., & Wingert, M. (1996). Creating the ideal group composition effects at work. In E. Witte & J. Davis (Eds.), *Understanding group behavior: Small group processes and interpersonal relations.* (Vol. 2, pp. 11–35). Mahwah, NJ: Erlbaum.

Nagda, B., Spearman, M., Holley, L., Harding, S., Balassone, M., Moise-Swanson, D., & Demello, S. (1999). Intergroup dialogues: An innovative approach to teaching about diversity and justice in social work programs. *Journal of Social Work Education, 35*(3), 433–449.

Pettigrew, T. (1998). Intergroup contact theory. *Annual Review of Psychology, 49*, 65–85.

Pettigrew, T., & Tropp, L. (2000). Does intergroup contact reduce prejudice? Recent meta-analytic findings. In S. Oskamp (Ed.), *Reducing prejudice and discrimination: Social psychological perspectives* (pp. 93–114). Mahwah, NJ: Erlbaum.

Rittner, B., & Nakanishi, M. (1993). Challenging stereotypes and cultural biases through small group process. *Social Work with Groups, 16*(4), 5–23.

Schein, E. (1979). Personal change through interpersonal relationship. In W. Bennis, J. Can Maanen, E. Schein, & F. Steele (Eds.), *Essays in interpersonal dynamics* (pp. 129–162). Homewood, IL: Dorsey Press.

Schoem, D., & Hurtado, S. (Eds.). (2001). *Intergroup dialogue: Deliberative democracy in school, college, community, and workplace.* Ann Arbor: University of Michigan Press.

Sherif, M. (1958). Superordinate goals in the reduction of intergroup conflicts. *American Journal of Sociology, 63*, 349–356.

Sherif, M. (1966). *Group conflict and cooperation.* London: Routledge & Kegan Paul.

Shipler, D. (1986). *Arab and Jew: Wounded spirits in a promised land.* London: Bloomsbury.

Stephan, W. (1985). Intergroup relations. In G. Lindzey & E. Aronson (Eds.), *Handbook of social psychology* (pp. 599–658). New York: Random House.

Stephan, W. (1999). *Reducing prejudice and stereotyping in schools.* New York: Teachers College Press.

Stephan, W., & Finlay, K. (2000). The role of empathy in improving intergroup relations. *Journal of Social Issues, 55*, 729–744.

Stephan, W., & Stephan, C. (1996). *Intergroup relations.* Boulder, CO: Westview.

Stephan, W., & Stephan, C. (2001). *Improving intergroup relations.* Thousand Oaks, CA: Sage.

Tajfel, H. (1982). Social psychology of intergroup relations. *Annual Review of Psychology, 33*, 1–39.

Tajfel, H., & Turner, J. (1986). The social identity theory of intergroup behavior. In O. S. Worchel & W. Austin (Eds.), *Psychology of intergroup relations* (pp. 7–24). Chicago: Nelson Hall.

Toseland, R., & Rivas, R. (1984). *An introduction to group work practice.* New York: Macmillan.

Toseland, R., & Rivas, R. (1995). *An introduction to group work practice* (2nd ed.). New York: Macmillan.

Yalom, I. (1985). *The theory and practice of group psychotherapy* (3rd ed.). New York: Basic Books.

Part V

Group Work in Organizational and Community Settings

$\mathbf{A}$s we stated in our introduction to Part II, the early practice models of group work were developed primarily for members who joined groups for their own enhancement. Because of the social philosophy embedded in social work and particularly in group work, these members were often helped to work for changes in systems outside of the group. Approaches to group work that most strongly emphasized this aspect were referred to as being related to a "social goals" model.

Group workers were aware that their understanding of group processes and ways of facilitating groups could and should be applied to groups that were formed to enhance the functioning of organizations and communities, often referred to as *macro* practice. The details of this kind of practice, however, were not well enunciated. In this book, we sought to present models for group work in macro practice, as well as to introduce the reader to some of the newer uses of groups in this context.

The first two chapters in this section, Chapters 18 and 19, examine some models that may not be familiar to social workers. These are termed *participatory research* because of an idea that originated several decades ago as a social science research concept, *action research* (Lewin, 1997). This type of research proposed what is still a radical idea: that research should be a partnership between social scientists and the persons who are the focus of the research; that the research should meet both the needs of the affected persons to change aversive aspects of their environments and the needs of social scientists to understand the processes of social change. This kind of activity should have special relevance to group workers, who should seek, in partnership with group members, to more fully understand the processes of change. In fact, throughout the history of action research, the focus was on groups of people who sought social change. Chapter 18 contributes ideas that can be used in group-based participatory research by members and practitioners to study the processes in which they are both engaged. Chapter 19 presents some of the emerging kinds of group activities that are oriented to social change and that lend themselves to this kind of research, namely popular education and popular theatre.

Chapter 20 considers the strategies utilized by groups when they are engaged in bringing about social change, primarily in a community organization context. This is usually termed "social action" and is defined in the chapter as "bringing people together to convince, pressure, or coerce external decision makers to meet collective goals either to act in a specified manner or to stop or modify certain activities." Chapter 21 focuses on how groups can help people in poverty to challenge those conditions that maintain their impoverishment.

Chapter 22 focuses on creating teams, groups that are designed to enable people from different professions or with different roles to coordinate their work toward a common end. Teams face special challenges, not the least of which are differences in terminology, status, and perspectives that must be resolved if the team is to accomplish its purposes.

It was impossible for us to mandate chapters on all of the other types of groups that exist in community and organizational settings. For Chapter 23, we asked the author to create a generic discussion of the kinds of knowledge and skills required of a practitioner in order to work with the variety of so-called "task groups" created in social work settings.

Chapter 24 presents the emerging practice of helping consumers of social work services to form their own groups to meet their needs. The example used throughout this chapter is of a consumer-led group composed of a family and members of its social network working together to meet the needs of the children in the family. This approach represents a new form of partnership between agencies and community members.

REFERENCE

Lewin, K. (1997). *Resolving social conflicts*. Washington, DC: American Psychological Association.

Chapter 18

Assessing and Strengthening Characteristics of Effective Groups in Community-Based Participatory Research Partnerships

AMY J. SCHULZ
BARBARA A. ISRAEL
PAULA LANTZ

In this chapter, we examine the literature on group dynamics and discuss implications for understanding and evaluating those dynamics within community-based participatory research partnerships. We include a discussion of the development and adaptation of an instrument that can be used to evaluate group dynamics within community-based participatory research partnerships. We close with a discussion of the potential, challenges, and areas for further investigation in the evaluation of partnership group dynamics and the use of such assessments to facilitate ongoing partnership enhancement. The authors' experience has been with partnerships that address the implications of inequalities for public health, and the examples on which we draw reflect that experience. However, the methods and instruments discussed are readily applicable to community-based participatory research partnerships that address a broad range of issues.

The complex and interrelated nature of many social issues has contributed to interest in the potential of community-based partnerships that bring together a wide range of groups and organizations that pool their resources to address jointly identified concerns. For example, the adverse effects of social, economic, and racial-ethnic inequalities in the United States have become more visible and more visibly intertwined as their contributions to a wide range of concerns has been documented, including their implications for childhood development (Chase-Lansdale, Gordon, Brooks-Gunn, & Klebanov, 1997; Jarrett, 1997); educational risk and attainment (Connell & Halpern-Felsher, 1997; Halpern-Felsher et al., 1997); adolescent behavior (Spencer, Cole, Jones, & Swanson, 1997) and achievement (Darling &

Steinberg, 1997); infant mortality (O'Campo, Xue, Wang, & O'Brien-Caughy, 1997; Roberts, 1997); physical health (Collins & Williams, 1999); and mental health (Williams & Harris-Reid, 1999). Reducing the inequalities themselves, as well as their negative effects on those with fewer social and economic privileges, is rightfully a high priority for researchers, service providers, funding agencies, and community groups concerned with education, development, social conditions, and physical and mental well-being. Increasingly, many groups are seeking mechanisms for addressing these complex social issues that engage multiple strands of this web of causation (Krieger, 1994; Stokols, 1996; Yen & Syme, 1999).

Partnerships offer one mechanism for addressing the complex array of factors that contribute to the adverse effects of inequalities, engaging organizations and individuals from multiple sectors (e.g., private, public) and perspectives (e.g., housing official, community resident) to address common concerns. For example, health service providers, housing organizations, community-based organizations, parents, environmental advocacy groups, and academic researchers may pool expertise, resources, and energies to address childhood asthma (Krieger & Higgins, 2002). Understanding the dynamics of such partnerships and how those dynamics may affect the partnerships' ability to work effectively toward their goals is a matter of intense interest to funding agencies, as well as those who contribute time, energy, and expertise toward partnership efforts (Butterfoss, Goodman, & Wandersman, 1996; Florin, Mitchell, & Stevenson 1993; Francisco, Paine, & Fawcett, 1993; Green & Kreuter, 1992; Lasker, Weiss, & Miller, 2001; Sofaer, 2000; Tarlov et al., 1987).

COMMUNITY-BASED PARTICIPATORY RESEARCH PARTNERSHIPS

The term "community-based research" is used in many ways, sometimes interchangeably with other terms such as "community-wide research," "community-involved research," and "community-centered research" (Israel, Schulz, Parker, & Becker, 1998). We use the term *community-based participatory research* (CBPR) to emphasize the active engagement and influence of community members in all aspects of the research process, including the integration of the knowledge gained with action to improve the well-being of community members (Israel et al., 2001; O'Fallon & Dearry, 2002).

Coalition approaches to intervention and research bring together partners with diverse perspectives and areas of expertise to work toward a common agenda, often within a defined geographic area, for example, a region or city (Butterfoss et al., 1996; Lasker et al., 2001). Community-based participatory research partnerships are one form of coalition in which representatives from communities of identity, professional researchers, and service providers work together to analyze and take action to address prioritized concerns (Israel et al., 1998).[1] Communities of identity may coincide with geographically defined areas (e.g., an urban neighborhood) or may transcend physical locations (e.g., the black community). The common thread is that members share an identity or sense of connection that provides a basis for analysis of collective concerns and generation of potential actions to address those concerns (Chaskin, 1997; Steuart, 1975).

Participatory approaches to research engage the partners involved both in the development of knowledge and in efforts to address mutually identified concerns. Thus, within CBPR partnerships, representatives from communities of identity are actively engaged in and influence all aspects of the research process, and professionals (including researchers) are part of the problem solving, as well as the action components, of the effort (Hatch, Moss, Saran, Presley-Cantrell, & Mallory, 1993; Israel et al., 1998; Schulz, Israel, Selig,

Bayer, & Griffin, 1998). Such partnerships share a number of fundamental assumptions, including the assumption that diverse partners contribute different perspectives, expertise, and resources in identifying and understanding community concerns and the assumption that these multiple perspectives and resources can be engaged to develop solutions to identified concerns (Israel et al., 1998). Lasker and colleagues (2001) use the term "synergy"—defined as the ability to "combine the perspectives, resources, and skills of a group of people and organizations" (p. 183)—to describe a group's ability to work effectively together toward common goals.

In the following sections, we briefly review characteristics of effective groups—or groups that have synergy—as these have been defined by Johnson and Johnson (1982, 1997, 2003). Next, we describe a conceptual framework that illustrates relationships among these characteristics and the outcomes of community-based participatory research partnerships. Finally, we describe an evaluation instrument and a participatory evaluation process that attempt to apply this conceptual framework in a manner that is consistent with principles for conducting CBPR (Israel et al., 1998; Schulz et al., 1998). This evaluation instrument and process can be used by partnerships to assess, discuss, analyze, and take action in addressing concerns related to the group's working relationships—that is, to facilitate the development of synergy within partnerships. To the extent that such instruments enable partnerships to assess their own group dynamics, they offer one mechanism to evaluate and improve the group dynamics that are essential for successful collaboration. For example, groups that identify ineffective leadership or lack of trust among members may take steps to address these concerns in order to strengthen their ability to reach long-term goals. We close with a discussion of the potential for use of such instruments to promote the development of characteristics of effective groups within community-based participatory research partnerships.

CHARACTERISTICS OF EFFECTIVE COMMUNITY-BASED PARTICIPATORY RESEARCH PARTNERSHIPS

Community-based participatory research partnerships explicitly seek to bring together groups of people who can combine their perspectives, resources, skills, and ideas to create solutions to community problems. Like any group that comes together with a function or goal, dynamics that unfold among members shape the partnerships' actions and ultimately its success in working together. The rich literature on group process and group dynamics is useful to those seeking to foster community-based participatory research partnerships. Partnership members, evaluators, and funders are, in the long run, concerned with the outcomes of CBPR partnerships—that is, their ability to achieve specific outcomes and objectives. However, those long-term objectives may become visible only after a period of years. Gaining insights into group dynamics that can contribute to or interfere with a partnership's ability to create the synergy necessary for achievement of its goals can help partnerships assess their own process as it unfolds. When necessary, such assessment offers opportunities to modify actions or adjust group dynamics to enhance the group's effectiveness in working together and, ultimately, to further develop its potential to achieve long-term objectives.

Characteristics of Effective Groups

Johnson and Johnson (2003) define an effective group as one "whose members commit themselves to the common purposes of maximizing their own and each other's success. . . .

[Members] believe that their success depends on the efforts of all group members" (p. 22). Based on an extensive review of the group dynamics literature, Johnson and Johnson (1982, 1997, 2003) identify the following characteristics of effective groups: mutual commitment of members to clearly defined operational goals; two-way communication; mutual leadership; appropriate decision-making procedures; shared power; the ability to challenge each other in a constructive manner; the ability to resolve conflicts effectively; mechanisms for mutual accountability; and the ability to appropriately engage the skills and expertise of group members.

Following from the identification of these characteristics, Johnson and Johnson (2003, pp. 12–14) suggest several guidelines for fostering them within groups, which we describe briefly here (see Table 18.1, left-hand column). Guideline 1 recognizes the importance of establishing clear goals for the group that can be defined and measured and that are relevant to the group and its members. These should be goals to which members can commit themselves and that they are unable to achieve by themselves, thus establishing positive interdependence among members. Guideline 2 recognizes that effective group work requires two-way communication that allows all members to participate in the exchange of information, as well as ideas and feelings. Guideline 3 emphasizes the importance of participation and shared leadership, with all members assuming responsibility for being involved in the collective work of the partnership and committed to implementing decisions that are made by the group as a whole. This guideline includes working toward the collective goals of the group, commitment to maintaining working relationships among members, and commitment to the development and growth of the group as a whole. Guideline 4 recognizes the importance of insuring that power is shared among group members on the basis of expertise, ability, and access to information. Such shared power can promote interdependence and mutual influence among members. Guideline 5 emphasizes the importance of diverse decision-making processes that are consistent with the needs of the situation. Determining the appropriate decision-making process for any given decision involves balancing the time and energy required for various forms of decision making (e.g., consensus vs. top-down) against the size of the decision and the commitment of group members necessary to put the decision into practice.

Guidelines 6 and 7 both have to do with the ability of the group to name, discuss, and resolve conflicts or controversies effectively. The ability to disagree, challenge, and discuss alternative perspectives on a given issue is fundamental to the ability to identify creative solutions that reflect diverse perspectives and values among group members. Similarly, although partnerships are based on defining shared interests and common goals, conflicts of interest and differences in priorities are inevitable within partnerships. For example, within any community-based participatory research partnership, there are likely to be differences among partners in terms of the relative weight to be placed on research and intervention activities, as well as individual- and community-level intervention efforts. The ability of the partnership to identify strategies to address such conflicts is an important aspect of effective group work.

Group Dynamics in CBPR Partnerships

Recognizing the important role of group dynamics in the success of community-based participatory research partnerships, many such partnerships have explicit objectives—in addition to their outcome objectives—related to partnership formation, dynamics, relationships among group members, and collective action (Israel et al., 1995; Sofaer, 2000). This empha-

TABLE 18.1. Guidelines for Creating Effective Groups and Sample Items for Evaluating Group Dynamics in Community-Based Participatory Research Partnerships

Guidelines for creating effective groups[a]	Sample items from survey instrument for evaluating group dynamics characteristics and intermediate measures of partnership effectiveness[b]
Guideline 1: Establish clear, operational, relevant group goals that create positive interdependence and evoke a high level of commitment from every member.	How much do you feel a part of the group (like you belong to the group)? How much do you have a sense of ownership over what the group does? How frequently do you think of severing your affiliation with the group?
Guideline 2: Establish effective, two-way communication within which group members communicate their ideas and feelings accurately and clearly.	How much do people in the group feel comfortable expressing their points of view? How much do group members listen to each others' points of view, even if they might disagree? How much is your opinion listened to in group meetings? How much are you willing to listen to others' points of view?
Guideline 3: Insure that leadership and participation are distributed among all group members.	How often do you suggest new ideas? How often do you point out ways to proceed when the group is stuck? How often do you invite other members to work with you on specific issues? How often do you place items on the agenda for discussion? To what extent are roles and tasks shared by members?
Guideline 4: Insure that the use of power is distributed among group members and that patterns of influence vary according to the needs of the group as members strive to achieve their mutual goals.	How much do you feel pressured to go along with decisions of the group even though you might not agree? Is your opinion listened to and considered by other group members? Does one person or group dominate the meetings?
Guideline 5: Match decision-making procedures with the needs of the situation.	Do certain individuals have more influence over the decision-making process than others? How true is it that it takes too much time to reach decisions? How true is it that everyone in the group has a voice in the decisions? How true is it that good decisions are made? How satisfied are you with the way the decision-making process is working? How much is the group able to make the necessary decisions in order to keep the project moving forward?
Guideline 6: Engage in controversy by disagreeing and challenging each other's conclusions and reasoning, thus promoting creative decision making and problem solving.	How well do you think the group has been able to work together to solve problems? In working together to solve problems, how well has the group been able to identify the important issues and generate several possible solutions? How satisfied are you with the way the group deals with problems that come up?
Guideline 7: Face conflicts and resolve them in a constructive way.	In your opinion, what (if any) have been the major points of conflict or disagreement within the group? How well do you feel that these conflicts were handled by the group?

[a] Johnson and Johnson (2003).

[b] Copies of the questionnaires used in the three projects highlighted in this chapter are available from Amy J. Schulz.

sis acknowledges relationships between a group's dynamics (process objectives), members' perceptions of the partnership itself (impact objectives), and improved community health outcomes (outcome objectives). In other words, the ability of a partnership to reach its long-term objectives is explicitly linked to the success of the group in mobilizing its individual and collective resources to reach its goals and to satisfy the needs of group members.

Figure 18.1 illustrates relationships among these three types of objectives within the context of a conceptual framework for assessing coalitions adapted from Sofaer (2000). Briefly, the model suggests that the ability of a partnership to reach its outcome objectives is shaped by intermediate measures of partnership success, influenced by the partnership's programs and interventions. These are, in turn, shaped by the group dynamics that are characteristic of the partnership (called "functional" characteristics by Sofaer, 2000), as well as characteristics of the environment. Group dynamics are also shaped by the structural characteristics of the partnership, including the members, and the environmental characteristics. The characteristics of effective groups described herein can be seen in Figure 18.1 in the box "Group-Dynamics Characteristics of Effective Partnerships." The "Intermediate Measures of Partnership Effectiveness" include, for example, members' perceptions of the effectiveness, benefits, and costs of participation in the partnership, the extent of member involvement, and members' perceptions of the ability of the partnership to achieve future objectives and goals.

The recent literature on assessing coalitions or partnerships has confirmed the importance of many of these group-process characteristics. For example, Butterfoss and colleagues (1996) have shown that community leadership and shared decision making are linked to member satisfaction and participation in coalitions. In a review of the literature on community partnerships, Lasker and colleagues (2001) also describe leadership (Lasker & the Committee on Medicine and Public Health, 1997), administration and management (Chaskin & Garg, 1997; Israel et al., 1998; Lasker et al., 1997), trust (Goodman et al., 1998; Himmelman, 1996; Kreuter, Young, & Lezin 1998), and conflict and power differentials (Forrest, 1992; Israel et al., 1998; Kegler, Steckler, McLeory, & Malek, 1998) as critical aspects of the ability of a coalition to develop synergy. Similarly, partners' perceptions of the relative benefits and drawbacks of participation have been linked to partnership dynamics and are described as key to understanding partners' level of commitment to and willingness to invest resources in the work of the coalition (Butterfoss et al., 1996; Lasker et al., 2001; Wandersman, Florin, Friedman, & Meier, 1987).

DEVELOPMENT, ADAPTATION, AND APPLICATION OF AN EVALUATION INSTRUMENT TO ASSESS GROUP DYNAMICS IN CBPR PARTNERSHIPS

The important role played by group-dynamics characteristics in the success of community-based participatory research efforts suggests that they are necessary, although by no means sufficient, conditions for the success of the partnership. We have developed and used an evaluation instrument that was designed to assess central characteristics of effective groups, as described previously, to assess group dynamics in several participatory research partnerships.[2] Each of these partnerships has drawn on results from the assessments to examine and develop more effective group processes. In this section we describe briefly the development and adaptation of this instrument in three distinct CBPR partnerships and its use as a tool for partnership growth and development. In so doing, we focus on this evaluation instru-

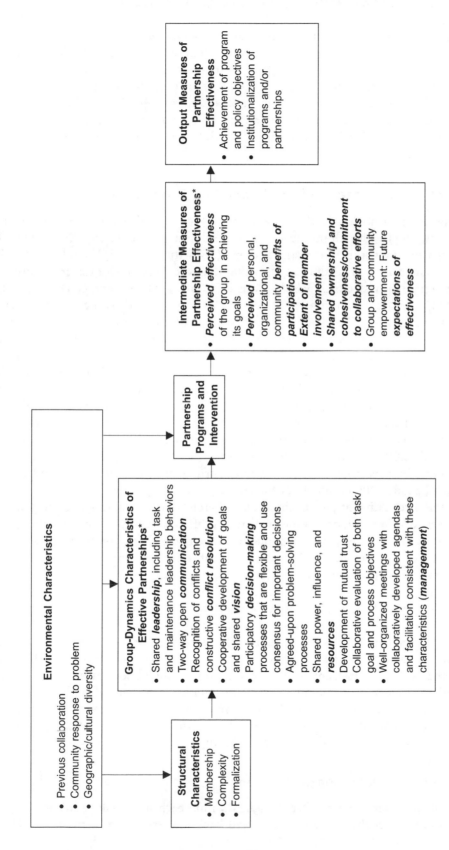

FIGURE 18.1. Conceptual framework for assessing group dynamics as an aspect of effectiveness of community-based participatory research partnerships. Adapted from Sofaer (2000). *From Johnson and Johnson (1982, 1997). *Italicized* and **bolded** items are derived from Johnson and Johnson and are also included in Sofaer (2000). Other items are derived from Johnson and Johnson and are not included in Sofaer's model.

ment as a component of a collaborative or participatory evaluation, one that enables groups to assess their process and progress toward intermediate and outcome objectives and to make modifications and improvements in their practices as necessary (King, 1998; King & Lonnquist, 1992; Nunneley, Orton, & King, 1997; Patton, 1997; Rossi, Freeman, & Lispey, 1999). The application described here is an example of one strategy that can be used to promote effective group dynamics within the context of community-based participatory research partnerships (Fox, 1987; Israel et al., 2001; Johnson & Johnson, 2003; Schwartz, 1994; Zander, 1982).

Development and Adaptation of the Evaluation Instrument

The evaluation instrument described here was initially developed within the context of a partnership for workplace health promotion (Israel, Schurman, & House, 1989) and subsequently adapted for use within two distinct community settings (Lantz, Vireull-Fuentes, Israel, Soffley, & Guzman, 2001; Schulz et al., 1998). Based on a review of the group process literature at the time the instrument was developed (Blumberg, Hare, Kent, & Davies, 1983; Bradford, 1978; Johnson & Johnson, 1982; Shaw, 1981) and a synthesis of the characteristics of effective groups described herein, specific aspects of group process were prioritized for assessment. The evaluation instrument includes items corresponding to each central-group process characteristic (e.g., leadership, participation, communication). Some of these indicators were drawn from existing questionnaires (Alexander, 1985; Burns & Gragg, 1981; Johnson & Johnson, 1982; Seashore, Lawler, Mirvis, & Cammann, 1983), and others were developed to operationalize dimensions for which existing measures were unavailable. The intent was to include items that would enable partnership members to evaluate themselves in light of characteristics of effective groups (Green & Kreuter, 1992; Israel et al., 1998; Israel et al., 2001; Mertens, 1999; Schulz et al., 1998). Table 18.1, right-hand column, shows sample items from these evaluation instruments and their correspondence to Johnson and Johnson's (2003) guidelines for creating effective groups.

Because the three different partnerships had different priorities and dynamics, the specific items or sets of items included in the evaluations differed slightly. Each partnership undertook a process to define the group-dynamics characteristics that were most important or salient to them (see Israel et al., 2001) and those characteristics were incorporated in the final evaluation instrument. For example, in one of the partnerships the distribution of power was particularly salient. Although each of the evaluation instruments included items designed to assess the distribution of power, the instrument was adapted for this partnership to include a more comprehensive set of items on various forms of influence (e.g., decision-making power, community empowerment, equitable distribution of resources) to insure that the evaluation adequately addressed the priorities of the members. Furthermore, within each partnership, the evaluation instrument described here was one of several methods of data collection (others included, for example, in-depth interviews conducted with partners or field notes collected at group meetings). Within each of the cases examined here, the instrument was revised and adapted over time to reflect concerns and priorities that were identified through these other, open-ended evaluation methods.

Application of the Evaluation Instrument

Just as the evaluation instrument differed slightly within each partnership, so did the processes used to administer the instrument and feed back the results (see Lantz et al., 2001, and Schulz et al., 2003, for more detailed discussions of these processes). In one case, the instrument was administered during a regular meeting of hourly and salaried employees of an automobile components manufacturing plant who participated in the project (Israel et al., 1989). In the other two cases considered here, the instrument was mailed to representatives from community-based organizations, health and social service providers, and academic institutions that were members of the group (Lantz et al., 2001). In each case, the researchers/ evaluators were responsible for administering the evaluation instrument to members of the partnership and for compiling and feeding back the results from the questionnaires on an annual basis.

Results were presented back to group members showing numbers and percentages for each question, along with a listing of the number of persons who made up the percentages presented (e.g., 50% = 10 persons). Results were also included for each previous year, allowing for comparison over time. Within each of the partnerships (workplace and the two community-based partnerships), results were presented at a formal partnership meeting with time dedicated to discussion of the findings, for example, agreement, disagreements, surprises, and interpretations. This opportunity for critical reflection on their process (i.e., formative evaluation) allowed partnership members to identify areas in which they might want to make changes in the way they worked together. For example, in one of the partnerships, first-year survey results indicated that approximately one-fourth of the partnership members felt "somewhat" pressured to go along with decisions of the group even though they might not agree. This finding resulted in a discussion about the group's earlier decision to use consensus decision making, and partners agreed that they needed to continue to discuss and revise decisions until they reached consensus (Israel et al., 1989). In another example, about one-third of committee members indicated that they felt that it was "somewhat true" that decisions that the partnership made did not get implemented. Based on this finding, the partnership discussed the lack of ongoing involvement of and support from top management in the organizations involved in the partnership and adopted strategies to try to more effectively engage those decision makers as a means to facilitate implementation of decisions made by the group.

In a final example of the use of partnership results to examine and implement changes in group-process dynamics, results from one partnership suggested that larger organizations had more consistent participation over time than smaller, community-based organizations, who often had less consistent participation and more frequent changes in representatives (e.g., due to staff turnover). In addition, the survey found that newer members of the partnership reported less ownership over team decisions; were less likely to suggest new ideas, express opinions, or point out ways to proceed when the team was stuck; were less likely to take leadership roles within the team; and were less satisfied with the amount of influence they had over decisions made by the partnership. The group discussed their concern that these findings suggested the possibility that high turnover and less frequent attendance by representatives from smaller organizations with fewer resources could exacerbate differences in influence and leadership between the larger and smaller organizations active in the partnership. The group discussed and implemented several strategies intended to support participation from smaller organizations in an effort to equalize influence and decision-making power between the involved groups. Reflecting on this process, one partner noted: "We became able to put the cards on the table. 'Let's do some brainstorming. Let's do some green-light thinking.' There are some tough questions that you can't resolve unless you have some really tough dialogues" (Schulz, 1998).

The different partnerships used a variety of techniques to identify specific issues to be raised for discussion based on the survey findings. In one partnership, an evaluation sub-committee worked with the staff evaluator to determine which issues should be brought to the full group for discussion (Lantz et al., 2001), whereas in the other partnerships, the evaluator presented results to the entire group, and the full partnership prioritized items for discussion (Israel et al., 1989). Criteria used by these partnerships to select items for discussion included issues raised repeatedly over two or more administrations of the survey, items that showed substantial change from one year to the next, or issues or concerns that influenced the ability of partners to participate and have influence in the decision-making process. As an example, when the results of the first survey in one partnership indicated that community partners were disproportionately unsure of how to place an item on the agenda, and thus were not satisfied with the degree of influence they had over what was discussed at partnership meetings, these results were prioritized for discussion among the partners. A frank discussion ensued about the meeting agenda-setting process and the importance of the ability of all members (not just a select few) to help craft meeting agendas. The group agreed on a process for getting items on the agenda that was better understood and more inclusive. Following implementation of this process, subsequent evaluations have indicated increased satisfaction with what is addressed at meetings and how meeting agendas are developed.

In each of the three partnerships considered in this chapter, presentation of results from the group-process evaluation regularly generated considerable discussion. The presentations have provided opportunities to discuss and refine both the process and the structure of the group, and partnership members have identified these discussions and the ensuing changes as key factors supporting the groups' achievements (Lantz et al., 2001). One partnership member noted: "The trust and relationships we've built have really launched the (partnership) and helped out with all of our accomplishments. What really helped was the trust and relationship building that was done" (Lantz et al., 2001). As data from the evaluation of the group processes were brought to the group, they provided opportunities for discussion and trust building among partners, as well as for the development of solutions to problems and challenges identified through the evaluation.

DISCUSSION AND LESSONS LEARNED

In each of the projects described in the previous section, the group-dynamics evaluation instrument provided a structure for discussion of members' perceptions, concerns, and interactions within the partnership. Annual data collection and feedback allowed regular identification and discussion of issues and concerns that would have been difficult to raise in the context of ongoing meetings, when task or content objectives were of primary concern. Based on these experiences, we discuss a number of principles and processes that may be useful for facilitating and evaluating the development of characteristics associated with effective groups within community-based participatory research partnerships. Given the critical role that evaluation can play in assessing and enhancing group dynamics, emphasis is placed here on suggested strategies for those involved in evaluation.

Equitable Engagement

Equitable engagement of all partnership members in all phases of the research/evaluation process does not necessarily mean that all partners engage in all aspects of the evaluation to an equal extent. A basic assumption behind a partnership approach is that each partner brings unique perspectives and skills and that the partnership is strengthened through the application of those diverse resources toward a common goal. Thus some members may bring considerable skill and/or interest in evaluation, and others may bring in-depth understanding of group dynamics, both of which contribute to building a strong group. It may not be an efficient, or even desirable, use of partnership resources to engage all members in actually administering questionnaires, entering data into a database, or conducting preliminary analyses of the results. All partners, however, have important perspectives and insights to share in interpreting the results of the evaluation and in thinking through ways to address issues and concerns that may be brought to light through the evaluation process.

In two of the three partnerships described in this chapter, discussions of evaluation goals and questions were conducted by the full boards and shaped the overall evaluation design (Israel et al., 1989; Schulz, 1998). In the third group (Lantz et al., 2001), a subcommittee was created to help develop the evaluation, and this subcommittee presented the preliminary evaluation plan to the full board for discussion prior to its finalization. Participatory development of the evaluation plan insured that it incorporated multiple perspectives and that the group agreed on priorities for evaluation of their process, impact, and outcomes. Once the evaluation plan had been mapped out, those with expertise in data collection and analysis applied their skills, bringing the results back to the larger group for discussion, interpretation, and decisions about action steps.

Furthermore, early in the development of each of the partnerships described here, members engaged in a discussion of the characteristics of groups that they had been members of in the past and that they considered effective or worthwhile groups (Israel et al. 2001). These discussions generated many of the same dimensions identified in a review of the literature on effective groups or coalitions that achieve synergy—mutual respect, shared leadership, effective governance. They also offered an opportunity for the group to collectively discuss which aspects of group dynamics they particularly valued and, in some cases, generated specific items to be included in the evaluation. Perhaps most important, these discussions provided an opportunity for the group members to "own" the questions included in the process evaluation document and laid the groundwork for later discussions of the results.

Selecting Items for Feedback to the Group

The length of the instrument described here argues against the verbal presentation and discussion of the full set of results. Complete results may be better shared in a written report made available to all members, in combination with presentation and discussion of selected results. The evaluator, evaluation subcommittee, or group as a whole may select particular items or sections for a more focused discussion. This selection may be done in a number of ways.

For example, items or issues that appear to have undergone substantial change between the preceding year and the current year could be highlighted. Discussion of change may help to identify precipitating causes and can contribute to the development of constructive suggestions for addressing (or sustaining) those changes. Conversely, in some instances stability in a set of indicators might be highlighted, for example, issues that surface in multiple waves of data collection or across multiple data collection methods (the group-dynamics instrument, field notes, and in-depth interviews). Decisions about which issues to highlight can be informed by regular participation of the evaluator in meetings and other partnership events, enabling the evaluator to develop insights into group dynamics, including issues that may arise at particular meetings or carry over as undertones through a series of meetings. Such dynamics may be very difficult to assess through closed-ended data collection strategies, which offer only a snapshot at a point in time, or with longitudinal data, repeated snapshots at particular points in time. Field notes provide important information that contributes to the interpretation of results gathered with a closed-ended instrument and can inform the selection of particular results for feedback and discussion by the group.

Finally, the group may choose to highlight differences in perceptions that occur across subgroups or constituencies within the partnership. For example, two of the three partnerships referred to in this chapter had representatives from a number of community-based organizations, health departments, and academic institutions. Central goals of the partnerships involved the development of equitable working relationships among these types of organizations, each of which brought qualitatively and quantitatively different resources. Therefore, perspectives on the way that the partnership was working together might reasonably be expected to differ—and, indeed, in many cases they did. Such differential results and perceptions provide a basis for conversation and discussion about mutual and reciprocal benefits and identification of actions that might be taken to address imbalances.

Some Considerations and Limitations

There are several limitations to the use of the group-dynamics instrument we have described here. First, this instrument focuses solely on group dynamics, that is, relationships among members of the partnership and the ways that they work together. As illustrated in Figure 18.1, there are other important dimensions of any particular partnership that may be considered. Furthermore, data are collected at specified points that may be influenced by recent events that could potentially overshadow longer term dynamics and trends. The use of closed-ended items on the instruments also may limit their ability to pick up new and emergent issues that are not reflected in the items included. For these reasons, as well as those previously described, we recommend that closed-ended survey instruments to assess group dynamics be used in conjunction with other methods of data collection. Those used by the partnerships described here have included in-depth interviews with partnership members, field notes of meetings, and document reviews (Israel et al., 1989; Lantz et al., 2001; Schulz et al., 2003).

The small numbers involved in most partnerships may preclude the use of anything but simple descriptive statistics in data analysis. Even with high response rates, these numbers may limit the use of tests of statistical significance to assess change over time. Rather, their utility lies in their ability to give an overall sense of critical group dynamics, especially when combined with other types of data that are collected simultaneously, and to stimulate and shape candid discussions regarding group process and the current state of the partnership among members. The results are not meant to stand alone as a metric of group dynamics.

One consideration is whether to track change in individual respondents over time or change in the group as a whole or some combination of these strategies. Simple aggregates of results from two points in time can be useful for obtaining a snapshot of group dynamics but fail to address the question of whether changes are due to events that may have unfolded in the group (history), changes in group composition, or some combination (for example, events that may have affected some group members more than others). Decisions about whether to present results for the group as a whole or for particular subgroups may be based on the particular question being asked, on the extent and nature of turnover in the group between the two points of data collection, or on issues identified through analysis of other data collection efforts (e.g., meeting field notes).

For example, it seems possible that individuals who participate in a partnership over longer periods of time may perceive that they have greater influence in the process and outcomes of the partnership than newer members, a result of skills and relationships that develop over time. This effect may be masked in examining aggregate data if, at the same time that some members develop an extended history with the partnership, new members join whose lack of history or experience within the partnership contributes to their feeling that they have little influence. To assess the effects of history and of turnover of members on the overall working relationships among the partners, the evaluator may wish to examine key process indicators by length of membership (and/or intensity of participation) in the partnership. Similarly, there may be differences in experiences and perspectives, for example, between representatives in community-based organizations and those in larger service-providing organizations or academic institutions. Dividing responses by relevant categories can allow the partnership to examine these differences in some detail and to gain greater clarity on both the processes that drive them and their implications for the group.

Evaluators must, however, take care not to identify or expose individual group members when presenting results, particularly when categories are quite small (for example, if there are only two representatives from health-care-providing organizations). Potential breaches of confidentiality or anonymity must be guarded against very carefully. In addition to violating basic tenets of research ethics, they also have important implications for working relationships among group members. Furthermore, once respondents have been divided into categories of interest, response summaries will be very sensitive to small changes in membership (e.g., new people), as well as small changes in the assessments offered by individuals (e.g., changing perceptions among long-term members). Group members must take care not to overinterpret changes in light of these sensitivities and at the same time be attentive to the potential implications of such changes.

CONCLUDING COMMENTS AND DIRECTIONS FOR FUTURE RESEARCH

The complexity of many current social issues has led to the development of partnerships that seek to bring together diverse resources, skills, and perspectives to address issues of common concern. A growing body of evidence argues that the ability of such partnerships to realize their potential to work effectively for change rests on the dynamics that emerge among group members. Group-dynamics characteristics described in this chapter are consistent with key factors identified in the community coalition literature as associated with the successful formation, implementation, and maintenance of coalitions (Butterfoss et al., 1996; Lantz et al., 2001; Lasker et al., 2001). Tools that enable partnerships to assess their own group dynamics offer one important mechanism for evaluating and taking action to improve the working relationships that are essential for effective collaboration.

Despite the limitations and caveats discussed in the preceding section, group-dynamics instruments such as the one described in this chapter can be a useful tool for groups whose success relies on the development of effective and equitable working relationships among members. As a formative evaluation tool used in an ongoing manner, such group-dynamics data collection instruments can provide a structured opportunity for group members to engage in discussion and collective problem solving, enhancing the groups' ability to meet its goals.

ACKNOWLEDGMENTS

This chapter was adapted from Schulz, Israel, and Lantz (2003). Copyright 2003 by Elsevier Science. Adapted by permission.

Support for this work was provided in part by the W. K. Kellogg Foundation Community-Based Public Health Initiative (Grant No. 922871), the Centers for Disease Control and Prevention's Urban Health Centers initiative (Grant No. U48/CCU515775), the National Institute of Alcohol Abuse and Alcoholism (Grant No. R01/AA06553), and the United Auto Workers/General Motors National Joint Committee on Health and Safety (No. 89-604). We wish to acknowledge the contributions of the Broome Team (Coalition for Positive Youth Development, F.A.C.E.D., Flint Neighborhood Coalition, Flint Odyssey House, Genesee County Community Action Agency, Genesee County Health Department, Pierson School Parent Club, University of Michigan Flint Campus, University of Michigan School of Public Health); the Detroit Community–Academic Urban Research Center (Butzel Family Center, Community Health and Social Services Center, Detroit Health Department, Friends of Parkside, Henry Ford Health System, Kettering/Butzel Health Initiative, Latino Family Services, University of Michigan Schools of Public Health and Nursing, and Warren Conner Development Coalition); and Sue Schurman and participants in the Stress and Wellness Project. In addition, we thank Sue Andersen for her contributions to the preparation of the manuscript.

NOTES

1. Again, although our focus here is on community-based participatory research partnerships to address health concerns, similar approaches may be applied to housing, transportation, the environment, or any number of other complex issues. The composition of the partnership and, particularly, the service providers involved may vary accordingly. However, the group-dynamics principles and general framework presented here are applicable across a broad range of outcomes.
2. The items are described in Table 18.1.

REFERENCES

Alexander, M. (1985). The team effectiveness critique. *Annual, Developing Human Resources, 14*, 101–106.

Blumberg, H. H., Hare, A. P., Kent, V., & Davies, M. F. (Eds.). (1983). *Small groups and social interaction* (Vols. 1 & 2). New York: Wiley.

Bradford, L. P. (Ed.). (1978). *Group development* (2nd ed.). San Diego, CA: University Associates.

Burns, F., & Gragg, R. L. (1981). Brief diagnostic instruments. *The 1981 annual handbook for group facilitators* (pp. 87–94). San Diego, CA: University Associates.

Butterfoss, F. D., Goodman, R. M., & Wandersman, A. (1996). Community coalitions for prevention and health promotion: Factors predicting satisfaction, participation, and planning. *Health Education Quarterly, 23*(1), 65–79.

Chase-Lansdale, P. L., Gordon, R. A., Brooks-Gunn, J., & Klebanov, P. K. (1997). Neighborhood and family influences on the intellectual and behavioral competence of preschool and early school-age children. In J. Brooks-Gunn, G. J. Duncan, & J. L. Aber (Eds.), *Neighborhood poverty, Volume I* (pp. 79–118). New York: Russell Sage Foundation.

Chaskin, R. J. (1997). Perspectives on neighborhood and community: A review of the literature. *Social Service Review, 7*(4), 521–547.

Chaskin, R. J., & Garg, S. (1997). The issue of governance in neighborhood-based initiatives. *Urban Affairs Quarterly, 32,* 631–661.

Collins, C., & Williams, D. R. (1999). Segregation and mortality: The deadly effects of racism?" *Sociological Forum, 14*(3), 495–523.

Connell, J. P., & Halpern-Felsher, B. L. (1997). How neighborhoods affect educational outcomes in middle childhood and adolescence: Conceptual issues and an empirical example. In J. Brooks-Gunn, G. J. Duncan, & J. L. Aber (Eds.), *Neighborhood poverty, Volume I* (pp. 174–199). New York: Russell Sage Foundation.

Darling, N., & Steinberg, L. (1997). Community influences on adolescent achievement and deviance. In J. Brooks-Gunn, G. J. Duncan, & J. L. Aber (Eds.), *Neighborhood poverty, Volume II* (pp. 120–131). New York: Russell Sage Foundation.

Florin, P., Mitchell R., & Stevenson, J. (1993). Identifying training and technical assistance needs in community coalitions: A developmental approach. *Health Education Research, 20*(4), 345–357.

Forrest, J. E. (1992). Management aspects of strategic partnering. *Journal of General Management, 17,* 25–40.

Fox, W. M. (1987). *Effective group problem solving: How to broaden participation, improve decision making, and increase commitment to action.* San Francisco: Jossey-Bass.

Francisco, V., Paine, A., & Fawcett, S. (1993). A methodology for monitoring and evaluating community health coalitions. *Health Education Research, 20*(4), 403–416.

Goodman, R. M., Speers, M. A., McLeroy, K., Fawcett, S., Kegler, M., Parker, E. A., et al. (1998). Identifying and defining the dimensions of community capacity to provide a basis for measurement. *Health Education and Behavior, 25*(3), 258–278.

Green, L. W., & Krueter, M. W. (1992). CDC's planned approach to community health as an application of PRECEED and an inspiration for PROCEED. *Journal of Health Education, 23*(3), 140–147.

Halpern-Felsher, B. L., Connell, J. P., Spencer, M. B., Aber, J. L. Duncan, G. J., Clifford, E., et al. (1997). Neighborhood and family factors predicting educational risk and attainment in African American and white children and adolescents. In J. Brooks-Gunn, G. J. Duncan, & J. L. Aber (Eds.), *Neighborhood poverty, Volume I* (pp. 146–173). New York: Russell Sage Foundation.

Hatch, J., Moss, N., Saran, A., Presley-Cantrell, L., & Mallory, C. (1993). Community research: Partnership in black communities. *American Journal of Preventive Medicine, 9,* 27–31.

Himmelman, A. T. (1996). Collaboration and the three Ts: Time, trust and turf constraints. *Health System Leader, 3*(10), 13–16.

Israel, B. A., Cummings, K. M., Dignan, M. B., Heaney, C. A., Perales, D. P., Simons-Morton, B. G., & Zimmerman, M. A. (1995). Evaluation of health education programs: Current assessment and future directions. *Health Education Quarterly, 22*(2), 364–389.

Israel, B. A., Lichtenstein, R., Lantz, P., McGranaghan, R., Allen, A., Guzman, R., et al. (2001). The Detroit Community–Academic Urban Research Center: Lessons learned in the development, implementation, and evaluation of a community-based participatory research partnership. *Journal of Public Health Management and Practice, 7*(5), 1–19.

Israel, B. A., Schulz, A. J., Parker, E. A., & Becker, A. B. (1998). Review of community-based research: Assessing partnership approaches to improve public health. *Annual Review of Public Health, 19,* 173–202.

Israel, B. A., Schurman, S. J., & House, J. S. (1989). Action research on occupational stress: Involving workers as researchers. *International Journal of Health Services, 19*(1), 135–155.

Jarrett, R. L. (1997). Bringing families back in: Neighborhood effects on child development. In J. Brooks-Gunn, G. J. Duncan, & J. L. Aber (Eds.), *Neighborhood poverty, Volume I* (pp. 48–64). New York: Russell Sage Foundation.

Johnson, D. W., & Johnson, F. P. (1982). *Joining together: Group theory and group skills* (2nd ed.). Englewood Cliffs, NJ: Prentice-Hall.

Johnson, D. W., & Johnson, F. P. (1997). *Joining together: Group theory and group skills* (6th ed.). Englewood Cliffs, NJ: Prentice-Hall.

Johnson D. W., & Johnson, F. P. (2003). *Joining together: Group theory and group skills* (7th ed.). Englewood Cliffs, NJ: Prentice-Hall.

Kegler, M. C., Steckler, A., McLeroy, K., & Malek, S. H. (1998). Factors that contribute to effective community health promotion coalitions: A study of 10 Project ASSIST coalitions in North Carolina. *Health Education and Behavior, 25*(3), 338–353.

King, J. A. (1998). Making sense of participatory evaluation practice. *New Directions for Evaluation, 80,* 57–67.

King, J. A., & Lonnquist, M. (1992). *A review of writing on action research: 1944–present.* Minneapolis, MN: Center for Applied Research and Educational Improvement.

Kreuter, M. W., Young, L. A., & Lezin, N. A. (1998). *Measuring social capital in small communities.* Atlanta, GA: Health 2000.

Krieger, N. (1994). Epidemiology and the web of causation: Has anyone seen the spider? *Social Science and Medicine, 39*(7), 887–903.

Lantz, P. M., Vireull-Fuentes, E., Israel, B. A., Softley, D., & Guzman, R. (2001). Can communities and academia work together on public health research? Evaluation results from a community-based participatory research partnership in Detroit. *Journal of Urban Health, 78*(3), 495–507.

Lasker, R., & the Committee on Medicine and Public Health. (1997). *Medicine and public health: The power of collaboration.* Chicago: Health Administration Press.

Lasker, R. D., Weiss, E. S., & Miller, R. (2001). Partnership synergy: A practical framework for studying and strengthening the collaborative advantage. *Milbank Quarterly, 79*(2), 179–205.

Mertens, D. M. (1999). Inclusive evaluation: Implications of transformative theory for evaluation. *American Journal of Evaluation, 20*(1), 1–14.

Nunneley, R. D., Jr., Orton, R. E., & King, J. A. (1997, March). *Validating standards for action research.* Paper presented at the annual meeting of the American Educational Research Association, Chicago.

O'Campo, P., Xue, X., Wang, M.-C., & O'Brien-Caughy, M. (1997). Neighborhood risk factors for low birth weight in Baltimore: A multi-level analysis. *American Journal of Public Health, 87*(7), 1113–1118.

O'Fallon, L. R., & Dearry, A. (2002). Community-based participatory research as a tool to advance environmental health sciences. *Environmental Health Perspectives, 110*(2), 155–159.

Patton, M. Q. (1997). *Utilization-focused evaluation* (3rd ed.). Thousand Oaks, CA: Sage.

Roberts, E. M. (1997). Neighborhood social environments and the distribution of low birthweight in Chicago. *American Journal of Public Health, 87,* 597–603.

Rossi, P. H., Freeman, H. E., & Lipsey, M. W. (1999). *Evaluation: A systematic approach* (6th ed.). Thousand Oaks, CA: Sage.

Schulz, A. J. (1998). *Broome Team evaluation report.* Unpublished report of the Kellogg Foundation for the Community-Based Public Health Initiative, University of Michigan, Ann Arbor.

Schulz, A. J., Israel, B. A., & Lantz. P. (2003). Instrument for evaluating dimensions of group dynamics within community-based participatory research partnerships. *Evaluation and Program Planning, 26*(3).

Schulz, A. J., Israel, B. A., Selig, S. M., Bayer, I. S., & Griffin, C. B. (1998). Development and implementation of principles for community-based research in public health. In R. H. MacNair (Ed.), *Research strategies for community practice* (pp. 83–110). New York: Haworth Press.

Schwartz, R. M. (1994). *The skilled facilitator: Practical wisdom for developing effective groups.* San Francisco: Jossey-Bass.

Seashore, S. E., Lawler, E. E., III, Mirvis, P. H., & Cammann, C. (1983). *Assessing organizational change: A guide to methods, measures and practices.* New York: Wiley.

Shaw, M. E. (1981). *Group dynamics: The psychology of small group behavior* (3rd ed.). New York: McGraw-Hill.

Sofaer, S. (2000). *Working together, moving ahead: A manual to support effective community health coalitions.* City University of New York, Baruch College, School of Public Affairs.

Spencer, M. B., Cole, S. P., Jones, S. M., & Swanson, D. P. (1997). Neighborhood and family influences on young urban adolescents' behavior problems: A multisample, multisite analysis. In J. Brooks-Gunn, G. Duncan, & J. L. Aber (Eds.), *Neighborhood poverty, Volume 1* (pp. 200–218). New York: Russell Sage Foundation.

Steuart, G. (1975). The people: Motivation, education, and action. *Bulletin of the New York Academy of Medicine, 51*(1), 174–185.

Stokols, D. (1996). Translating social ecological theory into guidelines for community health promotion. *American Journal of Health Promotion, 10*(4), 282–298.

Tarlov, A. R., Kehrer, B. H., Hall, D. P., Samuels, S. E., Brown, G. S., Felix, M. R. J., & Ross, J. A. (1987). Foundation work: The health promotion program of the Henry J. Kaiser Family Foundation. *American Journal of Health Promotion, 2,* 74–80.

Wandersman, A., Florin, P. F., Friedman, R., & Meier, R. (1987). Who participates, who does not, and why? An analysis of voluntary neighborhood associations in the United States and Israel. *Sociological Forum, 2*(3), 534–555.

Williams, D. R., & Harris-Reid, M. (1999). Race and mental health: Emerging patterns and promising approaches. In A. V. Horwitz & T. L. Scheid (Eds.), *A handbook for the study of mental health: Social contexts, theories and systems* (pp. 295–314). New York: Cambridge University Press.

Yen, I. H., & Syme, S. L. (1999). The social environment and health: A discussion of the epidemiologic literature. *Annural Review of Public Health, 20,* 287–308.

Zander, A. (1982). *Making groups effective.* San Francisco: Jossey-Bass.

Chapter 19

Participatory Research, Popular Education, and Popular Theater

Contributions to Group Work

Janet L. Finn
Maxine Jacobson
Jillian Dean Campana

In this chapter we examine the relationship of participatory research and popular education to the theory and practice of group work. We consider their relationship to one another and to social work more broadly and then examine the ways in which both interweave and diverge in the history and practice of social work with groups. Although a number of social workers have argued the case for the compatibility of popular education and participatory research principles to social work, few have examined their fundamental connection to group work. We make this connection and argue its importance in enriching and expanding the possibilities of group work. We attend to the linkage of theory and practice and ongoing collective processes of reflection and action for transformation that provide the foundation for both popular education and participatory research (Freire, 1970, 1998a, 1998b; Lather, 1986). This intimate linkage is at the heart of social group work, as well. As we discuss later, social work has a rich, if somewhat hidden, history of engaging those affected by oppressive social conditions in group efforts to understand those conditions, probe their causes and consequences, and organize collective action for change. We highlight moments in that history and draw lessons from history to inform group work practice today.

We address the role performance plays in popular education and participatory research and its relationship to group process. By "performance" we mean conscious human interaction in theater and other social contexts. The literature on social group work offers celebratory examples of the use of performance to evoke feeling, provoke dialogue, and promote action (Halperin, 2001; Kaplan, 2001; Middleman, 1983). However, there has been very little attention to the group processes through which these significant interactions contribute to consciousness raising (conscientization), capacity building, and change.[1] We forge direct links here to the concept of *popular theater*, a form of popular education that employs the performing arts as a means of critical reflection and catalyst for action (Boal, 1985; Kraii, MacKenzie, & Youngman, 1979). The concept of "popular" as used in this context refers to people living in conditions of poverty, oppression, or exploitation.[2] We turn to the work of Brazilian theater theorist and practitioner Augusto Boal, a key figure in popular theater and founder of the international movement of *theatre of the oppressed*, to better understand the practice of popular theater. We explore its relationship to participatory research, popular education, and group work.

We summarize ways in which social workers and other advocates for social change are currently engaging with participatory research, popular education, and popular theater and highlight some exemplary case studies. We address generative themes that link participatory research, popular education, popular theater, and group work. We conclude with a brief consideration of the future directions and possibilities for group work informed by these creative and critical approaches.

This chapter is the product of our dialogue and co-learning. Two of us (J. F. and M. J.) are professors of social work and have been engaged in ongoing work on the place of participatory inquiry and action in bridging social work and social justice (Finn & Jacobson, 2003). One of us (J. D. C.) is a professor of drama, has extensive background in popular theater, and has been engaged in research and curriculum development regarding the role of theater in social change. We have been jointly exploring the exciting theoretical and practice possibilities that emerge in the dialogical space between social work and theater.

MAPPING THE TERRAIN

Participatory Research

Participatory research can be described as a collaborative approach to research that integrates systematic investigation with education and political action (Cancian & Armstead, 1990; Maguire, 1987; Sohng, 1992, 1996). Participatory research calls for the meaningful involvement of people in the coproduction of knowledge to address the concerns that affect their lives; it challenges the separation of researcher and "subject," and it takes power and inequality as central themes. Participatory research is a form of praxis involving critical reflection and dialogue, development of critical consciousness, and democratized processes of inquiry among participants (Brown, 1985; Brown & Tandon, 1983; Gaventa, 1988; Lather, 1986; Maguire, 1987) Participatory approaches to research question positivist assumptions of objectivity and value-free inquiry. Participatory researchers make values explicit, expose personal assumptions and perspectives, and openly contend with the ways these influence their choice of methods and modes of analysis. They strive for critical awareness of their own subjectivity in the research process (Finn, 1994; Lather, 1986, 1991; Maguire, 1987; Park, 1993, 1997; Sohng, 1992, 1996).

Popular Education

Popular education has been defined as a strategy for social change in which people struggling under conditions of oppression come together to critically question and reflect on the conditions of their lives; become conscious of the social, political, and economic contradictions in which their social experience is bound; and take action to transform their social reality (Freire, 1970, 1998a, 1998b; hooks, 1994; Weiler, 1988). It emerged as a grounded approach to adult literacy education through which people come to know the word through knowing the world (Freire, 1970, p. 13). Through dialogue with others, people connect their personal troubles to broader structural problems in society and strive to rectify these conditions through collective action. The educational process is one of becoming critically conscious of one's social reality, historical and political positioning, and human agency (Freire, 1970, 1998a, 1998b; Poertner, 1994). Similar to participatory research, popular education starts from the assumption that education is not neutral. Popular education cannot be reduced to method and technique. Rather, it is grounded in historical, cultural, and political contexts and shaped by their "ruptures and flows" (Heaney, 1995).

Popular Theater

As introduced previously, *popular theater* is a form of popular education that uses performance as a tool for dialogue, conscientization, and transformation. Popular theater is an educational process that is available to everyone and can be performed anywhere. It covers a wide range of theatrical activities, including drama, dance, puppetry, and song. These theatrical techniques engage people in examination of the issues that affect their lives, facilitate communication and interaction that spark awareness of collective oppression, and encourage development of viable strategies for action (Bates, 1996; Boal, 1985; Srikandath, 1991). The content of popular theater is created by the participants, not mandated by an outside force (Kraii et al., 1979). The goal of popular theater is to research and respond via participatory performance to the social, economic, cultural, and political conditions that have shaped people's lives (DeCosta, 1992). Boal's practice of *forum theatre* exemplifies this. The forum theater process generates a scripted play that explores an identifiable, yet unsolved problem. After the play is presented to the audience, it is discussed and presented again. During several subsequent performances, any audience member may stop the action and come on stage to replace the protagonist. When audience members are invited on stage to demonstrate their ideas, they are engaged in an empowering process of simultaneously imagining and practicing change. In forum theater, both performers and audience are what Boal terms "spect-actors," at once spectators and actors.

Unifying Themes

Participatory research, popular education, and popular theater are not simply methods or techniques but modes of inquiry and action with a common philosophical base and political commitment. They share the epistemological assumption that knowing is a "permanent human process, not an individual event but a social one, an historical one, a cultural one" (Freire, 1985, p. 11). Knowledge of the world is co-created through critical dialogue about lived experience in the world. Participatory research, popular education, and popular theater see knowledge as power and seek to democratize practices of knowledge production. They challenge hegemonic notions of "power over" and promote alternative forms of power—power within, power with, power to do—among people living in conditions of oppression (Townsend, Zapata, Rowlands, Alberti, & Mercado, 1999). They are transformative processes that recognize ordinary people as protagonists of knowledge development and change. In so doing, they blur the boundaries between researcher and researched, teacher and learner, and actor and audience.

Participatory research, popular education, and popular theater are fundamentally *group* processes through which participants problematize their social reality and build collective capacity to challenge and change that reality. They recognize the group aspects of oppression along particular axes of difference, such as race, class, gender, age, and citizenship. They utilize group processes of listening, dialogue, assessment, decision making, action, and reflection that engage participants and help create in the group both awareness and power to act (Carroll & Minkler, 2000; Freire, 1970, 1998a; Poertner, 1994). They acknowledge the power of oppression to produce isolation and alienation. In response, they emphasize practices of mutual aid, trust building, crafting of group solidarity, and honoring of difference.

HISTORICAL PERSPECTIVE

As instruments of social change, participatory research, popular education, and popular theater developed from conditions of social, economic, and political discontent. A historical perspective is helpful in understanding these approaches and appreciating their political and ethical grounding.

Participatory Research

Historians of participatory research find the first use of the term in Tanzania in the early 1970s (Hall, 1981). A number of writers have linked the beginnings of the participatory research tradition to work with oppressed peoples in Latin America, Africa, and Asia, often in response to exploitative development projects and policies (Brown & Tandon, 1983; Hall, 1981; Maguire, 1987; Tandon, 1981). Hall (1981) contends, however, that long before participatory research was named, its principles and practices could be traced to early social investigations conducted by Engels (1968) and Marx in the mid-1800s and to the contributions of John Dewey, George Herbert Mead, and scholars of the Tavistock Institute in London who challenged positivist approaches to knowledge production.

Social work was also an early forerunner in participatory research methods, although this information has generally been erased from the social work canon. At the turn of the 20th century, settlement house workers teamed up with neighborhood residents to conduct investigations that linked research with social reform (Addams, 1910). Collectively, they investigated social conditions that plagued the working-class, immigrant-community residents and sought to influence policy makers by publicly displaying the results. In *Twenty Years at Hull House*, Jane Addams (1910) reflects on an investigation conducted by a group of neighborhood mothers. After Hull House residents presented them with the connection between sanitation conditions and high infant mortality rates in their neighborhood, the mothers set out to "carefully investigate the condition of the alleys" (Addams, 1910, p. 284). Ultimately, their efforts promoted systematic garbage removal, decreased infant death rates, and paved the way for other social investigations.

Social work research originated in the survey movement that began around the turn of the 20th century and gained momentum through settlement houses and their intimate connection to neighborhood conditions and concerns (O'Connor, 2002; Zimbalist, 1977). Social surveys were an integral component of community organizing, social work with groups, advocacy, and social reform (Malekoff, 1994; Wagner, 1991). Speaking about the Pittsburgh survey and its methodology, Paul Kellogg (1914, p. 492) remarked, "The staff included not only trained investigators—housing inspectors, sanitarians, lawyers, engineers, labor experts, and the like—but members of the immigrant races who make up so large a share of the working population."

Popular Education

Scholars often cite the work of Brazilian educator Paulo Freire and Latin American social movements of the 1960s and 1970s as a starting point for discussions of popular education. Freire developed his educational philosophy and practice through his 30 years of literacy work with impoverished people in Brazil. Freire's best-known work, *Pedagogy of the Oppressed* (1970), is a treatise on the philosophy and practice of popular education. The book received international recognition and created the basis from which others have sought to critique formal educational practices. Following its translation into numerous languages and its dissemination around the globe, *Pedagogy of the Oppressed* was widely discussed in the 1970s by academics, community organizers, educators, and politicians. At the same time, it was banned and burned in countries with authoritarian governments fearful of its implications, that is, that ordinary people have important knowledge to share and must be given a voice in the educational process (Schugurensky, 1998).

Although Freire's work is certainly the most well known, forms of popular education have evolved independently and created the momentum for social movements around the globe (Hurst, 1995). For example, roots of popular education can be found in the Danish folk school movement and the work of Nikolai Frederik Severin Grundtvig, a theologian, educator, and writer, who in the early 1880s fought against German imperialists who were attempting to eradicate the language and culture of the Danish people. Grundtvig struggled to retain the cultural identity of his people by promoting what he called "schools for life," in which ordinary people used their own language and collectively developed their own capacities to address problems of everyday living (Kohl, 1991, p. 40).

Danish folk school philosophy and practice spread to countries in Europe and distant continents initially through what Toiviainen (1995, p. 6) calls "traveler's tales," stories brought home about educational possibilities in other countries. This was certainly the case with the Highlander Folk School in Monteagle, Tennessee, founded in 1932 by community organizer and educator Myles Horton and several of his friends.[3] Discontent with the traditional educational system—namely, its failure to recognize and make use of the existing knowledge and experience of learners—Horton explored alternative educational structures. His quest led to Hull House in Chicago, where he visited Jane Addams and discussed the early days of the settlement house movement, and to Denmark in 1931, where he learned about the Danish folk school movement. Frank Adams (1972) recounts how Horton found his explorations wanting. Although he relished the early history of the settlement house movement and the Danish folk school, he found that their present operations had "lost their initial vitality and sense of purpose" (p. 501). Throughout his life, Horton insisted that Highlander was modeled after the people who came there to learn and teach others and that "education must come from the people and the situations they confront in their everyday lives" (Adams, 1972, p. 42). Given Horton's philosophy of "education growing out of the people" (Horton, 1999), Highlander has continued to transform itself throughout its 70–year history (Park, Brydon-Miller, Hall, & Jackson, 1993).

Popular education continues to be a key strategy for community change among oppressed peoples throughout the world. Its principles have informed empowering social work practice in diverse cultural and political contexts (see, for example, Bock, 1980; Brigham,

1977; Carroll & Minkler, 2000). However, its potential for informing and engaging social work, especially group work, has only begun to be tapped.

Popular Theater

It is difficult to locate precisely when and where theater became an instrument of social change. Performance is deeply woven into human cultural experience, as evidenced in collective ceremony and ritual (Turner, 1969). Diverse forms of performance have served as vehicles for promoting empowerment, creating and sustaining community, and enabling artist and audience to express emotion and thought. Popular theater likely emerged from these types of community performance, and it has continued to be shaped by political and social contexts. Western examples include the French Revolution and powerful leaders such as Boissy d'Anglas, who viewed theater as a strategy for political consciousness raising (Van Erven, 1988), and 19th-century German theater, which sought to be a "powerful stimulus to thinking about the great topics of the day" (Davies, 1977, as quoted in Van Erven, 1988, p. 9). More recent examples include political street theater, such as the radical American group, The Living Theatre, created by Judith Malina and Julian Beck in the 1950s, and the Vermont-based Bread and Puppet Theater, started by Peter Schumann in 1961. Schumann's goal was to unite communities through theater; fresh-baked bread was often shared with audiences during the performance.

Augusto Boal took the concept of popular theater further, making it truly theater *by* the people and *for* the people. Boal's Theatre of the Oppressed, named after Freire's *Pedagogy of the Oppressed* and incorporating its principles, uses the medium of popular theater as a tool for creating knowledge and initiating transformation among people living in conditions of poverty and oppression (Bates, 1996).[4] Participants make connections between their personal plights and structural inequalities and create realistic strategies for transformative action (Boal, 1985).

Augusto Boal participated in theater all his life, but it was not until he completed his doctorate in chemical engineering at Columbia University and returned to his native Brazil to become the artistic director of the Arena Theatre in São Paulo that he began to experiment with new forms of popular theater. In the 1960s Boal adapted a process whereby audience members could stop a performance to suggest alternative scenarios for the actors to carry out. In a now infamous production, a woman in the audience became frustrated that an actor could not understand her suggestion, and she came up on stage and entered the dramatic fiction to show the actor what she meant. This marked the birth of forum theater, which readily became incorporated into Boal's repertoire of techniques.

Popular theater has been embraced as part of many people's movements and grassroots change efforts. It is a mode of collective inquiry and action that remains largely foreign to social work.

Relationship to Group Work History

Group work was born from the same social, political, and economic conditions of discontent as participatory research, popular education, and popular theater. Andrews (2001), quoting Judith Lee (1991, p. 3), states that, "From its beginnings, group work practice and theory has been rooted in social reform, social responsibility, democratic ideals, and social action as well as social relatedness and human attachment." Group work at the turn of the 20th century was a product of humanitarian, democratic ideals that immigrated to the United States as intact, historical aspects of particular cultures. Jewish people, for example, formed groups founded on the principles of democracy to preserve culture and insure that oppressive regimes would have little room to grow in the new country.

Group work was also shaped by the tensions and contradictions of industrial capitalism, immigration, and urbanization. These shifts, accompanied by changing labor practices, low wages, poor living conditions, and fears of "difference," had profound effects on the family life, interpersonal relations, and physical and mental health of poor and working-class people. Groups were a haven amid this sea change. They provided security, support, and some semblance of stability through self-help, recreation, and informal education in immigrant centers, settlement houses, camps, and labor organizations (Andrews, 2001, p. 47). This same sense of collectivism was the dynamic that motivated group efforts at participatory research, popular education, and popular theater.

Unfortunately, as group work became incorporated into the field of social work, with its growing interest in professionalization, the focus on political commitment was overshadowed by a therapeutic, person-changing orientation. Group work as a strategy for participatory knowledge development, community building, and social change receded to the background as social work claimed an identity premised on professional helping and the "depoliticizing" of practice.

LEARNING FROM CONTEMPORARY PRACTICE

In recent years there has been a rekindling of interest in popular education and participatory research among progressive social workers. Perhaps this is a reflection of the struggles critical practitioners face as we grapple with the contradictions of social work practice in the face of globalization and its social consequences. Proponents point to the fundamental compatibility with the stated mission, philosophy, and values of social work and question the profession's drift from this foundation. For example, social workers articulating empowerment theory and practice have sought inspiration from Freire (Gutiérrez, 1990; Gutiérrez & Lewis, 1999; Lee, 1991; Simon, 1994). Carroll and Minkler (2000) argue that Freirian nonformal education and group methods, with emphasis on overcoming alienation, respecting culture, and orientation to change, resonate with the core historical, theoretical, and methodological underpinnings of social work. They address the compatibility of popular education with group and community practice and offer examples from diverse practice contexts (see, for example, Breton, 1989; Lee, 1991; Mann, 1987; Parsons, 1991; Sachs, 1991; Wallerstein, 1992). They note the significance of the shared teacher–learner role and the centrality of group process in developing mutual trust, dialogue, and individual and collective capacity. Similarly, Poertner (1994) addresses key themes of popular education drawn from South American contexts—cultural grounding, political intention, and bottom-up methodology—and argues their relevance for social group work in the North. Feminists have examined the common philosophical underpinnings of popular education, participatory research, and feminist methodology with emphasis on consciousness of collective oppression, power and inequality, everyday life experience, and political commitment and their significance for social work (Finn, 1994; Figueira-McDonough, Netting, & Nicols-Casebolt, 1998; Gutiérrez & Lewis, 1999; Maguire, 1987).

Over the past decade, a number of social work writers have specifically addressed the promise and limitations of participatory research and its compatibility with the philosophy and values of social work (Altpeter, Schopler, Galinsky, & Pennell, 1999; Alvarez & Gutiérrez, 2001; Carroll & Minkler, 2000; Finn, 1994; Healy, 2001; Sarri & Sarri, 1992; Sohng, 1992, 1996). Some social workers have turned to participatory methods in their practice with groups and communities (see, for example, Alvarez & Gutiérrez, 2001; Healy & Walsh, 1997; Malekoff, 1994; Mathrani, 1993; Sarri & Sarri, 1992; Sohng, 1992, 1996; Wagner, 1991). They have utilized citizen surveys, community forums, and focus groups involving those affected as coresearchers in program development, evaluation, and advocacy (Sarri & Sarri, 1992; Sen, 1994; Yeich, 1996). They have shown the capacity of historically marginalized groups to identify and collectivize problems, envision alternatives and name solutions, and advocate for systemic change (Gaventa, 1998; Gutiérrez, 1990; Johnson, Ivan-Smith, Gordon, Pridmore, & Scott, 1998; Maguire, 1987; Minkler, 1997; Sen, 1994). They have addressed challenges of team building, negotiation of power and difference, strategies for community ownership and oversight of the research, and possibilities for co-learning (Alvarez & Gutiérrez, 2001; Townsend et al., 1999).

Proponents of participatory methods also pose cautions. They note that participatory approaches are demanding in terms of time, resources, and energy (Alvarez & Gutiérrez, 2001; Healy, 2001; Sarri & Sarri, 1992). They recognize that participation does not necessarily result in empowerment and that power differences among participants need to be recognized and addressed on an ongoing basis (Finn, 1994; Healy, 2001; Whitmore & Wilson, 1997). They challenge romanticized notions of "the people" and "the community" and call attention to the need for ongoing negotiation of questions of meaning, power, and difference. Feminist researchers, in particular, have drawn attention to the gendered dimensions of power that need to be addressed in collective processes of investigation, education, and action (Gutiérrez, 1990; Gutiérrez & Lewis, 1999; Maguire, 1987; Townsend et al., 1999; Weiler, 1988). Proponents are also sensitive to the difficulties in engaging groups with long histories of oppression in processes of change. These processes threaten dominant interests and power relations and may pose very real risks to the participants. There are very few examples of the use of popular theater in the social work literature. Social workers have addressed the role of play and performance as components of group work (Halperin, 2001; Kaplan, 2001). Adult educators and community practitioners outside of social work have discussed the incorporation of popular theater in their change efforts (Hammond, 1999; Valla, 1994). Boal's *Legislative Theatre* (1998) has provided concrete evidence of the use of popular theater to change social policy. Legislative theater is a type of forum theater in which participants research social issues they want addressed and use performance as a means of education and advocacy. For example, the first law approved with the aid of legislative theater maintains that all municipal hospitals in Rio de Janeiro must have doctors on staff who specialize in geriatric health. Until this law went into effect in 1995, virtually no hospital in the city employed specialists in geriatrics. It is only in the recent contributions of Trevor Spratt, Stan Houston, Mark McCollum, and Tom Magill (Houston, Magill, McCollum, & Spratt, 2001; Spratt, Houston, & Magill, 2000) that we see a careful, in-depth articulation of the theoretical and practical relationship among popular theater, participatory research, and social work and the possibilities therein. We include their work among the case examples discussed in this chapter.

We focus here on a few select examples of participatory research, popular education, and popular theater that illustrate both the potential and the challenges for group work and community practice. We highlight themes and principles of practice that emerge from these examples. In closing, we suggest future directions for group work informed by this nexus of participatory research, popular education, and popular theater.

CHILDREN AND POPULAR THEATER

The Philippine Educational Theatre Association (PETA), founded in 1967, shares a vision of theater as a tool and a process that enables the development of people and society. PETA has initiated numerous theater groups and networks that operate, for example, in schools, entire communities, and migrant groups. PETA sees itself as an active part of a national theater movement whose vision is "nationhood, global understanding, respect for persons, democratization and greater participation of the people in theatre, culture and social change" (Cloma, 1998, p. 106).

One of PETA's drama groups is the Children's Theatre Collective, a group of artists and teachers who specialize in children's theater and whose vision concerns the development of the Filipino child. The group trains adults and children in how to produce children's plays with children as the actors. The process begins by consulting with an organization that wants to solve a problem that relates to the well-being of children or to their concerns regarding the community. Children are consulted on their interpretation of the issue. Next, the topic is researched, and relevant data is gathered to promote a deeper understanding of the issue. Children then weave together the story of the issue and create a play that may include singing, dancing, and other forms of visual representation in an effort to breathe life into the story for a developed theater production. The process combines fun and the development of new skills with the analysis of social problems. Cloma (1998) describes how a similar process was used to assist children from the Subanam tribe who had identified mercury pollution in the river as a key source of illness in their community. As they moved through the stages of the process, children interviewed elders in the community to arrive at a story and dramatic methods to represent the story back to the community. First children performed their play for the village people, and then they presented it at the municipal board meeting. The process is both empowering to individual participants and to the larger community.

GRASSROOTS RESEARCH WITH HOMELESS PEOPLE

Susan Yeich's (1996) case study of a Homeless Union project illustrates the linkage of participatory research and popular education. The project's goal was to empower homeless people in Lansing, Michigan, in struggles to fight homelessness in their community. The outcome of the research process was the formation of a union for and of homeless people, which, after 3 years, grew to include 350 people.

In describing how the union formed, Yeich breaks the process down into three components—research, education, and action. The research component consisted of gathering secondary data on the topic of homelessness, reviewing information, and bringing it back to the group for discussion. The education component was divided into three subparts: "creation of common knowledge, transfer of knowledge to the people, and development of critical awareness" (Yeich, 1996, p. 117). Forming the union brought people together to share their experiences of homelessness and the influence of poverty on their lives. In her role as advisor, Yeich shared her knowledge about unions and their formation. Participants, in turn, decided to form their own union. Developing critical awareness, in this case, meant linking structural forces with causes of poverty. Yeich describes how the development of critical awareness was a natural by-product of the investigative process, that is, learning more about the conditions that shape homelessness and learning from other participants through group interaction. The social action component evolved gradually over the course of the research process. The union and its membership took action to address cuts in social programs initiated by a new governor. Union members demonstrated, networked with other groups to form a more powerful base for change, and educated other citizens about the need to come to action.

Mujeres Unidas en Acción is a community-based program focusing on the education and empowerment of poor Latina women living in Dorchester, Massachusetts. The organization began as a low-income housing initiative in 1979. However, as organizers came to see the ways in which language barriers reinforced the oppression of immigrant Latina women in the area, they began a process of organizational transformation through ongoing dialogue, reflection, and action—responding to women's expressed concerns. Young and Padilla (1990) describe *Mujeres Unidas en Acción* as a "social incubator" dedicated to advocacy, skills sharing, capacity building, and community organizing by and for poor women of color.

Their literacy programs are grounded in a participatory approach to education and organization building wherein the curriculum emerges from women's expressed needs. Literacy is viewed as a right that the women, by virtue of gender, poverty, and citizenship, have been largely denied. Literacy education is culturally grounded, focusing first on literacy in the women's native Spanish and then in English. At *Mujeres Unidas en Acción*, literacy education is a group process in which women come together to name internal and structural oppressions, identify common experiences of oppression in their everyday lives, and find voice for their feelings and opinions in a context of safety and support. The group process of support and action is reproduced throughout the organization. In addition to literacy groups, *Mujeres Unidas en Acción* also sponsors support groups for battered women, minicourses and workshops, and forums on issues that affect women's lives. Moreover, *Mujeres* has adopted a collective administrative structure in which program participants have a meaningful role in organizational decision making.

Mujeres Unidas en Acción has specifically incorporated forum theater as part of their praxis. Women have used forum theater to tackle themes such as AIDS, violence, sexual identity, and the meaning of education in their lives. Participants have found the experience of dramatizing their problems, engaging as "spect-actors," and envisioning alternative possibilities to be personally and collectively empowering. *Mujeres* organizational praxis has effectively incorporated participatory research, popular education, and popular theater as mutually informing processes for individual, group, and organizational empowerment.

FORUM THEATER: COMMUNITY EMPLOYMENT PROJECT

Tom Magill, founding member and a current director of Creative Training Solutions in the United Kingdom, uses the methodology of *Theatre of the Oppressed* to " . . . offer social workers new ways of working that link critical analysis and creative expression" (Houston et al., 2001; Spratt et al., 2000). In December of 2000, Magill and Mark McCollum, coordinator of the Community Arts Company, worked on the government-funded Community Employment Project, which sought to reach poor, unemployed communities in rural Donegal County, Ireland. Their goal was "to use theatre as a means of enabling socially and economically marginalized communities to participate in wider society through a realization of their social and economic potential" (Houston, Magill, McCollum, & Spratt, 2001, p. 287). Magill and McCollum facilitated the group process by helping the project participants uncover common experiences of oppression and by offering the forum theater process as a method in which to work toward achieving critical consciousness.

The original project participants were unemployed adults and nonactors, and although their life experiences differed, through group dialogue it was revealed that they all shared the common experience of being bullied. The group chose to metaphorically replicate their adult experiences by locating the dramatic action of the forum in childhood, especially as the play was to be performed for Donegal County schools. Together the participants worked to create characters and a story line that displayed their shared experience of oppression to which their audience could relate. The result was a forum theater play in which a child seeks ways to join a group at school but is prevented from doing so by a bully. In the play the child turns to both his mother and father, who each offer inappropriate solutions to the problem. The bully convinces the child's class to steal his book bag, which contains his homework, and when the teacher discovers what has happened, she blames the entire class, punishing all of them. This action further victimizes the child because the class now views him as the reason they are in trouble. The play ends with the class physically beating up the child, after which one final action occurs: a prospective ally arrives in the form of a classmate who returns the stolen book bag to the victim.

In the school performances, the audience was informed that the play was not finished and that they would have to help write the ending. After watching the original story unfold, the audience was then transformed into spect-actors, and a variety of possible solutions to the protagonist's problem were offered and enacted by the schoolchildren. By becoming spect-actors, the audience of schoolchildren and the adult performers recognized that they were not alone in their oppression and, as a united group, they were then able to conduct their own research and then to use that research to "rehearse for reality," as Boal would say.

Spratt, Houston, and Magill (2000) have taken their pioneering work further to demonstrate the potential for cross-disciplinary work in social work, theater, and cultural studies. For example, they have utilized popular theater to engage social work students and practitioners in grappling with the contradictions in child protective service work and in envisioning positive and realistic strategies for change. They specifically speak to interrelated group practices of trust building, imaging, and sculpting through which participants identify and analyze oppressive bureaucratic structures and their dehumanizing effects and craft images of a child welfare system in which citizenship is fully enacted (Houston et al., 2001, p. 291).

GENERATIVE THEMES FOR PRACTICE

These examples share a number of common principles and practices that resonate with the unifying themes outlined previously. In the spirit of popular education, we highlight these as *generative themes* that speak to the mutually informing possibilities of participatory knowledge development, action, and group work.

1. *Linking culture, power, and history* (Dirks, Eley, & Ortner, 1994). These examples reflect an appreciation for the specific cultural, political, and historical contexts of human experience and for people's capacities as interpreters of their social reality. They recognize the structural forces that shape oppression, inequality, and subjectivity and the power of human agency to make and transform history.

2. *Dialogue.* Knowledge for action emerges through dialogue. Freire describes dialogue as an act of humility and love. Boal defines dialogue as the basic rule of humanity. Monologue, he argues, is the definition of oppression. In participatory processes we constitute ourselves as social beings and our knowledge of the social world through dialogue. As these examples illustrate, meaningful dialogue begins with listening to one another's stories, creating common knowledge, and drawing from that collective knowledge to weave together a larger story. Honest dialogue is a necessary condition for building relationships, and relationships must precede problem solving (Coughlan & Collins, 2001).

3. *Conscientization.* As people come together to create a collective story, they are better able to problematize their social reality, investigate the forces and conditions that shape their experience, and thus develop critical consciousness. In contexts of support, people are able to identify common experiences of oppression and express the ways in which they embody and live personal and structural contradictions. Conscientization also entails recognizing the possibility of alternative realities informed by an alternative common sense.

4. *Praxis.* The practice of reflection and action on the world in order to transform it is a recursive process of being, doing, and becoming (Kelly & Sewell, 1988). The concept of *performance* captures the dynamic fusion of awareness, embodiment, and movement that praxis entails. Praxis is an intellectual, aesthetic, and kinesthetic process—the joining of heads, hearts, and hands. This holistic engagement sustains and supports participation and organization.

5. *Transformation.* Finally, these participatory endeavors are fundamentally transformative in their intent. They challenge participants to move beyond the familiar, engage with ambiguity and uncertainty, talk back to hegemonic truths, and grapple with contradiction. The examples seek lasting, concrete change and see personal and social transformation as mutually constituting parts of the process. They speak of social incubators, organizations, and movements—the collective means for realizing transformative possibility. They speak to a geography of participation in which people come together in conscious action to transform sites of oppression into spaces of hope, places of relationship, and bases of action (Harvey, 2000; Kelly & Sewell, 1988).

FUTURE DIRECTIONS AND POSSIBILITIES

The linkages among participatory research, popular education, popular theater, and social group work expand and enrich future directions and possibilities for social work practice. In this section, we discuss a number of ways in which their interconnections open up new thought and practice in social work.

Blurring the Boundaries

The profession has much to gain from making disciplinary connections between social work and theater. The work of Spratt, Houston, and Magill (2000) and Houston, Magill, McCollum, and Spratt (2001), mentioned in an earlier case study, illustrates how forum theater can help child protection workers uncover the contradictions of their work, problematize those practices they take for granted, and understand better the standpoints of key players in the process. Their work prompts us to ask, "How might group work practice be transformed by opening a space for dialogue between social work and theater?" "How might we reconceptualize practice through the lens of performance?" For example, William Schwartz (1994) describes rehearsal as an integral part of the group process wherein participants try out new interactions in the safety of the group. In forum theater, we see the concept of rehearsal developed further. Participants not only rehearse the way things ought to be but also they create a dramatization of the way they are and of their vision for the future. Rehearsal speaks to the potential for multiple solutions sought through a collective process. Participants more fully experience their predicament and potential solutions, and group members learn vicariously from the work of others.

Houston et al. (2001, p. 286) encourage social workers to embark on the "messy and indeterminate nature" of theory in action projects and, thus, to bring creative thought to the integration of Boal's methodology with the practice of social work. They stress the commonalities between his work with socially marginalized people and social work. Furthermore, they remind us that social workers have basic group work practice skills that can be enhanced through Boal's techniques of democratic problem solving. We propose that social work can be "enlightened and enlivened" (Williams, 1996) by incorporating popular theater, thus bringing "it closer to the lifeworld of disadvantaged communities" (Houston et al., 2001, p. 292).

Rethinking Roles of Social Workers in Group Work

The philosophy and practice of participatory research, popular education, and popular theater challenge us to reconsider the roles of the social worker in supporting group processes for consciousness raising and transformative action. We briefly develop three roles—animator, *bricoleur*, and joker—that we see as central to group and community practice that is grounded in the values, philosophy, and political commitment of popular, participatory approaches.

The concept of animator "stresses the individual as a shaper of his or her own destiny" (Reisch, Wenocur, & Sherman, 1981, p. 115). The animator seeks to sustain action through facilitative skills that recognize the power of groups coming together to create change. The ultimate goal of animation is the liberation or empowerment of oppressed and marginalized people or groups. Thus the social worker as animator acts as a catalyst to spark consciousness that informs action and to facilitate the social relations and material conditions that enable people to act. Animators open up possibilities for meaningful participation; pose critical questions; coach participants through the processes of risk taking, skill building, and rehearsal; and validate their contributions. Animators do not impose problem definitions and directions for action. Rather, they encourage and nurture people's critical reflection on their own reality, validate the wisdom of lived experiences, and help people envision and plan their own journeys.

French anthropologist Claude Levi-Strauss defined a *bricoleur* as a "Jack of all trades or a kind of professional do-it-yourself person" (Levi-Strauss, 1966, p. 17, as cited in Denzin & Lincoln, 1994, p. 2). He saw people as *bricoleurs*, that is, cultural beings with the wherewithal, imagination, and sense of discovery and possibility needed to adapt and transform human and material resources in response to new challenges. We find the image of the *bricoleur* helpful in imagining the transformed role of the social worker engaged in the participatory process of investigation, education, and action. The role of *bricoleur* speaks to the creative, contextual, and culturally grounded practice of participatory, justice-oriented group and community work. The *bricoleur* is in ongoing engagement with other participants and with the resources and circumstances at hand to expand spaces of hope and invent new possibilities for action. Through participatory processes of education and action, the social worker also encourages participants to see themselves as *bricoleurs* and to engage accordingly. The practice of popular theater is, in effect, a practice of *bricolage*. Participants literally sculpt their vision of existing realities and possible alternatives. Drawing from the collective wisdom of the group, they reframe problems and possibilities and create new meanings from the resources at hand.

In the Theatre of the Oppressed, the master of ceremonies is known as the "joker." "The term derives from the joker (or wild card) in a deck of playing cards; just as the wild card is not tied down to a specific suit or value, neither is the Theatre of the Oppressed joker tied down to an allegiance to performer, spectator, or to any interpretation of events" (Schutzman & Cohen-Cruz, 1994, p. 237). When assisting the participants in the creation of plays or short workshop scenes, the joker does not mandate content, narrate story, or offer solutions; rather, she or he facilitates dialogue by providing a process and by encouraging the participants to think critically about the nature of the situation illustrated. The joker serves as the link between actors and spectators, providing commentary for the unfolding drama and inviting response and intervention. A joker avoids actions and statements that could sway or manipulate the participants' conclusions and subsequent actions. The job of the joker is to smooth the participants' progress and to keep the group on the track toward achieving critical consciousness. This characteristic of the Theatre of the Oppressed can be utilized outside of the theatrical arena; the joker can serve as a model for social workers interested in working with groups to facilitate participatory processes of planning, rehearsal, and action.

Centrality of Group Work to Social Work

As Gutiérrez, Reed, Ortega, and Lewis (1998) discuss, group work is critical to a transformative practice. Throughout this chapter we have argued that participatory research, popular education, and popular theater are fundamentally group processes that embrace social work's commitment to social justice and create possibilities for social transformation. We contend that the practice of group and community work can be strengthened through ongoing critical engagement with these possibilities. As Lewis (1988, p. 217) articulates, community work is group work, and group work is the location "in which the integration of personal and social foci can take place." We have the knowledge and resources at hand to claim the best of social work's history and revitalize the practice of group and community work in dialogue with others. To do so, we must move outside our comfort zones, stretch the boundaries of our professional knowledge base, and become engaged learners. Can we muster the courage, will, and humility to transform our practice and ourselves in the process?

NOTES

1. We note two exceptional articles that explicitly address the potential contributions of popular theater to social work (Houston, Magill, McCollum & Spratt, 2001; Spratt, Houston & Magill, 2000). We elaborate on their work later in this chapter.
2. The notion of "popular education" is not the same as "community education." Rather it means "of the people" and refers to those of the oppressed classes. The term as used by Boal and others draws on a Marxist understanding of class conflict and refers to those who sell their labor. We employ the broader interpretation of members of oppressed groups.

3. Myles Horton is rarely discussed in the social work literature, but his influence on generations of social activists outside the boundaries of social work provides inspiration and lessons for practice today. Horton's autobiography, *The Long Haul*, chronicles his life and the influences that guided his philosophy on education and life in general. It is important to note that Paulo Freire and Myles Horton were contemporaries. Their "talking book"(a transcription of their conversations) *We Make the Road By Walking* provides insights on the intersections and the divergences in their backgrounds and their educational philosophies and practices.

4. Like Freire, Boal was persecuted for the radical idea that common people could have a say about the issues that affect their lives. Both men were exiled during Brazil's military dictatorship. They continued to develop the possibilities of popular education and popular theater, taking their ideas to an international audience.

REFERENCES

Adams, F. (1972). Highlander Folk School: Getting information, going back and teaching it. *Harvard Educational Review*, 42(4), 497–520.

Addams, J. (1910). *Twenty years at Hull House.* New York: Crowell/Macmillan.

Altpeter, M., Schopler, J., Galinsky, M., & Pennell, J. (1999). Participatory research as social work practice: When is it viable? *Journal of Progressive Human Services*, 10(2), 31–53.

Alvarez, A., & Gutiérrez, L. (2001). Choosing to do participatory research: An example and issues of fit to consider. *Journal of Community Practice*, 9(1), 1–19.

Andrews, J. (2001). Group work's place in social work: A historical analysis. *Journal of Sociology and Social Welfare*, 28(4), 45–65.

Bates, R. (1996). Popular theatre: A useful process for adult educators. *Adult Education Quarterly*, 46(4), 224–236.

Bell, B., Gaventa, J., & Peters, J. (Eds.). (1990). *We make the road by walking. Myles Horton and Paulo Freire: Conversations on education and social change.* Philadelphia: Temple University Press.

Boal, A. (1985). *The theatre of the oppressed.* New York: Theatre Communications Groups.

Boal, A. (1992). *Games for actors and nonactors.* New York: Routledge.

Boal, A. (1998). *Legislative theatre.* New York: Routledge.

Bock, S. (1980). Conscientization: Paulo Freire and class-based practice. *Catalyst*, 6, 5–25.

Breton, M. (1989). The need for mutual aid groups in a drop-in homeless shelter for homeless women: The sistering case. In J. A. B. Lee (Ed.), *Group work with the poor and oppressed* (pp. 47–59). New York: Hawthorn.

Brigham, T. (1977). Liberation in social work education: Applications from Paulo Freire. *Journal of Education for Social Work*, 13(3), 5–11.

Brown, L. D. (1985). People-centered development and participatory research. *Harvard Educational Review*, 55, 69–75.

Brown, L. D., & Tandon, R. (1983). Ideology and political economy in inquiry: Action research and participatory research. *Journal of Applied Behavioral Science*, 19, 277–294.

Cancian, F., & Armstead, C. (1990). *Participatory research: An introduction.* Unpublished manuscript, University of California at Irvine.

Carroll, J., & Minkler, M. (2000). Freire's message for social workers: Looking back, looking ahead. *Journal of Community Practice*, 8(1), 21–36.

Cloma, E. (1998). The Children's Theatre Collective of Philippine Educational Theatre Association. In V. Johnson, E. Ivan-Smith, G. Gordon, P. Pridmore, & P. Scott (Eds.), *Stepping forward: Children and young people's participation in the development process* (pp. 105–109). London: Intermediate Technology.

Coughlan, F., & Collins, K. (2001). Participatory development research: A working model. *International Social Work*, 44(4), 505–518.

Davies, C. (1977). *Theatre for the people: The story of the Volksbuhne.* Austin, TX: University of Texas Press.

De Costa, E. (1992). *Collaborative Latin American popular theater.* New York: Peter Lang.

Denzin, N., & Lincoln, Y. (Eds.). (1994). *Handbook of qualitative research.* Thousand Oaks, CA: Sage.

Dirks, N., Eley, G., & Ortner, S. (1994). *Culture/power/history: A reader in contemporary social theory* (pp. 3–45). Princeton, NJ: Princeton University Press.

Engels, F. (1968). *The condition of the working class in England.* Stanford, CA: Stanford University Press.

Figueira-McDonough, J., Netting, F. E., & Nichols-Casebolt, A. (Eds.). (1998). *The role of gender in practice knowledge: Claiming half the human experience.* New York: Garland.

Finn, J. (1994). The promise of participatory research. *Journal of Progressive Human Services, 5,* 25–42.

Finn, J., & Jacobson, M. (2003). *Just practice: A social justice approach to social work.* Peosta, IA: Eddie Bowers.

Freire, P. (1970). *Pedagogy of the oppressed* (M. B. Ramos, Trans.). New York: Seabury/Continuum. (Original work published 1968)

Freire, P. (1985). The social worker's role in the process of change. In P. Freire, *The politics of education* (pp. 36–41). South Hadley, MA: Bergin-Garvey.

Freire, P. (1998a). The adult literacy process as cultural action for freedom. *Harvard Educational Review, 68*(4), 480–498.

Freire, P. (1998b). Cultural action and conscientization. *Harvard Educational Review, 68*(4), 499–521.

Gaventa, J. (1988). Participatory research in North America. *Convergence, 21,* 19–29.

Gutiérrez, L. (1990). Working with women of color: An empowerment perspective. *Social Work, 35,* 149–153.

Gutiérrez, L., & Lewis, E. (1999). *Empowering women of color.* New York: Columbia University Press.

Gutiérrez, L., Reed, B., Ortega, R., & Lewis, E. (1998). Teaching about groups in a gendered world: Toward curricular transformation in group work education. In J. Figueira-McDonough, F. E. Netting, & A. Nichols-Casebolt (Eds.), *The role of gender in practice knowledge* (pp. 169–204). New York: Garland.

Hall, B. (1981). Participatory research, popular knowledge and power: A personal reflection. *Convergence, 14*(3), 6–19.

Halperin, D. (2001). The play's the thing: How social group work and theatre transformed a group into a community. *Social Work with Groups, 24*(2), 27–46.

Hammond, J. (1999). Popular education as community organization in El Salvador. *Latin American Perspectives, 26,* 69–94.

Harvey, D. (2000). *Spaces of hope.* Berkeley: University of California Press.

Healy, K. (2001). Participatory action research and social work: A critical appraisal. *International Social Work, 44*(1), 93–105.

Healy, K., & Walsh, K. (1997). Making participatory processes visible: Practice issues in the development of a peer support network. *Australian Social Work, 50,* 45–52.

Heaney, T. (1995). When adult education stood for democracy *Adult Education Quarterly.* Retrieved April 16, 1998, from: *http://nlu.nl.edu/ace/Resources/Documents/AEQ-Highlander.html.*

hooks, b. (1994). *Teaching to transgress: Education as the practice of freedom.* New York: Routledge.

Horton, M. (1999) *The long haul.* New York: Teacher's College Press.

Houston, S., Magill, T., McCollum, M., & Spratt, T. (2001). Developing creative solutions to the problems of children and their families: Communicative reason and the use of forum theatre. *Child and Family Social Work, 6,* 285–293.

Hurst, J. (1995). Popular education. *Education and Social Change, 9*(1), 1–9. Retrieved February, 2002, from: *http://www-gse.berkeley.eud/Admin/ExtRel/educator/spring95texts/popular.educ.html.*

Kaplan, C. (2001). The purposeful use of performance in groups: A new look at the balance of task and process. *Social Work with Groups, 24*(2), 47–67.

Kellogg, R. (1914). Appendix EL: Field work of the Pittsburgh Survey. In Russell Sage Foundation, *The Pittsburgh District Civic Frontage* (pp. 492–515). New York: Survey Associates.

Kelly, A., & Sewell, S. (1988). *With head, heart, and hand: Dimensions of community building.* Brisbane, Australia: Boolarong Press.

Kohl, H. (1991, Winter). A tradition of radical education: Highlander in context. *Social Policy, 36–43.*

Kraii, Z., MacKenzie, B., & Youngman, F. (1979). *Popular theatre and participatory research.* Paper presented at the African Regional Workshop on Participatory Research, Mzumbe, Tanzania.

Johnson, V., Ivan-Smith, E., Gordon, G., Pridmore, P., & Scott, P. (Eds.). (1998). *Stepping forward: Children and young people's participation in the development process.* London: Intermediate Technologies.

Lather, P. (1986). Research as praxis. *Harvard Educational Review, 56,* 257–277.

Lather, P. (1991). *Getting smart: Feminist research and pedagogy with/in the postmodern.* New York: Routledge.

Lee, J. A. B. (1991). Foreword. In M. Weil, K. Chan, & D. Southerland (Eds.), *Theory and practice in social group work: Creative connections* (pp. 1–2). New York: Haworth Press.

Levi-Strauss, C. (1966). *The savage mind.* Chicago: University of Chicago Press.

Lewis, E. (1988). Social group work: A central component of social work education and practice. In M. Leiderman, M. Birnbaum, & B. Dazzo (Eds.), *Roots and new frontiers in social group work* (pp. 217–231). New York: Haworth Press.

Maguire, P. (1987). *Doing participatory research.* Amherst, MA: Center for International Education.

Malekoff, A. (1994). Action research: An approach to preventing substance abuse and promoting social competency. *Health and Social Work, 14*(1), 46–53.

Mann, B. (1987). Working with battered women: Radical education or therapy? In E. Pence (Ed.), *In our best interest: A process for personal and social change* (pp. 104–116). Duluth, MN: Minnesota Program Development.

Mathrani, V. (1993). Participatory research: A potential for in-depth understanding. *Indian Journal of Social Work, 53,* 345–53.

Middleman, R. (1983). *Activities and action in group work.* New York: Haworth Press.

Minkler, M. (1997). Organizing the elderly poor in San Francisco's Tenderloin District. In M. Minkler (Ed.), *Community organizing and community building for health* (pp. 244–258). New Brunswick, NJ: Rutgers University Press.

O'Connor, A. (2002). *Poverty knowledge: Social science, social policy, and the poor in twentieth-century U.S. history.* Princeton, NJ: Princeton University Press.

Park, P. (1993). What is participatory research? A theoretical and methodological perspective. In P. Park, M. Brydon-Miller, B. Hall, & T. Jackson (Eds.), *Voices of change* (pp. 1–19). Westport, CT: Bergin & Garvey.

Park, P. (1997). Participatory research, democracy, and community. *Practicing Anthropology, 19*(3), 8–13.

Park, P., Brydon-Miller, M., Hall, B., & Jackson, T. (1993). *Voices of change: Participatory research in the United States and Canada.* Westport, CT: Bergin & Garvey.

Parsons, R. (1991). Empowerment: Purpose and practice principles in social work. *Social Work with Groups, 14,* 7–21.

Poertner, J. (1994). Popular education in Latin America: A technology for the North? *International Social Work, 37,* 265–275.

Reisch, M., Wenocur, S., & Sherman, W. (1981). Empowerment, conscientization, and animation as core social work skills. *Social Development Issues, 5*(2/3), 108–120.

Sachs, J. (1991). Action and reflection in work with a group of homeless people. *Social Work with Groups, 14*(3/4), 187–202.

Sarri, R., & Sarri, C. (1992). Participatory action research in two communities in Bolivia and the United States. *International Social Work, 35,* 267–280.

Schugurensky, D. (1998). The legacy of Paulo Freire: A critical review of his contributions. *Convergence, 31*(1&2), 17–29.

Schutzman, M., & Cohen-Cruz, J. (Eds.). (1994). *Playing Boal: Theatre, therapy, activism.* New York: Routledge.

Schwartz, W. (1994). The social worker in the group. *Social Work with Groups, 8*(4), 7–27.

Sen, R. (1994). Building community involvement in health care. *Social Policy, 24*(3), 32–43.

Simon, B. (1994). *The empowerment tradition in American social work: A history*. New York: Columbia University Press.

Sohng, S. L. (1992). Consumers as research partners. *Journal of Progressive Human Services, 3*(2), 1–14.

Sohng, S. L. (1996). Participatory research and community organizing. *Journal of Sociology and Social Welfare, 23*(4), 77–97.

Spratt, T., Houston, S., & Magill, T. (2000). Imaging the future: Theatre and change within the child protection system. *Child and Family Social Work, 5,* 117–127.

Srikandath, S. (1991, May). *Social change via people's theatre*. Paper presented at the annual convention of the International Communications Association, Chicago.

Tandon, R. (1981). Participatory research in the empowerment of people. *Convergence 14*(3), 20–27.

Toiviainen, T. (1995). A comparative study of Nordic residential folk high schools and the Highlander School. *Convergence, 28*(1), 3–20.

Townsend, J., Zapata, E., Rowlands, J., Alberti, P., & Mercado, M. (1999). *Women and power: Fighting patriarchies and poverty*. London: Zed.

Turner, V. (1969). *The ritual process*. Chicago: Aldine.

Valla, V. (1994). Popular education and knowledge: Popular surveillance of health and education services in Brasilian metropolitan areas. *Educational Action Research, 2*(3), 403–414.

Van Erven, E. (1988). *Radical people's theatre*. Bloomington: Indiana University Press.

Wagner, D. (1991). Reviving the action research model: Combining case and cause with dislocated workers. *Social Work, 36*(6), 477–482.

Wallerstein, N. (1992). Powerlessness, empowerment and health: Implications for health promotion programs. *American Journal of Health Promotion, 6*(3), 197–205.

Weiler, K. (1988). *Women teaching for change: Gender, class and power*. New York: Bergin & Garvey.

Whitmore, E., & Wilson, M. (1997). Accompanying the process: Social work and international development practice. *International Social Work, 40*(1), 57–74.

Williams, L. (1996). First enliven, then enlighten: Popular education and the pursuit of social justice. *Sociological Imagination, 33*(2), 94–116.

Young, E., & Padilla, M. (1990). *Mujeres Unidas en Accion*: A popular education process. *Harvard Educational Review, 60*(1), 1–18.

Yeich, S. (1996). Grassroots organizing with homeless people: A participatory research approach. *Journal of Social Issues, 53,* 111–121.

Zimbalist, S. (1977). *Historical themes and landmarks in social welfare research*. New York: Harper & Row.

Chapter 20

Social Action Groups

LEE H. STAPLES

This chapter situates social action within community organizing, distinguishing it from other methods, such as community development. Social action groups can be organized around three different sets of interest domains—*geographic*, *issue*, and *identity* (Staples, 2000). Regardless of the interest domain, small groups are the primary vehicles through which community members engage in social action. Examples include organizing committees, house meetings, issue committees, negotiating teams, lobbying committees, leadership training sessions, and small groups for a variety of other organizational functions. Individuals typically are involved in social action groups as members, leaders, and/or organizers, with particular responsibilities and challenges attendant to each role.

COMMUNITY ORGANIZING

Community organizing entails collective action at the grassroots level to address common problems and to bring about social change. There is an extensive literature on organizing, community organization, and community practice (Alinsky, 1971; Bradshaw, Soifer, & Gutiérrez, 1994; Checkoway, 1995; Fisher, 1994; Grosser & Mondros, 1995; Hyde, 1986; Rothman, 1968, 1995; Rubin & Rubin, 1992; Staples, 1984; Weil, 1996). In much of this literature, community organizing is used interchangeably with a number of concepts, including advocacy, citizen participation, coalitions, community development, community economic development, planning, political action, program development, social action, and social movements. There are important differences in how assorted writers define and operationalize these practice modalities. It is not within the scope of this chapter to explore this conceptual variance. For purposes of this discussion, I will distinguish between two primary organizing approaches that are included in this list, social action and community development. In my opinion, the other concepts transcend, partially overlap, are distinct from, or are subsumed under community organizing.

Social action brings people together to convince, pressure, or coerce external decision makers to meet collective goals either to act in a specified manner or to stop or modify certain activities. This approach operates from the basic assumption that community members are disadvantaged or oppressed and that most of their problems are products of social injustice (Alinsky, 1971; Bobo, Kendall, & Max, 2001; Checkoway, 1995; Kahn, 1991; Rothman, 1968; Staples, 1984). There is a further assumption that attempts to bring about social change—thus altering relations of power—will be met by resistance from decision-makers in powerful institutions (Delgado, 1986; Hanna & Robinson, 1994; Fisher, 1997; Rothman, 1968; Staples, 1984). Therefore, collaborative strategies will not be effective until or unless the parties share a greater degree of consensus. Rather, organized collective action and self-advocacy (social action) will be necessary for the affected community members to develop the requisite power to change the behavior and actions of external decision makers. Depending on the degree of difference, organized community members will be required to employ either campaign strategies to persuade and convince decision makers to support their goals and objectives, or adversarial contest strategies to pressure and coerce concessions (Netting, Kettner, & McMurty, 2001; Warren, 1975).

Community development, on the other hand, involves participants in constructive activities and processes to produce improvements, opportunities, structures, goods, and services that increase the quality of life and build member capacities. There is an assumption that problems can be addressed successfully by strengthening relationships among community members and bringing people together to work cooperatively for common interests (Fisher, 1994; Pantoja & Perry, 1998; Rothman, 1968; Rubin & Rubin, 1992; Shragge, 1997). Self-help is central to this approach. If external institutions are engaged in change efforts at all, then typically either collaborative or mildly persuasive campaign strategies (Netting et al., 1993; Warren, 1975) are employed to enlist their assistance in cooperative activities.

Despite these important differences, both community organizing approaches share a number of common features, including the involvement of large numbers of the affected constituency taking action on their own behalf, the exercise of "people power" to resolve shared problems, a commitment to participatory democracy, the central role of indigenous leadership, the importance of developing effective organizational structures as vehicles for ongoing social change, and a dual emphasis on inclusive processes and successful outcomes.

Many community groups are organized to represent the interests of everyone living in a distinct geographical area—a neighborhood, a municipality, or even a whole region. Usually, such groups would address a range of community concerns, which might include housing, education, recreation, employment, environmental issues, transportation, or health care. The key is that the "turf" issues addressed are of concern to members of a specified geopolitical locale. So, for instance, the Coalition for a Better Acre is organized in the lowest income neighborhood of Lowell, Massachusetts, a blue-collar industrial city still suffering the effects of a declining industrial base. The residents of the Acre are predominantly Central American and Cambodian. These very disparate ethnic populations have joined together to improve their neighborhood, taking social action for more affordable housing, the creation of youth programs, and cleanup of the abandoned canals, once utilized to transport goods to and from the many vacant textile factories within or nearby the Acre.

A second way that community groups can be organized is according to a particular issue focus, such as clean elections, tax reform, women's rights, environmental justice, or elderly issues. The Green Space and Recreation Committee in Chelsea, Massachusetts, is involved in a wide variety of social action campaigns and community development activities, including organizing against corporate polluters, supporting a community garden, restoring the city's only salt marsh, establishing environmental education programs, and fighting for resident involvement in the city's planning process for development along Chelsea Creek. The Massachusetts Senior Action Council (MSAC), a statewide organization with a number of local chapters, has waged high-profile social action campaigns for improved maintenance and security in elderly public housing, for the nation's first state-subsidized prescription drug insurance program, for expanded state funding for pharmacy assistance for seniors and disabled persons, and for a managed-care patients' bill of rights.

A third dimension of interest is identity, for instance, ethnicity, religion, sexual orientation, or physical or mental disability. The Latino Immigrant Committee in Chelsea, Massachusetts, is composed primarily of recent immigrants from El Salvador, Honduras, Guatemala, Colombia, Chile, and Nicaragua. A core group of 30 people is most active and has engaged in social action focused on discriminatory treatment at the local branch of the post office, on worker safety at a local meat processing plant, on gang violence, on immigrant rights, and on increased participation in the political process. M-POWER (Massachusetts People/Patients Organized for Wellness, Empowerment, and Rights) is a member-run social action organization for deinstitutionalized mental health consumers. With chapters in three of the state Department of Mental Health's six regions, M-POWER has conducted successful campaigns for a Mental Patients' Bill of Rights, guidelines for the use of seclusion and restraints in mental hospitals, and creation of an Informed Consent Policy for psychotropic drugs.

SMALL GROUPS AND SOCIAL ACTION

Although social action may engender images of enormous meetings, rallies, and demonstrations, small groups and committees are the primary medium through which this type of organizing takes place (Gutiérrez & Lewis, 1997). The group setting is an ideal access point for most community members to engage in social action. Small groups maximize opportunities for participation in processes of discussion, analysis, consciousness raising, decision making, and planning. They provide a vehicle through which people can become more actively involved in organizational work. Usually, for every event with a large turnout, many smaller meetings are held for a range of purposes, including action research, leadership training, executive decisions, strategic analysis, community education, recruitment, action planning, negotiating, lobbying, and evaluation. An illustrative, but not exhaustive, set of examples follows.

Organizing Committees

The organizing committee is a time-tested mechanism for overseeing and conducting an initiative to build a new organizational structure or to revitalize an existing one. Ideally, 12 to 15 people who are well-respected opinion leaders will form such a committee, legitimating the organizing effort, neutralizing potential opposition, examining possible issues, and providing a consistent leadership core (Staples, 1984). ACORN (Association of Community Organizations for Reform Now), a multistate social action organization working in low- and moderate-income neighborhoods, sees the creation of an organizing committee (OC) as a critical step in its model for developing new chapters. Delgado (1986) describes the purposes of an ACORN OC's first meeting during an organizing drive as follows:

> (1) to specify the initial issue the organization will address and map out the steps of an organizing campaign; (2) to legitimate the organizing drive by developing an organizing letter, signed by all

of the participants in the meeting, which is then mailed to all neighborhood residents; (3) to collect dues, thus establishing the practice within the organization; (4) to involve members of the committee in contact work (petitions, doorknocking, phone calls); and (5) to prepare for the upcoming neighborhood meeting. (p. 68)

Clearly, the formation of an organizing committee during a first membership drive is designed to develop an action group, a leadership cadre that is willing and able to "own" the organizational structure that soon will follow. Because community organizations should do regular systematic member recruitment and outreach to replenish their numbers, to identify potential new leaders, to discover fresh issues, and to reconnect with their constituency, variations of organizing committees can be found regularly overseeing this activity with well-established groups.

House Meetings

These are small meetings (5 to 15 people is a typical attendance), which may be held in someone's home or also in a familiar place such as a church, school, library, or human services agency. House meetings usually are utilized either for recruitment or educational discussion about complex or controversial issues. Attendees can be recruited by the person hosting (friends, neighbors, colleagues, relatives), by word of mouth, or by knocking on doors, but there is a conscious effort to limit the number. The small meeting size and comfortable, informal format are designed to maximize participation. A number of roles (welcoming, presenting information, facilitating discussion, securing commitments for further participation) can be divided, providing opportunities for emerging organizational leaders to develop experience, confidence, and skills.

For instance, the Franklin Hill Tenants Association in Boston held a series of house meetings in every building of their large (more than 300 families) public housing development. The house meetings were used to recruit new participants in a social action campaign to force the Boston Housing Authority (BHA) to improve maintenance and make repairs as required by the state sanitary code. A slide show was employed to stimulate and focus discussion on a number of specific grievances. Slides depicted exposed wiring, leaky plumbing, crumbling walls, broken stairs, the lack of recreational facilities for youth, an empty basement space, unsecured common hallways, and a number of abandoned apartments that had become havens for drug dealers and violent gangs. The slides served to "rub raw the sores of discontent" (Alinsky, 1971), and both tenant leadership and organizing staff were quick to channel the attendees' dissatisfaction into discussions about taking collective action to confront the Housing Authority. A spirited social action campaign evolved from these preliminary house meetings, and ultimately the tenants group successfully pressured the BHA to make a number of changes. Repairs were made to individual apartments, a twice-weekly trash pickup was instituted, a youth program was developed, vacant units were rehabilitated and filled, locked doors to common hallways were put in place along with a buzzer system, and the basement now houses a child care program during the day and a range of community activities in the evenings.

Issue Committees

Often, members of social action organizations will have a variety of concerns relating to the institutions, organizations, and decision makers that affect their lives. A range of possible campaigns may exist, and the organization will need to choose new issues carefully and strategically. Issue committees can help meet this organizational need; typical activities include prioritizing goals, selecting new issues, conducting action research, engaging in strategic planning, developing action plans, implementing direct action, and evaluating the results.

Social action organizing entails aggregating and politicizing individual problems, and then "cutting" issues from the fabric of shared problems. As defined by *Webster's New World College Dictionary,* a problem is "a question, matter, situation or person that is perplexing or difficult" (Agnes, 2000), whereas matters "at issue" are "in dispute." Essentially, problems are broad concerns that generate dissatisfaction but not necessarily *action*. On the other hand, issues encompass controversial, and often competing, courses of action to address a problem or aspects of it. Thus the lack of affordable housing in a low- and moderate-income area may be a *problem*, whereas possible social action *issues* that could be cut might include the establishment of rent control, a housing trust fund, a condominium conversion ordinance, inclusionary zoning, a development linkage program, low-interest mortgages, creation of new housing, or expansion of subsidized housing. Depending on how the issue is cut, different parties will have positive or negative self-interests and will be more likely to engage in social action either as proponents or opponents. Identifying, prioritizing, and selecting issues often takes place in small social action groups or issue committees.

Cox (1991) offers a number of reasons that these groups are optimal for this activity:

> Small groups of individuals of like status provide a medium in which members can sort out the personal from the political aspects of their problems. Empowerment groups are helpful to individuals coping with and changing the internalized aspects of oppression/powerlessness in the following ways: (1) The group as a whole, through sharing experiences, can better describe the full impact of specific problems of the members' lives and the lives of their families and friends; (2) Members who have survived or overcome aspects of powerlessness can inspire and motivate others; (3) Members who have identified beliefs and/or behaviors of their own which reinforce their own oppression (i.e., belief that they cannot learn valued skills) are incapable of achieving higher status roles, or cannot have an impact on a social service agency), can confront their peers and in so doing facilitate the consciousness raising process; (4) Groups can provide a forum in which individuals can gain increased knowledge on the political dimension of their situation, and a better understanding of the origins of the personal dimensions of their problems. (p. 82)

When prioritizing goals and choosing a new issue, a strategic analysis helps committee members assess the potential for simultaneously winning a victory and developing organizational capacity. Questions that serve this analysis for social action groups follow (Staples, 1997):

- Is the issue consistent with the long-range goals of the organization?
- Will the issue be unifying or divisive?
- Will the campaign help the organization grow?
- Will the campaign provide a good educational experience for leaders and members, developing their consciousness, independence, and skills?
- Will the organization receive credit for a victory on the issue, improve its credibility, and increase its overall visibility?
- How will the campaign affect organizational resources?
- Will the campaign develop new allies and/or enemies?
- Will the campaign emphasize direct action and produce new tactics or issues?
- Will the campaign produce a significant victory?

Action research should not be the sole purview of professional staff. It is important to demystify and democratize information that may seem highly technical, esoteric, privileged, and beyond the intellectual grasp of average community members. When leaders and activists are involved in doing action research, they quickly develop even more ownership of issue campaigns and become more sophisticated about "handles" that can provide leverage on institutions that the group is trying to influence. Working as a committee to sift through background material, read relevant newspaper articles, study official reports, gather statistical data, learn about regulatory processes, and research the law can be very empowering for organizational leaders, enhancing their knowledge, increasing their confidence, and raising their consciousness. The group also enables a more natural division of labor, with members taking on responsibility according to their interests and talents. Discussion and dialogue among group members also enhances the learning process.

Strategic planning is a natural outgrowth of action research. Strategies are overarching systematic plans to achieve organizational goals, whereas tactics are specific methods, procedures, and techniques employed to carry out those plans. Warren's (1975) classic framework continues to be recognized as the definitive guideline for selecting the most effective strategy. Warren's basic operating principle holds that the level of agreement or disagreement between two parties is the key variable for determining the best strategy. For instance, when a community group reaches a consensus with an external institution, collaborative methods associated with community development will be most productive. If a difference of opinion exists but the potential is there to change the views of an institutional target, a persuasive campaign will be the best strategic option. Here the lines often blur between a community development approach (gentle persuasion through education or appeals for assistance; usually positive incentives) and social action (pressure to "do the right thing"; occasionally positive incentives, but often negative sanctions such as bad publicity, public embarrassment, loss of votes, loss of business, disapproval by significant third parties). And a contest approach will be necessary when the disagreement is so basic that the community group has no realistic possibility of winning over an institutional target.

The Massachusetts Senior Action Council (MSAC) was able to undertake a highly visible persuasive/pressure social action campaign to win passage of state health care reform legislation during the summer of 2000 by gathering signatures, presenting research studies, holding public media events, and lobbying state legislators. Several years earlier, MSAC won legislation to expand eligibility and benefits in the $30 million senior pharmacy program only after they used a contest strategy, picketing health maintenance organizations (HMOs) and packing a federal courtroom to defend the state law—originally passed largely through the efforts of MSAC—requiring HMOs to offer full prescription drug coverage. In both instances, MSAC issue committees provided the leadership for a number of large-turnout actions and events. Strategy and tactics were developed in numerous social action planning meetings. Immediately prior to the large collective actions, more small-group meetings were held to identify and allot roles and responsibilities, as well as to practice and rehearse specific assignments. Finally, after conducting each tactical step of these social action campaigns, the issue committees came together to evaluate their efforts and begin planning for their next actions.

On the other hand, the Chelsea Green Space and Recreation Committee's Salt Pile Campaign has utilized an adversarial contest approach, which has led to a community mediation process. A private company in a mixed residential and industrial area provides rock salt used to melt snow and ice on highways in most of the other cities and towns in Massachusetts, as well as in parts of several other New England states. The pile of more than

140,000 tons of salt is the largest in the eastern United States and towers to the height of a five-story building, dwarfing the nearby houses. Trucks that transport the salt out of Chelsea routinely spill part of their load as they travel over the city's bumpy streets. Most important, the pile is not properly covered, and rock salt that is exposed to sun and water releases a toxic chemical (ferocyanide) into the air. The uncovered salt pile is a clear violation of state law. Given that this neighborhood primarily is composed of Latino residents, Green Space members view the situation as a clear case of environmental racism.

Neither the company nor the state was responsive to the committee's repeated demands that the law be obeyed and enforced. Therefore, a strong direct action approach was undertaken. Green Space members staged angry protests at the company's headquarters and later disrupted several meetings of the Massachusetts Department of Environmental Affairs. These actions were covered prominently in the media, and the state Secretary of Environmental Affairs received significant negative publicity during a gubernatorial election year. Shortly thereafter, the state, the city of Chelsea, and the salt pile company agreed to fund a community mediation process. As of this writing, the Green Space Committee has entered into a "good faith effort" to resolve the issue, ever mindful that they will resist being co-opted or "bought off." Therefore, further social action remains a viable possibility if the mediation process proves to be unsatisfactory.

Lobbying Committees

Legislative lobbying goes hand in hand with social action at the municipal, state, and even national levels. Public officials are quick to recognize the potential voting power of organized community members. As Judy Meredith (2000, p. 4) notes, "Elected and appointed decision-makers make different decisions when watched by the affected constituents," and "Lobbying is simply getting the right information to the right person at the right time." Large numbers of organized people go right to the heart of the self-interest of public officials. Typically, the larger and better organized the group is, the greater the positive results secured.

For instance, the Greater Boston Interfaith Organization (GBIO) recently conducted a successful social action campaign to convince the Massachusetts state legislature to establish a $100 million trust fund to build affordable housing over a 5-year period. First, GBIO gathered more than 100,000 signatures on a petition to increase the state's funding for affordable housing. Next, the group held 11 "accountability sessions" in legislative districts in which hundreds of constituents pushed elected officials to make a commitment to support legislation establishing an affordable-housing trust fund. Following these local sessions, a huge rally with more than 3,000 people present pressured the legislative leadership to commit to moving the legislation through both house and senate. And, finally, small well-informed constituent groups lobbied their elected representatives to support the legislation. This last step—small groups directly interacting with their own representatives—was crucial to the success of this campaign. And, as discussed previously, each of the prior steps—gathering signatures, holding local accountability sessions, and conducting the large rally—was preceded and followed by numerous small-group planning and evaluation sessions.

Negotiating Teams

At times, social action may be designed to get the group to the bargaining table. In other instances, opponents may offer to negotiate, but such proposals may be made in good or bad faith. Splain (1984) has offered guidelines for determining whether or not community groups should engage in formal bargaining. He also lays out seven areas of planning, preparation, and training that should precede any negotiating session. These ground rules help clarify and establish the relationship between the bargaining committee or negotiating team and the larger social action organization:

1. The organization must determine the general makeup of the bargaining committee, as well as the specific election or selection process.
2. The organization, not just the bargaining committee, must reach consensus on the time limit allowed for bargaining to achieve its purposes before the membership reevaluates the basic decision to engage in negotiations.
3. An accountability mechanism must be established through which the committee will keep the membership informed on an ongoing basis and, on occasion, seek votes on various bargaining positions.
4. The basic formalization of demands and possible bottom lines is established by the membership, but the specific details of both are drawn up by the committee.
5. The question of nonbargaining campaign activity, such as use of the media during the negotiation period, should be resolved by the bargaining committee with input from the membership.
6. The committee must devote one or more preparatory sessions specifically to role playing, research, and record-keeping skills.
7. The committee must discuss and agree on specific roles for each individual member to play, including the organizer, as well as the use of caucuses for decision-making purposes.

Once issues of representation, mandate, responsibility, accountability, and roles are resolved, the negotiating team will be empowered to move forward with the bargaining process.

In 1996, M-POWER completed a protracted and ultimately successful negotiating process with the Massachusetts Department of Mental Health (DMH) to establish and implement a procedural policy for informed consent to treatment. This policy requires doctors to spend time with mental patients discussing and explaining all aspects of a proposed course of treatment, including the potential benefits, risks, side effects, dosages, alternative treatments, and the possible consequences of no treatment. After taking direct action to highlight the need for such a policy and to get to the bargaining table, M-POWER entered negotiations with the Deputy Commissioner of DMH and officials from its human rights office. Once DMH made the commitment to institute an informed consent policy, M-POWER entered a second round of negotiations to develop the actual guidelines and a timeline for implementation. The negotiating team reported back to the full M-POWER membership on a regular basis as this process unfolded.

Leadership Training

Kieffer (1984) examined personal empowerment for emerging leaders in grassroots organizations, which he described as "a necessarily long-term process of adult learning and development" that results in increased "participatory competence." Leaders in grassroots social action groups tend to learn most from direct experience, but formal training also can be of great value. Burghardt (1982) has distinguished between simply teaching organizational skills and developing the capacity for critical consciousness (Breton, 1995; Carroll & Minkler, 2000; Freire, 1968; Gutiérrez, 1995; Pecukonis & Wenocur, 1994), joining action and reflection about relations of power to one's own role in the process of social change. The strongest leadership development programs combine practical skills, personal growth, participatory competencies, consciousness raising, neopopulist democratic principles (Fisher, 1997), and strategies for collective empowerment (cultural, political, economic). And most formal training and education takes place in small-group settings in which participants easily can share experiences and insights, learning from one another, as well as from those leading the sessions.

Delgado (1997) has noted the expansion and long-term success of "training intermediaries" such as the Highlander Research and Education Center, Industrial Areas Foundation, Center for Third World Organizing, Midwest Academy, National Training and Information Center, Organizing and Leadership Training Center, and the Institute for Social Justice, which (to varying degrees and with different emphases) provide educational, analytical, and skill-building sessions that address an assortment of social action topics, including power analysis, the roots of oppression, recruitment techniques, mentoring less experienced leaders, conducting effective meetings, conflict resolution, researching community issues, strategic analysis, action planning, collective action tactics, working with the media, fund-raising, using information technology, building coalitions, general organizational development, and redistributing wealth and power. In addition to these large national training centers, a plethora of locally based programs offer similar services in communities all across the United States. Indeed, I have done considerable leadership development work with the Center for Civil Initiatives in the Balkans, and comparable support operations exist around the world. Typically, the leaders of well-established social action organizations, including all those cited in this chapter, have had the opportunity to participate in formal leadership training delivered in a small-group format.

Small groups are utilized by social action organizations for a variety of other functions, including media teams, long-range planning, grassroots fund-raising projects, special events (conventions, annual meetings, candidates' nights, festivals, etc.), developing bylaws, officers meetings, nominating committees, hiring staff, and evaluating virtually every aspect of organizational activities.

MEMBERS, LEADERS, AND ORGANIZERS

People may be involved in social action groups as members, leaders or organizers, with distinct roles and responsibilities for each. The role of members can vary from mere followers who take directions from the group's leadership to active participants in all group decisions and actions. And, of course, there can be wide variation in the degree to which individuals take part in the group, from regular to more casual participants. Leadership forms can range from a single individual in charge of all group affairs to several people sharing different roles to collective models in which theoretically all members are leaders. Leadership may be formal or emergent, and individuals may be first- or second-line leaders. Although leaders typically are out front guiding, directing, or showing the way for followers, organizers function to get *others* to take on more responsibility (Staples, 1984). Many social action groups formally acknowledge the role of organizer through paid staff positions, although Delgado

(1997) has noted that one person may function as a leader-organizer and that compensation frequently is not provided for this role in organizations in communities of color. Challenges associated with each of these three functions in social action groups are explored below.

Members

Insuring the active participation of group members always has and always will be a fundamental challenge for social action organizing. Large numbers of active participants are the primary means by which group goals are accomplished; the power of numbers is harnessed through an organizational structure to bring about social change. However, the involvement of community members also is an end in itself, giving participants ownership of decisions and processes, developing and deepening relationships, promoting active involvement, and building group solidarity. The most successful groups will have a commitment to enlisting new activists and a recruitment technology that may include knocking on doors, targeted home visits, house meetings, networking, presentations to various "captive audiences," community forums, and printed and electronic communications. The group should be inclusive and reflective of the potential participants with regard to race, ethnicity, religion, age, gender, social class, sexual orientation, and physical or mental ability. It will be useful to analyze involvement along dimensions of both breadth and depth—how many people are participants and how actively they are involved.

Although social action groups always have competed for people's time, a number of phenomena make this challenge even more difficult in the context of the current economy and culture in the United States. Today, more people than ever before are working more than one job just to make ends meet (Ehrenreich, 2001), and this economic reality leaves them with both scarce time and limited energy to engage in social action. This situation is compounded by increased individualistic behavior and a general decline in community involvement (Bellah, Madsen, Sullivan, Swidler, & Tipton, 1985; Putnam, 1995). Yet, in spite of these barriers, there has been a dramatic rise in social action organizing over the past several decades (Delgado, 1997; Pilisuk, McAllister, & Rothman, 1997), much of it concerning issues of social identity, culture, and economic self-interest.

During this same time frame, geographical communities have become more multicultural, and within-group ethnic diversity has grown apace (Daley & Wong, 1994), creating new challenges relating to members' differing expectations regarding group norms and processes. These differences can play out around a variety of issues, including but not limited to meeting sites, starting and ending times, whether children attend, provision of child care, if and when food is served, use of formal agendas (with or without time limits), note taking, dealing with latecomers, gender and age dynamics, degree of formality, chairing styles, comfort levels with intragroup conflict, and decision making by consensus or voting. As groups establish their norms and procedures for these and other matters, a group culture emerges, providing the members with formal and informal guidelines for conducting their business. Such a culture offers security and direction for group members, but often at the expense of being open and welcoming to nonmembers. The particular challenge for social action groups in diverse settings is to build enough cohesion and shared culture to establish the requisite solidarity necessary to engage in adversarial organizing campaigns while remaining permeable enough for newcomers to enter and sufficiently malleable for these new members to influence that very same culture.

Social action itself raises particular issues for some recent immigrants. Many may be uncomfortable confronting government officials, based on their experience with political repression in their countries of origin. Noncitizens, especially those who are undocumented, may fear being singled out and deported; and the growth of anti-immigrant sentiment in the wake of the 9/11 tragedy has done little to diminish these concerns. However, there are creative ways for dealing with these types of challenges. For instance, the aforementioned Chelsea Latino Immigrant Committee formed a community support committee for immigrant workers at a meat processing plant at which numerous severe violations of basic health and safety regulations existed. The group linked with the United Food and Commercial Workers Local 1445, Jobs for Justice, and MassCOSH (Massachusetts Committee for Occupational Safety and Health) to organize a rally and march with more than 200 people. A delegation entered the factory and confronted management. Since the rally, attorneys for the National Labor Relations Board (NLRB) have begun interviewing workers, the Chelsea Health Department has begun to make regular inspections citing violations at the plant, and the state Occupational Safety and Health Administration (OSHA) has become involved. An NLRB lawsuit is pending; some equipment has been added, repaired or replaced; workers report that they are being treated better; and an active union drive is under way.

Leaders

Bales (1970) identified two types of small-group leaders, those who provide instrumental leadership to accomplish the group's tasks and those who are concerned with group processes and members' feelings (socioemotional or affective leaders). Bales also found that it is unusual for a single individual to provide both types of leadership. Yet Burghardt (1979) has noted that both forms of leadership are essential for social action groups. Logically, several leaders, operating through a shared leadership model, provide a social action group with a range of strengths and areas of expertise that no one person can supply. Groups with a shared leadership structure are in the best position to operate consistent with the principles of participatory democracy and can avoid overreliance on one or two individuals.

There also will be opportunities and incentives for new leaders to emerge and take on increasing levels of responsibility. Shared leadership is most possible when clear division of roles and responsibilities exist between first- and second-line leaders, as well as the full membership. Essentially, a group's top leaders hold formal positions, such as president, chairperson, secretary, treasurer, or governance board member, whereas second-line leaders are neither elected to office nor appointed to head key organizational committees. They are core activists, who are regular participants in organizational meetings, activities, and events. Like "worker bees," they are industrious and indispensable for implementing the group's policies, procedures, and plans. They serve as links between the top leaders and the group's rank-and-file members, often infusing the group with energy, creativity, and fresh perspectives. New first-line leaders often come from their midst, and they may offer a healthy challenge to long-term top leaders, who may have a tendency to become entrenched. This process helps democratize the group and serves as a preventative for "groupthink" (Janis, 1972), a phenomenon in which healthy questioning and dissent is squelched.

Indeed, Robert Michels (1949), in a classic piece on organizational behavior, termed the tendency for power to become concentrated in the hands of a few leaders "The Iron Law of Oligarchy." Preventing this phenomenon from occurring remains a serious challenge for social action groups to this day. Oligarchic leadership often is vulnerable to co-optation and corruption. It also is contrary to the principles of participatory democracy, which is so intertwined with the power of numbers—the basic fuel of social action organizing. Second-line leaders help forestall (or slow down) the occurrence of oligarchic leadership. Therefore, it is essential to include these secondary leaders in any leadership training sessions in order to prevent this process from widening the gap (knowledge, skills, commitment) between the first-line leaders and the members. Whoever plays the role of organizer is responsible for finding and developing second-line leaders; the importance of this task in social action groups cannot be overemphasized.

Concern about the emergence of oligarchic leadership has led some groups, especially those committed to feminist principles, to experiment with collective structures that have no formal leaders. In another classic article, Jo Freeman (Joreen, 1972) described the "tyranny of structurelessness" as a phenomenon that usually occurs when unstructured or "leaderless" groups attempt to engage in social action. Freeman argued that the lack of formal leadership insures that a group will be controlled by informal and unacknowledged elites, which are neither responsible nor accountable for carrying out tasks. Ironically, this attempt to mitigate problems created by too much structure usually results in the concentration of power in the hands of an informal oligarchy. Freeman concluded by offering some very sound principles for democratic structuring:

1. *Delegation* of specific authority to specific individuals for specific tasks by democratic procedures.
2. Requiring all those to whom authority has been delegated to be *responsible* to those who selected them.
3. *Distribution* of authority among as many people as is reasonably possible.
4. *Rotation* of tasks among individuals.
5. *Allocation* of tasks along rational criteria.
6. *Diffusion of information* to everyone as frequently as possible.
7. *Equal access to resources* needed by the group.

The appropriate use of permanent and temporary committees also helps balance a social action organization's need for both experience and new leadership. Long-term standing committees have the advantage of giving the organizational structure continuity and stability; there is a minimal change in their membership over time. This relative permanence makes it possible for committee members to form a working team that can learn technical responsibilities together, such as finances, bylaws, or personnel policies, without constantly having to slow down while new activists master the learning curve.

Short-term ad hoc committees can be even more important, as they provide structural access points through which newcomers can become active. These temporary committees are suitable for issue campaigns, special events, or time-limited activities, and new participants often first get involved at this level. Having standing committees in these areas would make it more difficult for new people to plug in to a social action group's structure, because veteran activists might monopolize positions of influence and responsibility. The structural permeability of ad hoc committees keeps a steady flow of fresh "new blood" flowing into the organization, helping to prevent oligarchic concentration of power. Temporary committees also are suitable for projects such as developing a strategic plan, nominating new officers, or evaluating an organizational initiative, which may require members to have a higher degree of familiarity with the organization. But whether short-term committee members are veterans or newcomers, these structures exist for a specific purpose and are disbanded when their work is complete, helping to keep the group more dynamic and energized than standing committees, which may fall dormant between campaigns and projects, thereby contributing to organizational fossilization.

Organizers

When someone takes on the role of organizer, their primary responsibility is to engage community members to act on their own behalf. Organizers identify new activists and potential leaders, motivating them to become involved. They work closely with a social action group's leaders, supporting them as they develop both confidence and skills and preparing them for various organizational responsibilities. Organizers help leaders and members to formulate visions and goals, assist in developing strategies and action plans to achieve those ends, and facilitate processes to evaluate the results of the group's actions. Most important, they work to develop organizational structures (e.g., committees, governance boards, task forces, coalitions) through which collective action can be taken. Organizers who do not do their jobs effectively often are doing too much for both members and leaders—making decisions, advocating, brokering, speaking publicly, and negotiating on their behalf. This builds dependency and stunts the growth of the constituency's own leadership. Organizers should not be directing the group's positions, policies, programs, projects, or procedures, for that is the prerogative of members and leaders. Rather, the role of organizer—whether formally recognized or not—is to work with the group to motivate, recruit, educate, enable, facilitate, and catalyze others to take collective action for social change.

If a social action group retains an organizer in a paid staff position, more or less emphasis will be placed on whether she or he shares the same characteristics as the group's members along dimensions such as race, ethnicity, religion, class, gender, sexual orientation, age, and physical or mental ability, depending on the group's interest domain. Frequently, groups that are organized along identity interests (e.g., disabled people, single parents, ethnic refugees) will prefer, although not necessarily require, staff who have similar personal traits or experiences. Members of social action groups organized along geographical lines, especially where a particular ethnic group predominates, may favor staff of that ethnicity or residents of that community but may not feel as strongly as activists who focus on that very identity. For members of most groups working with issue interests, the staff's "insider" or "outsider" status vis-à-vis the majority of members is far less relevant (Staples, 2000).

In all three instances, regardless of similarities or differences with the constituency, it is crucial that organizers play a facilitative rather than a directive role. Although they may have a measure of expertise about the technology of building powerful social action organizations, they also will have much to learn from community members and leaders. To the extent that they have knowledge to impart, organizers should take on the role of "teacher-learners" and relate to group members as "learner-teachers," as articulated by Paulo Freire (1973). Bradshaw et al. (1994) offer further guidelines for organizers working with communities of color:

1. Develop a positive connection with the community.
2. Understand the minority community.
3. Develop self-awareness.
4. Build adequate leadership within the community.
5. Engender cohesiveness within and among communities of color.
6. Develop cultural competence.

But, in fact, these principles can be adapted and applied to any organizer working with a social action group in any community. Indeed, each of the groups cited as examples in this chapter has paid organizing staff who generally subscribe to these guidelines, whether they are "insiders" or "outsiders."

Thus members, leaders, and staff members each have their own particular responsibilities and challenges in the various types of small groups that operate within larger social action organizations. When each party works at an optimum level, the groups may approach a "democratic microcosm" (Ephross & Vassil, 1988), operationalizing a set of values that include "the worth of each individual group member, active participation by each member, each member's responsibility for actions and behaviors, respect for differences of background, ability, and personal characteristics among the members, and an awareness within each member of responsibility, to some extent, for the entire group" (pp. 44–45). At such times, these groups can perform both task and process functions successfully, and effective social action will be most possible.

REFERENCES

Agnes, M. (Ed.). (2000). *Webster's new world college dictionary* (4th ed.). Foster City, CA: IDG Books.

Alinsky, S. (1971). *Rules for radicals: A practical primer for realistic radicals.* New York: Vintage Books.

Bales, R. F. (1970). *Personality and interpersonal behavior.* New York: Holt, Rinehart, & Winston.

Bellah, R. N., Madsen, R., Sullivan, W. M., Swidler, A., & Tipton, S. M. (1985). *Habits of the heart: Individualism and commitment in American life.* New York: Harper & Row.

Bobo, K., Kendall, J., & Max, S. (2001). *Organizing for social change* (3rd ed.). Santa Ana, CA: Seven Locks Press.

Bradshaw, C., Soifer, S., & Gutiérrez, L. (1994). Toward a hybrid model for effective organizing with women of color. *Journal of Community Practice, 1*(1), 25–41.

Breton, M. (1995). The potential for social action in groups. *Social Work with Groups, 18*(2/3), 5–13.

Burghardt, S. (1979). The tactical use of group structure and process in community organization. In F. M. Cox, J. L. Erlich, J. Rothman, & J. E. Tropman (Eds.), *Strategies of community organization* (3rd ed., pp. 113–130). Itasca, IL: Peacock.

Burghardt, S. (1982). *The other side of organizing.* Cambridge, MA: Schenkman.

Carroll, J., & Minkler, M. (2000). Freire's message for social workers: Looking back, looking ahead. *Journal of Community Practice, 8*(1), 21–36.

Checkoway, B. (1995). Six strategies of social change. *Community Development Journal, 30*(1), 115–133.

Cox, E. O. (1991). The critical role of social action in empowerment oriented groups. In A. Vinik & M. Levin (Eds.), *Social action in group work* (pp. 77–90). New York: Haworth Press.

Daley, J. M., & Wong, P. (1994). Community development with emerging ethnic communities. *Journal of Community Practice, 1*(1), 9–24.

Delgado, G. (1986). *Organizing the movement: The roots and growth of ACORN.* Philadelphia: Temple University Press.

Delgado, G. (1997). *Beyond the politics of place.* Oakland, CA: Applied Research Center.

Ehrenreich, B. (2001). *Nickel and dimed.* New York: Owl Books.

Ephross, P. H., & Vassil, T. V. (1988). *Groups that work: Structure and process.* New York: Columbia University Press.

Fisher, R. (1994). *Let the people decide* (2nd ed.). New York: Twayne.

Fisher, R. (1997). Social action community organization: Proliferation, persistence, roots, and prospects. In M. Minkler (Ed.), *Community organizing and community building for health* (pp. 53–67). New Brunswick, NJ: Rutgers University Press.

Freire, P. (1968). *Pedagogy of the oppressed.* New York: Seabury Press.

Freire, P. (1973). *Education for critical consciousness.* New York: Seabury Press.

Grosser, C. F., & Mondros, J. (1985). Pluralism and participation: The political action approach. In S. H. Taylor & R. W. Roberts (Eds.), *Theory and practice of community social work* (pp. 154–178). New York: Columbia University Press.

Gutiérrez, L. (1995). Understanding the empowerment process: Does consciousness make a difference? *Social Work Research, 19*(4), 229–237.

Gutiérrez, L. M., & Lewis, E. A. (1997). Education, participation, and capacity building in community organizing with women of color. In M. Minkler (Ed.), *Community organizing and community building for health* (pp. 216–229). New Brunswick, NJ: Rutgers University Press.

Hanna, M. G., & Robinson, B. (1994). Lessons for academics from grassroots community organizing: A case study—The Industrial Areas Foundation. *Journal of Community Practice, 1*(4), 63–94.

Hyde, C. (1986). Experience of women activists: Implications for community organizing theory. *Sociology and Social Welfare, 13,* 545–562.

Janis, I. (1972). *Victims of groupthink.* Boston: Houghton Mifflin.

Joreen. (1973). The tyranny of structurelessness. In A. Kroedt, E. Levine, & A. Rapone (Eds.), *Radical feminism* (pp. 285–299). New York: Quadrangle/The New York Times Book Co.

Kahn, S. (1991). *Organizing: A guide for grassroots leaders.* Silver Spring, MD: NASW Press.

Kieffer, C. H. (1984). Citizen empowerment: A development perspective. In J. Rappaport & R. Hess (Eds.), *Studies in empowerment: Steps toward understanding and action* (pp. 9–36). New York: Haworth Press.

Meredith, J. C. (2000). *Lobbying on a shoestring* (3rd ed.). Boston: Massachusetts Law Reform Institue.

Michels, R. (1949). *Political parties: A sociological study of the oligarchical tendencies of modern democracy.* New York: Free Press.

Netting, E. F., Kettner, P. M., & McMurty, S. L. (2001). Selecting appropriate tactics. In J. Tropman, J. E. Erlich, & J. Rothman (Eds.), *Tactics and techniques of community intervention* (pp. 85–99). Itasca, IL: Peacock.

Pantoja, A., & Perry, W. (1998). Community development and restoration: A perspective and case study. In F. G. Rivera & J. L. Erlich (Eds.), *Community organizing in a diverse society* (3rd ed.). Boston: Allyn & Bacon.

Pecukonis, E. V., & Wenocur, S. (1994). Perceptions of self and collective efficacy in community organization theory and practice. *Journal of Community Practice, 1*(2), 5–21.

Pilisuk, M., McAllister, J., & Rothman, J. (1997). Social change professionals and grassroots organizing: Functions and dilemmas. In M. Minkler (Ed.), *Community organizing and community building for health* (pp. 103–119). New Brunswick, NJ: Rutgers University Press.

Putnam, R. D. (1995). Bowling alone: America's declining social capital. *Journal of Democracy, 6*(1), 65–78.

Rothman, J. (1968). Three models of community organization practice. In National Conference on Social Welfare, *Social work practice.* New York: Columbia University Press.

Rothman, J. (1995). Approaches to community intervention. In J. Rothman, J. L. Erlich, & J. E. Tropman (Eds.), *Strategies of community intervention* (5th ed., pp. 26–63) Itasca, IL: Peacock, pp. 26–63.

Rubin, H., & Rubin, I. (1992). *Community organizing and development* (2nd ed.). New York: Macmillan.

Shragge, E. (Ed.). (1997). *Community economic development: In search of empowerment* (2nd ed.). Montreal, Quebec, Canada: Black Rose Books.

Splain, M. J. (1984). Negotiations: Using a weapon as a way out. In L. Staples, *Roots to power: A manual for grassroots organizing* (pp. 164–170). New York: Praeger/Greenwood.

Staples, L. (1984). *Roots to power: A manual for grassroots organizing.* New York: Praeger/Greenwood Press.

Staples, L. (1997). Selecting and "cutting" the issue. In M. Minkler (Ed.), *Community organizing and community building for health* (pp. 175–194). New Brunswick, NJ: Rutgers University Press.

Staples, L. H. (2000). Insider/outsider upsides and downsides. *Social Work with Groups*, 23(2), 19–35.

Warren, R. (1975). Types of purposive change at the community level. In R. M. Kramer & H. Specht (Eds.), *Readings in community organization practice* (2nd ed.). Englewood Cliffs, NJ: Prentice-Hall.

Weil, M. (1996). Model development in community practice: An historical perspective. *Journal of Community Practice*, 3(3/4) 5–67.

Chapter 21

Accessing Resources, Transforming Systems

Group Work with Poor and Homeless People

E. SUMMERSON CARR

Because empowerment-oriented group work is directed at multilevel change, from the building of individual skills to the transformation of institutional, community, and state systems, it is a particularly effective approach for creating, accessing, or accruing resources. For example, an empowerment-oriented group may advocate for the community-based child care that would allow local parents to access gainful employment. Another such group might point to discriminatory hiring practices at the very same child care center, developing and activating a variety of strategies to redress them. The relative success of both of these groups relies on the integration of praxis,[1] that is, the extent to which the process of identifying problems through intensive dialogue and the goal of attaining needed resources are effectively coordinated.

In this chapter, I propose an empowerment-oriented model of group work aimed at accessing resources, housing, and/or employment. Because poor people, by definition, do not have ready access to basic resources,[2] empowerment-oriented groups must point to where resources are, develop and implement concrete strategies of how they can be attained, and work not only to hurdle but also to ultimately dismantle any barriers that may hinder access. I argue that empowerment-oriented groups aimed at the alleviation of poverty should combine traditional advocacy and social action approaches, thereby making exacting demands on the group worker, as well as on other group members. I further suggest that such a group's transformative potentials and effects can spread as resources are distributed beyond its immediate bounds. Thus empowerment-oriented groups should be evaluated not only to the extent to which they create resources and opportunities for group members but also to the degree to which they effect positive social change in relevant communities, institutions, and other systems.

This chapter is organized in three sections. In the first section, I delineate a theoretical frame by selectively drawing on a diverse body of scholarly work on empowerment-oriented groups (e.g., Breton, 1989a; Butler, 1991; Cox, 1991, 1997; Garvin & Reed, 1995; Gutiérrez, 1990; Lewis, 1991, 1992; Mullender & Ward, 1991; Shapiro, 1991). In the second section, I address how issues of poverty, especially as they intersect with gender, can raise particular challenges for psychosocial group work (e.g., Lee, 1986; Moldofosky, 2000; Subramanian, Hernandez, & Martinez, 1995). Then, in reference to my initial frame, I review select applications of an empowerment-oriented approach in working with groups of poor and homeless individuals (Breton, 1989b; Butler, 1994; Cohen, 1994a, 1994b; Lee, 1986; Sachs, 1991). This brief review demonstrates that a group's success is dependent not only on the realization of concrete goals, such as the acquisition of affordable housing, but also on the development of the interpersonal processes, such as acquisition of knowledge about local and state economies, by which those goals are reached and often extended.

In the third section, I illustrate an empowerment-oriented approach to group work with poor and homeless individuals by recounting my experiences as a group worker at a consortium of homeless service agencies in a small Midwestern city.[3] Within this consortium, I worked with women clients to establish a group aimed at (1) accessing immediately needed resources and (2) changing systems so as to ameliorate these needs in the future. Reflecting on my foibles and accomplishments as a group worker, I propose practice principles for group work with poor and homeless individuals, stressing the importance of combining advocacy and social action approaches.

GROUP WORK AND EMPOWERMENT: CONCEPTS AND CONNECTIONS

Many group work scholars have advocated for group work as an ideal modality for empowerment (e.g., Breton, 1989a, Chapter 4, this volume; Cox, 1991; Gutiérrez, 1990; Harrison & Ward, 2000). Despite such convincing rationales, group work's mission has changed from "that of instrument of social action to that of training ground for democracy," according to Shapiro's keen assessment (1991, p. 7). Critiquing current conceptualizations of the group as a microcosm of society, Shapiro advises that social group work should not aim to adjust individuals to the oppressive demands of their environment but instead should work to modify the environment in accordance with the demands of the individual. Indeed, group work that focuses exclusively on individual motivation and responsibility cannot adequately account for or respond to issues of poverty and oppression.

By definition, empowerment-oriented group work does not rely on the ideal liberal agent as an already empowered participant in a readily accessible marketplace of resources and instead focuses on how socioeconomics shape, stymie, and produce possibilities for acting and attaining in an often unjust world (e.g., Breton, 1989a; Lewis, 1991). For example, much empowerment-oriented group work begins with the premise that the economic circumstances of group members have infiltrated their ways of thinking and acting in the world, for better and sometimes for worse. Similarly, group workers influenced by feminist thought strive to discern the multifaceted dimensions of oppression, attending to how gender ideologies, for example, not only influence people's decision to participate in groups but also shape and style the composition of that participation (e.g., Butler 1991, 1994; Lewis, 1992). Thus feminist group workers and group members alike must account for socioeconomic and political forces that inflect every group process:

A feminist model indicates that members are expected to deal with issues related to oppression and sexism and to seek understanding of how personal, interpersonal, group, organizational, and societal issues relate to these. . . . Members also should explore how the personal and the political interact and, as a result of this, focus on the ways to change both personal and environmental barriers to overcoming oppression. (Garvin & Reed, 1995, pp. 56–57)

As Garvin and Glover Reed suggest, empowerment-oriented group work demands two inherently cyclical processes: intensive group dialogue, known as conscientization[4] or consciousness raising,[5] as well as concerted group action. Through the process of conscientization, individuals embark on a dialogical process in which the inherent connections between their personal lives and their political circumstances are explored, deciphered, and challenged. Such newly generated understandings provide the basis for both personal action and change, as well as the impetus for social action and change, effecting empowerment on both "micro" and "macro" levels.

This multilevel transformation is the stuff of empowerment-oriented group praxis. Through the formulation of ideas during group dialogue, the empowerment-oriented group critically transforms individual members' understandings and interactions. As such intragroup transformation is channeled into strategic planning for extragroup action, members begin to explore how their immediate influence and efficacy can be extended to larger systems (Breton, 1989b; Drysdale & Purcell, 2000; Mullender & Ward, 1991). When change occurs as a result of group action, members witness their collective and individual capacities, reflecting on past strategies and hatching plans for future action via, within, and beyond the group. Furthermore, the mutual-aid relationships established in the group serve as the core of more expansive networks as group members begin to identify and interact with others in relevant communities and systems to effect institutional or social change. In the case of empowerment-oriented groups aimed at the alleviation of poverty, social action aimed at transforming local resource distribution, for example, can clearly affect community, as well as group, members.[6]

POVERTY, RESOURCES AND
EMPOWERMENT-ORIENTED GROUP PRAXIS

People living in poverty lack access to a number of resources that many others take for granted, including shelter, nutritious food, and health care, as well as to the educational and employment opportunities that render resource acquisition less arduous. Other forms of oppression, such as racism and sexism, intersect with these deprivations, as is evidenced by the disproportionate number of people of color who live below the poverty line and the unrelenting feminization of poverty. Indeed, most of the nation's poor are women, and as most women are charged with primary child care responsibilities, they must worry about not only their own unmet needs but also those of their children.

Indeed, the fact that so much of the literature on group work with the poor is focused on all-women groups is testament to the intersecting oppressions that lead so many women to seek support outside family and community networks. Group practitioners who work with poor and homeless women must understand that members' lack of access to transportation and child care will necessarily affect any future group work. Responding appropriately by providing transportation or selecting a nearby meeting venue is essential to the long-term functioning of the group (Subramanian et al., 1995). For example, in planning for their work with low-income Hmong women, community-based researchers in Detroit understood that child care services must be provided if members were to participate in Saturday sessions (Yoshihama & Carr, 2003). Furthermore, group practitioners who work with poor and homeless individuals will want to exercise flexibility, understanding that long lines at the welfare office or a sick child can easily translate to missing or being late for group sessions (Mueller & Patton, 1995).

Group workers should also acknowledge that poverty often involves a lack of information about where resources are, how they are distributed, and how one might get hold of them, as well as a lack of resources themselves. Knowledge is in fact the most valuable resource that most empowerment-oriented groups will seek to acquire. Through mutual-aid relationships, members can share knowledge of local services and resources. However, in a society characterized by vast and systematic inequalities that render many resources unavailable to group members, mutual-aid schemas will likely involve tapping professional and institutional knowledge pools. The worker, who often has experiential knowledge of powerful systems and institutions that other group members likely lack, has a responsibility to share this information as the group works together toward benefiting from and/or transforming these systems. Yet, although the worker may be privy to information due to her relative privilege, she will soon also learn (if she hasn't already!) that poor and homeless individuals have accrued keen and critical knowledge of systems through the very experience of being oppressed, ignored, or mistreated by them.

Finally, group workers will want to understand that the experience of poverty often engenders a healthy mistrust of powerful persons and institutions. Many poor people have limited interplay with educational, market, and social supports and increased contact with institutions that involve implicit or explicit social control (such as the prison system, the child welfare system, social services, and drug treatment). Although the resulting mistrust often manifests itself as keen criticism that is the potential fodder of conscientization, it can also hinder poor people from joining an institutionally based group in the first place. When planning for a group with poor or homeless women, this reticence is one that workers will likely need to address up front.

Some practitioners who work with poor and homeless people have interpreted their members' reticence as sign of "learned helplessness" or low self-esteem and take a psychoeducational approach to remedy it. In fact, many group workers working with poor, homeless, and disenfranchised populations begin with the goal of psychological rather than socioeconomic change. Such approaches are often premised on what Johnson and Castengera (1994) refer to as the "conservative view" of poverty not as a matter of availability or distribution of resources but as a problem of people's ability to find or use them appropriately. In this view, change rests or at least begins not in unjust systems but instead in members' psyches, which are thought to suffer from a deep sense of inefficacy rather than learned mistrust. For example, in her work with clients at a food bank, Moldofosky (2000) takes a psychoeducational approach, teaching group members how to cook nutritious meals with donated materials. In recounting this group project, she notes:

> At the outset, the dominant feature in the recruiting phase was the negative attitudes of the clients of the food bank about joining the cooking class. This initial resistance was addressed by cognitive behavioral methods that were aimed at encouraging their participation. (p. 91)

Although Moldofosky's intentions were doubtlessly good and her project successful in its aims, by ignoring the institutional indices of clients "negative attitudes," she potentially overlooks both members' institutional critiques and an opportunity to work toward informed systematic rather than presumed psychic change. Furthermore, in addition to teaching people to cook more economically, such a project could have addressed institutional or social systems that make such remedial projects necessary in the first place.

Although Subramanian and colleagues (1995) suggest that psychoeducational groups' emphasis on teaching leaves less room for victim blaming, the emphasis on individual behavior modification implicitly places the onus for change on individual group members. When working with groups of poor and homeless people, this emphasis dovetails into the age-old philosophy that one's poverty is a simple matter of how hard one pulls on her own proverbial bootstraps. By contrast, empowerment-oriented group praxis combines action and reflection, attends simultaneously to the personal and the political, and explicitly addresses how oppressive forces affect members' ability to act and interact both within and outside the group. Because poverty is often thought of in individualist terms that focus on psychic or "cultural"[7] barriers to economic success, empowerment-oriented groups provide a practical anecdote. Such groups work not only to connect group members' circumstances with larger socioeconomic forces through conscientization but also to develop concrete collective strategies to resist and counter these forces.

In this light, group work with poor and homeless individuals aims beyond the immediate acquisition of resources toward the long-term goal of transforming distribution systems. For example, if group members are able to share experiences with and information about racial discrimination in the local housing market or in a social service institution, they will be more equipped to strategically respond to relevant parties, lobbying for fairer practices and services. Such actions, of course, not only increase the chances of group members' locating affordable and safe housing but also create change in the community at large, increasing their neighbors' chances of similar success.

Several group workers have recognized the efficacy of empowerment-oriented group work for critically addressing poverty and homelessness. For example, detailing his work with a social action group with homeless people, Jerome Sachs (1991) suggests that much of the group's early work aimed at overcoming political resistance to its very existence as a group. Similarly, Marcia Cohen (1994a) focuses on institutional resistance to an empowerment-oriented consumer advisory group in a small New England homeless services agency, suggesting that analyzing such barriers is an intrinsic element of the group process. Along the same lines, Butler (1994) describes a women's action group of mothers whose discussion about their children's problems soon led to a critical dialogue about the politics of poverty and the government's punishment of the poor.

Discussing her work with homeless women at a drop-in center in Toronto, Breton (1989b) not only addresses how group dialogue should be aimed to analyze such extragroup barriers, such as staff resistance, but also highlights its importance to intragroup functions. For example, Breton (1989b) describes how members' individual testimonies about personal health issues soon blossomed into a consciousness-raising session as they identified problems that were collective rather than individual. This critical dialogue served an educational role as group members exchanged information about health problems and relevant local resources. Furthermore, through the process of consciousness raising, the women at the drop-in center not only gained deeper insight into their collective problems but also moved toward engaging in social action, hatching the idea of writing to city officials about the health-related concerns they collectively identified (Breton, 1989b).

Moving from such critical dialogue to concerted action is a critical aspect of any empowerment-oriented group work, though one that is often not well addressed in the literature. Describing her group work efforts in a homeless shelter, Judith Lee (1986) discusses not only how "[t]he creation and support of primary group ties . . . [has] lasting effects [in] increased relatedness, competence, and actual support networks over time" (p. 260) but also how these dynamics were translated into concrete, positive changes at the shelter. Such changes included setting up a client pay phone, establishing an informational bulletin board, and forming linkages to job preparation programs. Although perhaps not revolutionary, these changes are indeed important preliminary actions toward accessing employment, housing, and other resources that group members needed, as well as evidence of real institutional change. As such, Lee's (1986) work demonstrates that empowerment-oriented social action group work with the poor wields both psychosocial and socioeconomic effects and thereby renders a too-strict theoretical dichotomy between psychosocial and social action approaches to group work spurious and ultimately unhelpful.

The aforementioned work illustrates both the complexities and the benefits of implementing empowerment-oriented group work among severely disenfranchised and oppressed populations. In reviewing this literature, I have outlined the relationship between group work and empowerment generally and assessed the applicability of empowerment practice principles to group work with poor people more specifically. The following section amalgamates and extends such practice principles in an effort to introduce a "new and improved" model of group work with poor and homeless women.

GROUP WORK WITH HOMELESS WOMEN: A CASE STUDY

Like Shapiro (1991), Garvin (1991) suggests that group work has strayed from its historical commitment to social action, but offers more immediate strategies for group practitioners seeking to reclaim activist roots. Primarily, Garvin (1991) argues that the group worker should expand her or his practice to include advocacy, mediation, negotiation, and brokerage, functioning as a "helpful resource" for the social action group (p. 72). Serving as an essential liaison between the group, the agency, and other relevant institutional and community contexts, the empowerment-oriented group worker acts primarily as an advocate, urging agencies to develop opportunities and create resource pools for group members. In doing so, group workers help establish a conducive context in which group members can successfully advocate for themselves in the future.

This delicate balance between performing traditional advocacy and supporting group members' own social action efforts is particularly important in work with disenfranchised groups. Advocacy on the part of the worker allows access to resources and knowledge to which group members, by virtue of their social position, are often not privy. However, although the group worker should capitalize on her or his relative privilege, she or he should also encourage group members to take advantage of all opportunities to successfully advocate for themselves. Determining how to strike this balance is a key component of the conscientization process, as both group worker and group members analyze their respective positions vis á vis the systems that they target. Furthermore, the array of skills required of the group worker, including self-reflection, facilitation, networking, advocacy, strategic planning, mediation, and brokerage, are learned skills that can be transferred to and among group members. Later I illustrate that the transfer of power from group worker to group members is the linchpin of empowerment-oriented groups with poor and homeless individuals. Ideally, this "transferring process" continues as group members teach others how to successfully engage in social action.

In the remainder of this chapter, I draw on my experience as a group worker with homeless women in an outpatient drug treatment program that I will call "Fresh Beginnings." The group, known as the Client Action Group, accomplished many goals over a 24-month period, including the establishment of an ongoing system of client representation on the program's key decision-making body (referred to hereafter as the "advisory board"), the reform of child care practices at the affiliated day care center, and the clarification of treatment contracts and protocols. However, as a project that best realized group empowerment, I recount the steps involved in establishing a client-run "clothes closet" in the basement of the treatment site.

Clothing is a basic resource to which many poor women and their children have limited access. Ill-sized or inadequate clothing cause an array of discomforts, and the lack of a warm jacket or proper shoes can pose significant health risks. Furthermore, because clothing plays a role in impression formation, it can easily affect poor women's ability to obtain gainful employment or to access other needed resources (Turner-Bowker, 2001). By soliciting, sorting through, and "selling"[8] good quality clothing, the Fresh Beginnings clothes closet facilitated members' ready access to this important, needed resource. The clothes closet also allowed clients in the program ownership over a piece of the organization, something that had hitherto been denied by an institutional structure that clearly differentiated staff and clients, charging the former with sole administrative power and responsibility. Furthermore, as the Client Action Group's first major project, the clothes closet created cohesion among the group and offered the opportunity for individual members to develop the skills associated with setting up a small business. Thus the group was successful both in accessing needed resources in an immediate sense and in developing abilities, networks, and strategies for future resource attainment.[9] This was evident in the fact that the clients' success in operating the clothes closet was soon followed by another victory: establishing a rotating client representative on the program's advisory board. In detailing the story of the Client Action Group and our clothes-closet project, I recount such successes, as well as foibles, in the hopes of providing some concrete practical guidance for groups aimed at the alleviation of poverty and the access of resources.

Steps for the Empowerment-Oriented Group Worker with Resource-Poor Groups

Engaging

Before initiating any group with poor and homeless individuals, the group worker is wise to "preplan" (Mullender & Ward, 1991), identifying sources of support and sites of resources toward which future group action might be aimed. This stage might best be described as a process of engagement as the group worker familiarizes him- or herself with the people who and systems that may participate in, support, or resist the group's efforts or very existence. The group worker should also conduct a preliminary but thorough local resource assessment so that this knowledge can be passed along to new group members. Another critical component of engagement involves the group worker's undertaking a personal inventory in which she determines her own position vis á vis these relevant systems and reflects on the principles that will guide her work.

INITIAL REFLECTION

As Butler (1991) notes, "Group work, both its practice and its theory, is a value laden enterprise. Attitudes and beliefs are there in worker's actions at every stage of the practice endeavor, whether they are aware of it or not" (p. 18). Therefore, it is critical that the empowerment-oriented group worker identifies, clarifies, and reflects on the principles that will guide her or his work before she or he initiates any logistical planning or engages with group members (Mullender & Ward, 1991). In groups of poor and homeless individuals, this initial inventory requires the worker not only to acknowledge her or his own experiences in relation to privilege and oppression but also to ascertain how these experiences relate to her or his desire and ability to work toward socioeconomic change. Sachs (1991) views such honest reflection as

> particularly important when one works with a group whose class interests, not to mention values, history, culture, race, gender, and lifestyle, are different from one's own and when one gains materially, however indirectly, from this difference, or when one's employment as a worker derives from the very existence of the social problem. (p. 189)

Determining the social position from which one perceives and acts in the world is essential to the understanding of oppression generally and of the related ways in which group efforts may be hindered or stymied more specifically.

When my proposal to start a Client Action Group at Fresh Beginnings was accepted by the advisory board to the program, my excitement was tempered only by an understanding of the formidable challenges the job would entail. First, I knew that the work I wanted to do might put me at odds with board members whose approach to social service was rather conservative but whose approval I sought as a fledgling social worker trying to further my career. Moreover, I was concerned about relationships with group members. Although I had come to Fresh Beginnings because of an ardent critical interest in the feminization of poverty, I knew that trust, effective communication, and working relationships would be harder to build with women with whom I shared little in common, at least in socioeconomic terms. I imagined my limited experience and relatively sheltered background immediately reflected on the disapproving faces of group members, but I forged ahead in the hopes that my tempered but tenacious enthusiasm would prove contagious.

ASSESSING SYSTEM BARRIERS

Several empowerment-oriented group practitioners who work with poor and homeless individuals document the organizational and community resistance to their work (e.g., Cohen 1994a; Sachs, 1991). Breton (1994) notes that social workers are often resistant to ceding professional expertise and power, rendering empowerment practice unpalatable. Butler (1991) adds that feminist groups may be particularly threatening in social service environments that operate on the basis of hierarchical practice protocols that clearly differentiate professionals and clients.

To the extent that it is possible, group workers should identify such potential sources of resistance prior to convening their groups, as such foresight can ultimately help prepare the group to face and negotiate these challenges in the future. Cohen (1994a) suggests employing force-field analysis and organizational change analysis to understand institutional resistance.[10] The use of ethnographic methods, such as participant observation, are also helpful in mapping the terrain of relevant systems. In addition to these methods, it is critical that the group worker carefully explain to relevant parties the concept and plan for the group and gauge their reactions.

Having participated on the Fresh Beginnings advisory board for several months prior to the initiation of the group, I had already identified some potential sources of resistance to empowerment-oriented group work within the organization. Generally, I had witnessed staff's rapport with clients, which, though well-intentioned and caring, often bordered on the patronizing. Moreover, I wondered how both staff and clients would make the transition from therapy groups, in which clients were encouraged to talk in monological, psychological terms about their problems, to the more dialogical process of connecting those very same problems to sociopolitical and economic circumstances.

Knowing that empowerment is possible largely to the extent that established power relations allow, on taking the job as the group facilitator, I designed an ethnographic project that, through participant observation and discourse analysis, sought to decipher the power dynamics within the treatment program. Soon I identified five discourses that staff members used to limit clients' participation in program decision making. This initial analysis proved to be helpful throughout the group process, as members and I successfully circumvented or challenged organizational resistance.

FINDING ALLIES AND MAKING CONTACTS

In addition to assessing environmental barriers to empowerment-oriented group work, it is equally important for group workers to find allies and make supportive contacts. Allies within relevant systems and communities can provide critical support for both the group and the group worker, supplying material resources, invaluable practical guidance, and encouragement. For example, such contacts can give excellent advice for recruiting group members, establishing local allies, or negotiating system barriers (Yoshihama & Carr, 2003). Aspiring group workers might also want to meet with a local consultant who has led social action or empowerment-oriented groups with poor and homeless individuals. These consultants can also provide the practical wisdom, experience, and support that aid workers in clarifying values, facilitating empowering group process, and meeting concrete goals.

My initial work at Fresh Beginnings was aided by a few critical allies who were affiliated with the program. I determined early on that one member of the advisory board shared with me the sociopolitical perspectives that differentiated us from many of our more psychosocially oriented colleagues. Initially, he was a vociferous advocate in support of my proposal for the group, and I continued to call on him when I needed to discuss group-related issues. Another system ally, who had long-term contact with both the staff and the clients, helped me to identify some potential sources of organizational resistance. Additionally, personal contacts within the program often lent encouragement although approaches and goals often differed significantly.

Because organizational separation between administrative staff and clients was an inherent feature of the organizational structure at Fresh Beginnings, I had little opportunity to meet with clients before I initiated the group. Such contact would have been extraordinarily helpful in preparing me for what was to come. On the other hand, my academic and community ties proved helpful as I relied on my mentor, a veteran group worker, as a consultant. Offering particularly good advice on how to handle staff resistance, she often helped me to negotiate the problems related to group development and planning by sharing her similar experiences.

BUILDING NETWORKS

Seasoned group practitioners suggest that in order to realize empowerment, the worker must help establish continuity between the group and the wider communities and systems with which it is affiliated (e.g., Drysdale & Purcell, 2000). This is particularly important in group work with poor and homeless people, who, by definition, experience significant disenfranchisement in relation to powerful parties and institutions (Johnson & Castengera, 1994). Workers can pass on knowledge about support systems and resources, building critical networks from which group members can draw.

My initial familiarity with local social services and community resources, such as domestic violence programs, food banks, thrift stores, housing, and psychological services, proved an important asset throughout the growth of the Fresh Beginnings group. Primarily, I was able to pass information to group members who later benefited from the services personally. As a group, we often gleaned support or borrowed ideas from these services and resources. For example, contacts at the local Welfare Rights Organization allowed contact with women activists who not only provided invaluable practical information to the group but also lent advice on successful organizing for social action. Other contacts in the community, such as a local activist/poet, provided inspiration for the group in its early stages. As we mapped the terrain of the community, group members also became increasingly aware of the lack of support and resources, thereby formulating potential goals for group action.

Initiating the Group

After the engagement stage, which includes self-evaluation, initial networking, and identification of sites of support, resistance, and resources, the empowerment-oriented group worker is ready to initiate the group. This is a busy and sometimes stressful time in which the worker must stay focused on his or her vision for the group and resist temptation to cut corners. Many logistics are required, such as finding an appropriate venue for the group, obtaining needed resources, and recruiting group members. It is also essential in the early stages of group development that the group worker establishes trust and collegiality with new group members who will eventually take over his or her role.

RECRUITING PARTICIPANTS

When planning any group, group workers must first weigh the pros and cons of selecting group members versus having open membership. Although there are substantial benefits to initiating open-membership groups, particularly in the inclusivity that it allows, it may be preferable to recruit a small number of participants in the initial stages of group development. These core members can then decide whether or not they will open the group to others. In either case, it is helpful to ask local community members' advice when determining the initial parameters of membership.

Substantial barriers may occur when trying to recruit members from oppressed or disenfranchised populations (Yoshihama & Carr, 2003). For example, flyers may not be an effective recruitment tool among those with limited literacy skills. Furthermore, flyers may not be posted by resistant local organizations or may be ripped down by hostile parties. Although some empowerment-oriented group workers suggest employing the help of relevant staff members when recruiting clients from institutions, group workers must be aware that staff members may recommend "compliant" or otherwise nonthreatening clients who share the perspective of the people and systems against which social action will be potentially directed. In the various social networks of group members themselves, word of mouth often serves as a potent recruitment tool, especially when working with populations who have a healthy distrust of "outsiders." Allies in these communities can effectively mobilize such hesitant individuals and promote participation in the group. In any case, outreach efforts must be consistently executed, as initial contacts with potential participants often require substantial follow-up protocol.

Meeting directly after the required Tuesday morning therapy group, all 10 Fresh Beginnings clients were invited to join the Client Action Group. However, without my knowledge, program therapists suggested to clients that membership in the group was "required," a misperception I quickly corrected. Clients were often burdened by meeting all the requirements of the program on top of the other burdens and chores of daily life that poverty and homelessness presented. Furthermore, I realized that some clients, who attended the program to meet parole or Child Protective Services requirements, may not be interested in joining a group that could potentially interfere, or even endanger, their tenuous position in the program. The group, after all, was intended to challenge such systems, including the treatment program itself. Although some clients decided not to join at first, in the end almost all clients participated in the group, though sometimes peripherally and selectively.

FINDING A VENUE AND OBTAINING NEEDED MATERIALS

Finding a venue and obtaining needed materials can be difficult when working with resource-poor groups. Due to systemic inequities, both the community and the social service environs of such groups are likely to be resource poor as well (a fact, in and of itself, that can be a poignant topic for early consciousness-raising discussions). Organizational resistance or discrimination can also be a barrier in finding an appropriate venue or obtaining materials for the group. The advice of group members, as well as group allies, can again be helpful in finding a nonalienating environment and in locating parties who might donate needed materials.

It is advisable to establish only a tentative meeting place for the initial meeting of the group. After that, group members can collectively decide a comfortable and readily accessible place to meet in the future. With resource-poor groups, difficulties with transportation must be acknowledged and ameliorated. Group workers should prepare the group to potentially meet in informal environs, such as group members' apartments or a local park. Even when group members are coping with serious economic deprivation, it is often possible to set up an elemental mutual-aid system in which each member makes a small contribution to the group resource pool. Taking control of these logistical matters allows members to establish collective ownership of the group early in its development.

Because the program provided both materials for the Client Action Group and a venue for the initial meeting, these were not formidable barriers in initiating the group. However, as the group developed—particularly after group members formulated collective critiques of the program and planned on confronting the board—some group members expressed discomfort with our meeting arrangements, suggesting that staff might overhear our deliberations. After some negotiation with staff, we were able to relocate our meeting venue to the basement of the program building, a change that immediately and substantially affected the degree to which members seemed to speak critically and openly about the problems they faced within the program and more generally.

BUILDING TRUST

Trust is always an essential element of successful group work. In empowerment-oriented groups with disenfranchised populations, group work cannot proceed until some degree of trust is established, not just among members who share a particular structural problem but between those members and the group worker, who is often relatively privileged in socioeconomic and political terms. Furthermore, when a worker is formally connected to an institution that is distrusted by group members, such as a university or state agency, further challenges can easily arise (Yoshihama & Carr, 2003).

The empowerment-oriented group worker builds trust with the group by openly and honestly expressing her or his own principles and perceptions, stressing how they are connected with her or his particular experiences, without trying to persuade or coerce. This group work principle has been elegantly developed by feminist group workers who advocate for transparency, in which the group worker clearly reveals her perceptions, demystifying herself as a "leader" (e.g., Butler, 1991; Garvin & Glover Reed, 1995). Maintaining an open attitude to diverging ideas and values facilitates group processes, which, in turn, enrich all group members' knowledge base and help guide the way to collective action. Through such practice, the group worker not only models the dialogical methods on which empowerment-group process relies but also allows members to understand her or his position in relation to the group and the social problems the group means to redress. The worker then can be seen as a helpful resource rather than as a directive leader.

My initial idea to start a Client Action Group was in good part inspired by the encouragement of a former Fresh Beginnings client, who said such a group would be heartily welcomed by other clients. However, such enthusiasm did not register on the wary faces of the six women I encountered when I first entered the group room to introduce myself. As I nervously began my introduction, telling of my interest in "women's issues," one group member ironically announced; "Oh, she's another one of these good-deed-doers from the university. Get ready." Her peers seemed to sneer in disapproving agreement.

Trust grew slowly and silently, and our first meetings were not productive in any material sense. Not without some pain and humiliation, I endured several hours of sometimes caustic teasing about my name, my style of speech and dress, and, of course, my "good deed doing." However, after about a month of meetings, a frustrated group member broached a problem—her lack of decent clothing for an upcoming job interview. She spoke to group members of all the beautiful clothes she jettisoned during a midnight departure from a home once shared with a violent husband. Other women chimed in to tell of clothes sold for drugs or food, worn to the point of deterioration, or stolen by shelter mates. Now, in treatment and seeking housing, education, and employment, all of the women expressed a need for appropriate and warm clothing. "Hey, can this group find a way to get us some clothes?" one group member asked to my glee. Our first task as a group was thereby born.

Though our success with this project eventually helped establish trust in the group, I quickly found that there was no way to expedite or solidify trust. It was a long and arduous process, complete with ebbs and peaks, especially as new members joined the group. However, word of mouth proved helpful as, for example, an old member told a new member,

"Yeah, she's cool. She's not just one of those good-deed-doin' students from the University. She is that, but she also hears what we're sayin'."

ESTABLISHING COLLEGIALITY

Although the group worker cannot erase the socioeconomic inequities that account for her relative privilege, by relinquishing the power of "expertise," a practice protocol Breton (1994) terms "collegiality," the group worker begins to work *with* group members, not just *for* them. Furthermore, group workers should practice collaborative, rather than patronizing, pedagogical styles, facilitating group processes in which group members can effectively share knowledge and skills.

Clearly, collegiality is stymied when group workers are not open to divergent ideas or try to control group process. However, collegiality does not mean that the group worker denies acquired or intuitive knowledge but instead that she accepts own her lack of knowledge and appreciates the knowledge of others in the group. Mullender and Ward (1991) draw a careful distinction between leadership that is directive and facilitation that is aimed at helping group members discover their own means to achieve group ends. They warn that empowerment-oriented group workers often fall too heavily in the direction of radical nonintervention, a move that can elicit mistrust and bitterness among group members who know that the worker has skills and resources to contribute. Thus it is important that the group worker continually mobilize her skills for the benefit of the group while establishing collegiality in facilitating group processes and achieving group goals.

Establishing collegiality with group members was a long-term process, especially considering the disparity between group members' and my own access to relevant information and other resources needed to achieve our newly set goals. As the Client Action Group started to seriously discuss the possibility of setting up a clothes closet in the basement of the Fresh Beginnings program, questions and comments were generally directed at me, and I sorted through them carefully. For example, when clients asked about how the agency processed donations, a question that I could readily answer based on my long-term affiliation with staff, I provided as much information as I could. I also volunteered information about potential allies among staff members and how we might most effectively go about broaching our plan of action to the board. However, when questions were posed that did not relate to my position within the program or access to resources, questions that all group members could answer, I deflected the question to other members accordingly. For example, when clients broached questions about how the clothes closet would be operated or how they might solicit donations, I would work to redirect them to other members, knowing that opinions abounded. As collegiality grew, I felt increasingly comfortable asserting my opinions on such matters as other group members did, but my basic role was that of an information giver, capitalizing on the knowledge and resources to which I had access by virtue of my professional status.

Facilitating the Group

Collegiality is one cornerstone of empowerment-oriented group facilitation, yet many other processes are involved. In order to sustain trusting and productive working relationships within the group, members do well to establish some protocols and ground rules for group interaction. Rather than restricting discussion, these protocols should engender the discursive process of consciousness raising, as well as aid in strategic planning for action.

ESTABLISHING GROUND RULES

Establishing ground rules is an essential group process that fosters members' sense of ownership over the group. When developed with collegiality, ground rules serve as an effective collective contract for group interaction and process. Although the group worker might suggest particular ground rules, his or her main role is to facilitate this initial group process, helping members negotiate their expectations and interests. Once ground rules are established and recorded, they not only help to guide group interaction but also help members to sort through inevitable conflicts. Because groups change and grow in various ways, a system by which ground rules can be revised is important.

The Client Action Group did not initially establish ground rules, and this proved to be a significant error. Conflicts that naturally arose in the course of our sometimes heated discussions could have been averted or ameliorated had we established collective rules of group comportment. Six months into meeting, we finally resolved to establish group rules, an arduous process that took two full sessions. During this process, old resentments about past conflicts arose (i.e., "well, remember when you left the room when I was talking, we shouldn't be able to do that"). At one point, we had to make ground rules for establishing ground rules! After much collective exasperation, we finally came up with a list of rules that were recorded in our meeting notebook, something that would have best been accomplished in our very first meetings.

FACILITATING CONSCIOUSNESS RAISING

The empowerment-oriented group worker's primary role is not to initiate topics for consciousness raising, but instead to facilitate critical discussion on issues broached by group members. Specifically, the group worker should encourage group members to draw connections between the problems that they identify as personal and the collective manifestation of these problems as political issues. Mullender and Ward (1991) suggest a strategy for facilitating empowerment-oriented group work by posing the questions *what* (is the collective problem?) and *why* (do group members share this problem?) As an anthropologist, I suggest adding the critical questions of "when" and "where," so that members may understand the historical and contextual dimensions of target problems and potential solutions. Accepting group members' own answers to these questions as they work to collectively define problems and solutions is essential, as it relays the worker's belief that members are quite capable of critically understanding the political nature of their circumstances (Gutiérrez, 1991).

Although the empowerment-oriented group worker takes a facilitating rather than directive approach to consciousness raising, she or he may feel it important to broach issues or perspectives that might not otherwise arise in the group. For example, members may persist with the presumption, common in contemporary American culture, that poverty is a matter of personal responsibility rather than systematic inequality, and the group worker may want to present evidence to the contrary. Or feminist workers might initiate discussion about how gender or race intersect with economic inequality and spark members to analyze the gender and race dynamics of their own group processes.

It was not long before the group's initial discussions regarding their common lack of adequate clothing branched into a more general exploration of the political circumstances (e.g., women's homelessness, violence against women, economic stratification) that framed their collective experience. For example, in reference to wardrobes abandoned in escape from an abusive partner, members asked each other, "Why do men do that shit?" Later in

*our planning, another member commented, "That store is for rich white folks . . . I went
there once and they were like waiting for me to lift something." Such talk of race and gender
arose spontaneously, warranting little facilitation, as members shared the expertise derived
from their uniformly tough but rich experiences.*

*Discussions such as these soon took more practical and directed form as we began to
plan for the clothes closet. When the question arose of who might be the best person to talk
with about the group's plan, I responded that the advisory board would be the most appropriate body. Most group members were totally unaware that this board existed, a fact that
became the kernel of an important consciousness-raising discussion and eventual action
plan. These early discussions were critical in allowing all of us to further understand the system within which we were working, particularly in terms of the structural divide between
"professionals" and "clients." The idea of a client-operated clothes closet, group members
recognized, would inherently challenge such a system. "We need something of our own in
this program," one group member declared to a circle of nodding heads. Thus, in planning
for the clothes closet, the group also began to discuss the question of why there was no client representation on the board. We also discussed what we wanted to do about it, and how
we wanted to proceed.*

SUPPORTING ACTION

To the degree that consciousness raising generates such critical dialogue, it is the necessary
precursor to any group action. Namely, it can help the group decide which problems it
wishes to address and how to best initiate action. The group worker serves to help the group
plan for and support social action, setting goals that are ambitious but within potential
reach.

Planning for and supporting action requires that group members identify sources of potential power and resources that could be utilized and/or attained through the group's efforts. Gutiérrez (1991) advises that this process should include identifying forgotten, innate,
or potential skills, such as personal skills of social influence, and making full use of group
support networks in relevant communities and institutions. Furthermore, the group worker,
who is often privy to information about target systems by virtue of her relatively privileged
position within those systems, should share and mobilize her knowledge to support the
group action. Finally, the group worker should serve as a steady source of encouragement
and support throughout the action-taking process, expressing confidence, congratulating
victories, and consoling defeats.

*The Client Action Group decided on two action goals: (1) to seek the authority to oper-
ate a collective clothes closet in the basement of the treatment site, and (2) to begin to advocate for a client representative on the program's advisory board. Collectively we prioritized
these goals, deciding that the members' need for clothes was more pressing. As we began to
understand the development of the current institutional structure by asking the critical questions of "when?" and "where?" (see "Facilitating Consciousness Raising"), we implicitly responded by establishing a tentative timeline and target for our action plans.*

*As a group, we began to think of how to most effectively present our plan for the
clothes closet, formulated during many weeks of group discussion, to the advisory board.
This discussion revolved around balancing advocacy and self-advocacy. Prioritizing the goal
of the clothes closet, we were operating within a system that had virtually no space for client
self-representation. In this light, several options were openly discussed: (1) client members*

of the group, en masse or individually, would attend the advisory board without invitation to represent their plan for the clothes closet, (2) the group would write a memo to the advisory board detailing our proposal, (3) they would send the memo with me, as a regular board member, so that I could advocate for the proposal in person. After much discussion, the group agreed that in light of both long- and short-term goals, sending me with the memo but allowing it to "speak for itself" best realized the group's ideals.

As a group, we created a memo that highlighted clients' need for clothes and emphasized the group's desire to operate the clothes closet without the help of or interference from staff. The memo was eloquent, detailed, and passionate. We decided to inform a couple of the "allies" we had identified on the board, hoping to garner their support in advance. Despite these efforts, soon after I distributed the memo at the board meeting, its primary premise was swiftly rejected; although board members thought the idea of the clothes closet was a good one, they were not comfortable with clients running the closet on their own. As a virtually silent messenger, I was not prepared for the board's counterproposal: a staff-run clothes closet in which clients gained "points" through meeting sobriety goals and program requirements. Feeling our idea had been usurped and twisted about, I returned to the Client Action Group disappointed and distressed.

ENCOURAGING PRAXIS

Paulo Freire (1993, p. 107) posited that "a revolution is achieved neither with verbalism or with activism alone, but rather with praxis, that is, with *reflection* and *action* directed at the structures to be transformed." Indeed, empowerment-oriented group work is a cyclical process, epitomizing the praxis ideal. Consciousness raising allows group members to identify, define, and redefine problems and to begin to formulate critical opinions and to plan for productive action. Social action follows to address the problems thereby identified. Such actions always produce change, whether positive or negative, expected or unexpected, relevant to the target system or confined to the group itself. The empowerment-oriented group worker helps the group deal with this array of outcomes by encouraging a process of collective reflection. Specifically, the group worker might pose the questions "What happened?", "Why?", "Where do we go from here?", and "How do we get there?" In answering these questions, group members reflect on their actions and reformulate previous definitions in order to take further action. However, in group work aimed at accessing resources, it is of continued essence that the group continue to see poverty as a manifestation of entrenched systems rather than the result of failed actors.

Realizing the principles of praxis, the Client Action Group met the bad news with reflection and plans for further action, as well as with bitter disappointment. We reviewed the staff's counterproposal and worked to analyze the nature of their objections to our plan. Group members agreed that the staff indeed seemed uncomfortable with ceding control of administrative functions, and although their need for clothes was pressing in the short term, they kept their eyes on the long term. The board's counterproposal for staff governance of the clothes closet was analyzed and soundly rejected. One group member saw the "point system" the board proposed as "just another way they try to control us." Other members agreed but expressed interest in the idea of "points" as a kind of currency. After much discussion, the group came up with a follow-up proposal, incorporating the advisory board's idea of a point system, but one that would be devised and overseen by clients rather than staff and remaining steadfast in the goal of client control of the project. Knowing that the board might want evidence that such a plan was feasible, the group included in our second memo detailed information about how the point system would work.

Carrying the memo, written as it was in the "group's voice," I attended the next board meeting. Though several members expressed admiration of the group's obvious efforts in the counterproposal, the board rejected the plan. Now, members expressed concern that such a project would "overwhelm" the clients, who, homeless and addicted, had "enough to worry about." The board's words rang eerily familiar, as I recalled the findings of my recently completed ethnographic research (see "Assessing System Barriers"). However, not wanting to respond in behalf of the group, still believing that group empowerment necessarily meant curtailed advocacy on my part, I returned to the group, once again disappointed.

Many members were dejected, and some insulted by the board's insinuation that they were too "overwhelmed" to carry through with the project. Some threatened to abandon the effort, saying, "These people just aren't gonna budge . . . they're stuck in their ways." These words gave me an idea: Why don't we point out to them how stuck in their ways they are? The advisory board always talked about empowerment, and this was a chance to realize it. "But they aren't listening to us anyway, Summerson," one group member protested, "do you think they are gonna hear that?" I responded that we try another way to get our message across. I suggested that, this time, I compose a memo as an advocate. The memo would draw from both our critical discussion in the group and my knowledge of the professional discourses in the program. I asked the group for permission to present and defend the memo at the next board meeting, and they, with some spark amid the general dejection, granted it unanimously.

The memo had two important effects. First, it changed the board's mind. With some dissension, the board voted to grant full custody of the clothes closet to the Client Action Group, with no interference from staff. Of course, the group was delighted to hear the news. However, the success of the memo belied another problem: that is, that the board was much more comfortable with advocacy (in the form of the memo I authored) than with empowerment (in the form of the memo written by the Client Action Group). Although we saw how advocacy was needed to reach our short-term goal, this information was used as the basis of reflection and strategic planning for our next major project: establishing a system of client representation.

Transferring Power

Breton (1994) notes that the most substantial challenge for the empowerment-oriented group worker is to transfer her or his professional power to allow group members to be the primary agents of their own successes. When working with poor and homeless individuals, who lack not only material resources but also often access to the pools of information, knowledge, and expertise by which those resources are distributed and managed, this transfer is all the more essential and difficult. Thus, the first step in attaining resources and effecting social change is to distribute among all members the knowledge, skills, and responsibility on which successful group work rests.

TRANSFERRING INFORMATION

In order to effectively distribute power among all group members, the worker must share his or her knowledge and pass information through nonhierarchical pedagogy. Feminist practitioners recognize that knowledge is the most potent form of power and suggest that the rendering of such knowledge should define all stages of group work (Butler, 1991). In group work with poor and homeless individuals, the first step in accessing resources can be pooling information about where those resources can be located. The group worker, by virtue of her or his professional training and experience, may have such essential information. However, it is at least equally important to tap into members' enormous reserves of knowledge about relevant systems, knowledge that is sometimes gleaned from their experiences of deprivation within those systems.

Throughout my work with the Client Action Group, I consistently passed on the information and knowledge I had gained through both my social work education and my position within the Fresh Beginnings program. Because of the organizational divide between clients and staff and my affiliation with the latter, I had gained much knowledge about the system that the Client Action Group worked to change. Therefore, I was able to suggest, for example, "we might want to go right to the director with that," explaining the intricacies of the organizational authority structure. Such bits of information allowed group members access to the kind of information that eventually helped them to advocate on their own behalf. Indeed, within a few months of establishing the clothes closet, one client was spontaneously placing phone calls to key program administrators, eloquently voicing clients' collective concerns about psychiatric care and hiring practices.

TRANSFERRING SKILLS

Teaching specific skills is an essential part of any empowering group work, but it is particularly important with groups with members who have had limited access to formal education. Though many of the skills needed to successfully run an empowerment-oriented group are intuitive and informal, skills training can be important in helping members to effectively plan, advocate, and attain resources. Group facilitation skills can also be taught both directly and through modeling. Due to her training, the worker herself will have skills to teach, but she should also work to facilitate skills sharing among members. By transferring these skills, the group members can successfully continue with their work without the worker's continued assistance.

Teaching skills was an important aspect of the continued success of the Client Action Group at Fresh Beginnings. While running the clothes closet, group members who had telemarketing experience helped others make phone calls to clothing shops to solicit donations. Similarly, another group member and I taught several group members basic word processing skills as we wrote memos and devised the point system. Those with bookkeeping skills took the lead in recording points and passed them along to others when they graduated from or left the program. These newly developed skills not only facilitated the establishment of the clothes closet and access to needed clothes but also served members in the future as they looked for employment.

Importantly, soon after obtaining the clothes closet, we established a cofacilitation model within the group. One natural group leader joined me in "running" the group, and I shared with her the lessons I had learned in both my formal training and experience as a group worker. Four months into our work together, I suggested that she was ready to take over the job as the lead facilitator, instituting a "train-the-trainer" model. Now, my cofacilitator took over primary duties of running the group and, before long, began working with another young member to train her in group facilitation skills. This cofacilitation model characterized the group for the remainder of its life.

TRANSFERRING RESPONSIBILITY

Finally, the group worker should prepare members for the responsibility that group facilitation entails. When working with disenfranchised groups whose lives can be extremely complicated by poor access to resources such as transportation or shelter, the transfer of responsibility should be undertaken with particular care. Thus, when passing on responsibility to group members, the worker works with the group to ascertain what resources are needed to insure continued group successes.

The cofacilitation model proved an important innovation in terms of passing on responsibility. First, with two members running the group in tandem at all times, responsibility over group functions could be effectively shared. Those without phones relied on their cofacilitator to make necessary communications, and car pools to board meetings were established once our client representation system was established.

Second, in a program in which many clients filtered through quickly, sometimes leaving town to go into an inpatient facility or to take advantage of Section 8 housing, responsibility for the group was sometimes explicitly fostered. After losing a cofacilitator, the group decided to record the responsibilities required of the cofacilitator and to vote as a group (rather than simply volunteer) to fill the job. In general, cofacilitators took the job quite seriously, working to nurture the group and move forward with collective action plans.

Wrapping Up

Knowing when and to what extent to withdraw from the group is perhaps the most formidable challenge that faces the empowerment-oriented group worker. Butler (1991) describes withdrawal as a potentially empowering act that allows members to develop skills, knowledge, and confidence that ultimately sustain the group. However, she also emphasizes that smooth transfer of power from worker to group members can be hindered by members' poor access to services and resources, an important reminder for practitioners working with poor or homeless individuals. Again, using one's advocacy skills to assure that the group has the resources needed to sustain itself without the continued, direct support of the group worker is of essence.

EASING OUT

For the group worker, leaving the group requires skill, intuition, and courage. Besides the practical and pedagogical skills of transferring power, analytical skill and intuition are needed in order to ascertain whether group members have the needed resources, knowledge, and skills to continue without the worker's direct support. Honed communication skills are also required, for it is important to discuss one's departure with other group members well in advance. Finally, the group worker needs the courage to know that empowerment-oriented group work is always aimed at the worker replacing him- or herself and that, despite failures and in light of successes, the group has healthily outgrown him or her.

With the cofacilitation model firmly in place, and the train-the-trainer model flourishing, I began to feel extraneous to the group. Attending the group less frequently, I saw that members continued to meet, to discuss problems within the program, as well as in their daily lives, and to set action goals regardless of my presence or absence. Several of our goals, including the long-term goal of establishing an ongoing client representative position on the board, had been accomplished. And though, after one year of successful administration of the clothes closet, clients' interest in it seemed to be waning, after a couple of months of exuberant cheerleading, I reminded myself that it was up to them to decide the fate of their first collective project. Most important, considering that the Client Action Group was an established aspect of the organization, with staff and clients now regarding it as an exemplar of empowerment practice, I assured myself that the group's life was far stronger than my connection with it. Explaining all of this to group members, I announced my intentions to officially resign from the group.

SATELLITE CONSULTANCY

After officially resigning in her or his original capacities, the worker ideally serves the group as a consultant, providing resources, support, and advice on an ongoing basis. Thus maintaining some level of proximity to the group, without interfering in the group's newly established processes, is often important, especially in groups of resource-poor members. As the worker-turned-consultant learns new information or discovers new resources, she or he can pass these along to group leaders, who may pass them along to the group. Furthermore, assuring that group members have a way to contact the consultant after her or his departure creates a sense of community support, a goal of every empowerment-oriented group.

Phone calls from group leaders were frequent, especially during crisis times. When the Client Action Group wanted to protest hiring decisions in the program or child care problems, they had little question of how to proceed (e.g., phone calls to the director; collectively or individually written letters), but they sometimes asked for advice about how they should deal with a new staff member. Once, members of the Client Action Group needed legal advice and called me to get a referral to a reliable source. Sometimes, members called just to relay the latest "scoop," much to my interest and delight. Most of the time, however, I was not informed of the group's decisions in advance, decisions that I sometimes thought were mistakes. One morning, after several months without a visit to the group, I approached the Fresh Beginnings building to see the contents of the clothes closet packed in two vans to be driven away to Goodwill. Panicking, thinking a staff member must be behind such an apparent debacle, I ran upstairs to the group room ready for group revolt. "It was our decision, Summerson," they calmly and collectively explained to me. "It just wasn't working anymore."

CONCLUSIONS: COMBINING ADVOCACY AND EMPOWERMENT IN GROUP WORK FOR THE ACCESS OF RESOURCES AND ALLEVIATION OF POVERTY

Perhaps there was something rather ironic about the group trying to comfort me as I watched the vans pull away with donated clothes piled in the back. At first, I couldn't help but regard the scene as one of failure, the beginning of the end. However, as group members worked to soothe me, answering my troubled queries in confident unison, I realized that the demise of the clothes closet was certainly not a sign of the demise of the group. Instead, as I listened to group members, I was reminded of and coached in the core principles of empowerment group practice. And, insofar as they delineated these principles, their wise comfort serves as an ideal conclusion here, a succinct guide for future practice with poor and homeless groups.

First, in talking with group members, I was reminded that empowerment-oriented

groups should be evaluated not only to the extent that they create resources and opportunities for group members but also to the degree that they effect positive social change in the
communities, institutions, and other systems with which they are involved. Group members
now had access to clothes vouchers and a number of community resources for clothing, rendering the clothes closet less necessary. Now, the women explained, the group's energies
were focused on representing their interests in policies and practices in the program that affected them. Through their concerted efforts, discharge and probation contracts had been
clarified, staff hiring and firing processes had been made more transparent, and the rotating
client representative had grown to be a respected and indispensable member of the board.
These changes not only made the program more accessible and client friendly—allowing
members to succeed in treatment and then move on to school, employment, and/or family
responsibilities—but also gave them experience in advocating for themselves and changing
the systems that contributed to their poverty. Furthermore, the Client Action Group ultimately changed the Fresh Beginnings program in ways that not only affected them as current clients in the program but also positively affected future clients and staff.

Group members' sage words also reminded me that empowerment-oriented groups
must discover resources, develop and implement concrete strategies to attain themed, and
work to hurdle the array of barriers that may hinder access. In the case of the clothes closet,
we not only negotiated and ultimately altered the institutional structures that hindered access to material resources (i.e., the clothes) but also did so in a way that ultimately gave
members resources that they could carry with them into the world (i.e., knowledge about
systems; skills in facilitation, administration, and advocacy; the pride of collective success).
Indeed, an empowerment-oriented group's success is dependent both on the realization of
concrete goals and on the development of the interpersonal processes by which those goals
are reached and often extended.

Finally, as group members spoke, I took some awkward comfort in the fact that our
roles had appropriately shifted, as their responsibility for the group came to include consoling a distressed, retiring worker. Indeed, the story of the Client Action Group exemplifies
that empowerment-oriented groups aimed at the alleviation of poverty should combine traditional advocacy and social action approaches, thereby making shifting demands on the
group worker, as well as on other group members. As indicated in the preceding procedural
guide, empowerment-oriented group work aimed at the alleviation of poverty requires many
skills on the part of both group worker and members. Group workers must develop and
pass along skills in self-reflection, facilitation, networking, advocacy, mediation, negotiation, and brokerage to insure the success of the group (Garvin, 1991; Gutiérrez, 1990).
However, the greatest challenge for the empowerment-oriented group worker is that of balance. As the story of the clothes closet keenly illustrates, knowing when to mobilize the
knowledge and skills gleaned from one's relatively privileged position can mean the difference between gaining or losing resources for the group. On the other hand, heavy-handed
intervention stymies the transfer of power that epitomizes the practice of empowerment. As
a kind of tightrope walk, empowerment-oriented group work requires acute attention to every step and much practice, as well as awareness that some stagnancy and falls are inevitable. This chapter is meant to help future empowerment-oriented group workers who work
toward the alleviation of poverty to strike this precarious balance.

In this chapter, I have proposed that empowerment approaches are particularly relevant
to group work with poor and homeless individuals to the extent that they (1) expose the
various dimensions and relations of power, both internal and external to the group, that can

facilitate, hinder, or even stymie access to knowledge and other resources; (2) recognize the inextricability of the personal lives of group members with the socioeconomic and political circumstances the group means to redress through social action; and (3) combine advocacy and self-advocacy both in attaining immediately needed resources and in working toward systematic change within and beyond the group's immediate institutional parameters. The future of group work with poor and homeless individuals is, therefore, the future of good empowerment practice.

NOTES

1. Praxis is a process that feminists and liberation theologists, for example, have adopted as a primary methodology in action-oriented group work and pedagogical practices aimed at social change. As an inherently collective endeavor, praxis implies that social action depends on a cyclical process of problem identification, problem deconstruction and redefinition, social action, and reflection (see Carr, 2003).
2. For the purposes of this chapter, I use the term "resources" not just to indicate material assets such as housing, income, or transportation. Recognizing that such things as information, professional stature, and institutional access are inextricably linked to acquisition of such material needs, I expand my working definition to include these less tangible resources as well.
3. In order to protect the anonymity of the program, as well as that of affiliated clients and staff, I use pseudonyms throughout the chapter and alter potentially recognizable details accordingly.
4. According to liberation theologians, conscientization is a process of uncovering the roots of group members' economic exploitation in class and colonial relations (Freire, 1970; also see Breton, 1989a; Gutiérrez & Lewis, 1999; Lewis, 1991).
5. Many second-wave feminists have suggested that through consciousness raising (CR), women can connect their experiences of oppression with those of other women and thereby see the political dimensions of their personal problems. However, because there are many "schools" of feminist thought, this statement calls for further qualification that extends beyond the scope of this chapter. For example, many contemporary feminist theorists have contested the seeming ideological determinism of CR, especially in regard to its implications of false consciousness (see Carr, 2003, for further discussion).
6. Anthropologist Carol Stack (1974, 1996) traced the intricate networks of resource exchange within poor African American communities in the urban North and rural South, demonstrating that the establishment and use of such largely female networks is a key strategy in surviving poverty, as well as in nurturing extended kin and community ties.
7. Culture-of-poverty arguments, outlined first in the early 1970s by anthropologists such as Oscar Lewis and popularized by politicians such as Daniel Moynihan, problematically assert that poverty is passed down through the generations like other cultural traits, assuming poverty to be a set of attitudes and inclinations rather than a set of historical, socioeconomic conditions. Thinly veiled racism often haunts these accounts as "culture" comes to stand in for "race" and the two ideas are mistakenly cast as interchangeable.
8. Operating on a "point system," devised and overseen entirely by the Client Action Group, clothes were "sold" only to Fresh Beginnings clients who had earned points through working in the closet.
9. Current research in substance abuse efficacy has highlighted the importance of clients' development of community networking, training, and employment through employment assistance programs (Reed, 1994). As a place in which clients developed management and communication skills, both within and outside the program, the clothes closet realized this kind of treatment practice.
10. Cohen (1994) further advises that even the most resistant staff members be included in the process of forming the empowerment-oriented group, purportedly with the hopes of neutralizing their resistance. However, I would counter that the group worker needs to be quite careful that such parties do not neutralize the group purpose itself.

REFERENCES

Breton, M. (1989a). Liberation theology, group work, and the right of the poor and oppressed to participate in the life of the community. *Social Work with Groups, 12*, 5–18.

Breton, M. (1989b). The need for mutual-aid groups in a drop-in for homeless women: The *sistering* case. In J. A. B. Lee (Ed.), *Group work with the poor and oppressed* (pp. 47–59). New York: Haworth Press.

Breton, M. (1994). On the meaning of empowerment and empowerment-oriented social work practice. *Social Work with Groups, 17*, 23–37.

Butler, S. (1991). *Feminist groupwork*. Newbury Park, CA: Sage.

Butler, S. (1994). All I've got in my purse is mothballs! The social action women's group. *Groupwork, 7*(2), 163–179.

Carr, E. S. (2003). Re-envisioning consciousness in empowerment theory through a feminist lens: The importance of process. *Affilia: Journal of Women and Social Work, 18*, 8–20.

Cohen, M. (1994a). Overcoming obstacles to forming empowerment groups: A consumer advisory board for homeless clients. *Social Work, 39*, 742–749.

Cohen, M. (1994b). Who wants to chair the meeting? Group development and leadership patterns in a community action group of homeless people. *Social Work with Groups, 17*, 71–87.

Cox, E. O. (1991). The critical role of social action in empowerment-oriented groups. *Social Work with Groups, 14*, 77–90.

Drysdale, J., & Purcell, R. (2000). Breaking the culture of silence: Groupwork and community development. In O. Manor (Ed.), *Ripples: Groupwork in different settings* (pp. 148–164). London: Whiting & Birch.

Friere, P. (1993). *The pedagogy of the oppressed* (M. B. Ramos, Trans.). New York: Continuum. (Original work published 1970)

Garvin, C. (1991). Barriers to effective social action by groups. *Social Work with Groups, 14*, 65–75.

Garvin, C., & Reed, B. G. (1995). Sources and visions for feminist group work: Reflective processes, social justice, diversity, and connection. In N. Van Den Bergh (Ed.), *Feminist practice in the 21st century* (pp. 41–69). Washington, DC: NASW Press.

Gutiérrez, L. (1990). Working with women of color: An empowerment perspective. *Social Work, 35*, 149–153.

Gutiérrez, L. (1991). Developing methods to empower Latinos: The importance of groups. *Social Work with Groups, 14*(2), 23–43.

Gutiérrez, L., & Lewis, E. (1999). The empowerment approach to practice. In L. Gutiérrez & E. Lewis (Eds.), *Empowering women of color* (pp. 3–119). New York: Columbia University Press.

Harrison, M., & Ward, D. (2000). Values as context: Groupwork and social action. In O. Manor (Ed.), *Ripples: Groupwork in different settings* (pp. 165–180). London: Whiting & Birch.

Johnson, A., & Castengera, A. R. (1994). Integrated program development: A model for meeting the complex needs of homeless persons. *Journal of Community Practice, 1*, 29–47.

Lee, J. (1986). No place to go: Homeless women. In A. Gitterman & L. Shulman (Eds.), *Mutual aid groups and the life cycle* (pp. 245–262). Itasca, IL: Peacock.

Lewis, E. (1991). Social change and citizen action: A philosophical exploration for modern social group work. *Social Work with Groups, 14*, 23–33.

Lewis, E. (1992). Regaining promise: Feminist perspectives for social group work practice. *Social Work with Groups, 15*(2–3), 271–284.

Moldofosky, Z. (2000). Meals made easy: A group program at a food bank. *Social Work with Groups, 23*, 83–97.

Mueller, M., & Patton, M. (1995). Working with poor families: Lessons learned from practice. *Marriage and Family Review, 21*, 65–90.

Mullender, A., & Ward, D. (1991). Empowerment through social action group work: The self-directed approach. *Social Work with Groups, 16*, 57–79.

Reed, B. G. (1994). Women and alcohol, tobacco and other drugs: The need to broaden the base within EAPs. *Employee Assistance Quarterly, 9*, 3–4.

Sachs, J. (1991). Action and reflection in work with a group of homeless people. *Social Work with Groups, 14,* 23–33.

Shapiro, B. Z. (1991). Social action, the group, and society. *Social Work with Groups, 14,* 7–21.

Stack, C. (1974). *All our kin.* New York: Harper & Row.

Stack, C. (1996). *Call to home: African Americans reclaim the rural South.* New York: Basic Books.

Subramanian, K., Hernandez, S., & Martinez, A. (1995). Psychoeducational group work for low-income Latina mothers with HIV infection. *Social Work with Groups, 18,* 53–64.

Turner-Bowker, D. (2001). How can you pull yourself up by your bootstraps, if you don't have boots? Work-appropriate clothing for poor women. *Journal of Social Issues, 57*(2), 311–322.

Yoshihama, M., & Carr, E. S. (2003). Community participation reconsidered: Feminist participatory action research with Hmong women. *Journal of Community Practice, 10*(4), 85–104.

Chapter 22

Group Process Dynamics and Skills in Interdisciplinary Teamwork

JULIE S. ABRAMSON
LAURA R. BRONSTEIN

Interdisciplinary teams were introduced in the 1940s and have been heavily used in health and mental health settings since the 1960s and 1970s as a means to call on the specialized knowledge of different categories of professionals (Julia & Thompson, 1994). Lately, such teams have been developed in school, child welfare, and other settings, as well, in which client problems are complex and require varied expertise for their resolution (Bronstein, 2003; Payne, 2000; Proenca, 2000). The dynamic interaction of specialized professionals on teams is assumed to promote an "expanded level of thinking" (Julia & Thompson, 1994, p. 39) or "generativity" (Lawson & Sailor, 2000), resulting in more creative, comprehensive, and effective problem solving. Teams are also grounded in the assumption that reliance on others for certain tasks and resources allows collaborators to spend their time doing what each knows and does best (Abramson & Rosenthal, 1995; Bronstein, 2003).

Despite some uncertainty in recent years about the contribution of teams to client outcomes and cost effectiveness and a surprising lack of empirical data about team functioning (Faulkner Schofield & Amodeo, 1999), the interdisciplinary team remains an integral part of many service delivery systems. As the population of this country expands in its numbers of immigrants, of members of racial and ethnic minority groups, and increasingly older adults, greater sophistication is called for in service delivery (Paris, Thompson, Riher, Quisenberry, & Cooper, 1996; Simmons, 1994).

Social workers are in an excellent position to assist teams in addressing such needs. Students do learn a variety of clinical and macro practice concepts and skills that can be easily adapted to work with teams (Hilton, 1995; Kovacs & Bronstein, 1999). These include: careful listening; beginning where the client is; respecting differences; maintaining a nonjudgmental stance; communicating empathically; reaching for feelings; and assessing individuals, groups, and organizations, among others (Abramson, 2002; Dana, 1983; Specht, 1985).Yet the relevance of these skills for teamwork is rarely articulated in the classroom or in the practice arena. Social workers often do not recognize or acknowledge that these skills are transferable to their work with colleagues, nor have they fully accepted that strategic and thoughtful interventions are needed in their collegial interactions (Abramson, 2002).

To draw on these skills successfully, social workers need to relinquish the false dichotomy between the skills they apply with clients and with colleagues. There is little basis for the often-held expectation that professionals can be counted on to "just act professionally." This assumption does not adequately acknowledge the personal and interprofessional differences that routinely obstruct teamwork processes. As Fatout and Rose (1995, p. 55) note, "A myth exists that all that is required for effective teamwork is a spirit of cooperation." Social workers also need to be clear about the importance of applying group work principles to team processes. After all, a team, whatever its primary function, is a group. If the dynamics of such a group are dysfunctional, then its client-focused objectives are less likely to be met. Teams are unique among task groups in the direct connection between their performance and the impact of their decisions on clients. Paradoxically, the teams that likely consider themselves client centered in that they attend primarily to client needs in their team meetings, may, in fact, be less so than those teams that also periodically address the team interaction issues that may be obstructing the development of better services to clients (Bronstein, 2002; Fatout & Rose, 1995).

Once social workers recognize their responsibility to address process issues in teams, they can draw on their group work knowledge base to assist teams in addressing these issues (Abramson, 1989). Kovacs, Bronstein, and Vega (2003) found that social workers in health care settings expressed comfort with their knowledge of groups yet claimed to need more knowledge and skills to work with teams. This finding suggests that workers are not translating their knowledge of group work to their participation on interdisciplinary teams. This chapter articulates critical issues in team functioning and identifies the key elements of group work practice that are most useful for addressing them.

DEFINITION OF A TEAM

Although the word "team" is used widely, some definitions of teams simply refer to the working together of professionals from different disciplines (sometimes referred to as a multidisciplinary approach). We assume that an effective interdisciplinary team will incorporate the following elements (Abramson, 2002):

- A group of professionals from different disciplines
- A common purpose
- Integration of various professional perspectives in decision making
- Integration of the client and family into team decision-making processes
- Active communication
- Role division based on expertise
- A climate of collaboration

Kagan (1992) describes the concepts of collaboration, coordination, and cooperation as a pyramid, with cooperation at the base, because it is "the most widespread and easiest to achieve" (p. 59). Collaboration, at the apex, is the most complex and difficult to actualize. "Here, joint goals and strategies are agreed on, resources and leadership are shared, and an identifiable durable collaborative structure is established" (p. 60). It is this last, collaborative model of teamwork that we believe is necessary to meet the needs of today's clients, families, agencies, and communities.

KEY INFLUENCES ON TEAM PROCESSES

Much of the literature on teamwork concentrates on the various obstacles to effective team functioning rather than on strategies to "make teams work" (Abramson, 1989). However, one cannot develop strategies without strong assessment capabilities in recognizing critical obstacles to successful teamwork. Table 22.1 lists the most commonly encountered obstacles. Many of these problems can be addressed through attention to the group process issues in teams that will be discussed later in this chapter.

Team Membership

There are few organizing principles for choosing members of a team; most often, the centrality of various professionals to a given client-care task determines the membership of a team. Teams of which physicians are members typically deal with the enduring dominance of physicians over team decision making (Abramson & Mizrahi, 1986; Faulkner Schofield & Amodeo, 1999; Freidson, 1970; Mizrahi, 1986; Opie, 2000; Watt, 1985). When present, physicians often take on or are looked to for leadership (Campbell-Heider & Pollack, 1987; Herrman, Trauer, & Warnock, 2002), and their higher status disproportionately influences team interaction, decision making, problem definition, and options for intervention on many teams (Abramson, 1989). Yet their preparation for teamwork is even less than that of other professions due to the continuing emphasis in medical training on self-reliance and autonomy (Koeske, Koeske, & Mallinger, 1993; Mizrahi, 1986). Other problems can arise

---

TABLE 22.1 Obstacles to Teamwork

- Continued dominance of higher status professionals
- Divided or conflicted commitment of participants to the team and to their respective affiliations
- Role competition or "turf" issues
- Excessive role blurring or lack of role clarity
- Differential professional socialization processes
- Inadequate organizational/administrative support and resources, including limited physical space for team meetings
- Difficulties resolving conflict
- Unclear responsibility for team leadership
- Unskilled team leadership
- Lack of experience with teamwork
- Personality difficulties among participants
- Time constraints
- Lack of shared professional language and technologies
- Emphasis on autonomy rather than training for teamwork in professional education

---

Note. From Abramson (2002); Abramson and Rosenthal (1995); Bronstein (2002); Bronstein and Abramson (2003); Drinka and Streim (1994); Faulkner Schofield and Amodeo (1999); and Lawson and Sailor (2000).

from team composition when the roles of different professions are not clearly defined so that either excessive role blurring or turf conflicts occur (Davidson, 1990; Herrman et al., 2002; Koeske et al., 1993).

A growing body of literature cites the importance of including clients and families as core members of teams (Bronstein, 2003; Graham & Barter, 1999; Lawson, 2003; Seaburn, Lorenz, Gunn, Gawinski, & Mauksch, 1996); yet in practice, if they are involved at all, clients and families primarily participate on a token basis whereby they receive the recommendations of professionals rather than share in the decision-making process. Therefore, it is important to recognize that many teams function without collaboration with or substantive input from clients and families.

Impact of Distinct Professional Socialization Processes on Teamwork

The capacity to arrive at consensus in decision making is an underlying premise of teamwork; therefore, it is essential to understand the profound impact of the varied professional socialization processes through which each profession inducts its trainees to its professional worldview (Cowles & Lefcourtz, 1992; Specht, 1985). Professional socialization shapes values, language, preferred roles and models of treatment, patterns of communication, methods of problem solving, and approaches to clients or patients (Bronstein & Abramson, 2003; Mizrahi & Abramson, 1985; Reese & Sontag, 2001; Waugaman, 1994). The process of becoming a professional often involves being mentored or responding to the support of superiors for certain behaviors and attitudes, as well as the formal imparting of professional ethics and knowledge. As an individual becomes a professional, perspectives particular to that profession become so ingrained that awareness of them diminishes; thus they often remain unexamined for their impact on teamwork and collaboration (Abramson, 2002).

Yet distinctions in professional beliefs and approaches to treatment are often at the root of disagreements among team members. Rather, the source of such difficulties is often ascribed to the personal qualities of the individual professionals involved, leaving a critical dimension of their collaborative relationship overlooked. Social workers can recognize this dynamic at work if they reflect on their often-judgmental reactions to colleagues' "lack of understanding of the client's right to self-determination."

Because professional education rarely educates students about the contributions made by other professions or about the tools and perspectives they use in their work (Drinka & Streim, 1994; Julia & Thompson, 1994; Lawson & Sailor, 2000; Waugaman, 1994), we suggest that social workers make concerted efforts to educate themselves about the socialization of other professionals through review of relevant literature and professional codes of ethics other than their own. Most important, social workers can compensate for the gaps in professional education through systematic, face-to-face discussions with their colleagues in other professions about the factors that have shaped their professional perspectives. See Table 22.2 for a list of questions that can serve as a guide for such discussions.

Clients and their families are also unlikely to understand the norms or socialization of professional team members; lack of such knowledge can put them at a considerable disadvantage when attending team meetings. Here it is incumbent on the social worker to prepare and guide the clients and families as to the professional orientations and roles of the different professionals. The social worker also can assist clients to communicate those aspects of their own culture and socialization that need to be taken into account in decision making; these can include the impact of their neighborhood, culture, country, race, values, religion, and socioeconomic status on their situation and preferences in problem solving.

Table 22.2. Understanding the Socialization of Other Professions

Questions to ask other professionals

- What is the structure and nature of their training?
- What is the primary focus of their code of ethics?
- What are the values that are most stressed in their training?
- What makes a good doctor, nurse, or occupational therapist, and so forth?
- What is most important to them in taking care of clients (or patients, students, inmates, etc.) or in doing their jobs?
- How do they see their role in relation to clients?
- To what model of treatment do they subscribe?
- What accountability mechanisms are common? What is their relationship to any administrative or supervisory structure?

Note. From Abramson (2002).

Communicating the Role of Social Work on Interdisciplinary Teams

Clear articulation of the social work role is a necessary precondition for effective collaboration by social workers with others on the team. Although social work educators have made a strong beginning in defining social work roles (Cournoyer, 1991; Germain & Gitterman, 1996), not enough has been done to define how these roles are delineated or described in collaboration with others (Specht, 1985). Studies of nursing and teaching professionals have found that a clear understanding and articulation of one's own role is a critical variable in successful teamwork (McKiel, Lockyer & Pechivlis, 1988; Mitchell & Scott, 1993). Yet clear role articulation is especially difficult for social workers because the social work profession has had difficulty defining itself; therefore, there is much ambiguity among the general public and other professionals as to what social workers "do" (Condie, Hanson, Lang, Moss, & Kane, 1978; Cowles & Lefcowitz, 1992; Gartner, 1976; Gibelman, 1995).

Social workers have often contributed to lack of role clarity through their reluctance to accord their resource-procurement and advocacy activities equal status with their counseling roles (Abramson & Mizrahi, 1994). Because the prior activities are often those most easily understood and appreciated by clients and other professionals (Cowles & Lefcowitz, 1992), social workers handicap their effectiveness on teams if they do not actively communicate the professional complexities of these activities. They also miss the critical opportunity to portray the uniqueness of social work's capacity to integrate traditional clinical skills with "systems" work, which provides more integrated services to clients (Abramson, 1993; Mizrahi & Abramson, 1985). Rather than bemoaning the poor understanding by others of their role, social workers need to accept responsibility for active and consistent education of their teammates about their contributions to client care on a case-by-case basis (Abramson, 1993; Abramson & Mizrahi, 1986; Bronstein & Abramson, 2003).

ATTENDING TO GROUP PROCESSES IN TEAMWORK

The team is a group; thus, group intervention principles can provide the foundation for addressing group-process issues that arise. It is reasonable to assume that any team, however well functioning, will encounter group dynamics that can undermine its effectiveness. Even when things are going well, consciousness of team dynamics will only serve to enhance the team's efficacy. We share the assumption of most teams that their primary function is to focus on those tasks that directly affect delivery of services to clients; such activities are the *raison d'etre* for the existence of teams. However, we recognize, as does Shulman (1982, p. 221), that often, "attention to the process leads directly to work on the task."

Certain tensions are inherent to teamwork and need to be accepted as normative rather than viewed as obstacles. Many of these very tensions contribute to the richness and creativity of the collaborative process, such as the range of professional perspectives or diversity of participants' language, culture, or race (Abramson & Rosenthal, 1995; Kane, 1975; Mizrahi & Rosenthal, 1992).

The remainder of this chapter identifies the group work–based intervention strategies and skills that team members and team leaders can draw on to facilitate team functioning.

Monitoring and Assessing Team Processes

Monitoring team processes is a critical team-maintenance task for all team leaders and team members; yet it is a responsibility often taken on reluctantly. Participants need the capacity to think simultaneously about treatment and team issues so that they are able to address those team-process issues that obstruct the client-centered goals of the team. Social workers are well prepared to assess those team dynamics that arise in a particular team meeting, those that are carried over from one team meeting to another, and those that may plague a team for an extended period of time. When working with client groups, they typically attend to interactions among clients while also addressing the topics being discussed; thus they can draw on similar skills in working with teams. Their systems orientation can assist them in evaluating organizational factors that impinge on team functioning, and their skills at tuning in to an atmosphere of tension or lack of productivity can position them to bring such issues to the attention of the team. Such interventions should be encouraged for all team members, but social workers come to teams with the skill repertoire to take on this role. The following example demonstrates such an intervention.

> At a team meeting in a rehabilitation hospital, the team leader, who was a physician, mentioned that he would begin interviewing applicants for the position of team psychologist. The former psychologist had been involved in some jurisdictional conflicts with the consulting psychiatrist, the nurse clinician and the social workers. The team leader did not seem to expect any discussion of his announcement and proceeded to review the patient roster for the week. Each team member presented a case for which the intake assessment had been completed. However, the usual exchanges about appropriate treatment approaches did not take place. The leader seemed baffled, asked team members for their opinions several times and then just made the decisions himself.
>
> Finally, one of the occupational therapists commented that everyone sure was quiet today. That remark created more silence. Then one of the social workers said that she didn't know if other people were also preoccupied, but she knew that her mind was on the possibility of a new psychologist and whether the same problems would exist with a new person. When several heads nodded in agreement, she suggested that it might be helpful, either now or later, to discuss the job description for this person. The team leader said he knew there had been some problems, but maybe he wasn't as aware of them as they were. Several people volunteered to meet with him after the meeting to discuss it further. (Abramson, 1989, pp. 49–50)

Contracting with Teams

It is all too rare for teams to have a formal discussion of how the team will operate in relation to membership, attendance, leadership, roles and allocation of responsibilities, decision making, and preferred models of treatment (Kahn, 1974). Rather, it is much more the norm for these aspects of teamwork to be established by default, by leader preference, or by tradition rather than selected because they make the most sense for a particular team (Abramson, 1989). New members typically "learn the ropes" and become socialized to team norms by observing rather than through any form of direct assistance, such as an orientation process (Sands, 1989). The discomfort of being an outsider frequently motivates new team members to adopt behavior that will be seen positively by the team (Levi, 2001; Sands, 1989; Werther & Davis, 1985). Thus the opportunity for the team to benefit from the ideas and experiences of new members is often lost. Clients and family members attending team meetings may also hesitate to share their perspectives or advocate for themselves before learning the norms of preexisting teams.

The most obvious time to develop a team contract is at the point of team formation or restructuring, although clarification or modification of the contract can be sought at any time. This contract then provides the baseline against which to measure the progress of the group; members and workers thus use their shared understanding of the contract to identify forces that may obstruct their efforts to accomplish their objectives or that "get in the way of the work" (Shulman, 1999).

It is a natural extension to apply contracting concepts used in group work to teamwork. However, concerted effort may be necessary to engage teams in contracting or recontracting processes because so few teams have approached their work in this way. Many of the difficulties faced by teams rest in unexamined assumptions and can be effectively addressed through a well-developed contracting discussion. An abbreviated version of such contracting can occur when new staff members, clients, or family members join the team or when other external forces have an impact on the teams' work.

A team that developed individual education plans (IEPs) for students at an urban elementary school functioned well together for many years in a somewhat static environment. Their unspoken contract for work was based on their assumptions about how to work with the population of students and families who had participated in the school for many years. Recently, however, individual team members had expressed feelings of frustration and a sense that they were not as successful in working with the students and their parents as they had been in prior years. After careful thought, the social worker assessed that neighborhood demographic changes over the previous two years had created new problems for the team. During that time, an increasing number of immigrants from Haiti had moved into this previously white working-class community, and their children were entering the school.

Team members had been feeling ineffective and were relieved when the social worker suggested that a new contract for work needed to be established, one that was based on the needs and strengths of the new population of students and families. The worker agreed to locate reading materials on Haitian culture to share with team members in helping to craft such a contract. She also agreed to plan a forum for dialogue with immigrant parents at a faculty meeting about the different educational expectations for students *and* parents in Haiti and in the United States. This new information then became the basis for a team contract regarding expectations and roles for professionals and families in the future IEP meetings.

Creating a Climate of Openness, Trust, and Group Cohesion

Group cohesion is difficult to describe, but most team participants would swear that they "know it when they experience it." Although team cohesion is generated from a number of sources, team members primarily experience it in an affective way, as a sense of belonging and ownership of the team's processes and outcomes (Keyton, 2000). Fleming and Monda-Amaya (2001) note that experiencing trust and respect for other team members, as well as comfort in sharing ideas, contributes to team cohesion. Cohesion has been identified as contributing to commitment to the team (Barrick, Stewart, Neubert, & Mount, 1998) and to its effectiveness (Fleming & Monda-Amaya, 2001). Commitment has also been found to be enhanced by highly collaborative teamwork styles, greater role clarity, and acceptance of team goals, values, and norms of performance (Lewandowski & GlenMaye, 2002; Nandan, 1997). These variables significantly affect satisfaction with the team as well, with respect for colleagues having a major impact on satisfaction (Abramson & Mizrahi, 1996; Bronstein, 2002; Lewandowski & GlenMaye, 2002).

A social worker wishing to facilitate the development of greater team cohesion would do well to focus on promoting mutual-aid processes within the team. Team members clearly need each other to accomplish their assigned responsibilities, and thus they are engaged in a mutual-aid process. Some key aspects of mutual aid likely to play out in team interactions include: mutual support; a mutual demand or expectation to accomplish the work of the group; sharing data; the development of the "all-in-the-same-boat" and "strength in numbers" phenomena; discussion of taboo areas; and joint problem solving (Bronstein & Kelly, 1998; Shulman, 1999).

Mutual support occurs when team members are "there" for one another as they deal with challenging patient/client circumstances and with the disappointments and struggles that are part of their daily work lives (Bronstein & Kelly, 1998). Such support provides the cushion that then allows team participants to assert their expectations of each other or make a "demand for work" (Schwartz, 1961). That same sense of support also makes the discussion of more taboo or painful topics possible (Shulman, 1999), and the sense of "strength-in-numbers" and that we are "all in the same boat" can encourage both staff and client/family team members to take on challenging or intimidating issues and tasks (Bronstein & Kelly, 1998).

Other strategies also increase trust and create a climate of openness. Some of these are most effective if they come from a team leader as the leader often has disproportionate influence on the development of team culture and norms. For example, the leader can mediate the tendency in many teams for higher status professionals to dominate decision making by promoting participation by others and supporting their contributions. At times, the leader may need to directly question an assumption or mode of operating of a higher status member whom others are hesitant to confront (Abramson, 1989). Team leaders can promote a sense of identification with the whole team, even in the face of sometimes contradictory professional ideologies and loyalties; however, to accomplish this, leaders must demonstrate evenhandedness in territorial disputes and must be careful not to overidentify with or overprotect members of their own profession. Finally, leaders can offer an optimistic vision of the team's potential for problem solving and working effectively together; communicating such a perspective evokes the energy, motivation, and capacity needed for successful teamwork (Abramson & Rosenthal, 1995).

Team members also can contribute to team cohesiveness and an atmosphere of respect and trust by modeling positive team behavior, even when a team leader has not created such norms. Support for others who take risks can be critical, as can building on or supporting another member's ideas. If a team member evaluates the idea of another member on its merit, without regard for the status or personal appeal of the individual or for his or her subgroup affiliations, others are more likely to do the same (Fisher & Ury, 1983). In a similar vein, it is essential that all team members maintain a "politeness ritual," because modeling a professional demeanor when dealing with strong professional or personal differences can activate norms of responsibility in others (Mikula & Schwinger, 1978).

Dealing with Conflict

Teams who can successfully manage conflict find their cohesion as a group greatly enhanced by their capacity to deal with differing points of view. The development of consensus in decision making and growth in team functioning often depends on the ability of group members to confront conflict within the group directly (Northen, 1988). The inability to deal with conflict within the team is perhaps the most critical obstacle to effective collaboration (Sands, Stafford, & McClelland, 1990). The following factors are likely to produce conflict (Abramson & Rosenthal, 1995):

- The participants have a history of adversarial relationships.
- The team includes ideologically diverse participants or those with different professional or organizational cultures.
- The outcome has the potential to shift dominance from those in power.
- The participants hold differing interests regarding the desired outcome.

Although many difficulties in addressing conflict in teams are encountered by individual team members and leaders, numerous tried and tested approaches exist that teams can draw on to manage conflicts. For example, efforts by "opposing" team members to recognize and understand the varied investments of stakeholders in a particular perspective can provide a foundation for "getting in others' shoes." Such assessment is the first step toward developing strategies to resolve conflict. Because these strategies are grounded in both an intellectual and an empathic understanding of another's perspective, there is greater likelihood that they will be effective. Most professionals are familiar with listening skills and apply them successfully when working with clients; however, once again, they often do not apply such skills with their colleagues or recognize the potency of this approach for collaborative interactions. However, the presence of clients and family members in team meetings may help to evoke the listening skills that most professionals possess.

Helping team members to acknowledge a conflict and express the reasoning behind conflicting opinions and alternatives can be a significant first step. When positions harden, it is useful to develop jointly agreed-on decision criteria or to identify the acceptable and unacceptable parts of each alternative; then it is often possible to combine the acceptable parts of several alternatives into one solution (Toseland & Rivas, 2001). Because resolving conflict inevitably involves some redistribution of power, it is important to avoid a total win-or-lose situation (Gouran, 1982). Common ground can be sought through reframing a contending perspective in terms of others' needs, ideology, or language. For example, a social worker interested in obtaining service for a client might stress the potential for learning from a specific case when presenting it at an intake meeting in a training setting (Abramson, 1989).

Much dissension or disagreement is expressed indirectly in team meetings through inattention, exchanges of glances, loss of eye contact, evidence of irritation or frustration in tone of voice, subgroup talking, sub-rosa or sarcastic remarks, eye rolling and even physical restlessness. It is essential to address these indirect communications of conflict (see Table 22.3 for conflict resolution strategies). Such behavior should stimulate other participants to seek out the underlying meaning. It is more effective to bring the behavior to the attention of the team through humor or use of one's own feelings rather than "accusing" others; in this way, defensiveness can be avoided, and others will be more likely to engage in an exploratory process (Abramson, 1989).

Developing Client-Centered Norms

At times, teams develop a culture or set of norms that can have a negative impact on clients and families. Teams that deal with client problems that are complex, overwhelming, and not easily addressed may find themselves using "black humor" or "client blaming" to deal with their frustrations (Fox, 1980). Teams and team members may lose the capacity to individualize certain categories of clients, especially those with a poor prognosis, those perceived as manipulative, or those for whom available interventions do not easily succeed. Such behavior may be less apt to occur overtly when clients and family members routinely participate in teams; however, it still may occur in informal or formal team discussions when they are not present or in subtle or nonverbal form when they are.

An alert team leader needs to identify such patterns and call the members' attention to them; an individual member also can raise such issues with other members and/or the team leader so that support is generated for addressing the problem. It can be helpful to use a retreat format, away from the pressures of client care, to reflect on the dynamics and resolution of the problem. The following example illustrates such a situation.

> Team members in an outpatient clinic for substance abusers had begun to set very limited treatment objectives for low-income clients. The team leader assessed this response as relating to a disproportionate number of treatment failures with this group of clients. She observed team members gradually withdrawing from this population and decided to raise the issue at the team meeting. After evoking much frustrated commentary from the team members, she suggested that

TABLE 22.3. Consensus-Building and Conflict-Resolution Strategies for Teams

- Emphasize points of consensus and broad, unifying themes.
- Deal with safer issues initially.
- Partialize conflicts into manageable parts and into areas in which there is common ground.
- Combine the acceptable and unacceptable aspects of each alternative into solution.
- Use decision criteria jointly agreed on.
- Gain consensus incrementally—a piece at a time.
- Reframe issues in terms of others' language or ideology.
- Demonstrate support and respect for differences—build culture in which difference is tolerated.
- Avoid self-righteousness.
- Separate the person from the issue.
- Emphasize unifying themes.
- Reach for indirect expression of difference.
- Don't paper over underlying but deeply felt disagreement.
- Recognize impact of socialization differences; develop strategies more relevant to those kinds of differences.
- Maintain a professional demeanor.
- Avoid a total win-or-lose situation.
- View conflict as a normal and helpful part of teamwork.

Note. From Abramson (1989, 2002); Graham and Barter (1999); and Toseland and Rivas (2001).

there might be other approaches that the team could develop to work more successfully with these clients. She proposed a workshop that would have components of specialized training with a consultant, followed by brainstorming sessions to integrate the consultant's input with the extensive knowledge already available within the team. (Abramson, 1989, p. 55)

Integrating Clients and Families into Teams

Although the inclusion of clients and families in teams has been discussed throughout this chapter, it is a complex process that deserves further discussion. Clients and families present their own unique set of challenges to team functioning, yet their involvement also opens up an array of possibilities that would not exist without their involvement. The two major challenges that result from including clients and families as core team members include their time-limited involvement and their perceived power deficit.

Even though team membership is often somewhat fluid, the time-limited involvement of the many clients and their families whose needs the team addresses poses particular challenges. However, as professional team members work together over time, they can develop ways to best greet, guide, and welcome the input of clients and families into their care planning. Strategies for incorporating clients and families successfully into teams include (1) preparing clients and families for team participation; (2) jointly developing meeting agendas; (3) limiting the number of professionals present; (4) avoiding technical language; and (5) keeping client/family concerns central (Opie, 2000). Social workers have revealed that more productive team interactions and outcomes have occurred when clients and families are involved in all stages of decision making (Bronstein, 2002).

The challenges inherent in the power differentials among team members were noted earlier; inclusion of clients and families in the team makeup can further complicate the team's power dynamics due to their status as recipients rather than providers of service. Social workers can help to empower clients and families such that their involvement goes beyond token status to actually holding teams accountable for providing the best possible care plan available. In some circumstances, clients and family members may be better able to challenge higher status professionals (i.e., physicians) than are social workers, nurses, and other professional "colleagues." In order to have an interprofessional team that truly serves clients' best interests, those clients and their self-defined family members need to be integral team members. Achievement of such an objective requires team members to value the input of clients and families as critical to the entire process of design, definition, development, and attainment of goals. Active participation by clients and families in teams can begin to make inroads into correcting the enormous imbalance of power between them and the professionals who so often make decisions of great consequence for their lives.

Future Directions in Teamwork

This chapter has examined those factors likely to affect team processes and identified the group work strategies most likely to improve team functioning. Given that teams are the primary mechanism for service delivery in many settings, developing teamwork approaches to enhance their effectiveness can only better serve clients and families. However, research on the work of interdisciplinary teams needs to be expanded. Although much clinical wisdom and many case studies exist to guide this work, we need to increase efforts to develop evidence-based models to define and guide best practices. A number of instruments exist in social work and related fields to assess teamwork, but these instruments rely largely on self-report (in social work, Bronstein, 2002; in nursing, Joy & Malay, 1992; in early childhood education, Garland, Frank, Buck, & Seklemian, 1995; and in organizational research, Kivimaki, Kuk, Elovainio, & Thomson, 1997, and Watson, Johnson, & Merritt, 1998). Specific areas cited in the literature as influences on teamwork should be empirically examined for their impact on team processes and outcomes—differential professional socialization, structural and organizational dimensions, contracting processes, the balance between task and process emphasis in teams, conflict management strategies, personal characteristics, and so forth (Bronstein & Abramson, 2003). Also, group workers in practice and in academia can add to the knowledge about teams with case studies, models, and research that looks particularly at dynamics that occur when clients and families are integral team members.

In addition to further research efforts, social work educators can make more explicit linkages between students' knowledge of group work and their work on interdisciplinary teams. This content should be required in foundation-level micro and macro practice courses, as well as in concentration-level courses in group work practice or interdisciplinary settings. Assignments in these courses can focus on collaborative as well as clinical work. Outside the classroom, field instructors can also foster this linkage in their supervision of students in the field. For example, field instructors can require that students produce process recordings of team meetings. If this aspect of their practice is elevated in importance to that given direct work with clients, and if students are evaluated on their performance in collaborative arenas, they will be eager to learn teamwork and collaborative skills. Field instructors will also need to articulate and consistently reinforce the connections between the group work skills that students are using in their clinical work and the skills they will need as team members.

Last, it is critical to keep in mind that interdisciplinary or interprofessional teamwork is only one "type" of collaboration; it is not exercised in a void and is best achieved when interlocking with a number of other "types" of collaboration. Payne (2000, p. 3) argues, "teams cannot just be about interpersonal group relations among professionals working together"; they "must also be a center of relationships within wider multi-professional, service user and community networks." These other forms of collaboration require the same skills necessary for interprofessional teamwork (Payne, 2000). Lawson (2003) categorizes these collaborative types as intraorganizational, interorganizational or interagency, and community based, among others.

Intraorganizational collaboration speaks to relationships within the same organization that stretch beyond the interprofessional team. This kind of collaboration is fostered in agencies in which professional and nonprofessional staff members share and feel empowered to support the agency mission. Intraorganizational collaboration occurs, for example, when a school bus driver, who is not a formal team participant, speaks to a teacher about something significant he has heard from a child on his bus. It is fostered when secretarial staff members at a mental health clinic, who are not usually part of the team, are included with professional staff in an in-service training session about ways to handle clients exhibiting upsetting behaviors in the waiting room. Collaboration that extends beyond the team lays a foundation for the advancement of team goals and processes by informally incorporating the contributions of other agency workers.

Interorganizational or interagency collaboration, often referred to as services integration, attempts to secure genuine engagement, shared responsibility and accountability, and coproduction capacities among two or more organizations (Lawson, 2003). These collaborations are most successful when agency relationships, policies and practices are formalized into clearly articulated agreements that go beyond what occurs when two or more agencies merely work together side by side on a shared initiative. For example, when hospitals have interagency agreements with community agencies, attendance by representatives of these agencies at team meetings to plan patient discharges can facilitate more seamless transitions for patients. In addition, such interagency relationships can extend the team's impact through the building of coalitions to address service gaps and local, state, or even national legislative and policy advocacy.

Community collaboration involves soliciting input, investment, and participation from lesser heard residents and service providers about local needs and initiatives. This involvement can enhance the interdisciplinary team in its work by providing resources and information not otherwise available. A wide consumer base can be garnered through community collaboration, which can broaden team goals and also provide support to the team in developing and advocating for a policy agenda that is truly grounded in community needs.

In addition to these kinds of collaboration, Lawson (2003) identifies other larger system levels as important in supporting successful collaborations for the interprofessional team. These include intragovernmental collaboration, intergovernmental collaboration, and international collaboration. The connections between these types of collaboration and teams need further exploration; however, it is safe to assume that governmental and global factors will have ever-increasing impact on services to clients and thus on the teams trying to provide care.

CONCLUSION

The purpose of this chapter has been to discuss the application of group work knowledge and skills to productive teamwork. However, this application cannot occur in a vacuum. It cannot be fostered without the assistance of researchers who build knowledge about productive teamwork processes or without social work educators who pass this knowledge on to students. And team processes cannot develop effectively without the contextual supports and other "types" of collaboration necessary to build and pave the road on which teams need to walk in their journey to serve clients. We count on teams to be a primary mechanism for service delivery, yet we provide little of the conceptual and skill-building supports necessary to do the job we expect of them. Here we suggest that some of the resources needed are available to social workers through their understanding of group processes and interventions with groups. We encourage teams to attend to their internal processes in the belief that such attention can make a significant contribution to improved team morale and to better outcomes for clients and families.

REFERENCES

Abramson, J. (1993). Orienting social work employees in interdisciplinary settings: Shaping professional and organizational perspectives. *Social Work*, 38(2), 152–157.

Abramson, J. S. (1989). Making teams work. *Social Work with Groups*, 12(4), 45–63.

Abramson, J. S. (2002). Interdisciplinary team practice. In G. Greene & A. Roberts (Eds.), *Social worker's desk reference* (pp. 44–50). New York: Oxford University Press.

Abramson, J. S., & Mizrahi, T. (1986). Strategies for enhancing collaboration between social workers and physicians. *Social Work in Health Care*, 12(1), 1–21.

Abramson, J. S., & Mizrahi, T. (1993). Examining social work/physician collaboration: An application of grounded theory methods. In C. Reissman (Ed.). *Qualitative studies in social work research* (pp. 28–48). Thousand Oaks, CA: Sage.

Abramson, J. S., & Mizrahi, T. (1996). When social workers and physicians collaborate: Positive and negative interdisciplinary experiences. *Social Work, 41*, 270–283.

Abramson, J. S., & Rosenthal, B. B. (1995). Interdisciplinary and interorganizational collaboration. *Encyclopedia of social work* (19th ed., pp. 1479–1489). Washington, DC: NASW Press.

Barrick, M., Stewart, G., Neubert, M., & Mount, M. (1998). Relating member ability and personality to work-team processes and team effectiveness. *Journal of Applied Psychology, 83*(3), 377–391.

Bronstein, L. R. (2002). Index of interdisciplinary collaboration. *Social Work Research, 26*(2), 113–126.

Bronstein, L. R. (2003). A model for interdisciplinary collaboration. *Social Work, 48*(3), 297–306.

Bronstein, L. R., & Abramson, J. S. (2003). Understanding socialization of teachers and social workers: Groundwork for collaboration in the schools. *Families in Society, 84*(3), 1–8.

Bronstein, L. R., & Kelly, T. B. (1998). Field education units: Fostering mutual aid in multicultural settings. *Arete, 22*(2), 54–62.

Campbell-Heider, N., & Pollack, D. (1987). Barriers to physician/nurse collegiality: An anthropological perspective. *Social Science and Medicine, 25*(5), 421–425.

Condie, C. D., Hanson, J. A., Lang, N. E., Moss, D. K., & Kane, R. A. (1978). How the public views social work. *Social Work, 23*(1), 47–53.

Cournoyer, B. (1991). *The social work skills workbook*. Belmont, CA: Wadsworth.

Cowles, L., & Lefcowitz, M. (1992). Interdisciplinary expectations of the medical social worker in the hospital setting (Part I). *Health and Social Work, 17*(1), 57–65.

Dana, B. (1983). The collaborative process. In R. Miller & H. Rehr (Eds.), *Social work issues in health care* (pp. 181–220). Englewood Cliffs, NJ: Prentice-Hall.

Davidson, K. (1990). Role blurring and the hospital social worker's search for a clear domain. *Health and Social Work, 15*, 228–234.

Drinka, T., & Streim, J. (1994). Case studies from purgatory: Maladaptive behavior within geriatrics health care teams. *Gerontologist, 34*(4), 541–547.

Fatout, M., & Rose, S. (1995). *Task groups in the social services*. Thousand Oaks, CA: Sage.

Faulkner Schofield, R., & Amodeo, M. (1999). Interdisciplinary teams in health care and human services settings: Are they effective? *Health and Social Work, 24*(3), 210–219.

Fisher, R., & Ury, W. (1983). *Getting to yes: Negotiating agreement without giving in*. New York: Penguin.

Fleming, J. L., & Monda-Amaya, L. (2001). Process variables critical for team effectiveness. *Remedial and Special Education, 22*(3), 158–172.

Fox, R. C. (1980). *The human condition of health professionals*. Durham: University of New Hampshire.

Freidson, E. (1970). *The profession of medicine*. New York: Dodd, Mead.

Garland, C., Frank, A., Buck, D., & Seklemian, P. (1995). *Skills inventory for teams*. Lightfoot, VA: Child Development Resources Training Center.

Gartner, A. (1976). *The preparation of human service professionals*. NY: Human Sciences Press.

Germain, C., & Gitterman, A. (1996). *The life model of social work practice* (2nd ed.). New York: Columbia University Press.

Gibelman, M. (1995). *What social workers do*. Washington, DC: NASW Press.

Gouran, D. (1982). *Making decisions in groups: Choices and consequences*. Glenview, IL: Scott, Foresman.

Graham, J. R., & Barter, K (1999). Collaboration: A social work practice method. *Families in Society, 80*(1), 6–13.

Herrman, H., Trauer, T., & Warnock, J. (2002). The roles and relationships of psychiatrists and other service providers in mental health services. *Australian and New Zealand Journal of Psychiatry, 36*, 75–80.

Hilton, R. (1995). Fragmentation within inter-professional work: A result of isolationism in health care professional education programs and the preparation of students to function only in the confines of their own discipline. *Journal of Interprofessional Care, 9*(1), 33–40.

Joy, L., & Malay, M. (1992). Evaluation instruments to measure professional nursing practice. *Nursing Management, 23*(7), 73–78.

Julia, M. C., & Thompson, A. (1994). Group process and interprofessional teamwork. In R. M. Casto, M. C. Julia, L. Platt, G. Harbaugh, A. Thompson, T. Jost, T. et al. (Eds.), *Interprofessional care and collaborative practice* (pp. 35–41). Pacific Grove, CA: Brooks/Cole.

Kagan, S. L. (1992). Collaborating to meet the readiness agenda: Dimensions and dilemmas. In Council of Chief State School Officers (Ed.), *Ensuring student success through collaboration.* (pp. 57–66). Washington DC: Council of Chief State School Officers.

Kahn, A. (1974). Institutional constraints to inter-professional practice. In H. Rehr (Ed.), *Medicine and social work: An exploration in inter-professionalism* (pp. 14–25). New York: Prodist.

Kane, R. A. (1975). *Inter-professional teamwork* (Manpower Monograph No. 8). Syracuse, NY: Syracuse University, Division of Continuing Education and Manpower Development.

Keyton, J. (2000). Introduction: The relational side of groups. *Small Group Research, 31*(4), 33–39.

Kivimaki, M., Kuk, G., Elovainio, M., & Thomson, L. (1997). The Team Climate Inventory (TCI)—four or five factors? Testing the structure of TCI in samples of low and high complexity jobs. *Journal of Occupational and Organizational Psychology, 70*(4), 375–390.

Koeske, G., Koeske, M., & Mallinger, J. (1993). Perceptions of professional competence: Cross-disciplinary ratings of psychologists, social workers and Psychiatrists. *American Journal of Orthopsychiatry, 63*, 45–54.

Kovacs, P., & Bronstein, L. R. (1999). Preparation for oncology settings: What hospice social workers say they need. *Health and Social Work, 24*(1), 57–64.

Kovacs, P., Bronstein, L. R., & Vega, A. (2003, January). *Goodness of fit: Social work education and practice in health care.* Poster session presented at the annual conference of the Society for Social Work and Research, Washington, DC.

Lawson, H., & Sailor, W. (2000). Integrating services, collaborating and developing connections with schools. *Focus on Exceptional Children, 33*(2), 1–24.

Lawson, H. A. (2003). Pursuing and securing collaboration to improve results. In M. Brabeck and M. Walsh (Eds.), Meeting at the hyphen: Schools-universities-communities-professions in collaboration for student achievement and well-being. In *The 102nd Yearbook of the National Society for the Study of Education* (pp. 45–73). Chicago: University of Chicago Press.

Levi, D. (2001). *Group dynamics for teams.* Thousand Oaks, CA: Sage.

Lewandowski, C. A., & GlenMaye, L. F. (2002). Teams in child welfare settings: Interprofessional and collaborative processes. *Families in Society: The Journal of Contemporary Human Services, 83*(3), 245–256.

McKiel, R. E., Lockyer, J., & Pechivlis, D. D. (1988). A model of continuing education for conjoint practice. *Journal of Continuing Education for Nurses, 19*(2), 65–67.

Mikula, G., & Schwinger, T. (1978). Intermember relations and reward allocations: Theoretical considerations of affects. In H. Brandslatter, J. Davis, & H. Schuler (Eds.), *Dynamics of group decisions* (pp. 229–250). Beverly Hills, CA: Sage.

Mitchell, D., & Scott, L. (1993). Professional and institutional perspectives on inter-agency collaboration. *Journal of Education Policy, 8*(5–6), 75–92.

Mizrahi, T. (1986). *Getting rid of patients: Contradictions in the socialization of physicians.* New Brunswick, NJ: Rutgers University.

Mizrahi, T., & Abramson, J. S. (1985). Sources of strain between physicians and social workers: Implications for social workers in health care settings. *Social Work in Health Care, 10*(3), 33–51.

Mizrahi, T., & Rosenthal, B. (1992). Managing dynamic tensions in social change coalitions. In T. Mizrahi & J. Morrison (Eds.), *Community organization and social administration: Advances, trends and emerging principles* (pp. 11–40). New York: Haworth Press.

Nandan, M. (1997). Commitment of social services staff to interdisciplinary care plan teams: An exploration. *Social Work Research, 21*(4), 249–259.

Northen, H. (1988). *Social work with groups* (2nd ed.). New York: Columbia University Press.

Opie, A. (2000). *Thinking teams/thinking clients: Knowledge-based teamwork*. New York: Columbia University Press.

Paris, W., Thompson, S., Riher, T., Quisenberry, M., & Cooper, D. K. (1996). A comparison of transplant patient and social work attitudes in regard to transplant patient psychosocial selection criteria, role expectations, and communication style. *Social Work in Health Care, 23*(1), 39–52.

Payne, M. (2000). *Teamwork in multi-professional care*. Chicago: Lyceum Books.

Proenca, E. J. (2000). Community orientation in hospitals: An institutional and resource dependence perspective. *Health Services Research, 35*(5), 210–218.

Reese, D. J., & Sontag, M. A. (2001). Successful interprofessional collaboration on the hospice team. *Health and Social Work, 26*(3), 167–175.

Sands, R. (1989). The social worker joins the team: A look at the socialization process. *Social Work in Health Care, 14*(2), 1–14.

Sands, R., Stafford, J., & McClelland, M. (1990). I beg to differ: Conflict in the interdisciplinary team. *Social Work in Health Care, 14*(3), 55–72.

Schwartz, W. (1961). The social worker in the group. In *New perspectives on services to groups: Theory, organization, practice* (pp. 7–34). New York: Columbia University Press.

Seaburn, D. B., Lorenz, A. D., Gunn, W. B., Gawinski, B. A., & Mauksch, L. B. (1996). *Models of collaboration*. New York: Basic Books.

Shulman, L. (1982). *Skills of supervision and staff management*. Itasca, IL: Peacock.

Shulman, L. (1999). *The skills of helping individuals, families, groups and communities* (4th ed.). Itasca, IL: Peacock.

Simmons, J. (1994). Community-based care: The new social work paradigm. *Social Work in Health Care, 20*, 30–46.

Specht, H. (1985). The interpersonal interactions of professionals. *Social Work, 30*(3), 225–230.

Toseland, R., & Rivas, R. (2001). *An introduction to group work practice* (4th ed.). Boston: Allyn & Bacon.

Watson, W., Johnson, L., & Merritt, D. (1998). Team orientation, self orientation and diversity in task groups. *Group and Organization Management, 23*(2), 161–188.

Watt, J. W. (1985). Protective service teams: The social worker as liaison. *Health and Social Work, 10*, 191–197.

Waugaman, W. (1994). Professionalization and socialization in inter-professional collaboration. In R. M. Casto, M. C. Julia, L. Platt, G. Harbaugh, A. Thompson, T. Jost, et al. (Eds.), *Interprofessional care and collaborative practice* (pp. 23–31). Pacific Grove, CA: Brooks/Cole.

Werther, W., & Davis, K. (1985). *Personnel management and human resources* (2nd. ed.). New York: McGraw-Hill.

Chapter 23

Group Work with Working Groups

PAUL H. EPHROSS
THOMAS V. VASSIL

This chapter discusses group work with working groups, those formed to produce a product or outcome external to the group itself. These groups seek to fulfill a specific function for the organization, community, or social movement of which they are part or which they represent. Others have used such terms as task groups, administrative groups, staff and administrative groups, groups for indirect services, groups in organizations, and citizens' groups to distinguish such groups from those whose primary purpose is to bring about change in the members themselves through the processes of group treatment or group therapy or through psychoeducational experiences (Ephross & Vassil, 1988, pp. 1–9).

The term "working groups" can be controversial. Treatment groups, those formed for the purpose of healing their members, also regard themselves as "working" in the sense that the group is addressing its therapeutic purposes. Others point out that certain phenomena are characteristic of all groups, regardless of their purpose (Hartford, 1972; Henry, 1992). Henry notes, however, that

> groups are an appropriate form for offering service to people with personal needs that are socially oriented. There are other kinds of needs, however, for which groups are an appropriate form of service. These are needs outside a person's individual needs, ones that can be met in some formal organization: boards, committees, and task-action groups, for task accomplishment; agency in-service training, supervision and staff development groups, for role performance, and consultation groups with decision and policy makers, with administrators, with direct service providers or with interdisciplinary teams, for improving the functioning of an organization. (1992, pp. 248–249)

All groups share characteristics, but there are different types of groups. In task-specific groups, work is defined by specific problem-solving activities that may range from creative to mundane (Thelen, 1958). These activities are meant to bring about change either in systems external to the group or in an organization or community of which the group is a part. Conscious of its limitations, we choose the term "working groups" as the most inclusive. Examples of working groups are:

- *Staff groups*—the staff employed by human service and health care organizations, paid and volunteer, composed of social workers or organized into multiprofessional teams.
- *Administrative groups within larger organizations*—committees or task forces charged to carry out a job or to provide a particular product for the entire organization or groups established and charged with responsibilities by statute or ordinance; often these are interagency bodies that prepare a budget proposal, or review and evaluate the performance of an organization, or investigate accusations of malfeasance.
- *Fiduciary groups such as boards of directors, electors, governors or trustees*— whether established by law, in the case of a governmental organization or corporation, or through bylaws, as in the instance of a voluntary not-for-profit or for-profit service delivery organization.
- *Well-established or ad hoc citizens' organizations*—these may involve citizens of a particular polity or residents of a neighborhood; members of one or many religious congregations or denominations or religious faiths; or persons representing one or many ethnic or racial groups or nationalities who are seeking help from a social worker who has the executive ability and skill to help them accomplish their purposes.
- *Groups defined by their own needs for a particular interest or activity*—for example, mothers or fathers of small children seeking to expand day care opportunities in their community.
- *Groups within advocacy organizations that represent and seek to advance the interests of particular populations*—these may be themselves or others, defined by geographical, demographic, or ethnoracial identities, religion, gender, age, health challenges, sexual orientation, political principles, history, nativity, or aspirations.
- *Groups within professional and multiprofessional organizations*—the former to advocate for the interests of the social work or other profession of which it is part, the latter generally concerned with a specific social or health problem—such as meeting the needs of young people with juvenile diabetes or the nutritional needs of older people or the job training needs of recent immigrants; revising the procedures through which children are assigned to foster homes is another example, as are groups within labor unions and coalitions of various unions.
- *Groups composed of organization representatives*—staffing such groups is often a responsibility of social workers employed by federations or associations of agencies, by the United Ways, or by various other kinds of councils of agencies or fund-raising and allocation agencies or even representatives of treatment agencies that serve the same local or metropolitan community.

Working groups are composed of a number of members. One of the members has a specialized role—namely, carrying executive responsibility for serving the needs of the group and helping the group implement its decisions. That person is charged with representing and working on behalf of the group as a whole—in many instances with working to achieve the purposes of the larger organization or community—and is generally paid for fulfilling the professional role, though volunteers are not unknown in this role. We prefer the term "staff person" to identify this individual to the term "worker." The latter term has little currency outside the profession of social work, whereas the alternative term, "facilitator," has become so broad as to render it meaningless in many organizations and settings.

WHAT IS DIFFERENT ABOUT WORK WITH WORKING GROUPS?

Social workers not only staff working groups but also participate in them as members and serve as their chairpersons and as members and chairpersons of subunits such as committees, subcommittees, and task forces. Much of the work of the social work profession itself is done in and by working groups. Thus group workers need skill not only in staffing but also in taking the roles of member and chairperson in working groups (Balgopal & Vassil, 1983; Henry, 1992; Bertcher, 1994; Toseland & Rivas, 1997).

Staffing working groups has long been a part of social work. The profession grew out of volunteer organizations, stimulated in part by the emergence of the Social Gospel movement in the various mainline Protestant denominations in the late 19th century and in part by the efforts of immigrant Catholics, Jews, and others to learn the English language and the skills to become Americans (Ephross & Vassil, 1988; Hartford, 1964; Siporin, 1986). In the early history of social work, much of this staffing responsibility fell to the chief staff member, variously known, over time and different organizations, as the general secretary, the executive secretary, the executive director, and now often as the chief executive officer (CEO) or the president, in imitation of business nomenclature. In the past, many social workers, devoted to direct practice, have shown a lack of interest in working with boards, committees, and community groups. An exception to this trend was, and still is, to be found in the settlement house–neighborhood center movement (Trattner, 1989). Staff members of these agencies have always understood the importance of working closely together with neighborhood and community groups.

Many contemporary group work textbooks devote a chapter to working groups (e.g., Brown, 1991; Garvin, 1997; Toseland & Rivas, 1997), whereas others (e.g., Northen & Kurland, 2001) view work with all groups through a common set of lenses, with only occasional references to working groups. It is interesting that community organizers and administrators, both of whom work extensively work with working groups, largely gloss over the question of group work skill. Three exceptions to this general comment should be noted. The first is an aging but still vital book by Steve Burghardt (1983), in which he devotes a major chapter to an account of the importance of working group skills for community organizers and the personal stresses and issues raised by community organization practice, especially in working with and in working groups. A second is the work of John Tropman, whose classic manual, *Effective Meetings* (1980), and later writings (e.g., Tropman, 1987), have emphasized the importance of skilled planning and use of self by the staff person in helping working groups accomplish their purposes. Tropman teaches the need to balance helping group members to meet their participatory needs with helping the groups of which they are part to accomplish their goals. A third exception is a chapter titled "Group Work in Context: Organizational and Community Factors" by Elizabeth A. Mulroy (2004), in which she relates the external turmoil of contemporary American economic and social contexts to the internal processes of groups within service delivery organizations.

Small groups can be viewed as the decision makers and framers of organizations (Lincoln, 1989). Small groups are incubators of organizational cultures, which, in turn, affect volunteers, staff members, and clients of service delivery organizations. It is in working group leadership and membership that careers are forged, maintained, or left to wither.

A cautionary note is in order. Not all collectivities or aggregations, whether inside or outside organizations, deserve to be called groups. There are many group-like collectivities that may be called "groupoids." Some look like functioning groups, and a few even sound like them. What makes them groupoids rather than groups, though, is their lack of adequate completion of the processes of group formation and development. The structures first taught us by Coyle and refined by the various useful and helpful stage/phase models from social work and cognate fields as to what is and what is not a group need to be borne in mind (Coyle, 1937, 1947, 1948; Garland, Jones, & Kolodny, 1965; Hartford, 1972; Sarri & Galinsky, 1985; Schiller, 1995; Schwartz, 1976; Tuckman, 1965; Tuckman & Jensen, 1977). Research into working groups and social work in working groups needs to come from studies "in the wild," studies of actual groups in their organizations and communities, what Frey (2003) has called "bona fide groups."

WORKING GROUPS AS DEMOCRATIC MICROCOSMS

More than 60 years ago, Erich Fromm (1941), then a refugee from a brutal dictatorship that sought his destruction and that of his people, argued that there is a human need to escape from freedom. What, after all, is so bad about an effective, humane dictatorship in a group? In our views and experience, what is so bad is that it prevents a group from forming as a democratic microcosm, keeps its members and its leadership from assuming responsibility for themselves and their work, and, in the end, prevents a group from being effective. It also funnels communication with the outside world through quasi-parental leadership figures, rather than promoting the development of open-system mechanisms for feedback from the other parts of the ecological system of which the working group is a part. Participatory democracy, within laws and a structure of rules, checks, and balances, is a requirement for group productivity. Modeling, teaching, and insisting on this participatory democracy is a prime function of the professional worker in groups.

This description may bring to mind a chaotic picture, but nothing is further from the atmosphere of participatory democracy than chaos. Civility and authority are prime requirements for democratic group function (Ephross & Vassil, 1988). Nothing positive takes place within a working group in the presence of fear, threats of retribution, violence directed at members, their group, and organization, or the threat of violence, scapegoating, or persecution. Helping to prevent the formation of a group culture based either on chaos and a lack of equanimity and civility or on interpersonal domination, fear, and scapegoating is a prime responsibility of the professional staff person in a group. Shulman (2001) suggested that the proper way to deal with a scapegoating process was preemptive intervention, whereas Northen and Kurland (2001) point out that the role of scapegoat in a group is an interactional role, not a one-way process imposed on one or more group members.

The staff person's role is to declare scapegoating unacceptable if the group is not able to get across this message by itself. Approaches need to be clear and based on the realities of the group's purpose. For example, statements such as, "We don't do that here," "This is not what we're here for," or "How will this help us get done what we need to?" can help a staff person to begin or end such a process.

The same may be said about discrimination and hate speech directed at members of those within or outside the group or organization because of their personal identities:

ethnoracial group, gender, immigrant status, political position, sexual identity, social class, religion, condition of handicap, or any other social characteristic. As much as civility and safety are requirements for working groups, so is the perspective that differences among members enrich groups and gives their decision making and consideration of issues an invaluable vitality and relevance to the social world outside the group. Authentic communication and honest disagreement are valuable to working groups, and freedom of speech deserves protection. Fostering intergroup hatreds is neither valuable nor worthy of protection. Staff persons and members need to decide where the line is in each specific instance.

Groups are and need to be systems in mutual aid. If group members cannot be of help to each other, then the very reason for groups' existence is undermined. Working groups are systems in mutual aid with a common purpose, tasks to perform, and often products to produce. If accomplishment of their tasks requires a mature working group, it is important for the organization of which the group is a part, the staff person, and the members to make the investment of time and energy that helping such a group develop requires. As we have noted elsewhere, a working group that is moving toward becoming a democratic microcosm and, we add, a system in mutual aid

> should be "our" group. It is never "their" group or "your" group. By these labels, we mean that each member of the group carries some responsibility for the totality of the group's functioning. Everything the group does is the business of every member. All suggestions should be welcomed, even those that cause problems for the group's leadership, because they represent an expression of concern and an input of energy from the member or subgroup offering the suggestions. (Ephross & Vassil, 1988, p. 52)

The concept of mutual aid has important implications for the professional role behavior of the staff member. Positive is better than negative, finding good in what members contribute is better than criticism and rejection; and the phrase "conscious use of self," so easy to say and often so difficult to enforce, is a prescription for a professional's behavior that is as old as group work itself. It is better to be real than to try to be perfect, for genuineness and authenticity on the part of a staff person invite trust, friendship, and participation, whereas presenting one's self as perfect both discourages trust and is doomed to fail.

A FRAMEWORK FOR UNDERSTANDING WORKING GROUPS

Many concepts provide a framework for understanding what goes on in working groups and guide group workers' participation and influence in such groups. We only list and briefly comment on some of these concepts. The reader is referred to fuller discussions elsewhere (for contracting, Shulman, 2001; for the others, Ephross & Vassil, 1988). These processes include the following.

1. *Contracting is especially important in working groups because, with few exceptions, members of such groups are there either as part of their work responsibilities or as part of their voluntary behavior as citizens.* In either case, it is important that there be agreement as to why they are there, what the purposes of the group are, what roles members will have, what risks, if any, come with membership in the group, and who has the ability and authority to decide on changes in the contract. All group contracts are subject to renegotiation by

the group in the course of its life, and part of the contract should specify who is responsible for implementing group decisions.

2. *Duration of the group is a significant consideration.* Short-term and long-term groups form and operate at different paces. An awareness of the available time frame seems to seep into working groups. A group that has a total of only four or five meetings to prepare an organizational budget that is due in the state capitol 6 weeks from now will tailor its use of time, its discussions, and its decision-making process so as to fit within the time available. The length of a group's life also has an effect, in our view, on the investment that members are willing to make in the group. One is likely to feel more committed when one undertakes a 3-year term on a board of directors, for example, than when one agrees to attend two meetings of a focus group. Another factor to consider about the length of a group's life is who makes the decision about how long a group will last. Sometimes, of course, this is not a decision that falls into the group's purview. But often, the decision can be made by a working group for itself. Bernstein, who was concerned with group self-determination throughout his long career, asked, "Whatever happened to self-determination?" (Bernstein, 1993). Like individuals and families, groups feel a sense of empowerment when they are able to control important aspects of their own lives and of disempowerment when they are not.

3. *The public and private sentiments of members have an important and ongoing impact on working groups.* Only a part of group members' feelings and therefore of their interactions with each other lies above the line of consciousness. This is to be expected and needs to be understood by other members, by the chairperson if there is one, and by the staff person as well. We select two examples from among many possibilities. Diversity of identity within a group and between group members and staff person are often present in working groups. The differences may concern gender, race, ethnic identity, social class, age, level of handicap, citizenship, sexual orientation, biography, having or not having children—the list is a long one. Members may be concerned with impressing other members for a variety of reasons. Interpersonal histories and loyalties, as well as past group experiences, may play a part. It is not unusual, for example, for community groups, as well as staffs, to contain two or more people who are related to each other. Not all of the private feelings that one member has toward another can be, or even should be, brought into the open or become topics for the entire group. This does not mean that sentiments derived from past experiences do not exist in the group. They do, and they should be expected by the staff person, though the direction that they take and their history is sometimes a surprise.

4. *The nature of interpersonal bonding is often different in working groups than in other types of groups.* The relationships formed may be quite intense as long as the group is working on a project dear to the hearts of some group members, but they may also be task specific and time limited. When they are not, issues of ethics and boundaries may be raised and need to be dealt with by the members involved or by the group as a whole, with or without the help of the staff person. For example, working together on a committee or subcommittee or coming to a meeting of such a body at someone's house may indicate to some group members an invitation to intimacy that is far from the intention of the subcommittee chair or the host or hostess.

Borrowing from the language of chemistry, we refer to interpersonal bonds in groups as "simple" when the exchange between people is largely or entirely informational. We label as "covalent" an interpersonal bond that is meaningful to two or more group members. We have in mind a situation akin to what writers from Schwartz (1976) to Northen and Kurland (2001) have termed "mutual aid" experiences. The latter authors write movingly about the difficulty that some group members have with accepting termination (2001, pp.

420–421), and their observations apply to some members' experiences in working groups, as well as to members of other kinds of groups.

Some interpersonal relationship experiences in working groups can truly be called transformative, for the members involved or sometimes for the entire group. We use the label "coordinate covalent" for such relationships, which may affect a change of roles within the group or in many areas of group members' lives far removed from the particular group (Argyris & Schon, 1974). We recall a good many such relationship experiences in groups ranging from a settlement house board of directors to a technical advisory committee for a demographic study of a community's population. For many people, experiences in working groups can trigger important changes in racial, ethnic, gender, and class-linked perceptions and attitudes. Though such experiences are not stated objectives of working groups, in the vast majority of cases, they are important and deserve empathic support from social work staff.

5. *Molar–molecular characteristics, another borrowing of terminology from the field of chemistry, are often important in groups.* These are part–whole relationships, as among subgroups—for example, between those who live east of the tracks and those who live to the west; between old residents and newcomers to the neighborhood; between the men who once held all of the places on the board of governors and the women who now make up half of the board. One place in which molar–molecular dynamics can often be seen is in councils, which are groups made up of representatives from other groups, or in coalitions that have gotten together because they share positions on a particular issue, though they and their memberships may differ widely on many other issues. An example may be a statewide coalition that includes many persons from faith-based organizations, which seeks to act on behalf of the needs of the state's children. That no child should go without medical care or enough food to eat may seem to be the only two things on which everyone on the steering committee of this coalition agrees.

Several of the aforementioned areas raise an issue for practice that causes a common conflict for staff persons. This conflict is often stated as *process* and (or versus) *product*. No matter how interesting and how rich in social importance, nor how engaging the discussion is for the staff member, at some point one must seek to limit the discussion because some important votes are needed on the budget, which is due in the state capitol next Tuesday. Despite the fact that there is tension among several subgroups, can the group progress toward its goal? Or should the staff person influence the group to stop working on its product and engage in a bit of self-analytic introspection to try to clear the air, as well as the members' minds? The specific answers to such questions also depend largely on the indigenous leadership of a specific group.

6. *Nothing in a working group is more vital nor more complex than leadership.* Some aspects of leadership are personality based, some situationally based; virtually all aspects have ethnocultural elements; many are linked to gender; some are linked to stability in group life, and some to crisis.

7. *Work, learning, and developmental stages of groups are crucial elements in most groups at one time or another.* Though stages of group development is a helpful concept, it must be kept in mind that stages are abstract ideas, whereas group members are persons who live and breathe, regress and progress, express their feelings or not, and sometimes regret whichever path they took. Groups do not progress in a straight line. Also, even though group members may be meeting the staff person for the first time, various dyads, triads, and larger subgroups may have known each other for a long time, may have worked together in other groups, may have gone to the same schools or colleges or worked together on the

same political campaigns, or may belong to the same civic and social organizations. A first meeting may be a first meeting in fact or may be a reunion for everyone in the room except the staff person.

8. *The organizational setting is a vital dimension in some groups and less so in others.* What varies greatly is the loyalty that group members bring to the group. Some are loyal to the organization overall, some to a specific part or branch or department, some to their own careers in the organization. Some members draw their personal authority and influence from "local" sources, that is, from sources within the particular organization that sponsors the group; others from "cosmopolitan" sources, that is, their broad experience in many organizations or in the world outside of the particular organization's emphasis (Wilson, 1985). For some group members, their technical skill is the important link to the group; for others, there is pleasure and/or gain in being associated with the other people in the group. For some group members, the group may be a step up from the point of view of social mobility, either within the organization or in the broader communities. For example, there may be a traditional family tie to certain boards or commissions or to public service in general, a sort of *noblesse oblige*, which spans generations and is a sort of marker of community social status.

9. *Group composition, group membership and citizenship, and the makeup of the group as a whole are characteristics that are always present, always important, and always foci of conflict, growth, or decay.* They constitute an important part—though not all, of course—of the identity of the group and therefore of its life. It is partly for this reason that the ability to hear—not just in the auditory sense but in the sense of communication—and to understand others in depth, which is correctly understood as a clinical social work skill, is also an important skill for members, leaders, and staff persons of working groups. In our view, participating in, leading, and staffing working groups demand finely honed skills that are essentially the same as those required for group work with other kinds of groups. Northen and Kurland (2001) quote approvingly Newstetter's definition of group work at the 1935 National Conference of Social Work, the conference at which group work was formally inducted into the social work profession:

> All group work has a dual set of objectives, working for social justice and working to meet the needs of the group members. The balance or proportion of effort that needs to be devoted to each of the purposes is what differentiates social work with working groups from social work with other kinds of groups. (Newstetter, 1935, quoted in Northen & Kurland, 2001, p. 9)

LEADERSHIP IN WORKING GROUPS

A distinction should be made between leadership as a function that needs to be performed in groups and the role of the social worker staff person. Members can and do capably provide part or all of their own leadership. One of the ways in which group workers can be helpful in working groups is to help the group identify, support, and work cooperatively with its own indigenous leadership. One of the strains that can arise for staff persons is the fact that group members and the staff person not only share a common human condition—this is, after all, the case in all groups—but also that frequently group members are as well or better educated than the staff member, have a variety of life experiences that the staff person may not have, speak in the idiom of the community or the organization that is the target of the group's actions, and may well have access to more and better resources than the professional does.

When the staff person carries some of the leadership responsibility, one should remember Kouzes and Posner's advice that: "Leadership isn't a place, it's a process . . . it's far healthier and more productive to start with the assumption that it's possible for everyone to lead. . . . Leadership is a relationship. . . . Leadership development is self-development" (Bennis, Spitzer, & Cummings, 2001, p. 85). Slater, in the same volume, points out, "People don't need to be controlled and manipulated to commit themselves to a heartfelt vision, and being controlled and manipulated tends to destroy that commitment. Those trained to a mechanistic world view often find it difficult to learn this" (p. 115).

Staffing a working group requires a capacity for aloneness, an ability to back off and see the group and its external environment in a thoughtful and perhaps a new way. It demands believing in the value of conflict and its nonviolent resolution, trusting the processes of the democratic microcosm, and fighting the natural tendency to do what feels good and to avoid what does not feel good.

ETHICAL AND MORAL ASPECTS OF SOCIAL WORK WITH WORKING GROUPS

Working effectively with working groups requires some sense of one's own and of others' dignity, but certainly not immunity from human failings. Like other people, social workers who work in working groups get tired, get annoyed, do not appreciate being the targets of blame, and are entitled to their hang-ups and feelings. All feelings are acceptable for professionals in groups. All behaviors certainly are not. Understanding and guarding strictly the boundary between feelings and behaviors is called professional skill. It is also called observing professional ethics. Two examples may make this point clearer. It is quite normal for professional staff to feel attracted to certain group members. It is not acceptable to act on these feelings, neither to favor some group members over others nor to undertake intimate relationships with a group member while one carries responsibility for maintaining a professional relationship. Conversely, it is normal for a professional to like some group members less than others, even not to like some group members. Again, the principle is that the feeling is acceptable, perhaps to be worked through by introspection, perhaps not. Hostile behavior toward such group members is not acceptable and flies in the face of professional ethics.

Effective group work with working groups requires taking seriously the entire body of ethics and morality of the social work profession and one's responsibility to it. It also requires a self-reflective stance, resiliency, and an ability to apologize for mistakes, together with a kind of indestructibility so far as the group is concerned. Operationally, indestructibility means that one tries hard not to lose self-control, regardless of the provocations; one does not engage in temper tantrums, in interpersonal violence, or in dramatic scenes involving leaving the group or returning to it. One bears in mind to the maximum extent possible that group successes are the group's, not the professional's, and that group failures likewise are the group's, not the professional's. Social work with working groups demands a sort of psychological sturdiness, a sense of not being able to be shocked or recruited into interpersonal conspiracies on the one hand and of being able to dampen one's mood swings on the other.

Working groups can be quite challenging for social workers. They require that one come to grips with one's own limitations on the one hand and with the profession's commitment to seeking social justice on the other. One must work toward a certain moral authority without denying one's own weaknesses. These groups require the ability to participate and the ability to learn, as well as the ability to lead and the ability to teach, all depending on the needs of the group, its members, and its tasks, rather than on needs that arise within the staff person.

Expertise in the content of the group has some importance. Knowing how to take a community's or an organization's pulse is an important skill, so ability and experience at quick, small-scale survey research can be a distinct asset. But because it is impossible for anyone, as a staff person, to have expertise in all areas that a group may need, and because there may well be someone in the group whose expertise surpasses the social worker's, it is important that the staff person not need to be an expert on everything that comes up in the group's life. An example that comes up in virtually every group at this time has to do with expertise in using computer technology. The competition that arises when group members compare their own experiences and the status that technological sophistication can give to a group member who may otherwise have little influence or power in the group are common trends at the beginning of the 21st century.

When he first laid out the functions of the group worker in his classic article, "The Social Worker in the Group," William Schwartz (1961) included among the functions of the group worker "lending a vision," a vision of how things could be, one that engendered hope for the future among the group members. It remains one of the major functions for a social worker in working groups. Unquestionably, the ability to provide staff leadership to a working group has something to do with personality, with experience, with maturity, with situational demands, and sometimes with accidental factors as well. From a moral point of view, we have noted:

> Various group members carry differential degrees of moral presence with them in groups. The presence . . . seems to be linked to a normative perception by group members that a particular individual is able to balance caring about the group's success, respect for the contribution of group members, and knowledge and skill at group processes, as well as the ability to help the group work with an atmosphere of "equanimity" (Thelen, 1981). . . . Moral presence also reflects a perception of others that a leader's own needs are sufficiently under control that they will not overwhelm a concern for the group's success. . . . To occupy a leadership position, one need not be an exceptional person, but one does need to be able to behave in specific patterns in a disciplined way. (Ephross & Vassil, in press)

These factors are close to those that have been identified as "moral involvement" in groups (Balgopal & Vassil, 1983). The importance of supporting and valuing differences in group composition have been touched on earlier. What also needs to be emphasized is the important of character, courage, and living with ambiguities in today's social milieu.

The past few years have brought authenticated news about personal and organizational immoral behaviors, such as diversion of philanthropic resources to personal enrichment and high living and embezzlement and fraud on the part of professional social workers, reflecting similar behavior on the part of organizational leaders in the for-profit sector of the economy (Axelrod, 2003; Pearlstein, 2003; Vogel, 2002–2003; "Sad chapter," 2003; Behr & Johnson, 2003a, 2003b; "Corporate scandals," 2003).

Such violation of the ethical code of the profession has been unthinkable, with only the rarest exceptions, in social work's history. In this atmosphere, we think it makes particular sense to teach, reinforce, and uphold the Code of Ethics (National Association of Social Workers [NASW], 1999). Northen and Kurland (2001) refer to relationship as the core of social work practice with groups. It should be superfluous, but apparently is not, to underscore that these relationships need to be based on trust, truth, and confidence between group members and professional social work staff.

EFFECTIVE METHODS FOR WORKING WITH WORKING GROUPS

Tropman (1980) has done a fine job of developing and discussing various rules and principles for conducting effective meetings. Without staking a group's existence on carrying out literally all of his many rules for meetings, one ignores his advice about agendas, time management, and related topics at great risk. Agendas, minutes, notices of meetings, reminders, schedules, follow-up with nonattendees—these are the day-to-day caretaking instruments for working groups.

For staffing working groups, the following is a list of techniques that, properly used and properly timed, can be effective.

1. *Silence*, not saying anything while behaving nonverbally in an accepting and interested way, is one way of permitting or even requiring group members to work on their tasks. Expressing empathy, sometimes in the form of sympathetically asking for clarification or more information, is a way of relating to individual members, a subgroup or the group as a whole.

2. *Mirroring or reflecting feelings*, as well as providing client feedback, can lead to group reassessment, to recentering, to clearing away obstacles and enabling the group to move ahead. One needs to be concerned with not overloading any one or small number of group members in this process. Social workers are not the only people who find taking criticism difficult at times.

3. *Exploring, probing, and questioning*, especially through using open-ended questions, is often useful for a variety of purposes in addition to the stated requests for information. For example, one way to involve group members who seem under- or uninvolved is to ask for their opinions. Sometimes it helps check out what appears to be unanimity but may just be hesitation on the part of some members to disagree with a predominant point of view or to risk others' disapproval.

4. It can be useful at times to *give directions or advice*. This is particularly the case when groups are clearly formed and have developed confidence in their own abilities. When one knows one's group thoroughly, it often makes sense to move right ahead with a piece of advice or a forceful suggestion. There is some danger, though, in the staff person playing the "politics of expertise" (Benveniste, 1972) too frequently. If a staff person gives direct advice more than twice in a particular meeting, that person should examine closely the motivations and effects of the behavior. *Universalizing*, and its close relative, *connecting points of view*, are ways to help groups move toward decisions made in a win–win rather than a win–lose manner.

5. *Confrontation* is a term that is often misused. The term actually means sharing with a group your view of where a particular action or inaction or decision is likely to lead. It does not necessarily connote interpersonal conflict, let alone hostility. Again, this term comes close here to Schwartz's (1961) concept, "lending a vision," but perhaps in the form of "lending an ego." Schwartz proposed that one of the functions of the worker was to share

with the group a view of future probabilities, based on extensive group experience, of outcomes that might result from the group's action. The counterpart term, "lending an ego," refers to the fact that the skill of being able to anticipate the future outcome of a present action is an ego function in those maps of personality that derive from psychoanalytic sources.

6. *Support* can refer to a variety of actions in a group. One can support a group member's right to express a point of view, one can support the point of view presented, one can support a group member while supporting his or her point of view, or one can support the manner in which a group has dealt with its member's suggestion.

7. *Modeling, coaching, and shaping*, as well as *role playing*, are all useful teaching techniques, ideally suited to rehearsing behaviors, choosing among alternative strategies, and the like. Care needs to be taken, when using role play as a technique that no one is forced or pressured into playing a role he or she does not want to play, nor one that can have destructive meaning at a particular time in the group member's life. It needs to be possible for a group member not to take part in a particular role play or, for that matter, in any particular activity or simulation.

8. *Supposals* are really another form of using imagination to solve problems and are a kind of mental role play. They are ways to practice looking ahead, thinking about possible outcomes of a course of action, at minimum risk. Supposals begin with the statement, "Let's suppose [we do this, we do that, we don't take a stand, we don't allocate money for this service in the budget, etc.]. What's likely to happen? Would we still have [a particular political figure's, say] support?"

9. *Summarizing and focusing, partializing, sequencing, pacing, and grading* are all ways of either putting together the bits and pieces of a problem to form a whole or taking apart a problem to better understand the bits and pieces.

10. *Decentering* and *setting limits* are the two sides of the same coin; the first refers to getting apathetic members, subgroups, and groups off dead center, the second to reinforcing limits for the sake of order, reducing noise level, or reducing the level of potential or actual danger. Another way of thinking about these techniques is that the first is geared toward increasing the activity level, and sometimes the anxiety level as well, within a group, whereas the second seeks to reduce one or both of these levels.

11. *Dividing into smaller subgroups*, sometimes called "buzz groups," may be a useful technique to get ideas and suggestions out into the open, to "brainstorm," and to seek alternative solutions.

12. Though most working groups operate informally most of the time, *a thorough knowledge of the concepts and techniques of parliamentary procedure* should be part of a staff member's armamentarium, to be called on and referred to with the group as needed (Ramey, 1993).

These are only some of the techniques that are applicable in working groups. They are potential elements in the professional role behavior of the staff person, though certainly any or all of them may be utilized by group members as well. There are also some aspects of staffing working groups that deserve mention, even though they cannot be found in most lists of techniques. Social workers in general and group workers in particular may often ignore their own interpersonal needs or, for that matter, their own needs for accomplishment, recognition, and even money. Ephross (1983) has suggested that this disregard is a strange form of macho behavior, particularly dissonant with the fact that social work's professional association membership is more than three-fourths (76%) female. The term "macho" here refers not to sexual identity but to the construction of a professional self that emphasizes service to others and concern with others but is silent on the subject of concern with one's own needs, aspirations, and life stage as a person.

Working effectively with others in groups requires, in our view, that one's own needs are being met to a reasonable extent. Yet, in some human service organizations, concern with the needs of staff is somehow judged to be illegitimate or a sign of weakness, of violating the ethics of the profession, when it is in fact the opposite, a way of fulfilling professional ethics. Given the burgeoning literature on the health needs of caregivers and the need to devote attention to avoiding tangled relationships (e.g., Haas & Malouf, 1995; Reamer, 2001; Scott & Hawk, 1986), social workers have a responsibility to members of groups they work with, to themselves, and to their own families and those significant in their lives to pay attention to meeting their own needs. There is an intensity to working with groups that can drain one's relationship capacity, one's psychic energy, and, at times, physical energy as well.

We conclude with brief considerations of two elements of professional practice with working groups—one common to work with all kinds of groups and one particular to social work practice in working groups. The common element is that all group work practice rests on *conscious use of self*. Each piece of professional behavior is a miniature research process, based on a hypothesis that the behavior will lead to a desired outcome, testing the hypothesis by the action, then concluding from one's data analysis that the hypothesis has been supported or supplanted by a revised or new hypothesis. For students and beginning practitioners, the process is apparent, sometimes painfully so. For experienced practitioners, it becomes almost second nature, and it is repeated at each group meeting, each contact with a group member between meetings, and each piece of planning on the part of the staff person.

The element that is distinctive to much work with working groups is the equality—sometimes the superior status—of group members vis-à-vis the staff person. As noted earlier, it is a common experience for one or more or all of the members of a working group to be equally as educated as the staff person, sometimes better educated; to be richer than the staff person (regrettably not usually difficult given the levels of many social work salaries), or to possess more expertise about particular problems facing a group or particular tasks that the group needs to accomplish. This relationship dynamic is an important one that should be part of the consciousness of social workers who work in and with working groups and one with which the social worker needs to be comfortable. The skills of group members should be viewed as sources of help for the group as a whole, not as problems or challenges for the professional staff member.

EPILOGUE

Some of the most important decisions and events in the career of a professional social worker take place in working groups, often in groups in which professionals serve as members, chairs, staff persons, or all three. As careers progress, even the most devoted clinical social work practitioners find an increasing proportion of their time and effort being spent in such groups. "Administration involves a large and crucial component of group participation and group leadership" (Ephross & Vassil, 1988, p. 3). Working groups, their processes, and their decisions are influential and important in the lives of citizens, as they are in the lives of professionals. Together, working groups constitute a significant part of the fabric of our society, and knowing how to work in them, lead them, staff them, and bring about change in them is essential to improving the effectiveness of social services and work toward the equity and social justice that are the goals of social work.

REFERENCES

Argyris, C., & Schon, D. A. (1974). *Theory in practice*. San Francisco: Jossey-Bass.

Axelrod, N. R. (2003, January/February). Looking inward after Enron. In *The WCA nonprofit agenda* (pp. 1–3). Washington, DC: Washington Council of Agencies.

Balgopal, P. R., & Vassil, T. V. (1983). *Groups in social work: An ecological perspective*. New York: Macmillan.

Behr, P., & Johnson, C. (2003a, May 1). More Enron charges expected today. *The Washington Post*, p. E-2.

Behr, P., & Johnson, C. (2003b, May 3). Enron prosecutions intensify. *The Washington Post*, pp. E-1, E-5.

Bennis, W., Spitzer, G. M., & Cummings, T. C. (Eds.). (2001). *The future of leadership*. San Francisco: Jossey-Bass.

Benveniste, G. (1972). *The politics of expertise*. Berkeley, CA: Glendessary Press.

Bernstein, S. (1993). Whatever happened to self-determination? In S. Wenocur, P. H. Ephross, T. V. Vassil, & R. K. Varghese (Eds.), *Group work: Expanding horizons* (pp. 3–15). New York: Haworth Press.

Bertcher, H. (1994). *Group participation: Techniques for group leaders and members* (2nd ed.). Newbury Park, CA: Sage.

Brown, L. N. (1991). *Groups for growth and change*. New York: Longman.

Burghardt, S. (1983). *The other side of organizing: Resolving the personal dilemmas and daily practical needs*. Cambridge, MA: Schenkman.

Corporate scandals: A user's guide [Editorial]. (2003, May 11). *The New York Times*, p. D2.

Coyle, G. L. (1937). *Studies in group behavior*. New York: Harper & Row.

Coyle, G. L. (1947). *Group experience and democratic values*. New York: Women's Press.

Coyle, G. L. (1948). *Group work with American youth*. New York: Harper & Row.

Ephross, P. H. (1983, Spring). Giving up martyrdom. *Public Welfare, 41*.

Ephross, P. H., & Vassil, T. V. (1988). *Groups that work: Structure and process*. New York: Columbia University Press.

Ephross, P. H., & Vassil, T. V. (in press). *Groups that work: Structure and process* (2nd ed.). New York: Columbia University Press.

Fromm, E. (1941). *Escape from freedom*. New York: Holt, Rinehart & Winston.

Frey, L. R. (Ed.). (2001). *Group communication in context: Studies of bona fide groups* (2nd ed.). Mahwah, NJ: Erlbaum.

Garland, J. E., Jones, H. E., & Kolodny, R. L. (1965). A model for stages of development in social work groups. In S. B. Bernstein (Ed.), *Explorations in group work* (pp. 17–31). Boston: Charles River Books.

Garvin, C. (1997). *Contemporary group work* (3rd ed.). Boston: Allyn & Bacon.

Haas, L. J., & Malouf, J. L. (1995). *Keeping up the good work: A practitioner's guide to mental health ethics*. Sarasota, FL: Professional Resource Press.

Hartford, M. E. (Ed.). (1964). *Working papers toward a frame of reference for social group work*. New York: National Association of Social Workers.

Hartford, M. E. (1972). *Groups in social work*. New York: Columbia University Press.

Henry, S. (1992). *Group skills in social work: A four-dimensional approach* (2nd ed.). Pacific Grove, CA: Brooks/Cole.

Kouzes, J. M., & Posner, B. Z. (2001). Bringing leadership. In W. Bennis, G. M. Spitzer, & T. C. Cummings (Eds.), *The future of leadership* (pp. 81–91). San Francisco: Jossey-Bass.

Lincoln, Y. F. (1989). *Organizational theory and inquiry: The paradigm revolution*. Newbury Park, CA: Sage.

Mulroy, E. A. (2004). Group work in context: organizational and community factors. In G. L. Greif & P. H. Ephross (Eds.), *Group work with populations at risk* (2nd ed.). New York: Oxford University Press.

National Association of Social Workers. (1999). *Code of ethics* (revised). Washington, DC: Author.

Northen, H., & Kurland, R. (2001). *Social work with groups* (3rd ed.). New York: Columbia University Press.

Pearlstein, S. (2003, April 30). A rigged market for CEOs. *The Washington Post*, p. E- 1.

Ramey, J. H. (1993). Group empowerment through learning formal decision making processes. In S. Wenocur, P. H. Ephross, T. V. Vassil, & R. K. Varghese (Eds.), *Social work with groups: Expanding horizons* (pp. 171–181). New York: Haworth Press.

Reamer, F. G. (2001). *Tangled relationships: Managing boundary issues in the human services*. New York: Columbia University Press.

Sad chapter on Wall Street [Editorial]. (2003, April 30). *The Washington Post*, p. A-22.

Sarri, R. C., & Galinsky, M. J. (1985). A conceptual framework for group development. In M. Sandel, P. Glasser, R. Sarri, & R. Vinter (Eds.), *Individual change through small groups* (pp. 70–86). New York: Free Press.

Schiller, L. Y. (1995). Stages of development in women's groups: A relational model. In R. Kurland & R. Salmon (Eds.), *Group work practice in a troubled society: Problems and opportunities* (pp. 117–138). Binghamton, NY: Haworth Press.

Schwartz, W. (1961). The social worker in the group. In *New directions in social work with groups* (pp. 7–29). New York: National Association of Social Workers.

Schwartz, W. (1976). Between client and system: The mediating function. In R. Roberts & H. Northen (Eds.), *Theories of social work with groups* (pp. 171–197). New York: Columbia University Press.

Scott, C. D., & Hawk, J. (Eds.). (1986). *Heal thyself: The health of health care professionals*. New York: Brunner/Mazel.

Shulman, L. (2001). *The skills of helping individuals, families, groups and communities* (5th ed.). Itasca, IL: F. E. Peacock.

Siporin, M. (1986). Group work method and the inquiry. In P. H. Glasser & N. S. Mayadas (Eds.), *Group workers at work: Theory and practice in the '80s*. Totowa, NJ: Rowman & Littlefield.

Slater, P. (2001). Leading yourself. In W. Bennis, G. M. Spitzer, & T. C. Cummings (Eds.), *The future of leadership* (pp. 103–116). San Francisco: Jossey-Bass.

Thelen, H. A. (1958). *Dynamics of groups at work*. Chicago: University of Chicago Press.

Thelen, H. A. (1981). *The classroom society*. New York: Halsted Press.

Toseland, R. W., & Rivas, R. F. (1997). *An introduction to group work practice* (3rd ed.). Boston: Allyn & Bacon.

Trattner, W. I. (1989). *From poor law to welfare state: A history of social welfare in America* (4th ed.). New York: Free Press.

Tropman, J. E. (1980). *Effective meetings: Improving group decision-making*. Beverly Hills, CA: Sage.

Tropman, J. E. (1987). Effective meetings: Some provisional rules and needed research. In R. W. Toseland & P. H. Ephross (Eds.), *Working effectively with administrative groups*. New York: Haworth Press.

Tuckman, B. W. (1965, June). Developmental sequence in small groups. *Psychological Bulletin, 63,* 384–399.

Tuckman, B. W., & Jensen, M. A.-C. (1977). Stages of small group development revisited. *Group and Organizational Studies, 2*(1), 419–427.

Vogel, D. (2002–2003). The split personality of corporate America. *The Responsive Community, 13*(1).

Wilson, E. K. (1985). What counts in the death or transformation of an organization? *Social Forces, 64.*

Chapter 24

From Agency Client to Community-Based Consumer

The Family Group Conference as a Consumer-Led Group in Child Welfare

GALE BURFORD
JOAN PENNELL

Social work with groups has a lengthy history of advancing the empowerment and well-being of individuals and communities in the face of market forces and government regulations (Simon, 1994). Listening closely to aspirations of community groups, we find that they have adopted a range of models, each pushing toward different relationships among members, between members and the social worker, and with the hosting organization and the wider community (Papell & Rothman, 1966). One model with increasing popularity is referred to as "consumer-centered groups." These are operated solely by, or with considerable involvement of, the service users or consumers themselves. They emphasize the principles of client self-determination and empowerment and stress the benefits to the consumers themselves of participation. In this context, the social worker moves from leader or facilitator to supporter or advocate of the group, and the auspices change from a human service agency to a community organization, commonly linked with a national or international social movement.

The term "consumer" signals a departure from agency-directed work and reframes populations in the lower echelons of a market economy as normal members of society. As consumers, they are translated from clients or patients into citizens who determine what services are provided and how they are delivered. In keeping with the social-goals model of group work (Papell & Rothman, 1966), these group settings foster the social responsibility for advancing a democratic society. Relabeling clients as consumers, however, leads down a forked path to decentralizing human services. One branch privatizes services, and consumers use vouchers to purchase services on the basis of their preferences. An alternative branch enlarges a civil society in which voluntary associations encourage noncoerced contributions on the basis of commitments (Cohen, 2001). Both branches seek to reduce bureaucratic controls and reinvent human services, the former through market mechanisms and the latter through community participation (Adams & Nelson, 1995; Schorr, 1997).

This chapter discusses how consumer-centered groups, because of their origins, philosophies, purposes, group format, and community context, primarily take this second branch. It begins by reviewing the fields in which consumer-centered groups have taken root, their interventive approach, and their relationship to other sectors of society, then delineates their main aims. Attention is also given to how specific forms of this group approach—consumer-driven and consumer-led groups—further advance the voice of their members. Next the theoretical orientation and evidential base for consumer-centered practice are explored, and potential benefits and dangers of this approach are identified. Because child welfare poses one of the greatest challenges to decentralizing human services and adopting a consumer-centered approach, an example from this field of practice is examined in depth. It is called "family group conferencing." This approach goes beyond consumer-centered groups by encouraging the leadership of the family in planning and provides an example of a consumer-led group within child welfare.

The overview of family group conferencing is based on a review of the international literature and on our long-term involvement with the model in child welfare. Detailed consideration is given to how a consumer-centered perspective is being embraced in a setting in which formal authorities must be involved because of the statutory nature of the service and the need to offer formal protections to some members of the group. The case is made that in these instances consumers are thought to be best served when the group is aligned with, or operated under the auspices or sponsorship of, a community-based governing structure working in partnership with formal authorities or mandated services. Suggestions for practice, dilemmas faced, and evidence to support the importation of empowerment and consumer-oriented philosophies into statutory services are discussed, along with the need for consumer leadership to be sustained by community-centered governance.

INTERVENTIONS

The idea of *client as consumer* is well recognized in the fields of developmental disabilities and mental health. Sustained, organized responses to promote self-determination in community-based, independent living arrangements and enhanced choice for service users are found in these fields (Frese & Davis, 1997; Staples, 1999; Tower, 1994). Taken from this view, a consumer-centered model is more than simply service coordination or integration of delivery. It requires the agreement or involvement of the consumers, their caregivers, and service providers at every stage, including needs assessment, program design, goal setting, implementation, governance, and evaluation (Bowers & Saucier, 1999).

Homan (1999) raises the concern that the word "consumer" suggests greater exercise of choice than many people utilizing human services can expect and overemphasizes their use of goods and services while playing down what they have to contribute. This is reflected in the advocacy work of the late Rae Unzicker (1999), specifically in the area of mental health services, in which, she argued, the use of the term should not apply unless consumers are granted the right to refuse treatment. Referring to services for people with disabilities, Nadash summarizes by saying that a "unifying force in the range of consumer-directed and consumer choice models is that individuals have the primary authority to make choices that work best for them, regardless of the nature or extent of their disability or the source of payment for their services" (Nadash, 1998, as cited in Simon-Rusinowitz, 1999, p. 3).

The literature on consumer-centered groups overlaps considerably with the self-help, mutual-aid, and empowerment literature (Kyrouz & Humphreys, 1997; Wituk, Shepherd, Slavich, Warren, & Meissen, 2000). It covers a rather wide range of groups, including those organized and operated completely by group members who share a problem or condition. These we would refer to as *consumer-driven groups*. Next are groups of people who are affected in some way by a common condition or social problem but who include the involvement of a professional advisor or local, state, or national advisory body and those co-led by a professional helper and a self-helper. These groups have the potential to be *consumer led* if they actively seek to advance the members' leadership with supports and protections from service providers. And finally there are those that are almost wholly organized by professionals who work to promote opportunities for empowerment with individuals who share a condition or problem. The latter groups are encompassed by the more generic term *consumer centered*. The "consumer movement," community and family-centered practice, social network theory, restorative justice, community partnership building, population health, and empowerment approaches have much in common with one another philosophically. Yet considerable difference is seen at the practice level in what is actually meant by these terms with respect to the principles used to guide groups to determine who administers the services, where they are located, and who provides needed resources. Innovations in this area draw on substantive and wide-ranging theoretical bases.

Although a wide variety of terms is used to describe practices, most terms are based on the notion that lasting efforts to prevent or intervene in complex social situations are efforts that involve the affected people in constructing solutions that fit for them and for their families and communities. Such involvement is thought to foster ownership of plans that are developed, thereby presumably heightening follow-through and successful completion of plans, while at the same time exponentially developing the overall capacities of the group for further self-directed effort. The hope is that participants will generalize the use of the skills and sustain their engagement at the civic level. By extension, these interests are predicated on the view that the maintenance of healthy and safe conditions for families and communities cannot and should not be the responsibility of any one social sector. Over and above mere cooperation or coordination of efforts, collaboration between members of formal and informal systems is required.

In general, consumer-centered groups are distinguished from therapeutic interventions by their emphasis on social goals rather than remedial goals. They also diverge because of their focus on participant leadership rather than expert, professional guidance. Nevertheless, overlap is found between consumer-centered groups and some approaches to family therapy (cf., McFarlane, 2002; Waldegrave, 2000) that have worked to integrate social and therapeutic goals.

The question of resources figures prominently in consumer-driven groups, from those that make do entirely with no support from government to those located within the auspices of government and reliant on public resources (Hardina, 2002; Hoehne, 1988). Concerns arise regardless of the level of government involvement. In the case of crime victims, Crawford (1997) suggests that community action may lack the authoritative means to mobilize resources. Historically, social movements have sometimes fallen prey to expropriation by government or corporate funders if groups depend on them for their survival. Strang (2001) argues that this is the case with the crime victims' movement in the United States.

In general, the aims of consumer-centered groups are for those who are affected to:

- Hold the right to say "no" to interventions.
- Organize the group or play a significant role in its direction.
- Set the goals, determine the solutions, and implement and refine the plan of action.
- Develop governance and funding structures that balance their autonomy with sustaining partnerships.
- Acquire competencies that can be more widely generalized to civic engagement.

PHILOSOPHICAL ROOTS

The consumer movement most often refers to people who are working together to make changes on their own behalf. The philosophical roots are common to the literature on self-determination, participatory decision making, and empowerment approaches in groups, community, social, and political movements (Day, 2002; Gutiérrez & Lewis, 1999; Gutiérrez, Parsons, & Cox, 1998; Kessler-Harris, 2001; Lerner, 2002; Simon, 1994; Wenocur & Reisch, 2002). Although the actual term "consumer" is most visible within the independent living and mental health rights movements, it can also be traced to the consumer movement's attempts to target corporations and to hold sellers and markets accountable to the power of a purchasing/spending public (Korten, 2001; Nader, 1973)—or at least to tie economic development together with social development (Midgley, 1997). The associated ideas and language have more recently been embraced by many who receive a wide range of human services. In particular, advocates from the antipsychiatry and women's movements called for changes in language away from depicting service recipients in terms associated with pathology and dependency. In this way, the consumer perspective has come to be associated with challenges to the imposition of expert models of diagnosis and intervention and to the domination of resources by corporate, including professional, interests and with the involvement of citizens in social planning efforts.

Specifically, the application of the term "consumer" to people receiving human services has been traced to the late 1960s and the modern beginnings of the self-advocacy movement. Tower (1994) points to the modern beginnings of the self-advocacy movement and the consumer rights movement as products of a number of complementary social movements that emerged in the United States in the 1960s and 1970s. In this connection, she identifies the civil rights movement and relevant legislation, the beginnings of self-help and mutual aid, demedicalization, deinstitutionalization of those with mental illness, and the independent living movement for those with developmental disabilities. To this we would add the influence of contemporary, market-oriented management philosophies and their apparent influence on the human services (Burford, 1994; Drucker, 1973, 1985; Osborne & Gaebler, 1992; Senge, 1992), introduced to social work through the administrative and management education tracks.

EVIDENTIARY BASIS

Given both the character of the work, which poses inherent challenges to the use of traditional methods of evaluation, and the complexity of efforts that embrace some common philosophical principles, it is unsurprising that few experiments utilizing randomized assignment to control and experimental groups have been carried out on the effectiveness of consumer-centered groups. As is the case in many other areas of social science research involving humans, longitudinal and comparison-group studies are less commonly employed than are exploratory, descriptive, single-group methods, and pre- and postintervention surveys of member satisfaction. From a consumer perspective, it is suggested that one way agencies and professional communities have of maintaining control over the emergence of consumer influence and other innovative approaches, especially ones that would curb or balance the power of entrenched programs and policies, is to require proof of their effectiveness that surpasses standards applied to existing, dedicated services.

Kyrouz and Humphreys (1997) note the important benefits of the effects of self-help/mutual-aid groups evidenced in the literature but point out a lack of clarity that results when researchers include findings from studies in which the group is led by a professional who does not share the problem of the group members. They point also to the lack of rigor of many studies. Their review of the literature included only studies of groups that were organized and/or led by the consumers themselves but that may have used professionals at most in either co-leadership or consultative capacities. They also selected studies that used experimental, comparative, and/or longitudinal designs. They report a variety of positive findings from self-help groups, including those for a variety of mental health concerns, weight loss, addiction recovery, bereavement, diabetes, infant and elderly caregivers, elderly persons, cancer support and survival, and chronic illness (Kyrouz & Humphreys, 1997). Other studies using experimental designs show benefits over treatment alone of integrating mutual-support groups with professional treatment in rehospitalization of discharged psychiatric inpatients (Gordon, Edmunson, Bedell, & Goldstein, 1979), engaging parents with their premature infants (Minde et al., 1980), and stopping smoking (Jason et al., 1987).

Considerable across-study consistency can be seen, however, in qualitative, process-oriented evaluations that focus on consumer satisfaction with a variety of related activities that emphasize consumer involvement, including self-help and mutual aid in a variety of contexts (Wituk et al., 2000). Further evidence is found in evaluations of mental health services (Lefley, 1996; Staples, 1999; Van Tosh & del Vecchio, 2000; Videka-Sherman, 1988), support for crime victims (Herman, 2001; Strang, 2001) and the elderly and disabled (Doty, Benjamin, Matthias, & Franke, 1999; Simon-Rusinowitz, 1999), research on client-run drop-in centers (Jackson, 2001), and corporate accountability (Braithwaite, 2002). These findings are similar to those of other scholars and researchers, who report that people are generally more satisfied with decisions when they feel they have had the opportunity to participate in making them (Boehm & Staples, 2002; Gastil, 1994; Itzhaky & York, 1994, 2000; Zimmerman & Rappaport, 1988).

Although little is written about the negative consequences of participating in consumer-centered groups, relevant concerns have been raised by individuals ranging from those who have had negative experiences in groups (Galinsky & Schopler, 1977, 1994; Plant et al., 1987; Schopler & Galinsky, 1981; Smokowski, Rose, & Bacallao, 2001; Smokowski, Rose, Todar, & Reardon, 1999) to those in groups in which outright exploitation of the aims of the group by professionals is the concern (Frese & Davis, 1997). The potential for harm from too little structure, from pressure to conform, from taking a critical stance, from tensions between self-help and advocacy emphases, and from exploitation would seem to be themes worth attending to in planning for or consulting with groups of consumers. We turn now to examining one consumer-centered group—the family group conference—for which structures have been developed to balance consumer leadership and professional input and in which high satisfaction has been reported by participants and some outcomes have been identified.

EXAMPLE: FAMILY GROUP CONFERENCES AS CONSUMER-LED GROUPS

Family group conferences (FGC) made their first legislated appearance in New Zealand in 1989 with the passage of the Children, Young Persons and Their Families Act (Department of Social Welfare, 1999; Hudson, Morris, Maxwell, & Galaway, 1996). The underlying analysis was consistent with concerns shared by social workers in other parts of the world, that is, that the issues surrounding the care and protection of children are too complex to be the domain of any one social agency or profession. No one is able to "go it alone." The approach has also appealed to advocates of the importance of cultural competence and participation in decision making. By involving extended family members and representatives of the same cultural community in making plans for the child, it is hoped that plans will be longer lasting, thereby providing stability for the children and strengthening vital connections between the members of families and their communities. Spreading rapidly, FGC have been used to involve families in situations of youth and adult offenders, family violence, children's mental health, and school-related issues in several countries (Burford & Hudson, 2000). The approach goes under various names, including "family group decision making" and "community conferencing," and shares much in common with family team meetings and other community- and family-centered approaches to child protection, including family unity meetings, Patch, peacemaking and healing circles, Wraparound, and others (cf. Burford & Hudson, 2000).

As used in child welfare, an FGC is a meeting of family members, along with their relatives, friends, and other close supporters, to make a plan for the care and protection of children seen to be at risk of abuse and neglect. These family and "like family" members form what is called the family group. They are the consumers at the center of the group. An FGC coordinator works with the family and the social worker to organize the conference and to insure that all participants, family and professional, are prepared to take part. These preparations are crucial to the family group who is exerting leadership at the conference and to orienting the professionals regarding their supportive and protective functions during the meeting. In addition to the referring child welfare worker, other service providers and community representatives may be present to give information and describe available resources. The conference has the following phases: an opening fitting the family's culture(s); information sharing about the family's situation and concerns to be addressed in the plan; the family's time, in which they deliberate in private to make a plan; and finalizing a plan that the protective authorities approve. Afterward comes the work of carrying out the plan and revising it as necessary. Establishing and maintaining an FGC program requires close attention to building partnerships among families, community groups, and public agencies. As explicated in this section, the conference is designed so that it advances the five main aims of consumer-centered groups set forth earlier while maintaining the statutory authority of child welfare. The following overview of FGC in child welfare follows the New Zealand model for conferencing and utilizes practice guidance that we developed in conjunction with other practitioners, trainers, and researchers (Burford, Pennell, & MacLeod, 1995; North Carolina Family Group Conferencing Project, 2002; Pennell & Anderson, 2004).

FGC Referrals: The Right to Say to "No" to a Child Welfare Intervention

Although practices vary somewhat, referral of a family for an FGC in a child protection matter is typically initiated by a representative from child welfare services (Lupton &

Nixon, 1999). A referral could be made at any time the social worker or the family wanted to see the family group brought together throughout the involvement of child welfare and at multiple times. Making the referral provides the social worker with an opportunity to communicate respect for the family and to encourage them to exercise influence in the process of group formation and later when they meet. The worker can raise the idea of a referral and tell the family representative enough about the process to stimulate their curiosity. The coordinator is described as an impartial person who will meet with the family and help them put together their conference.

Evidence from FGC implementation studies shows that social workers have been slow at the start to refer families (Marsh & Crow, 1998; Merkel-Holguin, 2000; Pennell & Burford, 1995; Sundell, Vinnerljung, & Ryburn, 2002; Walter McDonald & Associates, 1999). The hesitation is consistent with patterns of referral to psychiatric mutual-aid groups found by others. In summarizing research on the subject, Chinman, Kloos, O'Connell, and Davidson (2002) report that "despite the potential benefits, research has shown consistently that few professionals refer their clients to mutual support groups" (p. 352). Although workers with specific and more advanced training and experience were associated with more favorable attitudes toward mutual support, the researchers found a surprisingly low percentage of professionals who made referrals. They speculated that this situation may reflect the limited knowledge the workers have or attitudes about mutual support as being of little use or damaging. Either way, the researchers suggest that the absence of referrals from professionals supports the idea of "professional-centrism" and may have to do with "professionals underestimating the patient's abilities and willingness to participate in their own treatment" (Chinman et al., 2002, p. 353).

Similar findings are reported with respect to referrals of families for an FGC. In their study examining attitudes toward FGC and actual referrals made by social workers in Sweden and the United Kingdom, Sundell et al. (2002) reported that despite high levels of approval for the model, over half the workers did not refer a family over an 18-month period. They observed that workers who had been involved in local start-up efforts were more likely to refer than were workers who experienced the implementation as a "top-down" importation of the model. They also speculate that social workers may be reluctant to embrace participation in decision making unless they are assured that they will not be singled out for blame if things go wrong (Sundell et al., 2002).

In the child welfare context, the right to say "no" means that workers do not screen out families on the basis of their characteristics but instead screen out referrals on the basis of the families' situation. If the situation is too risky for individual members or if the agency has not yet substantiated child maltreatment, then screening out a referral makes sense. We recommend that vetoing a conference remain the responsibility of the FGC coordinator and the referring worker but that the decision be made in close consultation, particularly with victimized family members. We further recommend that individual family members do not hold the power or responsibility to veto the conference taking place, but are instead offered the opportunity to say "yes" or "no" to their own participation.

Preparation: The Significant Role of the Family Group in Organizing the Conference

There is considerable agreement that good preparation is crucial to having a successful child welfare FGC (Burford & Hudson, 2000). Implementation studies show that preparation typically takes between 20 to 30 hours of the FGC coordinator's time (Marsh & Crow,

1998; Pennell & Anderson, 2004) and that preparation is highly valued by both family members and involved professionals.

The FGC coordinator typically seeks the advice of the referring social worker about whom to contact first and whom not to contact, in the process of making contact with the family. The coordinator describes the conferencing process to the family members and discusses with each person his or her roles and responsibilities. Once set in motion, the process of contacting family members usually mobilizes considerable discussion within families. As the coordinator moves about and explores with parents, older siblings, children, and young people in the immediate family and members of the extended family, such as grandparents, aunts, and uncles, the family group suggests whom they think should be invited and how the meeting might best be organized.

The coordinator consults with the family group, as well as community resources, in making arrangements for the conference, with account being paid to issues of safety, privacy, comfort, accessibility, and cultural significance. Attention is given to where the family group wants the conference located, how it should be opened, what food to serve, and which roles various family members might play. In working to insure that the meeting is inclusive, the coordinator often is called on to bring messages from family members who cannot attend. If family members feel at risk during the conference, it is wise to help them select a support person to stay with them during the meeting. This is particularly crucial for abused young people and mothers, but it also serves as a mechanism for keeping perpetrators under control during the proceedings.

Preparation is not just for the family members. The coordinator works to help the service providers, especially those who have never attended a family group conference, prepare themselves to best support the family's decision making without compromising the seriousness of the matters about which they will speak. For professionals, typical concerns that surface during this stage include giving information that may jeopardize confidentiality, safety, or future investigations and possible prosecutions. They often need assistance on how to give information in a way that is respectful and clear and that encourages the family group to address the issues of concern.

Thus, throughout the preparation process, the coordinator plays the role of the broker who is organizing a conference for the family but who is also sensitive to family dynamics and the issues surrounding abuse in families. The question of how best to organize the meeting in such a way that family members will feel safe in coming together and speaking their minds freely while at the same time having sufficient influence over the process to feel as if they "own" the meeting is explored with everyone. The preparation process is seen as an opportunity to invite the family members to take up roles as experts on their family, including the various cultures represented.

The Conference and Follow-Through: Setting the Goals, Determining the Solutions, and Implementing and Refining the Plan of Action

Arrivals and Opening the Conference

In many instances, the family members may not have seen each other for a long time, if ever, and people typically experience a great deal of emotion in simply seeing for themselves who has come and who has not. They also are affected by the rituals associated with gathering together at the meeting place and ultimately arranging themselves physically in the seating circle. Especially when the group meeting is being held in some neutral space, where the family can move about in their own way and be catered to—as opposed to being controlled by the necessity for professionals to admit them through locked doors and so forth—the rituals of arrival and settling into the space are considered unique in the opportunities they present to dignify the meeting and imbue the event with significance. Some families also request a particular way of opening the conference. This might be a welcome by a senior family member, a prayer by a pastor, or simply passing around the children's photographs (Pennell & Anderson, 2004). By this means, the family group affirms its common heritage and connections.

The coordinator or the person chosen for the task clearly restates the purpose of the meeting (e.g., "we are all here for the same reason; that is to come up with a plan for keeping the children safe") and invites everyone to introduce themselves and say who they are in relation to the abused person(s) (e.g., "I'm Jane. Auntie to Sarah and Max and sister of their mom, Leona"). The coordinator also reviews the process for the day and, with the group, establishes guidelines for working together. By the time the conference coordinator or other designated person calls the meeting to begin, the family members and attending professionals have already had what is for most a new experience with one another that is typically emotionally laden with heightened expectations.

Giving Information (Not Solutions)

This stage has two parts. During the first, the coordinator invites the mandated authorities who have been involved with the family (e.g., child protection worker, police, correctional worker) to tell the group what has prompted their referral and what has been happening as far as the official record of abuse or neglect is concerned. The object of this stage is to make sure that the family members all have the same information and that they know what has happened to the person who has been abused or neglected. The effect of the family members hearing this together in the face-to-face group meeting deepens the feelings among group members and increases sympathy in the group for the abused person's experience. It is important that this information be available to family members in the language they speak, either by conducting the entire meeting in that language or by having interpretation available throughout any part of the meeting when any of the family members want it. The role of the professionals at this stage is to share the information respectfully and clearly, without resorting to professional jargon or introducing written materials that require detailed reading. The object is to address the family group members in such a way as to maximize the possibility that they will hear the professionals' presentations as a legitimate invitation to engage them in partnership.

Second, once the mandated authorities have completed their sharing of information and the family has had adequate opportunity to ask questions or react to the information, the meeting turns to presentations by invited guests, who give the family group information relevant to their relatives' situation and outline local resources that might be useful to include in their plan. During the preparations, the guests for a particular conference are identified in discussion between the coordinator and the family members after it is determined what might be most helpful. Examples of such guests are substance abuse counselors, domestic violence advocates, and tribal elders.

All of the information providers need to be clear, respectful, and succinct in their presentations to the family. Prolonging this stage of the group meeting or talking to the family pedantically can have the same effect it does on other groups placed in that position: It undermines the participants' beliefs that they are being seriously engaged for their knowledge and skills and reproduces the hierarchies that have contributed to a lack of success already. This part of the meeting presents, by its very organization, the opportunity for alliances of emotion and sympathy between family members and between family members and professionals. In particular, sympathy for the perspective of the abused person is typically increased, if it was not universally shared in the group beforehand. At this stage coordinators often arrange for letters from family members who could not be present to be read aloud.

Private Deliberations

The transition in the group from information giving to the family's private time is again marked by ritual, in this case the movement of the FGC coordinator, professionals, and other nonfamily members out of the immediate meeting room. The family group is on its own to consider what they have heard and to devise a plan or, more accurately, a recommended plan of action addressing the identified concerns. As a further demarcation, the family group often partakes of food together prior to beginning their more formal deliberations. Each family group has its own style of planning, in keeping with their ways of relating and the issues at hand. Some may actively confront relatives for their irresponsible behaviors; others may vent about "those social workers"; and others may jump right into writing down plans. During this stage it is not uncommon for a natural leader to emerge within the group. This individual may take charge by leading the discussion, making a flipchart of the plan, or lending support to family members.

The FGC coordinator remains close at hand and can be called back into the meeting to explain how the process works or to help to comfort a distressed family member. We encourage the child welfare worker to stay on site during the family's private deliberation time or, at a minimum, to stay in touch with the coordinator. Just being there sends an important message of support. The family may have some questions about the information that was presented or may want to clarify something.

Finalizing the Plan

Once the family group has drafted its plan, a member goes out to invite the professionals and other guests back to the group space to present their plan. It is most often the child welfare worker who is called on to approve the plan or negotiate parts of it and to supply resource support for certain things that may be needed for approved plans. The approval of the plan as an acceptable strategy for keeping the children safe needs to be separated from the issue of resources. At this time, the FGC coordinator plays an active role in insuring that the family group has the opportunity to outline its plan. The service providers can ask questions about specific items, the items are mapped out in a way that clearly establishes what is to be done and by whom, and a process for follow-through on plans is included. The latter involves specifying who is responsible for monitoring implementation and when and how the group will review progress and revamp the plan as necessary. Although the child welfare agency remains ultimately responsible for overseeing developments, it helps to have a monitor designated from within the family group to keep everyone working together. The research shows that most family groups come up with a plan, and usually the child welfare worker authorizes the plan (Marsh & Crow, 1998; Paterson & Harvey, 1991). The plans typically include tasks to be carried out by the family group, by community resources, and by the child welfare agency and incorporate both professional services and culturally relevant supports, such as from churches or tribal groups (Pennell & Burford, 1995; Shore,

Wirth, Cahn, Yancey, & Gunderson, 2002). The FGC coordinator should make sure that all participants receive a copy of the final plan (in their own language) to aid their taking part in its delivery.

Follow-Through

Plans are not usually carried out in their entirety (Lupton & Nixon, 1999). As long as the key items are, though, the family group is satisfied with the results (Burford & Pennell, 1998). Carrying out plans depends on whether all parties make their contribution, whether the agency holds to the agreement in the plan, and whether the family's situation remains sufficiently stable for the plan to continue to make sense. Given the very large difficulties faced by families referred to an FGC, it is not surprising that their lives do not hold still. What is important is to draw on the relationships cultivated during the course of the FGC to rework plans in a responsive and collaborative manner. For major changes, the coordinator should reconvene the family group; for lesser changes, the child welfare worker can call a family meeting to work out issues. In this way, the partnerships are respected and sustained during the follow-up period, and child welfare workers can integrate working with the family group into their general practice.

Governance and Funding Structures: Balancing Autonomy with Sustaining Partnership

Detailed guidelines for the development of community-based FGC projects have been developed (Burford, 2000; Burford et al., 1995; Pennell & Burford, 1995; Pennell & Weil, 2000), as have detailed descriptions of the issues that come up (Burford, 2000) and guiding principles for linking the use of conferencing to local governance. Two of those principles bear noting in this discussion of FGC as a consumer-led group.

First, it is understood to be essential for the FGC coordinator to be seen by the families as having a certain amount of independence from the social worker and other mandated authorities such as the police (Nixon, 2000). Second, the consumer-led philosophy will be well served in practice if the coordinator has a community-based advisory group who can provide consultation at any time of the conferencing process, but particularly during the referral and conference preparation stages. This is in line with other approaches to community-centered child and family practice (Aldridge, 2002; Center for the Study of Social Policy, 2001a; Dominelli, 1999; Kemp, Whittaker, & Tracy, 1997; Waldfogel, 1998).

Outcomes: Competencies for Wider Civic Engagement

The hope is that participation in consumer-led groups such as FGC will make possible the engagement of often marginalized populations in wider civic concerns, going beyond meeting the immediate needs of members. As noted earlier, this is the same outcome sought by one of the earliest models of social work with groups—the social-goals model—which aspires to hone a sense of social responsibility among the group membership (Papell & Rothman, 1966). Although FGC can be seen as in line with other models, such as self-help and mutual-aid groups, it is useful to view it in terms of the social-goals model in order to conceptualize its greater impact (Macgowan & Pennell, 2001).

Civic engagement is predicated on men and women participating as full citizens in their communities (Pennell, in press). For women to reach beyond their immediate involvements with family and paid work, domestic labor needs to be shared among men and women. The child welfare system, however, typically focuses on the deficiencies of mothers, with limited attention given to the "absent father." FGC goes against this pattern by including multiple generations and both genders and producing plans that go beyond the mother's responsibilities to those of the family group, community, and agency.

For children to grow into full participants, they require the nurturing, opportunities, limits, and respect for their heritage that help them grow. Observing the senior members of their family group engaging in planning on their behalf and seeing their elders' efforts taken seriously by the authorities go a long way to renewing the child or young person's sense of belonging to a worthwhile kinship network. As reported by both young and adult family members, one of the most beneficial outcomes of conferencing is its reknitting their connections and giving them a greater sense of pride in where they came from (Burford & Pennell, 1998). This outcome leads to an easing of conflicts between the professionals and the family, who are better enabled to work together.

Outcome studies have found that FGC leads to:

- Keeping children with their families or relatives (Burford & Pennell, 1998; Cashmore & Kiely, 2000; Crampton, 2001; Lupton & Stevens, 1998; Meredith, Mandell, & Sullivan, 2001; Robinson, Litchfield, Gatowski, & Dobbin, 2002; Shore et al., 2002; Sundell, 2000; Thoennes, 2003).
- Placing siblings together (Walter R. McDonald & Associates, 2000).
- Enhancing the stability of child placements (Marsh & Crow, 1998; Robinson et al., 2002; Shore et al., 2002; Walter R. McDonald & Associates, 2000).

There is also evidence that FGC promotes children's safety (Marsh & Crow, 1998; Quinnett, Harrison, & Jones, 2003; Shore et al., 2002; Thoennes, 2003) and that of their mothers (Pennell & Burford, 2000). All of this is crucial to advancing the well-being and sense of efficacy of developing children and teens and improving family stability and the health of communities.

FUTURE PROSPECTS

The prospects for the use of FGC in child protection cases are much the same as for other groups that emphasize empowerment and advocate self-determination for the clientele. Concerns include how to operationalize the concepts of empowerment, strengths, and group development at the community level (Staudt, Howard, & Drake, 2001). We need to develop good theory that goes back to the question of why people come together in the first place. Although there are promising research directions and some findings (Itzhaky & York, 2000; Speer, 2000; Zimmerman & Rappaport, 1988), being empowered to act does not necessarily lead to a positive change in behavior.

Perhaps most concerning is the challenge to social work to reconcile its own ambivalence about the use of groups and empowerment. Many social workers trained to be sensitive to issues of rights, social justice, strengths, and self-determination do not take the necessary steps to support their clients when it comes to empowerment. This challenge can be met in part by exploring ways to involve people who have had experience as consumers in family group conferences. The impact of mobilizing formal and informal social networks with this group approach is considerable; some even think of the group conference as an intervention into the system of services. It will surely involve, as Fisher (1991) points out, educating professionals in constructing new roles for social workers in which recursive practices allow for the inclusion of the voices of the consumers and taking responsibility within such a context. Stevenson, Wise, and Clark (as cited in Healy, 2000) point out that social workers must "situate their theorizing within the unavoidable obligation faced by statutory workers to use legal force if necessary to ensure minimum standards of well-being for the most vulnerable members" (Healy, 2000, p. 75).

Whether the consumer movement will or will not be well served by the extension of the philosophy and orientation to groups that bring members of the formal and informal systems into contact in the way that FGCs do remains to be seen. It depends in large measure on the extent to which balance can be maintained between the responsibilities of the state to protect and support families and the autonomy and privacy rights of the families. As Ruth Winchester (2001) points out about practice in the United Kingdom, "diluting the process to make it acceptable to the majority risks devaluing it altogether. Ultimately, the way FGCs are developed . . . will put our commitment to consumer-centeredness to the test" (p. 3).

REFERENCES

Adams, P., & Nelson, K. (1995). Introduction. In P. Adams & K. Nelson (Eds.), *Reinventing human services: Community- and family-centered practice* (pp. 1–14). Hawthorne, NY: Aldine de Gruyter.

Aldridge, M. J. (2002). Lessons learned from building collaborations. *Protecting Children, 17*(2), 2–11.

Boehm, A., & Staples, L. H. (2002). The functions of the social worker in empowering: The voices of consumers and professionals. *Social Work, 47*(4), 449–460.

Bowers, B., & Saucier, P. (1999, November). Guidelines for consumer centered integrated care systems serving dually eligible beneficiaries and other adults with special healthcare needs [Working draft]. Retrieved from the New England States Consortium website: *http://www.ahcpr.gov/news/ulp/ulpchrn2.htm*

Braithwaite, J. (2002). *Restorative justice and responsive regulation.* New York: Oxford University Press.

Burford, G. (1994). Getting serious about humanism in administration: The real unsolved mystery. *Journal of Child and Youth Care, 9*(3), v–viii. Retrieved from: *http://www.cyc-net.org/Journals/jcyc9-3.html*

Burford, G. (2000). Advancing innovations: Family group decision making as community-centered child and family work. *Protecting Children, 16*(1), 4–20.

Burford, G., & Hudson, J. (2000). *Family group conferencing: New direction in community-centered child and family practice.* Hawthorne, NY: Aldine de Gruyter.

Burford, G., & Pennell, J. (1998). *Family group decision making: After the conference—Progress in resolving violence and promoting well-being: Outcome report* (Vols. 1–2). St. John's: Memorial University of Newfoundland School of Social Work.

Burford, G., Pennell, J., & MacLeod, S. (1995). *Family group decision making: Manual for coordinators and communities.* St. John's, Memorial University of Newfoundland, School of Social Work, Family Group Decision Making Project. Retrieved from: *http://social.chass.ncsu.edu/jpennell/fgdm/Manual/index.htm.*

Cashmore, J., & Kiely, P. (2000). Implementing and evaluating family group conferences. In G. Burford & J. Hudson (Eds.), *Family group conferencing: New directions in community-centered child and family practice* (pp. 242–252). Hawthorne, NY: Aldine de Gruyter.

Center for the Study of Social Policy. (2001a). *Building capacity for local decision making: A series of learning guides* (Nos. 1–6). Retrieved from: *www.cssp.org.*

Center for the Study of Social Policy. (2001b). *Community partnerships for protecting children.* Washington, DC: Clearinghouse on Community Based Approaches to Child Protection. Retrieved from: *www.cssp.org*.

Chinman, M., Kloos, B., O'Connell, M., & Davidson, L. (2002). Service providers' views of psychiatric mutual support groups. *Journal of Community Psychology, 30*(4), 349–366.

Cohen, J. L. (2001). Civil society. In P. B. Clarke & J. Foweraker (Eds.), *Encyclopedia of democratic thought* (pp. 67–71). London and New York: Routledge.

Crampton, D. S. (2001). *Making sense of foster care: An evaluation of family group decision making in Kent County, Michigan*. Unpublished doctoral dissertation, University of Michigan, Ann Arbor.

Crawford, A. (1997). *The local governance of crime: Appeals to community and partnerships*. Oxford, UK: Clarendon Press.

Day, P. (2002). *A new history of social welfare* (3rd ed.). Boston: Allyn & Bacon.

Department of Social Welfare. (1999). *Children, young persons and their families act 1989 (amended 1994): Information pack for NZCYPS staff*. Wellington, New Zealand: Author.

Dominelli, L. (Ed.). (1999). *Community approaches to child welfare: International perspectives*. Brookfield, VT: Ashgate.

Doty, P., Benjamin, A. E., Matthias, R. E., & Franke, T. M. (1999, April). *In-home supportive services for the elderly and disabled: A comparison of client-directed and professional management models of service delivery*. Washington, DC: U.S. Department of Health and Human Services and the University of California, Los Angeles.

Drucker, P. (1973). *Management: Tasks, responsibilities, practices*. New York: Harper & Row.

Drucker, P. (1985). *Innovation and entrepreneurship: Practice and principles*. New York: Harper & Row.

Fisher, D. D. V. (1991). *An introduction to constructivism for social workers*. New York: Praeger.

Frese, F. J., & Davis, W. W. (1997). The consumer-survivor movement, recovery, and consumer professionals. *Professional Psychology: Research and Practice, 28*(3), 243–245.

Galinsky, M., & Schopler, J. H. (1994). Negative experiences in support groups. *Social Work in Health Care, 20*(1), 77–95.

Galinsky, M., & Schopler, J. K. (1977). Warning: Groups may be dangerous for your health. *Social Work, 22*, 89–93.

Gastil, J. (1994). A meta-analytic review of the productivity and satisfaction of democratic and autocratic leadership. *Small Group Research, 25*(3), 384–410.

Gordon, R. E., Edmunson, E., Bedell, J., & Goldstein, N. (1979). Reducing rehospitalization of state mental patients: Peer management and support. *Journal of the Florida Medical Association, 66*, 927–933.

Gutiérrez, L. M., & Lewis, E. A. (1999). *Empowering women of color*. New York: Columbia University Press.

Gutiérrez, L. M., Parsons, R. J., & Cox, E. O. (1998). *Empowerment in social work practice: A sourcebook*. New York: Brooks/Cole.

Hardina, D. (2002). *Analytical skills for community organization practice*. New York: Columbia University Press.

Healy, K. (2000). *Social work practices: Contemporary perspectives on change*. Thousand Oaks, CA: Sage.

Herman, S. (2001). A role for victims in offender reentry. *Crime and Delinquency, 47*(3), 428–445.

Hoehne, D. (1988). Self-help and social change. In F. Cunningham, S. Findlay, M. Kadar, A. Lennon, & E. Silva (Eds.), *Social movements/social change: The politics and practice of organizing* (pp. 236–251). Toronto, Ontario, Canada: Between the Lines.

Homan, M. S. (1999). *Promoting community change: Making it happen in the real world* (2nd ed.). Pacific Grove, CA: Brooks/Cole.

Hudson, J., Morris, A., Maxwell, G., & Galaway, B. (Eds.). (1996). *Family group conferences: Perspectives on policy and practice*. Annandale, New South Wales, Australia: Federation Press.

Itzhaky, H., & York, A. S. (1994). Different types of client participation and the effects on community-social work intervention. *Journal of Social Service Research, 19*(1/2), 85–98.

Itzhaky, H., & York, A. S. (2000). Sociopolitical control and empowerment: An extended replication. *Journal of Community Psychology, 28*(4), 407–415.

Jackson, R. L. (2001). *The clubhouse model: Empowering applications of theory to generalist practice.* Stamford, CT: Brooks/Cole.

Jason, L. A., Gruder, C. L., Martino, S., Flay, B. R., Warnecke, R., & Thomas, N. (1987). Work site group meetings and the effectiveness of a televised smoking cessation intervention. *American Journal of Community Psychology, 15*, 57–72.

Kemp, S., Whittaker, J., & Tracy, E. (1997). *Person–environment practice: The social ecology of interpersonal helping.* Hawthorne, NY: Aldine de Gruyter.

Kessler-Harris, A. (2001). *In pursuit of equity: Women, men, and the quest for economic citizenship in 20th-century America.* New York: Oxford University Press.

Korten, D. (2001). *When corporations rule the world* (2nd ed.). Bloomfield, CT: Kumarian Press.

Kyrouz, E., & Humphreys, K. (1997). A review of research on the effectiveness of self-help mutual aid groups. *International Journal of Psychosocial Rehabilitation, 2*, 64–68.

Lefley, H. P. (1996). Impact of consumer and family advocacy movements on mental health services. In B. Levin & J. Petrila (Eds.), *Mental health services: A public health perspective* (pp. 81–96). New York: Oxford University Press.

Lerner, G. (2002). *Fireweed: A political autobiography.* Philadelphia: Temple University Press.

Litchfield, M. M., Gatkowski, S. I., & Dobbin, S. A. (2003). Improving outcomes for families: Results from an evaluation of Miami's family decision making program. *Protecting Children, 18*(1–2), 48–51.

Lupton, C., & Nixon, P. (1999). *Empowering practice? A critical appraisal of the family group conference approach.* Bristol, UK: Policy Press.

Lupton, C., & Stevens, M. (1998). Planning in partnership? An assessment of process and outcome in UK family group conferences. *International Journal of Child and Family Welfare, 2*, 135–148.

Macgowan, M., & Pennell, J. (2001). Building social responsibility through family group conferencing. *Social Work with Groups, 24*(3/4), 67–87.

Marsh, P., & Crow, G. (1998). *Family group conferences in child welfare.* Oxford, UK: Blackwell Science.

McFarlane, W. R. (2002). *Multifamily groups in the treatment of severe psychiatric disorders.* New York: Guilford Press.

Meredith, G., Mandell, D., & Sullivan, N. (2001, December). *Final evaluation report: Toronto family group conferencing project.* Etobicoke, Ontario, Canada: George Hull Center.

Merkel-Holguin, L. (2000). Diversions and departures in the implementation of family group conferencing in the United States. In G. Burford & J. Hudson (Eds.), *Family group conferencing: New directions in community-centered child and family practice* (pp. 224–231). Hawthorne, NY: Aldine de Gruyter.

Midgley, J. (1997). *Social welfare in a global context.* Thousand Oaks, CA: Sage.

Minde, K., Shosenberg, N., Marton, P., Thompson, J., Ripley, J., & Burns S. (1980). Self-help groups in a premature nursery: A controlled evaluation. *Journal of Pediatrics, 96*, 933–940.

Nader, R. (with Carper, J.) (Eds.). (1973). *The consumer and corporate accountability.* New York: Harcourt Brace Jovanovich.

Nixon, P. (2000). How can family group conferences become family-driven? Some dilemmas and possibilities. *Protecting Children, 16*(3), 22–33.

North Carolina Family Group Conferencing Project. (2002). *Family group conferencing in child welfare: Practice guidance for planning, implementing, training, and evaluation.* Retrieved from North Carolina State University, Social Work Program website: *http://social.chass.ncsu.edu/ jpennell/ncfgcp/pracguid.*

Osborne, D., & Gaebler, T. (1992). *Reinventing government: How the entrepreneurial spirit is transforming the public sector.* New York: Plume.

Papell, C. P., & Rothman, B. (1966). Social group work models: Possession and heritage. *Journal of Education for Social Work, 2*(2), 66–77.

Paterson, K., & Harvey, M. (1991). *An evaluation of the organisation and operation of care and protection family group conferences.* Wellington, New Zealand: Department of Social Welfare.

Pennell, J. (in press). Restorative practices: Toward family welfare in an inclusive society. *Journal of Social Issues.*

Pennell, J., & Anderson, G. (2004). *Widening the circle: The practice and evaluation of family group conferencing with children, young persons, and their families.* Washington, DC: NASW Press.

Pennell, J., & Burford, G. (1995). *Family group decision making: New roles for "old" partners in resolving family violence: Implementation report* (Vols. 1–2). St. John's: Memorial University of Newfoundland School of Social Work.

Pennell, J., & Burford, G. (2000). Family group decision making: Protecting children and women. *Child Welfare, 79*(2), 131–158.

Pennell, J., & Weil, M. (2000). Initiating conferencing: Community practice issues. In G. Burford & J. Hudson (Eds.), *Family group conferencing: New directions in community-centered child and family practice* (pp. 253–261). Hawthorne, NY: Aldine de Gruyter.

Plant, H., Richardson, J., Stubbs, D., Lynch, D., Ellwood, J., Slevin, M., & de Haes, H. (1987). Evaluation of a support group of cancer patients and their families and friends. *British Journal of Hospital Medicine, 37,* 317–322.

Quinnett, E., Harrison, R. S., & Jones, L. (2003). Empirical research on the San Diego model of family unity meetings. *Protecting Children, 18*(1–2), 98–103.

Robinson, S., Litchfield, M., Gatowski, S., & Dobbin, S. (2002). Family conferencing: A success for our children. *Juvenile and Family Court Journal, 53*(4), 43–48.

Schopler, J., & Galinsky, M. (1981). When groups go wrong. *Social Work, 26,* 424–429.

Schorr, L. (1997). *Common purpose: Strengthening families and neighborhoods to rebuild America.* New York: Anchor.

Senge, P. (1992). *The fifth discipline: The art and practice of the learning organization.* New York: Random House.

Shore, N., Wirth, J., Cahn, K., Yancey, B., & Gunderson, K. (2002, September). Long-term and immediate outcomes of family group conferencing in Washington state. Retrieved from International Institute for Restorative Practices website: *www.restorativepractices.org.*

Simon, B. L. (1994). *The empowerment tradition in American social work: A history.* New York: Columbia University Press.

Simon-Rusinowitz, L. (1999, October). *History, principles, and definition of consumer direction: Views from the aging community.* College Park: University of Maryland Center on Aging.

Smokowski, P. R., Rose, S., Todar, K., & Reardon, K. (1999). Postgroup-casualty status, group events, and leader behavior: An early look into the dynamics of damaging group experiences. *Research on Social Work Practice, 9*(5), 555–574.

Smokowski, P. R., Rose, S. D., & Bacallao, M. L. (2001). Damaging experiences in therapeutic groups: How vulnerable consumers become group casualties. *Small Group Research, 32*(2), 223–251.

Speer, P. W. (2000). Intrapersonal and interactional empowerment: Implications for theory. *Journal of Community Psychology, 28*(1), 51–61.

Staples, L. H. (1999). Consumer empowerment in a mental health system: Stakeholder roles and responsibilities. In W. Shera & L. M. Wells (Eds.), *Empowerment practice in social work: Developing richer conceptual foundations* (pp. 119–141). Toronto, Ontario, Canada: Canadian Scholars' Press.

Staudt, M., Howard, M. O., & Drake, B. (2001). The operationalization, implementation, and effectiveness of the strengths perspective: A review of empirical studies. *Journal of Social Service Research, 27*(3), 1–21.

Strang, H. (2001). The crime victim movement as a force in civil society. In H. Strang & J. Braithwaite (Eds.), *Restorative justice and civil society* (pp. 69–82). New York: Cambridge University Press.

Sundell, K. (2000). Family group conferences in Sweden. In G. Burford & J. Hudson (Eds.), *Family group conferencing: New directions in community centered child and family practice* (pp. 198–205). Hawthorne, NY: Aldine de Gruyter.

Sundell, K., Vinnerljung, B., & Ryburn, M. (2002). Social workers' attitudes towards family group conferences in Sweden and the United Kingdom. *International Journal of Child and Family Welfare*, *5*(1–2), 28–39.

Thoennes, N. (2003). Family group decision making in Colorado. *Protecting Children*, *18*(1–2), 74–80.

Tower, K. D. (1994). Consumer-centered social work practice: Restoring client self-determination. *Social Work*, *39*(2), 191–196.

Unzicker, R. E. (1999, October). *History, principles, and definitions of consumer direction and self-determination*. Paper presented at the National Leadership Summit on Self-Determination and Consumer Direction and Control. Retrieved from: *http://www.ohsu.edu/selfdetermination/unzicker.shtml*.

Van Tosh, L., & del Vecchio, P. (2000). Consumer-operated self-help programs: A technical report. Rockville, MD: Center for Mental Health Services. Retrieved from *http://www.mentalhealth.org*.

Videka-Sherman, L. (1988). Meta-analysis of research on social work practice in mental health. *Social Work*, *33*, 325–338.

Waldegrave, C. (2000). "Just Therapy" with families and communities. In G. Burford & J. Hudson (Eds.), *Family group conferencing: New directions in community-centered child and family practice* (pp. 153–163). Hawthorne, NY: Aldine de Gruyter.

Waldfogel, J. (1998). *The future of child protection: How to break the cycle of abuse and neglect*. Cambridge, MA: Harvard University Press.

Walter R. McDonald & Associates. (1999). *The Santa Clara County family conference model: Strategy for system change*. Sacramento, CA: Author.

Walter R. McDonald & Associates. (2000). *The Santa Clara County family conference model year one process evaluation report*. Sacramento, CA: Author.

Wenocur, S., & Reisch, M. (2002). *From charity to enterprise: The development of American social work in a market economy*. Champaign, IL: University of Illinois Press.

Winchester, R. (2001, April 6). *Keeping it in the family*. Retrieved from *www.communitycare.co.uk*.

Wituk, S., Shepherd, M., Slavich, S., Warren, M., & Meissen, G. (2000). A topography of self-help groups: An empirical analysis. *Social Work*, *45*(2), 157–165.

Zimmerman, M. A., & Rappaport, J. (1988). Citizen participation, perceived control, and psychological empowerment. *American Journal of Community Psychology*, *16*(5), 725–750.

Part VI

Group Work Research and Evaluation

$\mathbf{A}$s we have stressed in the introduction to this book, we believe that progress in group work practice and theory requires a partnership between researchers and practitioners. For this reason, we have devoted this section to research on group work practice. The authors of these chapters recognize that research and evaluation in group work is a challenging task for many reasons. A critical issue pertains to the many systems levels involved in group work: the individual member, the practitioner, the subgroups within the group, the group as an entity, the organizational sponsor of the group, and the community and other environmental systems with which the group and its members interact. Depending on the research or evaluation question, any or all of these systems must be considered, and a research design strategy must be developed to accommodate the participation of actors in these systems. Another challenge is to devise an approach to measurement that will be feasible for respondents and that presents a valid answer to the research or evaluation questions. Chapter 25 is devoted to design; Chapter 26 to measurement, both quantitative and qualitative; and Chapter 27 to evaluation.

Chapter 25

Very Good Solutions Really Do Exist for Group Work Research Design Problems

AARON M. BROWER
ROBIN G. ARNDT
ANNEMARIE KETTERHAGEN

Conducting research on social work groups is difficult. As researchers and scholars, we must contend with design problems inherent in all small group research (such as how to handle individual- vs. group-level data) *and* the problems inherent to treatment research (such as ethical problems related to randomly assigning participants to experimental vs. control conditions). Several articles have been written over the past 10 years identifying the research design problems inherent to group work and small groups in general; we decided to use this chapter to examine how researchers have recently dealt with these problems.

We reviewed the past 5 years' worth of articles in the leading journals on social group work and small group research, and our main finding was that group work researchers have not changed their methods to address design problems and limitations, despite statistical and methodological advances available. And it was not only social workers who have not changed their research practices; we found little evidence that researchers in any field have changed how they conduct their research to better address the design and methods problems inherent to small-group research.

Thus, with the hope that this chapter can make the promising advances in group work research methods even more accessible to researchers, we present here exemplars of how group work design problems have been addressed. For this chapter, we considered "design problems" to be those due either to decisions made in the research design or in the research methods: Design problems, per se, are those that arise from the design of the research—

those, for example, that are due to the way hypotheses are specified, how samples are selected, how variables are defined, or how behavior is captured. Methods problems are those that arise from the methods used to construct the research design or that arise from the methods used to analyze data gathered. It is our sincere hope that a review of the small-group and group work research literature 5 years from now will show great changes in how group work researchers address their research design and method problems.

THE FUNDAMENTAL GROUP WORK RESEARCH PROBLEM

The fundamental problem in doing small-group research of any kind lies in trying to capture the essential "groupness" of groups—in trying to capture their complex dynamics and their somewhat unpredictable evolution. Furthermore, social group work researchers study small group dynamics not for their own sake but to harness these dynamics to affect change at a number of system levels (Toseland & Rivas, 1998).

But how do we capture a group's complexity and unpredictability using methods that require us either to take snapshots of an ongoing process or to focus our attention on some aspects of the group and not others? How do we study cohesion, for example, without examining this one process within the context of membership or group goals or any number of structural elements of the group (setting, time, etc.)? How do we examine individual outcomes, for example, without examining any number of interpersonal and group-level dynamics that contribute directly and indirectly to these outcomes? How do we even examine something like the interaction of member gender and leadership, for instance, knowing that this interaction itself is dependent on any number of other factors (such as structure, development, group purpose, and even current political and social climate)?

Capturing and harnessing the essential "groupness" of groups is one issue taken up by several of the chapters in this volume. And although the groupness of groups makes them special and wonderful to work with—and makes their format uniquely suited to many aspects of social and individual change—it also presents itself as a true paradox for researchers, because any attempt at study by reducing or dissecting group dynamics also fundamentally changes them. This is the fundamental problem of doing group work research: Studying a group changes the object of our study.

Some argue that the essential groupness of groups is literally impossible to capture using quantitative methods from a logical positivist perspective. Groups are "living" systems that change over time; group members do not interact in predetermined ways. As Frey (1994) argued recently, and as Papell and Rothman stated almost 40 years ago (Papell & Rothman, 1966), group researchers need to use more naturalistic paradigms to study groups because these paradigms more easily match the processes of interest in small groups. These writers argue that accurate descriptions of group processes or specific variables will never result from approaches that hold certain variables or aspects of the group constant in order to study one or two other variables. Instead, these writers argue, qualitative and naturalistic approaches should be used to study groups.

Our position is that although there may be some truth to this assertion, it is not true that quantitative methods can tell us nothing about groups. Quantitative and qualitative approaches each have their advantages and disadvantages, their strengths and their limitations. No one method can be applied without problems because inherent design and methods problems exist regardless of how small groups are studied—which brings us back to the purpose of this chapter. Selecting a research design and method, we believe, should be driven more by what one wants to know rather than by ideology. And above all, we are certain to learn nothing if we apply quantitative or qualitative methods poorly, and if we do not acknowledge and try to address the inherent problems that each method contains.

READING THE PAST FIVE YEARS OF GROUP WORK RESEARCH

Our objective for this chapter is to catalogue what is new and interesting about how researchers address methodological and design problems when studying group work. We did not intend to comprehensively examine the research results and new knowledge development within small groups as such. We refer readers to several excellent small-group review articles for that information (Ettin, 2000; Levine & Moreland, 1990). In addition, we did not intend for our review to uncover new methodological problems facing small-groups researchers—most of the methodological and design problems have been amply catalogued elsewhere (for example, see Brower & Garvin, 1989; Forsyth, 1998; Keyton, 1994). We did hope to find articles that described how researchers dealt with design problems, and we planned to report them to provide a guide for future research.

Because we wished to comprehensively review how small group and group work researchers addressed design and methods problems, we chose to review those journals that either focused on small-group research or on social group work. We reviewed all articles from 1996–2001 in the journals *Social Work with Groups*, *Small Group Research*, *Group Dynamics*, and the "Interpersonal Relations and Group Processes" section of *Journal of Personality and Social Psychology*. These journals were selected because the majority of their published articles deal with small group research or social group work and also because their intended audience is researchers of and practitioners in small groups. Reviewing the social psychology journals took us beyond social work's typical small-group journals, but these were selected because they form the literature base for many social group workers.

Several other journals were considered but ultimately rejected. Some were no longer in print (such as *Human Relations*), some did not primarily publish research and also did not focus on social group work (such as *Group* and *Group Processes and Intergroup Relations*), and some published very little research that was related to small groups (such as *Research on Social Work Practice*, *Social Work Research*, or *Group and Organizational Management*).

In our review of the four journals we selected, we were primarily interested in how the researchers (1) handled the problems inherent to small-group research, (2) discussed the design choices they made, and (3) discussed the limitations encountered. Our training for reading and capturing these dimensions in the research included several steps: First, we all read a set of three articles to calibrate our judgments and systematize the notes taken on each article. Coding consisted of taking notes, in two or three sentences, about each of the three dimensions of interest. Second, we each read independently three new articles and then afterward discussed them together to find areas of similarity and discrepancy in our judgments. We repeated this step until we agreed 90% of the time on our judgments about the articles. The remaining articles were divided between two of us (R. A. and A. K.). Finally, about halfway through the reading of the articles, we again read one article together to assess "coder shift." Agreement was found to remain at better than a 90% level.

One encouraging initial finding to report is that a lot of small-group research took place during the past 5 years. That is very good news: The fields of small-group research and social group work research appear to be thriving. A total of 326 articles were reviewed for this chapter. The increase in the number of articles we found that focused on small-group research concurs with Hoyle, Georgesen, and Webster (2001), and with Feldman (1987) before them, who found continual increases in the number of group research articles published over the past several decades. And not only has the total number of articles researching small groups increased, but we also noticed the same trend found by Garvin (2001) and Hoyle et al. (2001), who have observed an increase in research being done on "true" group processes and variables (those that exist because of the group environment, such as cohesion, development, leadership, and followership) rather than on processes or variables that just happen to take place in groups (such as task completion studies or those that evaluate individual outcomes in structured treatment programs that do not take advantage of the group environment).

CATEGORIES OF DESIGN PROBLEMS

As was stated in the beginning of this chapter, group work researchers must address problems from two fronts: They must contend with design challenges inherent to small-group research and with those inherent to treatment research. Some of the challenges for small-group research are how to handle power problems when doing group-level analyses; alternatively, how to handle individual-level data within the group setting; how to keep track of the different ways participants react to the same set of group conditions; and how to isolate variables of interest when each group changes or develops along its own specific path. Challenges for treatment research include ethical problems caused by withholding treatment from people who need it in order to create control conditions; treatment integrity problems when dealing with clients who present problems in idiosyncratic ways; and balancing a practitioner's desire to create the best conditions for successful treatment with a researcher's desire to systematically change conditions to test hypotheses. And, finally, both small-group researchers and group work researchers must contend with capturing and harnessing group dynamics that fundamentally change when they are isolated and examined.

Many of these challenges for both small-group and treatment researchers can be addressed with large enough samples; that is, if pools of participants were unlimited, research designs could be developed that allow for any type of variation that exists. But, of course, financial and other pragmatic constraints limit our ability to find large enough pools of participants.

Reviews by Brower and Garvin (1989), Forsyth (1998), and Keyton (1994) analyzing how small-group and group work research is most often conducted found three general categories of design problems that researchers must address:

- Problems associated with random assignment and the creation of control groups.
- Resource difficulties encountered when studying "naturalistic" group processes.
- Statistical difficulties encountered when studying "naturalistic" group processes.

The remainder of this chapter examines these categories of research design problems, the pitfalls that they present, and some suggestions for how to address them based on what appeared promising from our review of the past 5 years of literature in group work and small-group research.

Problems Associated with Random Assignment and the Creation of Control Groups

Randomly assigning participants to research conditions allows one to rule out several confounds that severely limit the validity of research findings. However, two main problems exist when using random assignment for group work research. First, as with all treatment research, ethical problems exist in withholding treatment from participants who are randomly assigned to control conditions. Second, random assignment to small groups is made difficult because group composition is often an important variable in the research design, meaning that the group worker often wants to populate groups strategically rather than randomly.

One solution to the ethical complication of withholding treatment is to delay treatment for participants in a control condition. Most often, this research uses a design that places participants into wait-list control groups, in which the person is put on a waiting list and not contacted until his or her group begins. Another solution is to give participants an alternative treatment, either by assigning them to another treatment that is the primary comparison to the one being tested or by assigning them to a "holding group" that may function much like a self-help group. A final common strategy is for researchers to screen out the participants who are in most need of treatment so these most needy individuals can be given treatment separate from the research project.

Finding solutions to the problem of composing groups strategically rather than randomly is somewhat harder. Often, the solution is to identify the one or two conditions of most interest to the researcher (such as participant gender, ethnicity, diagnosis, or referral source) and then stratify the random assignment process along these conditions. What results are groups strategically composed along one dimension and randomly composed otherwise. Of course, the more one composes groups along dimensions of interest, the less random are these groups.

Over the past 5 years, in the journals we reviewed, eight studies used random assignment when studying group processes—occurring in groups that were allowed to unfold more or less on their own. Eight additional studies used random assignment, though these studies used groups of "confederates" (research assistants posing as group members) to expose participants to either experimental or control conditions. An example of the use of random assignment with confederates could be seen in the study by Hart, Stasson, and Karau (1999), in which participants rated graduate school applicants in group settings created to foster either high or low influence over decision making.

Of the eight studies that did use random assignment to study more naturally unfolding group processes, two of them focused on treatment groups. Barrow, Burlingame, Harding, and Behrman (1997) were interested in whether professionally trained versus nonprofessional therapists—those who went through a structured and intensive therapist training program versus those who were given a treatment manual without actual instruction—were better able to generate "focus" in their groups. They randomly assigned 102 participants to treatment groups led by either professional or nonprofessional leaders or to a no-treatment control group. They were not interested in member effects, so they did not have to stratify their sample in any way, and to address ethical issues of withholding treatment, they first excluded 60 additional clients from their study—these clients met other research protocol criteria but were given treatment directly instead of via the study.

In the other study (Shechtman & Ben-David, 1999), group treatment for aggressive children was compared with individual treatment. The sample of 101 was stratified by age of child to create balanced numbers of groups of similarly aged children, and then participants were randomly assigned to either group or individual treatment. Using this design, no child was denied treatment for the sake of the research.

Resource Difficulties Encountered When Studying "Naturalistic" Group Processes

Groups change over time, and the variables that are of interest, and particularly their interactions, will likewise change over time. "Natural" groups differ in the time they take for a variety of processes and dynamics to unfold. Honoring these naturalistic processes requires "naturalistic" designs and methods, which are often expensive, cumbersome, or both.

One strategy for capturing the natural unfolding of groups is to describe the group as a case study, and, in fact, the case study approach is one of the oldest designs used to study groups. Interestingly, however, only four studies, all with a social group work focus, were found to use a case study approach out of the 5 years of articles we reviewed. A classic example of the case study design was used by Racine and Sevigny (2001). This study describes a board game devised by the researchers to generate both solutions to life situations and research data with women living in a homeless shelter in Montreal. In their study, Racine and Sevigny describe how the women used their game to solve problems in their lives and how their group interactions changed as a result of their participation. Characteristic of this type of research study is its careful attention to detail in its descriptions of the sample, the group setting, researcher objectives and biases, and the range of interactions that took place over the life of the group. This level of detail is important in these types of studies for two reasons: It allows readers both to evaluate the quality of the work being described and to determine the study's generalizability. In other words, case studies use descriptive detail to determine both internal and external validity.

Another strategy that captures group processes as they naturally occur is to use videotaping and act-by-act scoring systems; Brower and Garvin (1989) speculated that the use of these approaches would increase as the technologies that drive them became less expensive. The basic strategy for this approach is to videotape each group session and then use some sort of system to code each "act" (sometimes defined as each utterance in the group, and sometimes defined as each transaction between one person and another) displayed in the group. SYMLOG is one such common system (Bales & Cohen, 1980). Over the past 5 years in the group research journals that we read, 12 studies used videotape to record sessions, and 4 of these used SYMLOG to code group behaviors. The remainder of the articles coded specific behaviors of interest using coding systems created specifically for that study. An example of this type of study was done by Sonnentag (2001), who counted frequency of member utterances in a study of participation rates in software development teams.

Three additional studies are worth describing, as they used videotaping in interesting ways. Bavelas, Coates, and Johnson (2000) looked at the relationship between storytellers and their audiences, describing the listeners as "co-narrators" because storytellers changed their stories based on the responses they got from their audience. This study analyzed videos of small-group storytelling sessions and found that storytellers elaborated specific aspects of their stories in direct response to reactions from listeners while telling other aspects of the story in more "generic" ways when no response was elicited. Videotaping allowed the researchers to identify the specific sequences of interaction between storyteller and listeners when high or low engagement was found.

Miller and Donner (2000) videotaped race dialogue groups—public and structured small-group conversations about race and racism. In addition to documenting these dialogues and the group processes, the videos were played publicly to bring a wider audience into the discussions. Because more than one group was videotaped, the public presentation of the tapes also led to discussions about how these race dialogue groups were different and similar on a variety of themes, processes, and issues related to group development and racial identity.

Finally, Dutton (2001) showed her group its own videotapes of prior meetings as a way to help the members evaluate their own growth and development. Members in her group were urban adolescents, mixed in age and racial identity, who came together to stage a theater production. Each production meeting was videotaped, and the group members watched their own tapes at regular intervals to deepen their discussions about how they acted with each other and how they made decisions as a group. Through this self-referential analysis, the research and evaluation aspects of the project became another element of group process and development.

Statistical Difficulties Encountered When Studying "Naturalistic" Group Processes

Even if natural group processes are captured on videotape, the mountain of data generated—both the sheer number of variables to keep track of and the multidimensional relationships among them—is difficult to sort through. Act-by-act coding systems, such as SYMLOG, manage this problem by focusing attention on a handful of categories of variables, thereby allowing researchers to "see" aspects of group development and change through a conceptual filter. Another way to handle this problem is more typical but less desirable: obtaining member ratings of their perceptions or attitudes about the group after each session and then manipulating and aggregating them in a variety of ways to examine group-level processes and trends. The problem with using member ratings in this way is that it violates a basic statistical assumption of observational nonindependence, which in turn inflates Type 1 error, making it harder to know whether our findings are real or not.

Observational nonindependence can show up in groups in at least three ways. First, once group members know each other, it is difficult to determine whether members rate group items similarly because they view their group in similar ways or because they are influencing each others' judgments erroneously. Second, if one wants to measure group trends by asking members for group ratings in each session, observational nonindependence is a problem because members may base one session's rating on a previous session rather than on their judgment of that day's group. Third, we often want to say something about the group as a whole by aggregating ratings from individual members—perhaps the most blatant violation of observational nonindependence, as this method obscures important aspects of the member observations, such as their distribution and error variance.

Many multidimensional statistical methods exist to handle complex relationships among variables, and many of these methods can be successfully adapted to handle the types of problems and requirements of small-group research. A good general reference on these methods is Collins and Sayer (2001). However, two newer statistical methods—*structural equation modeling* and *hierarchical linear modeling*—are described briefly in this chapter because they are so well suited to capturing complex relationships using data generated by small-group research. Additionally, structural equation modeling specifically addresses the observational nonindependence problem endemic to small-group data.

Structural Equation Modeling and Complex Relationships

One statistical method that can handle the complex relationships in groups is based on the use of LISREL software and structural equation modeling (SEM; Joreskog & Sorbom, 1993). SEM is conceptually similar to a factor analysis in that the statistical technique is used to identify which variables "go" with other variables and is also conceptually similar to regression in that it can be used to show how variables are predicted by other variables. However, SEM can be used to create "paths" of relationships among variables, showing the paths of direct and indirect causal influence that variables have on each other, including the "latent" constructs that might undergird the relationships among variables. Thus SEM allows us to capture the rich and complex web of direct and indirect relationships that exist among group variables.

The most commonly used software to implement SEM is LISREL, and LISREL is fairly data intensive. To use it with confidence, the common guideline is to have a ratio of cases or observations-to-variables of about 10:1, or about 10 observations per variable. Others suggest that one must have at least 100 cases total in the sample. LISREL can be used with smaller data sets or with a smaller ratio of cases to variables, but this will greatly raise the likelihood that results are unique to the data set or artifacts of the data. LISREL also needs independent observations, so it does not solve the observational nonindependence problem that plagues group research when data are obtained from individual group members. Nevertheless, it is a statistical procedure that lends itself very well to capturing the richness of group relationships, and therefore it could be used productively to advance our research efforts.

Carless and de Paola (2000) used LISREL to study the relationships among group cohesion, work team effectiveness, and team performance for workers in retail stores. They surveyed 84 retail outlets, with one to four employees filling out surveys at each outlet. They measured group cohesion, team effectiveness, and work satisfaction through self-report; team performance was assessed by asking the regional manager to rate that retail store on various outcomes. A typical non-SEM analysis would have used bivariate methods to identify how each measure was related to each other, or at best used multiple regression to try to identify how a set of variables related to the outcome. Instead, these researchers constructed a variety of path models of the relationships among these measures and then tested each one using LISREL. Their results found that none of their models was a good fit to these data, allowing the researchers to conclude that group cohesion might not be an important factor in work group outcomes.

Hierarchical Linear Modeling and Group Trends

As we have discussed, observational dependency is a problem for small-group research, and one example of this problem occurs when trying to use member observations of each session to create a picture of group trends over time. Typical ways to chart trends in groups have been to use graphing techniques with visual inspection or to compare group means derived by lumping together sessions from arbitrarily determined beginning, middle, and end phases of the group. Hierarchical linear modeling (HLM) is a statistical method that hierarchically "nests" sets of observations within other sets (Bryk & Raudenbush, 1992) and that therefore does not need to make assumptions about observational nonindependence. Instead, it allows for the determination of individual-level and group-level effects to be assessed together and individually. It can be used to nest individual-level observations within the groups to which individuals belong as a way to address the individual level–group level unit of analysis problem. HLM can also be used to nest sequences of sessions together to assess group trends using a procedure called growth curve estimation.

We describe how HLM can be used to address the individual level–group level unit of analysis problem in the next section. What follows is a study that used HLM and growth curve estimation, using session-by-session group observations, to determine group trends.

Kivlighan and Lilly (1997) used HLM to explore how dimensions of group climate affected counseling outcomes. Climate was assessed using the Engaged, Conflict, and Avoidant scales of the Group Climate Questionnaire (ECQ); members completed this instrument after each session. The Target Complaints form was used to help members identify their group counseling goals. HLM was used to nest members' session observations within their group to create trends for each group that were then compared with counseling outcomes. Results showed interesting trends related to outcome: a high-low-high pattern for group engagement, a low-high-low pattern for group conflict, and a cubic pattern for group avoidance. Importantly, when these researchers compared "snap shot" scores on the GCQ (i.e., at the beginning, middle, or end) to outcomes, no significant results were found. It was the trend itself that appeared to make a difference, not the level of the scores per se.

HLM (and Other Methods) and the Unit-of-Analysis Problem

Problems associated with aggregating individual-level observations to say something about group-level phenomena are so common that statistical solutions have appeared in the literature repeatedly for the past 20 years (Hoyle, Georgesen, & Webster, 2001; see also Glisson, 1987). Yet, despite the repeated appearance of solutions to these problems and the appearance of powerful and easy-to-use software to compute the statistics required (Bryk & Raudenbush, 1992), recent reviews continue to find that researchers are ignoring these solutions. In a review done in 1994, Burlingame, Kircher, and Taylor (1994) found that almost 90% of group psychotherapy research published between 1980 and 1992 analyzed individual-level data without correcting for, or sometimes even acknowledging, the nonindependence problem. In a replication of this review, Hoyle and his associates (Hoyle et al., 2001) found only a modest improvement. By 1997, one-third of the articles reviewed still failed to either acknowledge this problem or to use a statistical strategy to correct for it. And of those that did address this problem, the most frequently used solution was not to use the powerful statistical approaches available but instead to simply use the group as the unit of analysis and therefore try to sidestep the problem altogether.

But we need not sidestep this problem, because several articles exist that can serve as blueprints for the use of HLM and other statistical procedures to address observational nonindependence. Hoyle and his associates (Hoyle et al., 2001; Hoyle & Crawford, 1994), Nezlek and Zyzniewski (1998), and Pollack (1998) all outline (sometimes in step-by-step detail) how to use HLM to study small groups. All of these articles are easy to follow and will greatly increase the validity of our results. If one wishes to continue to use ANOVA, Burlingame and his associates (Burlingame, Kircher, & Honts, 1994) outline a "bootstrapping" correction procedure to handle nonindependent observations. And, finally, if one wants an even less statistically inclined way to correct for this problem, Moritz and Watson (1998) and Glisson (1987) describe how to compare within-group to between-group variance—essentially allowing us to simulate a "multilevel" analysis that helps us determine how great an effect nonindependence is having on one's data. But whatever solution is used, we strongly urge researchers to use one. They are readily available and easy to apply.

One study we reviewed serves as a good illustration of why it is important to address nonindependent observations. Terry et al. (2000) studied the relationships between perceptions of cohesion on sports teams and mood of the athletes. They administered a mood scale, the Profile of Mood States—Children (POMS-C), and a group environment questionnaire to more than 400 adults who belong to rugby, rowing, and netball teams in England. Before correcting for nonindependence, they found substantial differences in the role of cohesion based on the sport played. After correcting, they realized that the primary findings cut across sports: The more cohesive the athletes perceived their teams, the more positive and the less anxious, angry, and depressed they felt. In their study, the cohesion measure and its relationship to other variables was inflated due to nonindependent-observation error.

CONCLUSION

Clearly, small groups are complex and present vexing design problems to which there are no simple answers. But just as clearly, these problems have been known almost since the time small groups were first studied—and many unambiguous and trustworthy solutions now exist in the literature. And in particular, the ubiquitous nonindependence problem can be easily addressed using a variety of readily available statistical methods. We hope through this chapter to have made some of these solutions more easily accessible.

However, given that many of these solutions have existed in the literature for years, why have we not made more frequent use of them? It cannot be that we do not take our own limitations seriously or that we do not feel our research findings are important enough to need to correct for statistical violations. It certainly cannot be that we are not well read enough to know that these solutions exist!

One might criticize the problems and solutions identified in this chapter as piecemeal; they provide technical solutions to "symptoms" in how we continue to study small groups. This critique would say that the research design problems identified will continue to plague us as long as we continue to "shoehorn" group work research into a logical positivist tradition (Papell & Rothman, 1966). Instead, researchers should use more naturalistic paradigms to study groups because these paradigms more easily match the processes of interest in small groups (Frey, 1994).

There may be wisdom in this logical positivist critique, and the literature is beginning to showcase new naturalistic paradigms that might allow for truly new discoveries in group work research. For example, Fuhriman and Burlingame (1994) describe how chaos theory— a science of "process rather than of state"—can be applied to groups. Because this theory puts at its center the interconnectedness of complex processes through time and space, it appears very well suited to the study of this same type of interconnectedness that is at the center of the groupness of groups.

But although a logical positivist perspective might have inherent limitations, we need not abandon its quantitative methods altogether to find holistic solutions to advance group work research. For example, Brower and Garvin (1989) argued more than 10 years ago that the field needs to standardize its dimensions of study—agreeing on variables and methods to measure these variables—to create a "grid" or matrix that would allow us to build up our knowledge about groups in a systematic way. By doing so, we could then systematically vary aspects of groups (outcomes, membership, processes of interest, etc.) to slowly but surely fill in the grid. However, we would need stronger leadership in our field for this solution to take hold.

This chapter's review found that small-group research, as a whole, is healthy and growing—we are producing more small-group research than ever before. But sadly, as a whole, we also appear to be only very slowly changing the way we conduct our research, *even though solutions to our design and methods problems exist*. We continue to make the same design mistakes we always have or only reluctantly embrace changes that are readily available for use.

If, as George Homans said half a century ago, the small group is at the very center of our lives as human beings (Homans, 1950), then knowledge of small groups should be at the very center of every discussion of human behavior. Those of us who continue to produce small-group research have the power to make this happen—and to do so means addressing our own fixable research design limitations in order to make our work as top quality as it can be.

REFERENCES

Bales, R. F., & Cohen, S. P. (1980). *SYMLOG: A systems for the multiple level observation of groups*. New York: Free Press.

Barrow, S. H., Burlingame, G. M., Harding, J. A., & Behrman, J. (1997). Therapeutic focusing in time-limited group psychotherapy. *Group Dynamics, 1*(3), 254–266.

Bavelas, J. B., Coates, L., & Johnson, T. (2000). Listeners as co-narrators. *Journal of Personality and Social Psychology, 79*(6), 941–952.

Brower, A. M., & Garvin, C. D. (1989). Design issues in social group work research. *Social Work with Groups, 12*(3), 91–102.

Bryk, A. S., & Raudenbush, S. W. (1992). *Hierarchical linear models*. Thousand Oaks, CA: Sage.

Burlingame, G., Kircher, J., & Honts, C. R. (1994). Analysis of variance versus bootstrap procedures for analyzing dependent observations in small group research. *Small Group Research, 25*(4), 486–501.

Burlingame, G., Kircher, J., & Taylor, S. (1994). Methodological considerations in group psychotherapy research: Past, present, and future practices. In A. Fuhriman & G. Burlingame (Eds.), *Handbook of group psychotherapy: An empirical and clinical synthesis* (pp. 41–80). New York: Wiley.

Carless, S. A., & de Paola, C. (2000). The measurement of cohesion in work teams. *Small Group Research, 31*(1), 71–81.

Collins, L. M., & Sayer, A. G. (2001). *New methods for the analysis of change*. Washington DC: American Psychological Association.

Dutton, S. E. (2001). Urban youth development—broadway style: Using theatre and group work as vehicles for positive youth development. *Social Work with Groups, 23*(4), 39–58.

Ettin, M. F. (Ed.). (2000). The future of group psychotherapy in the 21st century (Pt. 2) [Special issue]. *Group, 24*(2/3).

Feldman, R. A. (1987). Group work knowledge and research: A two-decade comparison. In S. D. Rose (Ed.), *Research in group work* (pp. 7–14). New York: Haworth Press.

Forsyth, D. R. (Ed.). (1998). Methodological advances in the study of group dynamics [Special issue]. *Group Dynamics, 2*(4).

Frey, L. R. (1994). The naturalistic paradigm: Studying small groups in the postmodern era. *Small Group Research, 25*(4), 557–578.

Fuhriman, A., & Burlingame, G. M. (1994). Measuring small group process: A methodological application of chaos theory. *Small Group Research, 25*(4), 502–519.

Garvin, C. D. (2001). The potential impact of small-group research on social group work practice. In T. B. Kelly, T. Berman-Rossi, & S. Palombo (Eds.), *Group work: Strategies for strengthening resiliency* (pp. 51–70). New York: Haworth Press.

Glisson, C. (1987). The group versus the individual as the unit of analysis in small group research. In S. D. Rose (Ed.), *Research in group work* (pp. 15–30). New York: Haworth Press.

Hart, J. W., Stasson, M. F., & Karau, S. J. (1999). Effects of source expertise and physical distance on minority influence. *Group Dynamics*, *3*(1), 81–92.

Homans, G. C. (1950). *The human group*. New York: Harcourt, Brace & World.

Hoyle, R. H., & Crawford, A. M. (1994). Use of individual-level data to investigate group phenomena: Issues and strategies. *Small Group Research*, *25*(4), 464–485.

Hoyle, R. H., Georgesen, J. C., & Webster, J. M. (2001). Analyzing data from individuals in groups: The past, the present, and the future. *Group Dynamics*, *5*(1), 41–47.

Joreskog, K., & Sorbom, D. (1993). *LISREL 8: Structural equation modeling with the SIMPLIS command language*. Hillsdale, NJ: Erlbaum.

Keyton, J. (Ed.). (1994). Research problems and methodology [Special issue]. *Small Group Research*, *25*(4).

Kivlighan, D. M., & Lilly, R. L. (1997). Developmental changes in group climate as they relate to therapeutic gain. *Group Dynamics*, *1*(3), 208–221.

Levine, J. M., & Moreland, R. L. (1990). Progress in small group research. *Annual Review of Psychology*, *41*, 585–634.

Miller, J., & Donner, S. (2000). More than just talk: The use of racial dialogues to combat racism. *Social Work with Groups*, *23*(1).

Moritz, S. E., & Watson, C. B. (1998). Levels of analysis issues in group psychotherapy: Using efficacy as an example of a multilevel model. *Group Dynamics*, *2*(4), 285–298.

Nezlek, J. B., & Zyzniewski, L. E. (1998). Using hierarchical linear modeling to analyze grouped data. *Group Dynamics*, *2*(4), 313–320.

Papell, C. P., & Rothman, B. (1966). Social group work models: Possession and heritage. *Journal of Education in Social Work*, *2*(2), 66–77.

Pollack, B. N. (1998). Hierarchical linear modeling and the "unit of analysis" problem: A solution for analyzing responses of intact group members. *Group Dynamics*, *2*(4), 299–312.

Racine, G., & Sevigny, O. (2001). Changing the rules: A board game lets homeless women tell their stories. *Social Work with Groups*, *23*(4), 25–38.

Shechtman, Z., & Ben-David, M. (1999). Individual and group psychotherapy of childhood aggression: A comparison of outcomes and processes. *Group Dynamics*, *3*(4), 263–274.

Sonnentag, S. (2001). High performance and meeting participation: An observational study in software design teams. *Group Dynamics*, *5*(1), 3–18.

Terry, P. C., Carron, A. V., Pink, M. J., Lane, A. M., Jones, G. J. W., & Hall, M. P. (2000). Perceptions of group cohesion and mood in sports. *Group Dynamics*, *4*(3), 244–253.

Toseland, R. W., & Rivas, R. F. (1998). *An introduction to group work practice* (3rd ed.). Boston: Allyn & Bacon.

Chapter 26

Measurement Issues

RANDY MAGEN

Examining groups from a systems perspective may be natural for contemporary social workers. The systems perspective, or group-as a-whole orientation, provides a solid conceptual foundation for understanding groups (Agazarian, 1992). However, to engage in evidence-based group work practice or to conduct research on groups requires that abstract systems concepts be described and operationalized "in terms of specific indicators by assignment of numbers or other symbols to these indicants in accordance with rules"; this is the process of measurement (Monette, Sullivan, & DeJong, 2002, p. 103). This chapter discusses measurement issues in groups. It offers an appraisal of both qualitative and quantitative instruments for studying group conditions and outcomes.

GROUP WORK IN THE CONTEXT OF MEASUREMENT

It is an ethical mandate for social workers to "protect clients from harm" (National Association of Social Workers, 1999, p. 9). Research has pointed out the potentially harmful effects of participating in a group (Coyne, 1999; Lieberman, Yalom, & Miles, 1973; Smokowski, Rose, Todar, & Reardon, 1999). It is only through systematic evaluation that practitioners can understand the effects of their groups and be able to, in the least, refute the claim that the group caused harm. Measurement generates the data necessary to systematically evaluate a group. Garvin (1997) also points out that evaluation is necessary in our current political climate, which stresses accountability.

Critics of the use of measures in social work practice argue that measurement is reductionistic and has little relevance to the complexities of social work practice (Goldstein, 1992; Witkin, 1996). Opponents of evidence-based practice argue that the focus on data devalues clinical experience (Williams & Garner, 2002). However, Gibbs (2003, p. 16) writes that measurement is not a substitute for practitioner judgment but rather lies at the "intersection between experience, the client's preferences and current best evidence."

447

Measures are tools for the group work practitioner to utilize in collecting data to understand the effects of a group. There are two general types of effects that can be measured. The first are the effects of the intervention on members' goals—measurement of the outcome of the group. Generally the question being asked of the data collected through the use of outcome measures is, Did the client change? The second type of effects are measures of the group conditions, often referred to as measures of group processes. The main question being asked of data collected from group process measures is, Do the group conditions exist that are necessary for group members to work toward achieving their goals? The general failure in the literature to link group processes with outcomes is a long-standing and serious problem. Methodologically, group processes can confound outcome. Rose, Tolman, and Tallant (1985) point out that differences between two interventions may be misattributed to content differences when in fact the differences were due to a failure to achieve optimal group processes in one condition.

In individually based practice, what can be measured is limited to the client, the practitioner, and the interactions between the practitioner and the client. In groups, what can be measured expands geometrically with every group member because each individual, dyad, triad, and so on can be the target of measurement. For example, in a group of six people in which one of the members is the designated leader, there are six individuals, 15 dyads, 20 triads, 15 subgroups of four members, 6 subgroups of five members, and the entire group of 6 that can be the focus of measurement. This assumes, of course, that measurement of the dyads, triads, or subgroups is meaningful and useful.

Like any tool, measures can be used carelessly and foolishly. Using measures that are a burden because of their complexity, length, or relevance is foolish. Similarly, using measures without a clear idea of how they will be used to assist clients or leaders is careless. Two general principles in the use of measurement are parsimony and simplicity.

INTERVENTION

The use of measures in groups is not limited to any particular approach to group work. As I show later, qualitative and quantitative measures have been utilized in psychodynamic and behaviorally oriented groups, in remedial and reciprocal model groups, and in leader-centered and self-help groups. However, some types of measures are more syntonic with specific approaches to group work. For example, Kurtz (1997) advises that qualitative methods and participatory action research are best suited to self-help groups.

EMPIRICAL EVIDENCE AND THEORETICAL BASE

Five issues need to be addressed before using any measure in groups. These issues are related to the unit of analysis, definitions of concepts, individualization of measurement, reliability, and validity.

Unit of Analysis

The unit-of-analysis issue may be the most commonly ignored methodological quagmire in group work research. The basic idea is that the unit measured (typically individuals) should be the unit analyzed. However, it is common for group work researchers to collect data on individuals yet analyze and report the data in terms of the group. There are many dangers with this practice. The first danger involves what have been termed the ecological fallacy and the reductionist fallacy (Monette, Sullivan, & Dejong, 2002), wherein data collected from one level (e.g., individuals) are used to infer something about a different system level (e.g., dyads, triads, or a group). Furthermore, if we believe conceptually, based on systems theory, that the group is more than the sum of the parts, then we need data in addition to those collected at the individual level to accurately describe the group. Another problem with using individual data to describe the group as a whole relates to errors in aggregating the data. It is common practice for group workers to report the mean of the group members' individual scores as the score for the group. Glisson (1986) pointed out the dangers of this approach: Depending on the distribution of individual scores, this procedure can either overestimate or underestimate the group score.

An additional problem in analyzing individual scores to draw conclusions about the group is that statistical analyses assume that data values are independent. Group practitioners believe that part of the power of the group is that members influence each other; thus scores on measurement instruments are affected by what other group members say and do—the data are not independent observations. The violation of the assumption of independence can lead to bias in standard error estimates and erroneous results in statistical tests (Barcikowski, 1981; Pollack, 1998). Although statistical analyses to deal with this problem are beyond the scope of this chapter, two solutions that have been suggested are using nested designs (Morran, Robison, & Hulse-Killacky, 1990) and hierarchial linear modeling (Pollack, 1998).

In some group work research, the individual level of analysis may be less important than other levels. For example, Maton (1993) proposed an ecological paradigm for understanding self-help groups within the context of communities and other large systems. In this model, if self-help groups are conceptualized as community organizations (Kurtz, 1997), then community-level variables such as human service budgets, prevalence of focal problems, and population stability affect group effectiveness and need to be measured.

Finally, the practice of aggregating individual scores as measures of group process is also suspect on conceptual grounds, given that almost all definitions of group processes are linked to the group rather than to individuals. However, there are also difficulties in relying on definitions of group processes.

Definitions of Concepts

Measurement does not start with the selection of an instrument but rather with clear definitions of the concepts to be measured. Bednar and Kaul (1994, p. 633), in reviewing 50 years of group research, were highly critical of the state of measurement in group work research. Instead of more rigorous research designs, they called on researchers and practitioners to carefully observe and describe groups so that specific measurement tools could be created. Bednar and Kaul's (1994) critique should be seen as a warning to anyone measuring aspects of group work. The usefulness of any measure is dependent on the clarity of the concept it is describing.

In group work practice and research, the difficulty in defining concepts is most pronounced in measures of group process. Although there have been rich descriptions of various group processes, little agreement exists about even the most basic phenomena. For example, on the one hand, there is widespread agreement that cohesion is a necessary group process for the functioning of effective groups. High cohesiveness has been linked to therapeutic change (Dies & Teleska, 1985, p. 120), whereas low cohesiveness has been shown to correlate highly with members dropping out of groups (Lieberman et al., 1973). On the other hand, there is little agreement about how to define cohesion, as illustrated by the following definitions:

- The total field of forces which act on members to remain in the group (Festinger, Schachter, & Back, 1950, p. 164).
- Attraction to the group (Lieberman et al., 1973).
- The composite of member–member, member–therapist, and member–group relations (Fuhriman & Barlow, 1982).
- The degree of members' involvement in and commitment to the group and the concern and friendship they show for one another (Moos, 1986, p. 2).

Kaul and Bednar (1986, p. 707) remark on the "lack of cohesion in cohesion research" and go so far as to say the research is a "spectacular embarrassment."

For group work researchers and practitioners, the first step in measurement is a clear conceptual definition of the concept. This leads directly to the operationalization of the concept.

Individualization of Measurement

A common research design for investigating the effect of a group intervention tests the hypothesis that the group members' mean score on an outcome measure is significantly different from pretest to posttest or is significantly different from scores of members in control or comparison groups. For example, to test whether a cognitive-behavioral group reduces members' levels of depression, a researcher could administer the Beck Depression Inventory prior to the beginning of the group and again at the end of the group. The researcher could then perform a matched-pairs t-test, assuming adequate sample size, to reject the null hypothesis that there was no difference in scores on the Beck Depression Inventory from pretest to posttest. In this research design, the goal is to offer a nomothetic explanation that cognitive-behavioral group intervention can reduce depression. The purpose of this type of research is to develop knowledge that can be generalized beyond the group being studied.

One advantage of this approach to research is that utilizing a norm-based instrument, such as the Beck Depression Inventory, allows researchers and practitioners to compare their samples to various published norms. The practitioner reading the report about the cognitive-behavioral intervention has a standard against which to evaluate the level of group members' depression. Measures that allow comparison to norms are referred to as nomothetic measures.

Nomothetic measures and explanations also have disadvantages. First, norm-based measures are often indirect proxy measures of client troubles and, as a result, are difficult to use in evaluating individual reactions, as well as the importance participants attach to their difficulties. Norm-based measures are often insensitive to small changes. Nomothetic explanations that rely on tests of sample means provide us with little or no information about what happened to an individual client. Average scores can underestimate clinically significant changes when the effect of treatment is variable within treatments (i.e., when there is large within-subject variability). Furthermore, the imposed significance levels associated with statistical tests often have little relevance to clinical practice (Jacobson, Follette, & Ravenstorf, 1984). In fact, with a large number of participants, results can be statistically significant even when the effectiveness of an intervention is "weak" (Barlow, Hayes, & Nelson, 1984). An adjunct to the use of nomothetic measures and explanations is ideographic measures and explanations.

Ideographic measures are precise and sensitive indicators of individual change. Although not commonly reported in group work research, ideographic measures can be found in the behavioral literature associated with single-system research designs. Ideographic measures allow clients to select indicators of important problems and determine how to measure a successful outcome. Furthermore, some ideographic measures can measure progress, as well as success. Ideographic measures of outcome, discussed later, include goal attainment scaling and individualized rating scales (Bloom, Fischer, & Orme, 1999).

Researchers and practitioners often want to know not only whether a group intervention is effective but also for whom it was most effective. Clinical significance tests following statistical significance tests are a method for obtaining ideographic explanations of outcome. Several statistical tests have been suggested for evaluating clinical significance (Christensen & Mendoza, 1986; Jacobson, Follette, & Ravenstorf, 1984, 1986; Jayaratne, 1990). The most useful of these statistics is the SC suggested by Christensen and Mendoza (1986), which yields a score, in standard deviation units, that indicates the magnitude of an individual subject's change on a measure. The SC statistic, used in conjunction with nomothetic explanations, can tell us not only whether the group was effective but also which individual members benefited most from the intervention.

Reliability

A synonym for reliability is consistency. There are many different ways to assess the reliability of a measure; the most common of these are test–retest, split-half, internal consistency, and multiple forms. For measures involving observation, the assessment of reliability refers to the consistency between raters, known as interrater reliability. Three methods for computing interrater reliability are Cohen's kappa, the interclass correlation coefficient, and the percentage of agreement.

By convention, the agreed-on standard for a reliable measure is .80, or 80%. Clearly, the higher the reliability the better, but in practice researchers commonly use measures with reliabilities considerably lower than .80. In fact, for several of the measures used in group work research, little published data are available on the reliability of the instrument. It is important for researchers and practitioners to understand the reliability of any instrument utilized. At a minimum, basic reliability statistics should be calculated and reported.

Validity

Valid measures are accurate measures. There are two questions associated with evaluating the validity of a measure. First, is the instrument measuring what it is suppose to measure? Second, how well does the instrument measure what is intended? Valid measures are reliable, but reliable measures are not necessarily valid. As with reliability, there are many methods for assessing the validity of a measure. These methods include face validity, content validity, criterion validity (concurrent and predictive), and construct validity (convergent, discriminate, and convergent). Assessing the validity of a measure is a complex and difficult task involving both clear concepts and careful empirical research. Measures are never completely valid nor completely invalid. Generally, the more information that is available about the validity of a measure, the more faith the researcher or practitioner can have in its use.

Again, as with reliability, for many measures used in group research limited published validity information exists.

EXAMPLES

Measures of Outcome

To select an outcome measure, the group practitioner or researcher needs to decide (1) what to measure, (2) how to measure it, and (3) who will collect the measurement data (or where they will be collected). This process of selecting outcome measures can be conceptualized as a three-dimensional cube, with each question corresponding to one dimension of the cube. Within each dimension are specific domains to be measured, methods of measurement, or source of the data (see Figure 26.1). There are many ways to conceptualize the elements within each dimension, the elements identified in Figure 26.1 are one example. The conceptualization of elements within each dimension is influenced, at a minimum, by the purpose of the group and the clients' needs. Other considerations in conceptualizing what to measure, how to measure, and who will collect the measurement data include theoretical orientation, practicality, and feasibility.

The metaphor of the cube is also helpful in identifying whether data collection is multimethod and multisourced, what qualitative researchers refer to as triangulation (Berg,

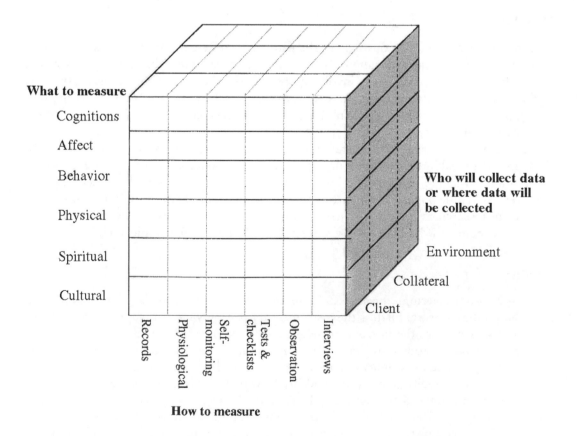

FIGURE 26.1. Triangulation matrix for selecting outcome measures.

1998). Measures that are triangulated will be indicated by multiple blocks within the cube containing data. However, not all measures can be triangulated; for example, some outcomes are covert, such as a change in cognitions. As a result, the cells in Figure 26.1 that correspond to cognitions can be collected only from the client. However, the measure of cognitions can be done by means of self-monitoring, via tests and checklists; through analog observations; or by way of interviews. Furthermore, the measure of cognitions can be either quantitative or qualitative.

In reality, practitioners and researchers rely on a few common methods for measuring client outcomes. Perhaps the most common of these tools are tests and checklists, primarily norm-based instruments. Empirical research studies, in particular, rely on norm-based measures. Highly touted and extremely practical, but less utilized, are rapid assessment instruments such as those developed by Hudson (1990a, 1990b).

Another type of instrument, commonly used in children's social skills training groups, is sociometric ratings (see, e.g., Hepler, 1994). Originally developed by J. L. Moreno, the father of psychodrama, these checklists have high face validity and some evidence of reliability. In a school setting, children would be asked to rate, on a Likert scale, the likelihood of their playing with every other member of the classroom. The scores from the classroom would then be used to identify those children most isolated, as well as those most popular. These sociometric ratings are an assessment tool that can be used to compose groups that are heterogeneous. The sociometric ratings can also be repeated after the end of the group to test either ideographically or nomothetically for changes.

Two methods for obtaining ideographic measures of change are individualized rating scales (IRS) and goal attainment scaling (GAS). IRS, as described by Bloom and colleagues (1999), use a single scale with descriptive anchors to operationally define target problems. For example, a client in a support group for people who have breast cancer might use such a scale to rate the intensity of fears about chemotherapy. The practitioner and client would work together to develop the labels for the 5 to 9 points found on the typical IRS. The client would then use this scale on a regular basis (e.g., weekly) to measure fears about chemotherapy.

Similar to IRS, GAS is frequently discussed in texts on measurement but rarely reported in the group work literature. GAS and IRS share many similarities. Both involve individualized ratings of a particular target. However, GAS is usually constructed on a scale from -2 to +2, with the level 0 being the client's current level of functioning. GAS, like IRS, can be used to measure not only outcome but also progress toward the ultimate goal (see, e.g., Magen & Rose, 1994).

Observation of group members' behavior within the group has long been used as material for social workers' progress notes. Systematic observation of group members' behavior both in and outside of the group has been reported infrequently as a means of assessing outcome. One of the more common applications of systematic observation has been parent–child interactions (see, e.g., Whipple, 1999), in which structured observational systems are available for both researchers and practitioners. Observation of classroom behavior as reported by a teacher has also been used to assess outcome in some skills training groups. Finally, analog measures of behavior through role playing have been used both during group sessions and outside of the group as measures of outcome.

In the biopsychosocial perspective of social work, the biological realm often receives less attention than the psychological or social realms. As a result, scant attention has been given to the use of physiological measures of outcome in the group work literature. The one exception to this has been in the field of substance abuse, in which urinalysis is employed to supplement self-reports of abstinence. Several other simple physiological measures can be used to measure agitation or stress, such as heart and respiration rates. More complex measures of stress, such as cardiac output, have been used in social support and stress management groups by O'Brien and his colleagues (see, e.g., Anthony & O'Brien, 2002).

Self-monitoring as a method for obtaining outcome measurement is easily implemented but can have low reliability due to problems with adherence. It is useful for practitioners and researchers to follow guidelines for enhancing adherence when implementing self-monitored outcome measurements. For example, to improve self-reports of sexual behavior in HIV research, Weinhardt, Forsyth, Carey, Jaworski, and Durant (1998) suggested building in techniques that improve the recall of behavior, such as appointment books or calendars, and placing the burden of denial on the client. Rather than having participants record "if" a behavior occurred, the researchers asked them to record how many times a behavior took place. From a research perspective, the reactive nature of self-monitoring can present a problem; however, in practice, this reactivity has been taken advantage of to strengthen an intervention. For example, in smoking cessation groups, monitoring the number of cigarettes smoked can help to reduce smoking.

Social workers are well trained in techniques of interviewing. Systematic collection of data during an interview can be used as a baseline for assessing outcome when compared with postgroup interview data. Interviews allow for the collection of rich qualitative data that cannot be obtained from other measurement methods. For example, to understand the effect of a self-help group in preventing drug use and improving client's lives, Felix-Ortiz (2000) and her colleagues interviewed 7 of 14 members participating in a self-help group at a methadone maintenance clinic. Whereas drug use and quality of life can be measured using other methods (e.g., tests and checklists), these interviews provided data on what the clients perceived to be the value of the group in contributing to their personal changes, a link that would be difficult to make using written measures.

Existing records may contain all the types of data listed here, as well as time-series data. Intake forms and other routinely collected agency records may be the only empirical data that exist to evaluate change for some group members. There are problems with the reliability of data in records, particularly if the records were contributed to by multiple practitioners. However, practitioners and researchers should not neglect this relatively easily obtained source of data.

Measures of Group Process

Measures of group process are designed to illuminate what is occurring within the group and to identify and assess the factors that are necessary for the functioning of an effective small group. A number of variables have been identified in the literature as belonging to the phenomenon of group process, but no one constellation of variables has received universal acceptance. Thus each measure of group process described in this section constitutes a slightly different subset of group process variables. Furthermore, a definitive list of group processes is probably not possible, given that group processes are influenced by the group work approach, by the stage of the group's development, by forces outside of the group, and by individual differences within the group.

A number of different tools have been developed to measure group processes or, more generally, group conditions. The tools discussed here were selected based on the following criteria: (1) their use has been discussed in peer-reviewed professional literature; (2) they have utility for both researchers and practitioners; (3) they are relatively low in cost and require little training to use. The reader is also referred to a recent book by Beck and Lewis (2000) that offers a comprehensive review of nine approaches developed over the past 50 years to study small groups. The systems of analysis presented focus on observations of group interaction from a psychodynamic perspective. Two of the instruments presented in the Beck and Lewis book, which may be of most interest to readers of this chapter, are the Hill Interaction Matrix and the Individual Group Member Interpersonal Process Scale (IGIPS). Readers are also referred to the annotated review of 26 group process instruments by Fuhriman and Packard (1986).

Perhaps the most widely known conceptualization of group process is Yalom's therapeutic factors (1995). To empirically explore these 12 therapeutic factors, which were developed based on his and others' experience with group psychotherapy, Yalom developed 60 statements, 5 for each of the 12 therapeutic factors. Patients, and in some cases group psychotherapists, were asked to perform a Q-sort on these 60 statements using seven categories, from most helpful to least helpful. The original Q-sort has been replaced by a self-administered checklist, on which Yalom's 60 statements are ranked on a 4-point Likert scale, with 0 corresponding to "not helpful" and 3 to "very helpful" (Butler & Fuhriman, 1983).

A variety of studies have demonstrated that clients view the presence of these factors as important to their group experience. However, the relative importance assigned to each factor has varied by the group studied. For example, research has consistently shown that cohesion and universality are perceived as important in the group experience of clients in self-help groups (Heil, 1992; Lieberman & Borman, 1979), psychotherapy groups (Bednar & Kaul, 1994), and cancer support groups (Weinberg, Uken, Schmale, & Adamek, 1995).

More than 40 separate studies have reported empirically on the use of the Yalom therapeutic factors questionnaire. Peer-reviewed data on reliability and validity have been published, including a factor analysis of the questionnaire; Yalom (1995) lists references to these in his book (see also Fuhriman, Drescher, Hanson, Henrie, & Rybicki, 1986). A critique of the therapeutic factors questionnaire and an alternative instrument based largely on the same concepts has been offered by MacNair-Semands and Lese (2000). However, this new questionnaire has not been as widely adopted as the original Yalom questionnaire.

Clearly, the advantage of the Yalom therapeutic factors questionnaire is its widespread adoption by both the practice community and researchers. Furthermore, the 60-item questionnaire is relatively easy to administer to adults. One disadvantage of the therapeutic factors questionnaire is that it measures participants' perceptions of the *importance* or *value* of each of the therapeutic factors but not whether the factor was actually present in the group (MacNair-Semands & Lee, 2000).

Another self-report instrument for measuring group conditions, developed by Rudolph Moos, is the Group Environment Scale (GES; 1986). The GES is a 90-item, true–false instrument. Conceptually, the GES consists of three domains: relationship, personal growth, and system maintenance/system change. Each domain is measured by 1 of the 10 subscales that constitute the GES. In the relationship domain, subscales measure cohesion, leader support, and expressiveness. The personal growth domain is measured by the independence, task orientation, self-discovery, and anger/aggression subscales. The system maintenance/system change domain is measured by the order and organization, leader control, and innovation subscales. The manual for the GES contains a conceptual and operational definition for each of the subscales, as well as normative data from 148 groups. The normative data is further broken down by type of group: task-oriented, social-recreational, and psychotherapy/

mutual-support groups. Data are provided on the reliability and validity of the scale. Finally, the manual for the GES contains references to more than 25 studies that have used one or more of the subscales.

Unlike Yalom's therapeutic factors questionnaire, which grew out of practitioners' experiences, the GES's development was guided by the application of systematic psychometric methods. Although the GES has been used with a wide variety of groups, from committees to support and psychotherapy groups, most of the current research appears to be focused on task-oriented groups and is found in the organizational management literature.

A number of relatively simple methods for collecting data on group conditions have been suggested by Rose (1984). Relevant to the discussion of tests and checklists, Rose proposed the use of a postsession questionnaire (PSQ) administered at the end of every group session. The questionnaire collects both qualitative and quantitative data on group member's perceptions of the usefulness of the group, satisfaction with the group, cohesion, and self-disclosure. There are no published data on the reliability or validity of the PSQ, and no norms exist; thus the PSQ should be used ideographically. Although the postsession questionnaire has been used in a variety of studies by Rose and his colleagues (e.g., Magen & Rose, 1994; Rose & Edleson, 1987; Whitney & Rose, 1989), as well as by others (e.g., Anthony & O'Brien, 2002), its utility is as a simple, easy-to-use tool for practitioners.

A qualitative instrument for collecting data on group conditions is the critical incident report. Like the postsession questionnaire, the critical incident methodology asks group members at the end of a group session to:

> Please describe briefly the event that was most personally important to you during today's session. This might be something that involved you directly, or something that happened between other members, but made you think about yourself. Explain what it was about the event that made it important for you personally. (MacKenzie, 1987, p. 31)

Mackenzie had clinicians categorize the critical incidents into categories that roughly corresponded to Yalom's therapeutic factors. A similar critical incident methodology, but one with a different conceptual coding system, has been used in the study of task group behavior (see, e.g., Taggar & Brown, 2001). The advantage of the critical incident report is that group members' words are not filtered through preconceived questions or limited to specific response categories. A disadvantage of this approach is that participants must possess the cognitive and writing skills to clearly explain the critical incident.

A relatively new instrument developed by Macgowan (2000) is the Groupwork Engagement Measure (GEM). In this instrument, engagement is conceptualized as a multidimensional construct across seven dimensions: attendance, contributing, relating to worker, relating with members, contracting, working on own problems, and working on others' problems (Macgowan & Levenson, 2003). The GEM has 37 items scored on a 5-point Likert scale from 1, "rarely or none of the time," to 5, "most or all of the time." Macgowan has subjected the GEM to tests of validity and reliability with various populations and types of groups (see also Macgowan, 1997). The GEM is a relatively short instrument, which makes it easy to use both in practice and research. There is a growing body of evidence to support the psychometric properties of this instrument. Furthermore, the multidimensional construct of engagement emerges both from practice with groups and from research on group conditions.

Rose (1984) also suggests several easy-to-implement observational coding systems for use in groups. A simple measure of attendance in group sessions is logically related to outcome, although, as Feldman, Caplinger, and Wodarski (1983) indicated, group members who drop out, who successfully complete treatment, and who unsuccessfully complete treatment are three distinct groups. Similarly, records of promptness to group sessions can be used to measure time in the group. The marketing wisdom that people vote with their feet also applies to groups; these simple measures of attendance and promptness can indicate to what degree people are voting with their feet.

Observational measures of participation in the group can be as straightforward as tally marks to record the frequency of group member participation. Rose (1984) recommends recording who in the group is speaking every 10 seconds. Somewhat more complex observational systems record the patterns of speaking, such as whether members are addressing the group, the leader, or one particular member. These measures of participation, much easier to learn and use than other observational systems such as the Hill Interaction Matrix, systematize what many group leaders and researchers treat as anecdotal data.

FUTURE DIRECTIONS

The knowledge and tools to measure outcomes for members participating in groups have advanced, both in the research and in the practice arenas. Although a number of tools exist for assessing group processes, they have not been subjected to the same rigorous use or testing as measures of outcome. The larger problem, however, is that the conceptual definitions of group conditions are still amorphous. Progress has been made; for example, Bonito (2002) tackled the methodological and conceptual issues involved in understanding and analyzing participation in groups. This is a good first step for one of the multitude of variables that have been identified as relevant to understanding groups. Similarly, researchers too often conduct rigorous studies in which a group is the context for the intervention but no measures are made of the group condition. This ignores both the context of the intervention and the possible confounding nature of group variables on outcome. Finally, there are a number of new and complex statistical techniques for analyzing nonlinear and dependent data. Although these statistical techniques offer researchers tools for analysis, their complexity may create a further divide between research and practice.

The *Oxford English Dictionary* (2003) lists one of the earliest uses of the word "measurement" in the 17th century. One of the definitions is "a magnitude, quantity, or extent calculated by the application of an instrument or device marked in standard units." This chapter has discussed the instruments as applied to groups. Measurement need not be a complex undertaking, but it needs to be systematic, with a set of associated standards. Measurement is necessary for understanding what is occurring in groups and with group members. The choice is what to measure and how, not whether to measure.

REFERENCES

Agazarian, Y. M. (1992). Contemporary theories of group psychotherapy: A systems approach to the group-as-a-whole. *International Journal of Group Psychotherapy, 42,* 177–203.

Anthony, J. L., & O'Brien, W. H. (2002). The effects of a group-based social support intervention on cardiovascular reactivity. *Small Group Research, 33*(2), 155–180.

Barcikowski, R. S. (1981). Statistical power with group mean as the unit of analysis. *Journal of Educational Statistics, 6,* 267–285.

Barlow, D. H., Hayes, S. C., & Nelson, R. O. (1984). *The scientist practitioner*. New York: Pergamon Press.

Beck, A. P., & Lewis, C. M. (2000). *The process of group psychotherapy: Systems for analyzing change*. Washington, DC: American Psychological Association.

Bednar, R. L., & Kaul, T. J. (1994). Experiential group research: Can the canon fire? In A. E. Bergin & S. L. Garfield (Eds.), *Handbook of psychotherapy and behavior change* (4th ed., pp. 631–663). New York: Wiley.

Berg, B. L. (1998). *Qualitative research methods for the social sciences* (3rd ed.). Boston: Allyn & Bacon.

Bloom, M., Fischer, J., & Orme, J. G. (1999). *Evaluating practice: Guidelines for the accountable professional*. Boston: Allyn & Bacon.

Bonito, J. A. (2002). The analysis of participation in small groups: Methodological and conceptual issues related to interdependence. *Small Group Research, 33*(4), 412–438.

Butler, T., & Fuhriman, A. (1983). Level of functioning and length of time in treatment variables influencing patients' therapeutic experience in group psychotherapy. *International Journal of Group Psychotherapy, 33*, 489–505.

Christensen, L., & Mendoza, J. L. (1986). A method of assessing change in a single subject: An alteration of the RC index. *Behavior Therapy, 17*, 305–308.

Coyne, R. K. (1999). *Failures in group work: How we can learn from our mistakes*. Thousand Oaks, CA: Sage.

Dies, R. R., & Teleska, P.A. (1985). Negative outcome in group psychotherapy. In D. T. Mays & C. M. Franks (Eds.), *Negative outcome in psychotherapy and what to do about it* (pp. 118–141). New York: Springer.

Feldman, R. A., Caplinger, T. E., & Wodarski, J. S. (1983). *The St. Louis conundrum: The effective treatment of antisocial youths*. Englewood Cliffs, NJ: Prentice-Hall.

Felix-Ortiz, M., Salazar, M. R., Gonzalez, J. R., Sorensen, J. L., & Plock, D. (2000). Addictions services: A qualitative evaluation of an assisted self-help group for drug-addicted clients in a structured outpatient treatment setting. *Community Mental Health Journal, 36*, 339–350.

Festinger, L., Schachter, S., & Back, K. (1950). *Social pressures in informal group: A study of human factors in housing*. Palo Alto, CA: Stanford University Press.

Fuhriman, A., & Barlow, S. H. (1983). Cohesion: Relationship in group therapy. In M. J. Lambert (Ed.), *A guide to psychotherapy and patient relationships* (pp. 263–289). Homewood, IL: Dow Jones, Irwin.

Fuhriman, A., Drescher, S., Hanson, E., Henrie, R., & Rybicki, W. (1986). Refining the measurement of curativeness: An empirical approach. *Small Group Behavior, 77*, 186–201.

Fuhriman, A., & Packard, T. (1986). Group process instruments: Therapeutic themes and issues. *International Journal of Group Psychotherapy, 36*(3), 399–425.

Garvin, C. D. (1997). *Contemporary group work* (3rd ed.). Boston: Allyn & Bacon.

Gibbs, L. E. (2003). *Evidence-based practice for the helping professions: A practical guide with integrated multimedia*. Pacific Grove, CA: Brooks/Cole.

Glisson, C. (1986). The group versus the individual as the unit of analysis in small group research. *Social Work with Groups, 9*, 15–30.

Goldstein, H. (1992). Should social workers base practice decisions on empirical research? No. In E. Gambrill & R. Pruger (Eds.), *Controversial issues in social work* (pp. 114–120). Boston: Allyn & Bacon.

Heil, R. A. (1992). A comparative analysis of therapeutic factors in self-help groups (Alcoholics Anonymous, Overeaters Anonymous). *Dissertation Abstracts International, 53* (08), 4373B. (UMI No. AAG9226528)

Hepler, J. B. (1994). Evaluating the effectiveness of a social skills program for preadolescents. *Research on Social Work Practice, 4*(4), 411–435.

Hudson, W. W. (1990a). *MPSI starter kit*. Tallahassee, FL: WALMYR.

Hudson, W. W. (1990b). *WALMYR classroom training package*. Tallahassee, FL: WALMYR.

Jacobson, N. A., Follette, W. C., & Ravenstorf, D. (1984). Psychotherapy outcome research: Methods for reporting variability and evaluating clinical significance. *Behavior Therapy, 15*, 336–352.

Jacobson, N. A., Follette, W. C., & Ravenstorf, D. (1986). Toward a standard definition of clinically significant change. *Behavior Therapy, 17*, 308–311.

Jayaratne, S. (1990). Clinical significance: Problems and new developments. In L. Videka-Sherman & W. J. Reid (Eds.), *Advances in clinical social work research* (pp. 271–285). Silver Springs, MD: National Association of Social Workers.

Kaul, T. J., & Bednar, R. L. (1986). Experiential group research: Results, questions, and suggestions. In S. L. Garfield & A. E. Bergin (Eds.), *Handbook of psychotherapy and behavior change* (3rd. ed., pp. 671–714). New York: Wiley.

Kurtz, L. F. (1997). *Self-help and support groups: A handbook for practitioners.* Thousand Oaks, CA: Sage.

Lieberman, M. A., & Borman, L. D. (1979). *Self-help groups for coping with crisis: Origins, members processes, and impact.* San Francisco: Jossey-Bass.

Lieberman, M. A., Yalom, I. D., & Miles, M. B. (1973). *Encounter groups: First facts.* New York: Basic Books.

Macgowan, M. J. (1997). A measure of engagement for social groupwork: The groupwork engagement measure (GEM). *Journal of Social Service Research, 23*(2), 17–37.

Macgowan, M. J. (2000). Evaluation of a measure of engagement for group work. *Research on Social Work Practice, 10* (3), 348–362.

Macgowan, M. J., & Levenson, J. S. (2003). Psychometrics of the group engagement measure with male sex offenders. *Small Group Research, 34*(2), 155–160.

MacKenzie, K. R. (1987). Therapeutic factors in group psychotherapy: A contemporary view. *Group, 11*(1), 26–34.

MacNair-Semands, R. R., & Lese, K. P. (2000). Interpersonal problems and the perception of therapeutic factors in group therapy. *Small Group Research, 31*(2), 158–174.

Magen, R. H., & Rose, S. D. (1994). Parents in groups: Problem solving versus behavioral skill training. *Research on Social Work Practice, 4*(2), 172–191.

Maton, K. I. (1993). Moving beyond the individual level of analysis in mutual help group research: An ecological paradigm. *Journal of Applied Behavioral Science, 29*, 272–286.

Monette, D. R., Sullivan, T. J., & DeJong, C. R. (2002). *Applied social research: Tool for the human services* (5th ed.). Fort Worth, TX: Harcourt.

Moos, R. H. (1986). *Group Environment Scale manual* (2nd ed.). Palo Alto, CA: Consulting Psychologists Press.

Morran, D. K., Robison, F. F., & Hulse-Killacky, D. (1990). Group research and the unit of analysis problem: The use of ANOVA designs with nested factors. *Journal for Specialists in Group Work, 15*, 10–14.

National Association of Social Workers. (1999). *Code of ethics.* Washington, DC: Author.

Oxford English Dictionary. (2003). Retrieved May 10, 2003 from: *http://dictionary.oed.com.*

Pollack, B. N. (1998). Hierarchical linear modeling and the "unit of analysis" problem: A solution for analyzing responses of intact group members. *Group Dynamics: Theory, Research and Practice, 2*, 299–312.

Rose, S. D. (1984). Use of data in identifying and resolving group problems in goal oriented treatment groups. *Social Work with Groups, 7*, 23–36.

Rose, S. D., & Edleson, J. L. (1987). *Working with children and adolescents in groups: A multimethod approach.* San Francisco: Jossey-Bass.

Rose, S. D., Tolman, R., & Tallant, S. (1985). Group process in cognitive-behavioral therapy. *Behavior Therapist, 8* (4), 71–75.

Smokowski, P. R., Rose, S., Todar, K., & Reardon, K. (1999). Postgroup-casualty status, group events, and leader behavior: An early look into the dynamics of damaging group experiences. *Research on Social Work Practice, 9*, 555–574.

Taggar, S., & Brown, T. C. (2001). Problem-solving team behaviors: Development and validation of BOS and a hierarchical factor structure. *Small Group Research, 32*(6), 698–726.

Weinberg, N., Uken, J. S., Schmale, J., & Adamek, M. (1995). Therapeutic factors: Their presence in a computer-mediated support group. *Social Work with Groups, 18*(4), 57–69.

Weinhardt, L. S., Forsyth, A. D., Carey, M. P., Jaworski, B. C., & Durant, L. E. (1998). Reliability and validity of self-report measures of HIV-related sexual behavior: Progress since 1990 and recommendations for research and practice. *Archives of Sexual Behavior, 27*(2), 155–180.

Whipple, E. E. (1999). Reaching families with preschoolers at risk for physical child abuse: What works? *Families in Society, 80*, 148–160.

Whitney, D., & Rose, S. D. (1989). The effect of process and structural content on outcome in stress management groups. *Journal of Social Service Research, 13*, 89–104.

Williams, D. D. R., & Garner, J. (2002). The case against "the evidence": A different perspective on evidence-based medicine. *British Journal of Psychiatry, 180*, 8–12.

Witkin, S. (1996). If empirical practice is the answer, then what is the question? *Social Work, 46*, 109–119.

Yalom, I. D. (1995). *The theory and practice of group psychotherapy* (4th ed.). New York: Basic Books.

Chapter 27

Evaluation of Group Work

Larry M. Gant

This chapter describes the evaluation of various group approaches found in published academic and professional literature. First presented is a general statement of the task, followed by a brief overview of the distinctions between program evaluation and clinical research paradigms. A strategy for selecting a focused sample of published evaluation accounts of group work intervention is presented. The remainder of the chapter is devoted to a discussion of evaluation approaches and findings across published accounts of group work interventions. The chapter concludes with an assessment of the current state of the art of evolution of group work interventions and suggestions for future directions.

STATEMENT OF THE TASK

In an age of declining fiscal resources for social supportive services, program and service providers are increasingly requested to justify the funds for social programs by reporting the effectiveness of the programs. Calls for "research-based practice" or "evidence-based practice" mandate—in ways never before seen—that program providers demonstrate significant change beyond chance computation (the purview of clinical research) or at the very least provide evidence that answers the question, "does it work or not," without the trappings of randomized clinical trials (the purview of evaluation). Calls for time-limited interventions further underscore the emphasis. Indeed, there is little evidence that the social service professions and their respective funders will return to earlier times of funding programs that "should" and "ought" to work; programs will need to demonstrate effectiveness or face some kind of sanction. Some argue that very few programs are actually terminated due to demonstrated program ineffectiveness (e.g., D.A.R.E. and Empowerment Zone reconstruction). It is not surprising that this holds even more true for programs with some champion in influential places than for programs with no such champion. It appears to be a statement of some accuracy that group-level interventions have few visible champions or spokespersons of influence. Hence the greater vulnerability, and thus the greater importance of demonstration of effect.

DISTINGUISHING PROGRAM EVALUATION
FROM CLINICAL RESEARCH

There is no more confusing conflation of terms to lay audiences involved in the "evidence-based practice" debate than that of program evaluation with clinical research. Perhaps evaluators have done a better task of speaking to each other than to other populations. Nonetheless, a brief discussion of evaluation here complements the superb discussion of clinical research found elsewhere in this volume.

The purpose of evaluation, according to Rossi (1999, p. 4) is to "investigate the effectiveness of social intervention programs." Program evaluation is generally used to (1) decide whether to accept a new program or service; (2) decide whether to continue, change, or eliminate an existing program or service; (3) examine the uniformity of program implementation with program plan; (4) assess the overall value of a program; or (5) help funders and stakeholders determine the ways in which issues are being solved or needs met (Piontek, 2003). More specifically, program evaluation "is the systematic collection of information about the activities, characteristics and outcomes of programs to make judgments, and/or inform decisions about future programming" (Piontek, 2003, p. 4). *Formative evaluation* is typically conducted during the operation of a program, providing information useful in improving and enhancing the program. *Summative evaluation* is conducted at the end of a program and provides a judgment about the effectiveness, worth, or merit of a program or activity.

Program evaluation differs from basic scientific research in at least two important ways: (1) the purpose of data collection and (2) the standards for judging validity. As to the *purpose of data collection*, program evaluation is done with an intent to inform decisions, clarify options, specify improvements, and provide information about programs and policies within the social and political context. Research is done to seek out new knowledge, engage in theory testing, confirm or disconfirm hypotheses, and generalize findings (Piontek, 2003; Rossi, 1999).

For the purposes of this discussion, validity can be operationally defined as the work being accepted as accurate, reliable, and exact. The validity of scientific research relies primarily on the methods of design, data collection, and analysis strategies used. The validity of program evaluation includes not only the methodology of the work but also the approach of the evaluation, the role of the evaluator, and the presentation of results and findings. The evaluation and the evaluator must both be perceived as reliable for the evaluation to be of optimal value.

Evaluations of group work can be quite complex; group-level interventions can be evaluated on a number of levels. For example, the evaluation can be taken from the perspective of the client, the group leader, or both. The evaluation can focus on individual change, group process, or the influence of the leader on the group interactions. Finally, group work evaluations can vary in foci, including accreditation, compliance, effectiveness, efficiency, equity, process, and impact (Patton, 1997, pp. 192–194).

DISCUSSION OF METHOD:
A SELECTIVE INQUIRY, NOT A META-ANALYSIS

We set the reader's mind at ease—but risk distress as well—with our intent to review a selection of evaluation studies of group work. This chapter is clearly not intended to be either a comprehensive review of all group work evaluation or a meta-analysis of the same. There certainly exist meta-analyses of social work practices with some emphasis on group work, and we refer the reader to these (e.g., Black, Tobler, & Sciacca, 1998; Borman & D'Agostino, 1996; Lipsey & Wilson, 1993; Witt & Crompton, 1996). Meta-analyses properly aggregate studies that have at least aspects of rigorous research design, including but not limited to random assignments to experimental and control conditions, systematic assignment to comparison groups, rigorous experimental designs, sample size computations, statistical analysis, and multiple data collection intervals (Rossi, 1999). Ironically, the exacting nature of most meta-analyses results in a greatly delimited number of clinical studies. Not surprisingly, as group-level interventions tend not to be funded by large research grants or research institutes, the methods for evaluation are not equivalent to the rigorous experimental designs or analyses required by many forms of meta-analysis.

We instead selected a different direction. What does an informed, somewhat more specific identification and review of studies evaluating group interventions—using any type of evaluation approach or design—yield beyond a call for more rigorous meta-evaluations?

Conceptualization of Group Work Tasks, Approaches, and Theoretical Models

The search for group work intervention studies was informed by conceptualization of group approaches, relevant change theories, and the group-level intervention task at hand. We were aided by adapting Garvin's (1997) work in group work classification with Prochaska and Norcross's (1994) transtheoretical model of change. Although controversial, Prochaska's model allows an efficient classification and coordination of intervention tasks and therapeutic approaches. Although the model has received ongoing change and modifications, we use the more classic spiral classification articulated by Prochaska, Norcross, and DiClemente (1994) (see Table 27.1).

Types of Intervention Tasks

Groups are used to help people address a variety of intervention tasks. The following tasks are illustrative and representative:

1. *Identifying problem to be solved.* Groups can increase personal awareness of problems or issues without personal accusation or prejudgment and with a normalization and destigmatization of the issue. Depending on the approach, groups can facilitate the personal location of problem cause, problem resolution, or both.
2. *Deciding to solve the problem.* In groups, people with low motivation to resolve problem issues can find ways and support to increase motivational levels to address the problem or issue.
3. *Planning for problem solving.* Persons learn in groups how to identify problems and employ problem-solving methods to generate, assess, and implement solutions.
4. *Active problem solving.* Groups can provide a wide variety of strategies for change, along with ways to implement and monitor the change efforts.
5. *Maintaining problem-solving strategies.* Groups can be more effective than individuals in working to sustain and support personal change efforts. Groups can also provide support in the face of personal lapse or relapse.

TABLE 27.1. Group Work Types of Intervention Tasks and Approaches

Types of intervention tasks	Group work approaches
Identifying problem to be solved	Consciousness raising Helping relationships Social liberation
Deciding to solve the problem	Emotional arousal Self-reevaluation
Planning for problem solving	Self-reevaluation Commitment Social support
Active problem solving	Countering Environmental control Reward Social support
Maintaining problem-solving strategies	Social support

Note. After Prochaska, Norcross, and DiClemente (1994).

Group Approaches

These approaches can be used in group work, with some approaches more directly applicable to certain types of intervention tasks than others (Prochaska, Norcross, & DiClemente, 1994):

- *Consciousness raising.* The most common of change processes, characterized by efforts to raise level of awareness, by increasing amount of useful information provided, and by improving the likelihood of intelligent decisions concerning the problem.
- *Social liberation.* The availability of new alternatives in the local environment that provides impetus to change behaviors, such as no-smoking areas as an alternative atmosphere for nonsmokers and those working to attain nonsmoking status. Social liberation not only makes actions related to change possible but also increases self-efficacy as people come to believe in their own ability to change.
- *Emotional arousal.* Efforts and techniques designed to create an emotional experience related to the current problem. The goal of such approaches as psychodrama or role play is to increase awareness and depth of feeling as an individual moves toward some type of change.
- *Self-reevaluation.* These processes require the generation of a considered or thoughtful reassessment of the problem and an assessment of how the person changes when the behavior is changed.
- *Commitment.* These activities result in the acceptance of responsibility for changing patterns of thought and behavior. Also termed "self-liberation," groups can support the acknowledgement of personal commitment for personal change.
- *Social support.* Efforts to secure external supports to review, apply, and reinforce processes and techniques of personal change.
- *Countering.* Active processes and strategies for substituting healthy responses for unhealthy responses. Also known as counterconditioning.

- *Environmental control.* Action efforts for restructuring personal environments to reduce probability of problem-causing events.
- *Rewards.* Actions and strategies that reward successful efforts to change behavior.

How the Sample of Studies Was Selected

We used a combination of methods to (1) identify journals publishing evaluation reports of group interventions and (2) systematically review selected journal articles. Although the strategies are certainly open to criticism and debate, we were nonetheless able to generate a useful set of articles for review and discussion.

Identifying Journals

Our task was to identify journals that publish evaluation reports of group interventions. We settled, somewhat arbitrarily, on evaluation reports published within the 2 years (2001–2003) previous to the writing of this chapter. We then identified two general academic and professional disciplines within social science that would likely yield relevant journals and articles: those of program evaluation and social work. We then accessed the Institute for Scientific Information (ISI) *Journal Citation Reports (JCR), Social Sciences Edition*, located within the ISI Web portal, Web of Knowledge. The *Social Sciences Edition* contains data from roughly 1,500 journals in the social sciences.

After identifying the fields of social work and program evaluation, we ranked the reported journals in each area by "impact factor." Briefly, the journal impact factor is a measure of the frequency with which the "average" article in a journal has been cited in a particular year. This helps evaluate the relative importance of a journal compared with others in the same field. We calculated the impact factor by dividing the number of current citations of articles in the journal in the 2 years we selected by the total number of articles published in the 2 years.

This allowed us to generate a ranking of the 20 most influential journals in social work and program evaluation. We then took these lists and ranked them by number of published evaluations of group work interventions. Unfortunately, this second ranking identified in only one journal (*Research on Social Work Practice*) that reported more than one published article on group work evaluation within the time frame identified, among either program evaluation or social work journals.

We then consulted leading group work texts, reviewing all chapters that addressed research and evaluation of group work programs. We also reviewed the entries on group work in the latest edition of the *Encyclopedia of Social Work*. This second effort was significantly more successful. We identified the following journals as having published at least three evaluation articles within the 2001–2003 time period: *Small Group Research* (four evaluation studies), *Research on Social Work Practice* (three evaluation studies), *Social Work with Groups* (six evaluation studies), and *Journal of Specialists in Group Work* (five evaluation studies).

In many respects, these articles were sound and well written. Although we were pleased to find journals publishing group work evaluation studies, we noted with some concern that only one of them—*Research on Social Work Practice*—was ranked within the top 20 social work journals as determined by the impact factor (ranked no. 14). The other journals were not even part of the *JCR Social Sciences* database. It seems all too likely that these reports may be somewhat difficult to find, and therefore to integrate into practice, unless a motivated individual knows precisely what to look for and how to obtain it.

Reviewing Journal Articles

Both Rossi (1999) and Piontek (2003) specify guidelines for the review of program evaluations, and we incorporated these. These guidelines are capably articulated by Royse (1999), who outlines the following criteria of published evaluation articles:

- Clear explanation of the problem and program response.
- Thorough literature review of the problem and program response.
- Stated reliability and validity of measures and data collection.
- Clear discussion of client recruitment.
- Detailed methodological procedures.
- Accessible statistical data analysis and presentation.
- Explicit implications for practice.

We also reviewed studies within the context of the Program Evaluation Standards—accuracy, feasibility, propriety, and utility (Joint Committee on Standards for Educational Evaluation, 1994). Table 27.2 provides a summary of these standards.

Each of the articles was reviewed, assessed, and discussed by three readers (one professor and two master's students) using the eight criteria listed. Each of the articles was categorized very simply as to the presence or absence of each criterion in each article. Thus the minimum rating possible was 0, and the maximum rating possible was 8. Each of the articles was also reviewed, to the extent possible, using the program evaluation standards. The list of articles reviewed is given in Table 27.3.

For the purposes of this chapter, we generated two clusters of articles. Articles in Cluster 1 reflected at least six of the eight items in the Royse (1999) checklist. Articles in Cluster 2 contained less than three items from the checklist. Generally speaking, articles in the clusters tended to reflect the same items; for instance, the Cluster 2 articles tended to reflect the same three checklisted items across all articles. We report the clusters in Table 27.4.

Table 27.5 presents a simple categorization of journals by cluster type. Not surprisingly, all articles published in two journals that explicitly solicit manuscripts with a research base,

TABLE 27.2. Program Evaluation Standards

Standards	Description
Accuracy	To insure that an evaluation will reveal and convey technically adequate information about the features that determine worth or merit of the program being evaluated.
Propriety	To insure that an evaluation will be conducted legally, ethically, and with due regard for the welfare of those involved in the evaluation, as well as those affected by its results.
Feasibility	To insure that an evaluation will be realistic, prudent, diplomatic, and frugal.
Utility	To insure that an evaluation will serve the information needs of intended users.

Note. After Joint Committee on Standards for Educational Evaluation (1994).

TABLE 27.3. Articles Reviewed

Journal of Specialists in Group Work (2001)
- "The Qualitative Exploration of Process-Sensitive Peer Group Supervision" (Christensen & Kline, 2001)
- "Prevention Groups for Angry and Aggressive Children" (Schechtman, 2001)
- "Team Brothers: An Afrocentric Approach to Group Work with African American Male Adolescents" (Franklin & Pack-Brown, 2001)
- "Using the Group for the Prevention of Eating Disorders Among College Women" (Sapia, 2001)
- "Providing Mental Health Services to Southeast Asian Adolescent Girls" (Queener & Kenyon, 2001)

International Journal of Group Psychotherapy (2001)
- "Treatment of Non-Incarcerated Sexually Compulsive/Addictive Offenders in an Integrated, Mulitmodal and Psychodynamic Group Therapy Model" (Lothstein, 2001)

Social Work with Groups (2001, vol. 24, nos. 1–4)
- "Enhancing Psychosocial Competence among Black Women" (Jones & Hodges, 2001)
- "Camps as Social Work Interventions" (Mishna & Mickalski, 2001)
- "The Effectiveness of Self-Help Groups in a Chinese Context" (Mok, 2001b)
- "Using Group Therapy to Enhace Treatment Compliance" (Miller & Mason, 2001)
- "Dreaming Their Way into Life" (Goelitz, 2001)
- "Divorce Support Groups" (Oygard & Hardeng, 2001)

Research on Social Work Practice (2002)
- "The Effectiveness of an Integrated Treatment Approach for Clients with Dual Diagnoses" (DiNitto et al., 2002)
- "Couples Who Care: The Effectiveness of a Psychoeducational Group Intervention with HIV Serodiscordant Couples" (Pomeroy & Green, 2002)
- "An Evaluation of Men's Batterer Treatment Groups" (Tutty & Bidgood, 2001)

Small Group Research (2002)
- "The Effects of a Group-Based Social Support Intervention on Cardiovascular Reactivity" (Anthony & O'Brien, 2002)
- "The Relationship of Group Process Variables and Team Performance" (Jordan et al., 2002)
- "Children's Learning Groups: A Study of Emergent Leadership, Dominance, and Group Effectiveness" (Yamaguchi, 2001)
- "Cancer Self-Help Groups in China: A Study of Individual Change, Perceived Benefit, and Community Impact" (Mok, 2001a)

Small Group Research and *Research on Social Work Practice*, were located in Cluster 1. All other journals were located in both clusters. At the very least, it is clear that evaluations of varying quality can be found in journals identified as having a group focus and that higher quality evaluations of group work are probably more consistently found in the two research-based journals.

FINDINGS

Cluster 1

The articles in this cluster reflect exemplars of published evaluations of group interventions. Consistently across the articles, readers were presented with clear context, detailed explanations of rationale, purpose, methodology, and analysis, ending with clear implications for practice implementation. The articles provide good evidence for tangible outcomes. Mok's (2001a,b) surveys of self-help group participants in mainland China provide clear cultural and historical context for the concepts of self-help, and clearly identify the roles and func-

TABLE 27.4. Articles by Identified Clusters

Cluster 1

- "The Effectiveness of an Integrated Treatment Approach for Clients with Dual Diagnoses" (DiNitto et al., 2002)
- "Cancer Self-Help Groups in China" (Mok, 2001a)
- "Couples Who Care: The Effectiveness of a Psychoeducational Group Intervention for HIV Serodiscordant Couples" (Pomeroy & Green, 2002)
- "The Effects of a Group-Based Social Support Intervention on Cardiovascular Reactivity" (Anthony & O'Brien, 2002)
- "Divorce Support Groups: How Do Group Characteristics Influence Adjustment to Divorce?" (Oygard & Hardeng, 2001)
- "An Evaluation of Men's Batterer Treatment Groups" (Tutty & Bidgood, 2001)
- "The Qualitative Exploration of Process-Sensitive Peer Group Supervision" (Christensen & Kline, 2001)
- "Using Groups for Prevention of Eating Disorders Among College Women" (Sapia, 2001)
- "Enhancing Psychosocial Competence Among Black Women" (Jones & Hodges, 2001)
- "Using Group Therapy to Enhance Treatment Compliance in First Episode Schizophrenia" (Miller & Mason, 2001)
- "The Effectiveness of Self-Help Groups in a Chinese Context" (Mok, 2001b)
- "Camp as Social Work Interventions: Returning to our Roots" (Mishna & Mickalski, 2001)

Cluster 2

- "Prevention Groups for Angry and Aggressive Children" (Schechtman, 2001)
- "Dreaming Their Way into Life: A Group Experience with Oncology Patients" (Goelitz, 2001)
- "TEAM Brothers: An Afrocentric Approach to Group Work with African American Male Adolescents" (Franklin & Pack-Brown, 2001)
- "Providing Mental Health Services to Southeast Asian Adolescent Girls: Integration of a Primary Prevention Paradigm and Group Counseling" (Queener & Kenyon, 2001)

---

tions of the self-help groups for cancer survivors (Mok, 2001a) and for participants in self-help groups for individuals with chronic physical and emotional diagnoses (Mok, 2001b).

Oygard and Hardeng's (2001) study of divorce support groups correlates participants' identification of characteristics of successful support groups with self-ratings of psychosocial adjustment (using nonstandardized rating scales) and control by gender. A thoughtful collection of participation variables (e.g., size of group, frequency of meetings, facilitator style, and group support) provides contextual analysis. Findings and implications complete a very accessible evaluation of the program. Sapia's (2001) evaluation of a group interven-

TABLE 27.5. Journal Representation in Identified Clusters

Cluster	Title	Total number of articles	Total number of articles in cluster
Cluster 1	*Research on Social Work Practice* (2002)	3	3
	Small Group Research (2002)	4	4
	Social Work with Groups (2001, vol. 24, nos. 1–4):	6	4
	International Journal of Group Psychotherapy (2001)	1	1
	Journal of Specialists in Group Work (2001)	5	2
Cluster 2	*Social Work with Groups* (2001, vol. 24, nos. 1–4)	6	2
	Journal of Specialists in Group Work (2001)	5	3

tion for prevention of eating disorders among college women provides a succinct literature review and background of the problem and delineates the theory of action behind the group intervention.

Experimental and quasi-experimental designs are also represented—perhaps proportionately—in the Cluster 1 evaluations. We have noted elsewhere the distinctions between research and evaluation. Yet we found two evaluations that used randomized clinical research designs (Anthony & O'Brien, 2002; DiNitto, Webb, & Robin, 2002). Interestingly, these were the two studies that revealed null effects between interventions and control conditions. Anthony and O'Brien (2002) found no differences between client outcomes of physical and psychological stress and assignment to social support or wait-list control interventions. In DiNitto et al. (2002), clients with dual diagnoses of substance abuse and mental illness were randomly assigned to psychoeducational or standard group interventions; outcomes were nonsignificant. In this study, a quasi-experimental nonequivalent control group design with random assignment into groups is supplemented with a brief discussion of measures used (but with no discussion of psychometric properties). The intervention and procedures are clearly described, with a brief but efficient presentation of statistical analysis and computed effect size.

Tutty and Bidgood (2001) provide an evaluation of 104 participants in 15 treatment groups for male batterers. The theoretical underpinnings of the group intervention are well articulated, with multiple data collection points. Psychometric properties of outcome measures for self-esteem, social support and isolation, abusive behavior, attitudes toward marriage and the family, and social desirability are clearly explained. Percent of variance explained (due to the intervention) ranges from 6 to 30%, with no difference in effect between court-mandated and non-court-mandated participants.

Mishna and Mickalski's (2001) study of camp interventions for 96 youths with learning disabilities and psychosocial problems provides a rich discussion of the role of camps in social work interventions with children and youths. The intervention is provided in considerable detail. Data for 48 children (ages 10–13) and 48 youths (ages 14–18) were collected in a traditional pre-and post-intervention follow-up design, with 3 weeks between pre- and posttests and a 6- to 8-month follow-up period. Three standardized measures of self-esteem, social skills, and social isolation were used, with reports of measure reliability and validity. Children completed two measures, and their parents completed a third. Findings are summarized in narrative fashion without tables or charts, which makes interpretation challenging but not impossible. Findings and conclusions flow clearly from the data analysis.

Although the majority of Cluster 1 evaluations were quantitative in approach and analysis, three evaluations reflected a clearly qualitative design. Two of the evaluations (Christensen & Klien, 2001; Yamaguchi, 2001) began with a grounded theory approach that obtains both information and concepts for theory construction from interviews with program participants (Lincoln & Guba, 1985). The approach utilizes established techniques and procedures reflecting substantial degrees of precision, verification, and rigor (Strauss & Corbin, 1990). Using this approach, Yamaguchi (2001) examines the effects on youths of performing math tasks in mastery or performance conditions. Yamaguchi details context, procedures, and findings and provides a comprehensive explanation of qualitative methods in content analysis. Christensen and Kline's (2001) analysis of process-specific peer-group supervision provides a denser presentation of qualitative methods but delineates the content analysis procedure in reasonable detail and provides lucid context and implications of program impact and future evaluation. Jones and Hodges's (2001) qualitative assessment of a psychoeducational program for African American women is capably identified as a case study, distinguishing this approach among other qualitative strategies. Clearly identified as a formative evaluation, Jones and Hodges's work provides a rationale for such programs and outlines a preliminary set of conceptual and implementation issues via two vignettes.

We note that several of these Cluster 1 evaluations included measures of effect size or percent variance explained (Anthony & O'Brien, 2002; DiNitto et al., 2002; Pomeroy and Green, 2002; Sapia, 2001; Tutty & Bidgood, 2002). As all three articles were published in *Research on Social Work Practice*, it is possible that the authors responded to an editorial request. Regardless of the source of the request, the evaluators had the data and the resources to generate these effect size scores and variance ratios. We also found three published well-designed studies of null findings (Anthony & O'Brien, 2002; DiNitto et al., 2002; Tutty & Bidgood, 2002 [partial null findings]), which we hope suggests the increasing willingness of evaluators to submit studies with null findings and the willingness of journal editors to publish them, countering the bias of evaluators and journals toward publishing reports of only effective interventions and programs.

Finally, we note the predominance of university researchers as authors of these evaluations. As reflected in the published accounts, the conceptual and technological resources needed to deploy such a high level of evaluation work are more likely found in such research institutes and less so outside of academic institutions.

Cluster 2

Group work evaluation articles in this cluster differed substantially from those in Cluster 1 in three specific ways. First, the evaluation articles listed in Cluster 2 reported far less detailed procedures than did the articles in Cluster 1. For example, Franklin and Pack-Brown (2001) explained the historical and cultural perspectives of being African American but did not discuss procedures of the group intervention. Second, these articles reported almost no discussion of the reliability and validity of the test and measures used in the evaluations. Third, the evaluations reflected a lack of discussion of either methodology or data analysis or both.

Queener and Kenyon's (2001) evaluation of a group-based mental health psychoeducational program for Southeast Asian adolescent girls reflects an impressive discussion of the cultural and gender-related issues in this population, with capable discussion of the access barriers to mental health services. The composition of the two groups by acculturation and language proficiency is clearly discussed, with reasonable explanation of the measures used to assess acculturation (Cultural Identity Survey) and language proficiency (self-report). Psychometrics of the Cultural Identity Survey are not reported. The six sessions that make up the group intervention are described in depth. The evaluation of the intervention consisted of completion of a nonstandardized 6-item Likert-type scale. The evaluation is limited, with a focus on discussions of the challenges facing white facilitators of group intervention sessions for Southeast Asian female youths with varying degrees of acculturation and English-language fluency.

Similarly, Franklin and Pack-Brown's (2001) discussion of a school-based group empowerment intervention for African American teen males (2001) is strongest in establishing the need for the program and description of the TEAM Brothers intervention. Outcomes of the 23 session program were assessed by teachers' pre- and posttest ratings using a Teacher Evaluation of Students' Classroom Behaviors (TESCB) instrument. Psychometric properties were unreported. Data were presented for nine participants clustered in two groups: regular attendance (at least 21 sessions attended) and sporadic attendance (7–12 sessions attended).

The small sample size prevents statistical analysis, although percent changes between pretest and posttest scores are reported, with average decreases in behavioral reports of 40% for regular attendees and 10% for sporadic attendees.

Schechtman's (2001) evaluation of prevention groups for angry and aggressive elementary school children uses extremely small groups ($n = 4$). The context and procedures of the group and group process are well described. The empirical results are provided in two small paragraphs; Shechtman presents scores from standardized measures of childhood empathy and aggression with a very delimited explanation of findings.

Miller and Mason (2001) provide an extensive discussion of background information about nonadherence to medication regiment and the relationship to dropout rates and effectiveness of group intervention. However, the researchers provide a very preliminary analysis, demonstrating the far lower dropout rates of 65 clients in group treatment (15%) compared with 12 clients in individual treatment (67%). To their credit, the researchers provide extensive delimitations of the study.

Goelitz's (2001) study of group dream work interventions for cancer survivors (2001) provides details on background and significance, a good discussion of the three-session intervention and group configuration (5 participants), and an interesting if nonempirical presentation and interpretation of member dreams and resultant therapeutic work. The conclusion about the effectiveness of dream work as an intervention tool seems unsupported by the evidence.

The challenge with Cluster 2 evaluations lies in an appreciation of context. Despite their titles, the reports are far less evaluations and more narrations and descriptions of context and program response in group work. These studies should be considered for what they provide and not critiqued for what they are not (evaluations). It is very possible that these studies, which share very few characteristics with Cluster 1 evaluations, were not intended to serve as exemplars of evaluation. We offer a modest suggestion to journal editors and reviewers that future reviews of such reports warrant article titles that do not connote the conduct of an evaluation per se.

A CODA ON SOCIAL JUSTICE AND EQUITY

Arguably, at least some social work traditions encourage interventions promoting social justice and equity as contextual, independent, or dependent variables (Garvin & Seabury, 1997). The notions of social justice are also articulated in an approach to evaluation known as empowerment evaluation (Fetterman, 2001). A social justice perspective in program evaluation can be addressed in two ways: evaluations that are *socially just* and evaluations done for the purpose of *social justice*. Tutty and Bidgood (2001) provide a prime example of a socially just evaluation. In their evaluation, the group method used a feminist theoretical model in order to combat men's trauma histories but also "the cultural, sociopolitical context that influences men's attitudes and gender roles [that] establish conditions that condone men abusing their partners" (Tutty & Bidgood, 2001, p. 647). Therefore, this intervention not only targets individual behavior but also targets and combats patriarchy. " Franklin and Pack-Brown (2001) is another socially just evaluation because it addresses the negative odds for African Americans in schools by empowering the participants through historical and cultural information about themselves.

With regard to evaluations done for social justice, Mok (2001a) develops his evaluation in such a way that he supports the historical and potential current-day use of self-help groups for social change and political activism. Additionally, DiNitto et al. (2002) give substantial information that advocates for the need for integrated approaches when dealing with mental illnesses and substance abuse. The evaluative model of this article promotes a harm reduction model. Such models endorse social justice, as harm reduction contextualizes understanding of an individual's social condition (e.g., substance abuse) as reflecting both personal and systematic/institutional dynamics while placing problem resolution as one largely of personal response. This evaluation report is also socially just in explaining the complexity and realities of relapse among substance abusers.

ASSESSMENT AND FUTURE TASKS: WHAT MAKES A GOOD EVALUATION OF GROUP WORK PRACTICE?

After carefully examining all of the articles, we find a bit of good news with some basic cautions. We were pleasantly surprised to discover the presence of a corpus of published evaluations of group work interventions. Most published accounts that we reviewed provided reasonable documentation of evaluation effectiveness. These articles reflected a clear rationale for the intervention and explained the methods, data collection, and analysis in understandable ways. We note the relative lack of discussion of validity and reliability of standardized measures and encourage the consistent reporting of these as a standard practice. Statistical analyses reflected simpler, main effects with some interactions reported. We were also pleased to note the increased availability of computed effect sizes. From a scientific perspective, group work evaluations are varied in the information that they provide, but they are by and large empirical. There also seems to be a need for more discussion on the reliability and validity of measures to properly assess the scientific significance of the evaluation results.

The driving forces of accountability, managed care, and quality assurance of services push the methodological standards of program evaluation. Clearly, the targets of evaluations continue to increase in importance. Thus program evaluation is ever more pushed toward adopting the gold standard of clinical research design—the randomized clinical trial. Randomized clinical trials provide the only robust response to the special set of internal validity threats with which evaluators of group work interventions must contend. Among these threats are nonequivalent controls, unit of analysis (group vs. individual member), and the consideration of group process as a variable (Garvin, 1997). The evaluations—particularly Cluster 1 evaluations—provided interesting and useful responses to these threats. Random assignment renders the issues of nonequivalent control groups and client matching moot (Anthony & O'Brien, 2002; DiNitto et al., 2002). Measures of group participation and process exist and can be incorporated as independent, moderating, or mediating variables according to theoretical placement (Oygard & Hardeng, 2001). Program effect can be reported at both the group and individual level, using effect sizes or percent of variance explained for group differences (Anthony & O'Brien, 2002; DiNitto et al., 2002; Pomeroy & Green, 2002; Sapia, 2001; Tutty & Bidgood, 2002).

There is no question that the problems plaguing the evaluation of group work interventions can be reasonably solved or at the very least considered. The less sanguine reality is that the required methodology is expensive and requires expertise not typically available in community-based organizations or agencies. Beyond this, the deployment of randomized clinical trials in natural settings of communities and organizations is extremely difficult and time-consuming. It is not inexpensive nor easy to do; it requires trained personnel and demands a high level of continuous oversight and monitoring. High-quality evaluations are thus possible but expensive and resource intensive. Funders and other audiences demanding clinical research designs need to understand this and provide funds for the very necessary, difficult, and expensive types of evaluation designs they demand. There are no short cuts to quality evaluation.

What, then, constitutes good group level evaluation? There is very little surprise in generating a minimum set of components of good group evaluation. At the very least, the evaluations in Cluster 1 suggest a classic list:

- Background and significance.
- Clear procedures and methodology, including:
  - Stated reliability and validity of measures and data collection
  - Clear discussion of client recruitment
  - Operationalization of organizational process
  - Detailed methodological procedures.
- Accessible and appropriate qualitative/quantitative data analysis and presentation, including effect size or percent variance explained.
- Clear connections between findings, analysis, and evaluation questions.

Although the preceding list can be used for either qualitative or quantitative analysis, and although we endorse the use of both forms of inquiry, we make the uncomfortable statement that quantitative methods have priority—at least here and now—in the ultimate empirical determination of program effect. Increasingly, qualitative methodologies can be quantified, analyzed (Christensen & Kline, 2001; Yamaguchi, 2001), and incorporated as quantitative variables in analysis. We leave to wiser heads the extensive and unresolved discussion of the merits and demerits of quantifying qualitative data (Strauss & Corbin, 1990).

Quasi-experimental designs—the hallmark of most program evaluation (Rossi, 1999)—have extraordinary merit, value, and worth. They should continue to be used extensively and supplemented with sophisticated statistical analysis and good, solid evaluation questions. At this time, however, the most definitive assessment of effect continues to be best answered with randomized clinical designs.

CONCLUSION

The empirical investigations of group research, characterized by randomized clinical studies, is discussed elsewhere (Brower, Arndt, & Ketterhagen, Chapter 25, this volume). The evaluation of group research continues apace, perhaps with fewer studies than are desirable, but with studies nonetheless. Although too few yet exist for any meaningful generalizability, the evaluation approaches persist across a continuum from formative to summative, with rather more summative than the former. At the very least, a tradition of evaluation of group work approaches exists and the work appears well done, with findings closely derived from analyses. The effect of group work approaches appears nicely demonstrated, with the more rigorous gold standard of randomized clinical trials awaiting greater technical sophistication, greater rigor, and, alas, more funding. In the final analysis, gold-standard evaluation and research comes neither cheaply nor easily. At the present, the level of analysis of group work evaluations is sufficient to offer a qualified "yes" to the question, "is group work intervention effective?" However, group work in general yet awaits better answers (perhaps with baited breath) to the follow-up question, "but compared to what?"

ACKNOWLEDGMENT

Thanks and appreciation to Tisha Fowler and Cindy Slagter, MSW students who provided extensive help in collecting and reviewing the articles.

REFERENCES

Anthony, J. L., & Brien, W. H. O. (2002). The effects of a group-based social support intervention on cardiovascular reactivity. *Small Group Research*, *33*(2), 155–180.

Black, D. R., Tobler, N. S., & Sciacca, J. P. (1998). Peer helping/involvement: An efficacious way to meet the challenge of reducing alcohol, tobacco, and other drug use among youth? *Journal of School Health*, *68*(3), 87–93.

Borman, G. C., & D'Agostino, J. V. (1996). Title I and student achievement: A meta-analysis of federal evaluation results. *Educational Evaluation and Policy Analysis*, *18*(4), 309–326.

Christensen, T. M., & Kline, W. B. K. (2001). The qualitative exploration of process-sensitive peer group supervision. *Journal for Specialists in Group Work*, *26*(1), 81–83.

DiNitto, D. M., Webb, D. K., & Rubin, A. (2002). The effectiveness of an integrated treatment approach for clients with dual diagnoses. *Research on Social Work Practice*, *12*(5), 621–641.

Fetterman, D. M. (2001). *Foundations of empowerment evaluation*. Thousand Oaks, CA: Sage.

Franklin, R. B., & Pack-Brown, S. (2001). TEAM brothers: An Afrocentric approach to group work with African American male adolescents. *Journal for Specialists in Group Work*, *26*(3), 237–245.

Garvin, C. D. (1997). *Contemporary group work* (3rd ed.). Boston: Allyn & Bacon.

Garvin, C. D., & Seabury, B. A. (1997). *Interpersonal practice in social work : promoting competence and social justice*. Boston: Allyn & Bacon.

Goelitz, A. (2001). Dreaming their way into life: A group experience with oncology patients. *Social Work with Groups*, *24*(1), 53–67.

Joint Committee on Standards for Educational Evaluation. (1994). *The Program Evaluation Standards: How to assess evaluations of educational programs* (2nd ed.). Thousand Oaks, CA: Sage.

Jones, L. V., & Hodges, V. G. (2001). Enhancing psychosocial competence among black women: A psycho-educational group model approach. *Social Work with Groups*, *24*(3/4), 33–52.

Jordan, M. H., Feild, H. S., & Armenakis, A. A. (2002). The relationship of group process variables and team performance: A team-level analysis in a field setting. *Small Group Research, 33*(1), 121–150.

Lincoln, Y. S., & Guba, E. G. (1985). *Naturalistic inquiry.* Beverly Hills, CA: Sage.

Lipsey, M. W., & Wilsom, D. B. (1993). The efficacy of psychological, educational, and behavioral treatment: Confirmation from meta-analysis. *American Psychologist*, *48*(12), 1181–1209.

Lothstein, L. M. (2001). Treatment of non-incarcerated sexually compulsive/addictive offenders in an integrated, multimodal, and psychodynamic group therapy model. *International Journal of Group Psychotherapy*, *51*(4), 553–570.

Miller, R., & Mason, S. E. (2001). Using group therapy to enhance treatment compliance in first episode schizophrenia. *Social Work with Groups*, *24*(1), 37–51.

Mishna, F., & Mickalski, J. (2001). Camps as social work interventions: Returning to our roots. *Social Work with Groups*, *24*(3/4), 153–171.

Mok, B. H. (2001a). Cancer self-help groups in China: A study of individual change, perceived benefit, and community impact. *Small Group Research*, *32*(2), 115–132.

Mok, B. H. (2001b). The effectiveness of self-help groups in a Chinese context. *Social Work with Groups*, *24*(2), 69–89.

Oygard, L., & Hardeng, S. (2001). Divorce support groups: How do group characteristics influence adjustment to divorce? *Social Work with Groups*, *24*(1), 69–87.

Patton, M. Q. (1997). *Utilization-focused evaluation: The new century text* (3rd ed.). Thousand Oaks, CA: Sage.

Piontek, M. E. (2003). *An introduction to classroom assessment and program evaluation.* Ann Arbor, MI: University of Michigan, Center for Research on Learning and Teaching.

Pomeroy, E. C., & Green, D. L. (2002). Couples who care: The effectiveness of a psychoeducational group intervention for HIV serodiscordant couples. *Research on Social Work Practice, 12*(2), 238–252.

Prochaska, J. O., & Norcross, J. C. (1994). *Systems of psychotherapy: A transtheoretical analysis* (3 rd ed.). Pacific Grove, CA: Brooks/Cole.

Prochaska, J. O., Norcross, J. C., & DiClemente, C. C. (1994). *Changing for good.* New York: Avon Books.

Queener, J. E., & Kenyon, C. B. (2001). Providing mental health services to southeast Asian adolescent girls: Integration of a primary prevention paradigm and group counseling. *Journal for Specialists in Group Work, 26*(4), 350–367.

Rossi, P. H. (1999). *Evaluation: A systematic approach* (6th ed.). Chicago: Nelson-Hall.

Royse, D. D. (1999). *Research methods in social work.* Chicago: Nelson-Hall.

Sapia, J. L. (2001). Using groups for the prevention of eating disorders among college women. *Journal for Specialists in Group Work, 26*(3), 256–266.

Schechtman, Z. (2001). Prevention groups for angry and aggressive children. *Journal for Specialists in Group Work, 26*(3), 228–236.

Strauss, A., & Corbin, J. (1990). *Basics of qualitative research: Techniques and procedures for developing grounded theory.* Newbury Park, CA: Sage.

Tutty, L. M., & Bidgood, B. A. (2001). An evaluation of men's batterer treatment groups. *Research on Social Work Practice, 11*(6), 645–670.

Witt, P. A., & Crompton, J. L. (1996). Major themes emerging from the case studies. In P. A. Witt & J. L. Crompton (Eds.), *Recreation programs that work for at-risk youth* (pp. 7–33). College Station, PA: Venture.

Yamaguchi, R. (2001). Children's learning groups: A study of emergent leadership, dominance, and group effectiveness. *Small Group Research, 32*(6), 671–697.

Part VII

The Uses of Technology to Create Groups

There is only one chapter (Chapter 28) in this section, devoted to a newly emerging area of group work practice. Increasingly, workers utilize the telephone and/or the computer to help people obtain the benefits of groups. This typically occurs when it would be difficult or impossible for them to meet face-to-face for such reasons as the geographical dispersion of the members or their physical status.

A growing body of experience and research is available that can help the practitioner determine the effects of such groups on members, the ways these groups may be created, the interventions that are utilized to facilitate such groups, and how they may be evaluated. There are differences in each of these phenomena that depend on the media utilized, such as whether members interact in the same time period or whenever they wish to do so; whether the communication device is a phone or a computer; and how members are "known" to each other. Chapter 28 provides detailed information on these and many other relevant issues.

Chapter 28

Technology-Mediated Groups

ANDREA MEIER

Since the early days of the settlement houses, social workers have been guided by the principle that people can face life's challenges better when they can draw on the support of a group than by going it alone (Sundel & Glasser, 1985). Now, innovations in telephone and Internet services are expanding our notions of "community" and "group." Until the advent of the Internet, the word "community" denoted groups of people who live near each other in physical space and share common interests (Coate, 1998). As Internet-mediated communication (IMC)[1] has become more universal, our notions of community have expanded to include relationships that provide a sense of belonging, regardless of geographic location (Coate, 1998; Hampton & Wellman, 2001). In the same way, we can now "meet" in groups in many more ways than just face-to-face gatherings. These rapidly and widely accepted changes in group communication technologies offer social workers novel ways to provide group services. They also challenge practitioners to expand their understanding of how therapeutic groups function when member interactions are mediated by telecommunications technology.

The statistics on technology-mediated communication (TMC) are impressive. Nearly 95% of Americans have access to a telephone. Although not as universal as the telephone, the Internet has been widely adopted. A Harris poll conducted by telephone in the spring of 2002 estimated that 137 million American adults (66%) had Internet access (Nua Internet Surveys, 2002); approximately half of all these Internet users had access from home (Fox et al., 2001). In a typical day, more than half (53%) of all Internet users go online, nearly half (46%) send e-mail messages, and nearly one-third (29%) surf the Web. Of those who do not currently have Internet access, nearly half (47%) report that they plan to get connected to the Internet within the next 6 months.

How are social workers using these technologies? Many routinely use telephone conference calls for case management and, increasingly, e-mail to coordinate agency teams (Marson, 1997) and for community mobilization (Blundo, Mele, Hairston, & Watson,

479

1999; Menon, 2000; Nartz & Schoech, 2000). Social workers have been somewhat slow in adopting and adapting TMC for therapeutic purposes (Marson, 1997; McCarty & Clancy, 2002). Their apparent reluctance to adopt communication technologies for interventions may be attributed partly to the lack of existing research evidence to guide them in designing and implementing technology-mediated (TM) therapeutic groups. Other factors may further dampen their enthusiasm, such as concern about inequities in consumers' access to technology-based services; or the costs to agencies of implementing and maintaining the technological infrastructure needed for technology-based groups (Galinsky, Schopler, & Abell, 1997; White & Dorman, 2001). Some social workers may be deterred by potential risks to their clients' privacy and confidentiality or their own liability if they use these tools in practice. Many already overloaded practitioners may be daunted by the prospect of learning the new skills they will need to conduct TM groups.

Even when they recognize the opportunities, organizations and practitioners must make hard decisions about the potential cost effectiveness of TM group services. Clinical licensing boards and insurance companies continue to discourage the use of all TM interventions by limiting practitioners to offering TM therapy in the states in which they are licensed (American Psychological Association, 1997; Childress, 1998; Clinical Social Work Federation, 2001; Jakobsen, 2002; National Association of Social Workers [NASW], 1999). Uncertain about intervention effectiveness and fearful of liability, third-party payers are not reimbursing practitioners for TM services, regardless of where they are offered (Grinfeld, 1998). For now, at least, the only consumers who can benefit from professionally facilitated TM groups are participants in research studies or those who are willing to risk the uncertainty and can afford to pay the fees themselves.

As the world grows increasingly reliant on TMC, social workers must overcome these barriers and become active agents in inventing ways to use these technologies therapeutically—particularly for therapeutic group work. To do this, we must be informed about the different types of TM groups and the research on how these groups are being used for self-help and as professionally facilitated interventions. We must think through how our practice models for face-to-face (F2F) treatment groups should be modified to take advantage of TM group processes.

With those aims in mind, we begin with a typology of TM groups so that readers understand the key features of each type of group. The second section summarizes the research evidence about the processes and outcomes of short-term, facilitated telephone and Internet-mediated (IM) treatment groups of the kind that social workers might expect to lead. In the third section, we suggest ways that social workers can expand the range of their group services by adapting their practice models for F2F groups to TM groups. The chapter concludes with a brief discussion of future prospects for TM group work.

TYPES OF TM GROUPS

TM groups differ according to the type of telecommunications technology members use to communicate; the timing of their message sending and receiving; the skills they need to participate in their groups; and the ways they can communicate and things they can do once they are connected. TM group members may communicate by phone or by using computers that are hooked up via modems to Internet services. When communication takes place over the Internet, it can be "text-based" or "Web-based." Text-based communication is limited to alphanumeric data (i.e., information that can be expressed only in letters and numbers).

With Web-based IM communication (IMC), users communicate using alphanumeric data, but they can also enrich their messages with graphical, audio and video data, and links to other websites.

Synchronous and Asynchronous TM Communication

Another key difference among TM communication channels is the timing of members' sending and receiving messages. When all users must be connected electronically at the same time to exchange messages, "synchronous communication" (often referred to as "real time" communication) takes place. "Asynchronous communication" occurs when message senders and their intended recipients do not have to be connected at the time when the message is sent.

Group members can communicate synchronously by telephone or with IM "chat." Except for the absence of visual cues, group communication using these media is casual and spontaneous, similar to F2F conversations in informal groups. Telephone groups can be conducted over speaker phones or using inexpensive conference call services. In a therapeutic context, telephone communication has the dual advantages of low equipment and transmission costs and high accessibility. Almost anyone who can communicate verbally can use a phone, regardless of their education level, socioeconomic status, or physical capacity.

With IM chat, group participants must use a specialized Internet site called a "chat room." Two forms of IM chat communication are widely in use: text-based Internet Relay Chat (IRC) and Web-based chat. For IRC, users must first download a special program to access a chat room. With Web-based chat, group members simply go to a specialized website where chat rooms have been implemented.

IRC and Web-based chat differ in their ease of use. IRC users must use a specialized programming language to manage their interactions with others in the chat room and the content of their messages. In Web-based chat, users can type their comments as usual in an onscreen data entry window. Apart from these differences, there are some key similarities between IRC and Web-based chat. At the start of a session, participants can sign in using "aliases," nicknames that protect their privacy while giving them identifiers to use during the session. All IM chat communication uses a "play script" screen format. When a member starts transmitting a message, his or her alias will be displayed first. The message will appear next to the name, displayed word by word as the text is transmitted. Web chat uses the same play-script screen format as IRC chat, but it is much simpler to use. Participants know who has signed on because their nicknames are displayed in a small on-screen window.

Asynchronous TMC occurs only over the Internet, but asynchronous IM groups can be text- or Web-based. One of the main advantages of asynchronous IMC is that message recipients do not have to be online at scheduled times to receive their messages. Members can write as much as they want, whenever they want, without fear of interruption, and other members can retrieve their messages at their convenience.

Text-based electronic bulletin board systems (BBS), USENET newsgroups and listservs, and Web-based discussion forums are the most common types of asynchronous TM groups. The major difference among them is whether members must use specialized programs (USENET newsgroups and BBS) to correspond with others in the group or whether messages are sent automatically to the members' e-mail in-boxes (listservs). On the Web, members can participate in asynchronous discussion "boards" or "forums" by submitting "forms" at a website or sending in e-mail messages to be posted via a Web browser. Members must go to the website to read the responses.

Listserv groups are easy to implement and are considered one of the most convenient forms of IM group communication. Members send their e-mail messages to the listserv's host computer, which then distributes them automatically to all of the other members' e-mail in-boxes. Because e-mail is the most commonly used Internet function, listserv members are more likely than BBS or newsgroup members to see their messages and respond. Probably because of these advantages, studies of IM therapeutic groups to date have usually used listserv groups.

User Skills

Members of each type of TM group must possess specific skills in order to participate. Telephone group members must be able to distinguish between different voices and interpret speech without visual cues. When members communicate by phone or IM chat, they must learn to take turns in expressing their views and allow each other to complete their thoughts. For all IM groups, members must be able to express their thoughts and feelings in writing and be able to interpret others' written messages accurately. IM chat group members must be able to compose their thoughts and type quickly so they can complete their comments before other members break in. Members of Web-based groups must also know how to "navigate" on the World Wide Web and use the various Web page functions and links.

Single- and Multifunctional IM Groups

Groups conducted over the Internet can be further classified according to whether they are single-function or multifunctional groups (Finfgeld, 2000). In single-function groups, members can participate in only one kind of group (e.g., listserv, newsgroup, Web-based asynchronous discussion, or chat group) at a time. Multifunctional groups are conducted over specially designed stand-alone computer programs and websites (also known as "Web portals") that offer users access to asynchronous discussion groups and chat support or self-help groups. Using these systems, members can access other services, such as information pages that address members' focal concerns, online decision support tools, self-assessment tools, behavior modification exercises, and private online consultations with group facilitators and experts. With this summary of TM group formats as a context, the remainder of this chapter focuses on how the technology has been—and can be—used to offer group treatment.

TM GROUP INTERVENTION RESEARCH

In this section, I review the research that has been done on facilitated telephone and IM therapeutic groups. The discussion within each category of group types examines the populations served, the problems addressed, and miscellaneous feasibility factors. Intervention outcomes are also reported, including participant satisfaction, social support, and intervention effectiveness.

Telephone Groups

For more than 50 years, social workers have used their telephones as tools for crisis intervention and outreach (Grumet, 1979). Group workers have found this familiar and ubiquitous way of communicating particularly appropriate for people with restricted mobility due to disability and/or age. Researchers have reported on two different kinds of telephone-mediated group interventions: telephone conferences and groups conducted over speakerphones. Studies of telephone conference groups are the most common, possibly because they are the most convenient to run. In these groups, group leaders and members can call in from wherever they are at the time of the session. In speakerphone groups, some members meet together for face-to-face sessions and talk, via speakerphone, with other members who cannot attend in person. In the studies reviewed here, all the telephone-mediated groups were small (four to six members). Typically, they were conducted over 9 or 10 weeks, with 60- or 90-minute sessions.

Telephone-Conference Groups

The first reported use of a semistructured telephone conference group was to alleviate social isolation among homebound elderly in rural Australia (Tropp, 1987). Since then, researchers have explored the benefits of connecting other populations of homebound, elderly women in various settings (Brown et al., 1999; Heller, Thompson, Trueba, Hogg, & Vlachos-Weber, 1991; Kaslyn, 1999); visually impaired elders (Evans & Jaugreguy, 1982); and people with multiple sclerosis (Stein, Rothman, & Nakanishi, 1993). Other studies have been conducted with groups of family caregivers of patients with spinal cord injuries (Houstra & Mallon, 1999) and Alzheimer's disease (Goodman & Pynoos, 1988). Telephone conference support groups have also been used with stigmatized populations such as gay and bisexual men (Roffman, Beadnell, Ryan, & Downey, 1995), adults and children living with HIV (Rounds, Galinsky, & Despard, 1995; Rounds, Galinsky, & Stevens, 1991; Stewart et al., 2001; Weiner, 1998; Weiner, Spencer, Davidson, & Fair, 1993), and family members who were caring for them (Meier, Galinsky, & Rounds, 1995).

Speakerphone Groups

One study (Springer & Stahmann, 1998) and one case report (Wilson, 2000) by psychodynamically oriented researchers demonstrate that F2F therapeutic groups can use speakerphones to continue their work when an absent member can be only "virtually" present. In their study, Springer and Stahmann explored whether family therapy sessions conducted over a speakerphone were feasible and perceived by participants as satisfying and beneficial. In this study, the psychiatrist met face-to-face with adolescent children at a residential psychiatric facility and communicated by speakerphone with their parents, who were at home.

Intervention Feasibility

In the early stages of intervention design and development, much of the work is devoted to testing the feasibility of intervention components and methods used to study them (Comer, Meier, & Galinsky, 1999; Rothman & Thomas, 1994). Overall, these studies and case reports have shown that the telephone-mediated treatment groups are feasible and that they provide members with accessible, flexible, and convenient support (Smokowski, Galinsky, & Harlow, 2001). Despite these clear benefits, telephone groups also have their limitations. Telephones use a synchronous TM channel, so groups must be kept small, limiting member diversity (Kaslyn, 1999). When group members participate from home, they may have problems arranging for undistracted time and the privacy they need to participate in their groups

(Kaslyn, 1999; Meier et al., 1995; Stein et al., 1993). Some members may be reluctant to acknowledge to the group that they are having difficulty hearing or distinguishing among different speakers (Kaslyn, 1999). Physically disabled or elderly group members may become exhausted by having to hold phone receivers to their ears for an hour-long group session (Kaslyn, 1999; Stein et al., 1993).

Group leaders must keep a friendly and inviting tone in their voices and be mindful that group members' impressions of them are based mainly on their words (Hines, 1994). Group leaders must be more active than they might be in F2F groups, keeping track of who has spoken, concentrating harder on what members say, and seeking clarification about the meaning of their silences (Hines, 1994; Houstra & Mallon, 1999; Kaslyn, 1999).

Outcomes

SOCIAL SUPPORT

There is considerable evidence that telephone group members receive social support through their groups. Members report that they felt accepted and validated in their experiences (Meier et al., 1995), less isolated and lonely (Evans, Fox, Pritzl, & Halar, 1984), and grateful to have others to talk with about the existential meaning of their situations (Evans et al., 1984; Meier et al., 1995).

PARTICIPANT SATISFACTION

In general, group members have reported that they were satisfied with their group experiences (Meier et al., 1995; Rosenfeld, 1997; Stewart et al., 2001). Few studies report on how group leaders reacted to the telephone groups they led. Rosenfeld (1997) commented that, based on her experience as a trainer, some leaders may initially feel uncomfortable not having visual cues to draw on. These concerns may be due mostly to inexperience with the TM group format (Schopler, Galinsky, & Abell, 1997). They usually diminish when group leaders have opportunities to role-play telephone group simulations (Kurtz, 1997) and accumulate experience with the group (Rosenfeld, 1997).

THERAPEUTIC EFFECTS

Only three studies of telephone groups have used experimental or quasi-experimental designs to assess their interventions' effectiveness (Brown et al., 1999; Goodman, 1990; Roffman et al., 1997). All three found that groups were effective to some degree in achieving targeted outcomes. Roffman et al. (1997) compared the effects of a 14-session structured cognitive-behavioral telephone group counseling intervention on risky sexual behaviors with gay and bisexual men with a wait-list control group. Compared with the control group, telephone group participants showed a significant and sustained reduction in the frequency of unprotected anal sex. They also showed significant improvements in key attitudes and expectancies related to risk reduction, including positive outcome expectancies for condom use, higher internal locus of control, increased self-efficacy for safer sex, and increased confidence in being able to cope with unsafe situations.

Brown and her colleagues (1999) assessed member satisfaction and changes in mood in a telephone support group for urban and rural family caregivers of with patients spinal cord injury. The study found significant improvements in measures of participants' mood states.

Goodman (1990) compared the effects of 12-week facilitated telephone support groups and an informational lecture series accessed over the phone on family caregivers' use of informal supports, perceived social support, mental health status, and information about Alzheimer's disease. Telephone support group participants reported that their psychological distress had decreased, and their levels of perceived social support and their satisfaction with that social support had increased, despite the fact that their relatives with Alzheimer's disease had become increasingly impaired since the beginning of the group.

Internet Groups

Research suggests that IM groups may be most appropriate for people who cannot or will not attend face-to-face therapeutic groups because they are living with stigmatized conditions, such as HIV, or are socially isolated due to restricted physical mobility or caregiving obligations (Smaglik et al., 1998; Smokowski et al., 2001). The discussion of research on IM treatment groups offers examples of such groups, following the typology of single-function and multifunction groups introduced earlier.

Single-Function Groups

Finfgeld's (2000) review of the literature on therapeutic online groups identified many studies of facilitated, single-function IM groups in which health care professionals served as passive facilitators who participated only occasionally. To date, there have been relatively few reports of single-function groups with active facilitators. One of the earliest case reports of this kind of group was a 3-month-long psychodynamic group composed of eight members run over a BBS (Colon, 1997). Since then, Meier has conducted three exploratory studies of facilitated short-term listserv-based support groups for social work students (Meier, 1997), practicing social workers (Meier, 1999), and spouses of colon cancer patients (Meier, 2003). Barak and Wander-Schwartz have compared the processes and outcomes of a 7-week psychodynamic Web-based chat group to those of face-to-face psychodynamic groups for Israeli university students and a nontreatment control group (Barak & Wander-Schartz, 1999). Colon (1997), Meier (1999), and Barak and Wander-Schartz (1999) all deliberately designed the groups they used in their studies to parallel the structure of short-term face-to-face groups in duration (from 6 to 12 weeks) and size (6 to 13 members).

To date, there have been only two evaluations of single-function IM support groups. One was a randomized, controlled trial of a large (211 members), listserv-based, facilitated support group for people with chronic back pain that lasted 12 months (Lorig et al., 2002). This study compared the effectiveness of the treatment group on members' pain, disability, role function, and health distress with a similar-sized, nontreatment control group. The second study, the "Bosom Buddies Project" (Winzelberg et al., 2003), was a wait-list-controlled study of Web-based asynchrononous 12-week structured cognitive-behavioral support groups for women with breast cancer. In addition to their discussion groups, members could post photographs and brief autobiographies. They could also write in their private on-line journals and read personal stories from other breast cancer survivors, without sending messages to their groups.

INTERVENTION FEASIBILITY

Early studies of single-function IM group interventions investigated how big groups should be, how long they should last, and what kinds of participation norms are reasonable.

Groups ranged in size from 6 (Meier, 1997) to 19 members (Meier, 1999). Colon's (1997) psychodynamic group had 8 members, and in the three studies conducted by Winzelberg and colleagues (1997, 1998, 2003), treatment groups ranged in size from 10 to 15 members. Meier (1997, 2003) found that a listserv-based group with 6 members was too small to keep members engaged, whereas a 19-member group produced more messages than many members could manage (Meier, 1999). In Meier's 1999 study, members were most satisfied when only 13 members were active contributors. Although more research on the relationship between group size and viability is needed, these studies suggest that short-term listserv-based groups should consist of between 8 to 15 members—roughly the size of face-to-face therapeutic groups.

OUTCOMES

Participant Satisfaction. In these early feasibility studies, participant satisfaction was a key outcome. In Barak and Wander-Schwartz's (1999), Colon's (1997) and Meier's (1997, 1999, 2003) studies, participants reported high levels of satisfaction and a willingness to recommend on-line group interventions to others. In the Bosom Buddies study, the investigators noted that "participants expressed a level of enthusiasm and concern for one another that was not captured by the self-report measures" (Winzelberg et al., 2003, p. 1170). Group leaders in Barak's and Wander-Schwartz's (1999), Colon's (1997) and Meier's (1997, 1999, 2003) studies also reported that the overall experience was satisfying and that the groups were positive and constructive, albeit extremely labor intensive.

Participant satisfaction is often an indicator of group cohesion. The Meier (1999, 2003) and Winzelberg et al. (1998) studies all demonstrated that IM group communication could promote emotional bonding. In all three studies, members decided to continue on independently as peer-led groups after their respective projects ended.

Therapeutic Outcomes. Neither Barak and Wander-Schwartz nor Meier found that participation in their groups was associated with statistically significant improvements in desired outcomes. Lack of significant findings is common in the early stages of intervention research, in which small-scale pilot studies are used to explore research design and intervention feasibility issues.

The larger studies conducted by Lorig et al. (2002) and Winzelberg et al. (2003) showed greater therapeutic effectiveness. In both studies, participants improved significantly in at least some intervention outcomes. Compared with the control group, participation in the back-pain group was associated with diminished pain, disability, and health distress (Lorig, 2002). Participants reported improved role functioning, along with a decline in visits to physicians. Participation in the breast cancer groups (Winzelberg et al., 2003) was associated with medium effect sizes for improvements in depression, posttraumatic stress disorder, and perceived stress compared with members of wait-list control groups. Participation in those groups was not, however, associated with reduced anxiety or improved adjustment to or efficacy in coping with breast cancer.

Multifunctional Groups

Multifunctional Web portals offer participants contexts for their groups that are richer than single-function groups in information and opportunities for other activities related to group goals. The first studies of multifunctional groups conducted in the early 1990s, Computer-

Link and the Comprehensive Health Enhancement Support System (CHESS), used support systems that were computer-mediated but not run over the Internet. Instead, participants were provided with computers to use at home that had specialized, stand-alone programs for accessing text-based project services that included facilitated support groups, decision support tools, "electronic encyclopedias," and community services information. Computerlink was designed to address the support and information needs of Alzheimer family caregivers (Brennan, Moore, & Smyth, 1992), and of people living with AIDS (Brennan & Ripich, 1994). In the CHESS study, computer-mediated facilitated groups and other services were offered to women with breast cancer (Gustafson et al., 2001).

As Web technologies advanced, researchers studying text-based TM multifunctional group interventions adapted them to take advantage of the new technologies. CHESS, for example, has changed completely, from a computer-based stand-alone system to a comprehensive Internet-based information and support system designed to help people cope with specific health concerns, make health decisions, and adopt healthy behavior changes. Web-based CHESS modules have since been developed to support people who are living with breast or prostate cancer, asthma, or heart disease. Other modules have been developed for adults and adolescents who are trying to stop smoking, women coping with menopausal symptoms, and caregivers of dementia patients.

The Israeli project, SAHAR,[2] is another example of a multifunctional Web-based group intervention. SAHAR's Web portal offers IM support for distressed or suicidal people (Barak, 2001). Users have access to facilitated on-line Web discussions and chat rooms for children, adults, and users who want to express their feelings through poetry, stories, and art. Besides those groups, members can participate in on-line counseling sessions with paraprofessional counselors.

In another project, a team of researchers has systematically developed and evaluated a multifunctional IM group treatment for undergraduate women students with eating disorders (Winzelberg, 1997; Winzelberg et al., 1998; Zabinski, Pung, et al., 2001; Zabinski, Wilfley, et al., 2001). They first pilot-tested a group treatment component that combined a 7-week structured cognitive-behavioral IRC-chat group with four members that met for 1 hour a week with a peer-led listserv group. Each week, participants were e-mailed a single page of information about the topic of the week to read before the session and "homework assignments" to do afterward. Group members could access the listserv group any time between their weekly chat sessions to discuss past chat sessions, readings, and homework assignments.

The same research team then developed and tested a more comprehensive multifunctional IM intervention, which they named "Student Bodies." The intervention combined a professionally facilitated listserv support group with an interactive software program composed of audio and video presentations about eating disorders, health weight regulation, nutrition, and exercise (Humphreys, Winzelberg, & Klaw, 2000). In the group, members could discuss their struggles with weight control, diet, and body image. The group leader was not very active but did periodically reflect members' concerns and offered suggestions consistent with the ideas taught in the program's educational components.

INTERVENTION FEASIBILITY

All of the studies of IM multifunctional groups described here attest to their feasibility, with IM support groups as core functions. When properly designed, even naïve users—and those with relatively little education—can and will use them to access social services (Barak, 2001;

Brennan & Fink, 1997; Gustafson et al., 2001); however, how they use the portal's features is highly variable. For example, minorities may use these kinds of services as much as nonminorities (Gustafson et al., 2001), but they tend to use information services more than they do groups (Boberg et al., 1995; Gustafson et al., 2001).

OUTCOMES

In general, participants reported that the groups in the multifunctional portals were good "places" to share experiences and to give and receive emotional support. In the CHESS breast cancer study (Boberg et al., 1995), women reported that the computer-mediated support group was an added source of support that helped them to face their illness. In a personal communication, SAHAR founder Azy Barak reported that SAHAR counselors' supportive counseling and direct crisis interventions have prevented deeply depressed people from acting on their suicidal impulses (Azy Barak, personal communication, August 5, 2002).

Outcome studies of ComputerLink and CHESS showed that participants improved significantly on a number of key outcomes. CHESS participants reported improved functional well-being, quality of life, perceived social support, and more efficient use of health care services (Gustafson et al., 1994). Participants in ComputerLink reported that they felt less isolated (Brennan, 1998). The early "Student Bodies" studies found moderate but significant improvements in members' attitudes about their body images but no differences between intervention and control groups in levels of improvement on other standardized eating disorder measures (Winzelberg et al., 1998). A subsequent controlled study with greater member participation showed significant improvements in body image and diminished eating-disorder symptoms (Zabinski, Pung, et al., 2001).

Although they are still largely untested, multifunctional intervention portals represent the leading edge of development in IM group interventions. Research still needs to be done to tease out the benefits attributable to group experience from other services available on these portals. Nonetheless, the studies described here show that this kind of IM support and information service can provide users with easy access to information and significant social support. Health care provider organizations have recognized their potential and have already begun offering them to consumers. It remains to be seen how many—and how soon—social workers in public agencies and community organizations will recognize the advantages and have the resources to adopt these technologies.

SOCIAL WORK PRACTICE
WITH TECHNOLOGY-MEDIATED GROUPS

The studies of facilitated telephone- and Internet-mediated support groups described here confirm that such groups are feasible and suggest that their therapeutic benefits are similar to those of F2F groups (Smokowski et al., 2001). What group workers need now is practical guidance to help them organize and conduct their own TM groups. Over the past decade, social work researchers have begun to adapt theoretical and practice models developed for F2F groups for TM groups. Schopler, Abell, and Galinsky (1998) did one of the first comprehensive reviews of TM group interventions and produced a conceptual practice-oriented framework for social workers. Grounded in open systems theory, their framework reminds practitioners of the importance of considering differences between these types of groups at three system levels: the individual, the group, and the organizational environment in which the group takes place. Meier has proposed an integrative framework that summarizes the interpersonal, intrapersonal, and social network effects of different TM channels and how they play out in therapeutic and support groups (Meier, in press). A research team at the University of North Carolina adapted Sarri and Galinsky's (1985) 5-stage model of group development to telephone-mediated support groups for people with AIDS (Galinsky, Rounds, Montague, & Butowsky, 1993; Potts & Verbiest, 1993) and their caregivers (Meier, 1993; Meier et al., 1995).

TM INTERVENTION GROUP DEVELOPMENT

Drawing on this foundation of social work theory and practice models, I now describe what group workers must do to plan and organize their TM groups and keep them viable.

Planning

Before deciding to sponsor a TM group, organizers must determine whether there are enough consumers who are appropriate for a TM group intervention and who are interested in this new type of service. Workplace telephone conferences and the proliferation of IM self-help groups have familiarized many people with these ways of communicating and may make them more receptive to the idea. One strategy for targeting new TM group services is to identify consumers who could benefit from group support but who cannot or will not attend F2F support groups.

Technical Implementation

Assuming there is sufficient consumer demand, organizers must then decide which kind of TM group to offer, taking into consideration what technologies consumers have access to, ease of use, and cost. Until recently, for example, group workers may have been deterred from doing telephone conferences because of the cost and complexity. Now, national telephone conferencing services make these groups affordable and easy to access through local-access or toll-free numbers (Telebridge, 2002). Consumers who are interested in participating in IM groups usually already have computers and access to the Internet through local phone lines, so participating in a group would not add to their technology costs. Organizers can help those who do not have their own computers to access the Internet using computers provided in public libraries, schools, or other community technology centers (Mark, Cornebise, & Wahl, 1997). Alternatively, organizers may decide that the best way to provide clients with IM support would be to provide them with Internet-ready computers to use during the group. Or they could subsidize both Internet service fees during the group and the purchase of inexpensive computers that members can keep.

Organizers must also decide which mode of TMC best meets the needs of targeted group members. IM group organizers should survey potential participants to see whether they would prefer the simplicity of a text-based group or a more sophisticated Web-based group. Before the group starts, group leaders and members should be informed about what to do if their equipment fails or there is a problem in their local telephone systems or Internet services (Meier, 1999; Meier et al., 1995).

Recruiting

Organizers' choice of recruiting strategies depends on the type of TMC used for the group and the target audience. If they are recruiting locally for telephone groups, they can use agency client lists, referrals, flyers, published announcements, and announcements on the agency website (Meier, 1997; Toseland & Rivas, 2001). If they are planning IM groups for people coping with relatively rare conditions, organizers may need to recruit nationally or internationally and collaborate with national on-line support associations. They can post announcements on association websites and to the IM self-help groups that the associations sponsor. Using IMC exclusively for recruiting can result in low response rates, so organizers should plan to use both F2F and TMC communication whenever possible (Comer, Meier, & Galinsky, 2002; Meier, 1999; Meier & Campbell, 2002).

Assessment

TMC offers group organizers more options for conducting assessments besides in-person in-terviews. They can collect baseline information by phone, e-mail, instant messaging, chat, or even video conferencing (Suler, 2001a). On-line standardized assessment procedures have been found to be equivalent to paper-and-pencil-administered versions (Pinsoneault, 1996). If the technical resources are available and members have the appropriate IMC skills, orga-nizers can speed up assessment data collection by putting their organization's assessment instruments and forms on-line through a secure website. Respondents may be more willing to disclose sensitive information on-line than through conventional F2F assessment methods (Kiesler & Sproull, 1986).

How should group members be assessed for TM groups? Apart from standard clinical case information, organizers also need to gather information about participants' experiences with TMC. Although there is continuing debate over the appropriate designs for assessment protocols to be used in IM therapies (Suler, 2001b), there is some consensus on how to assess group participants' prior experience with IM communication. Practitioners should confirm that group members do not have physical or cognitive conditions that would inter-fere with their use of the group's mode of TMC and that they have the necessary technical skills.

Even with all the information from these assessments, the group organizers may still not be certain whether a given individual would be appropriate for a specific TM group. Currently, there is no consensus among clinicians about the personality types, presenting complaints, and mental health diagnoses that would make a potential participant appro-priate or inappropriate for a facilitated TM group (Fenichel et al., 2002; Suler, 2001b). The International Society for Mental Health Online (ISMHO; Fenichel et al., 2002), along with researchers King and Moreggi (1998), argue that people with severe patholo-gies (including eating disorders) or who are at risk of doing violence to themselves or oth-ers are not appropriate for on-line therapy. IM text-based communication may exacerbate problems with poor reality testing and strong transference reactions. People with border-line personality disorders, who are challenging enough in F2F groups, are likely to be even more difficult to work with in on-line group settings (Suler, 2001b). On the other hand, the SAHAR project has reported success in serving severely depressed people through its groups. The "Student Bodies" research team was somewhat successful intervening with women with students with eating disorders (Winzelberg, 1997; Winzelberg et al., 1998; Zabinski, Pung, et al., 2001).

Risk Management

The possibility that a TM therapeutic group may include members with severe psychological problems raises the issue of risk management. Professional associations and licensing boards, insurance companies, and clinical ethicists across the clinical professions have expressed concern about the potential risks of TM therapeutic interventions (American Psychological Association, 1997; NASW, 1999; National Board of Certified Counselors, 2002; Oxley, 1996; Reamer, 1986). Their major concerns differ somewhat according to the type of TM communication used. Practitioners in any TM group cannot intervene directly in the event of an emergency in the group because they are not physically present. In IM groups in which the group leader has other no other kinds of contact with members, such as F2F or telephone assessments, there is always the risk that members may misrepresent themselves and their problems or that a member is a minor.

Agencies and practitioners should adopt strategies for reducing these risks. Participants must give their informed consents by signing a paper form, but agencies can post descriptions of their groups and the informed-consent statements on their websites to inform clients who are considering the group about the purpose of the group and its risks and benefits (Meier, 1999; Meier & Comer, in press; NASW, 1999). During the recruitment period, group organizers can use the telephone, e-mail, or on-line chat to discuss participants' concerns and answer their questions. As part of the assessment process, organizers should gather information about the settings in which members will be accessing the group and determine whether they will have access to the phone or Internet when they need it and sufficient privacy to protect all member communications.

Agencies should modify their release-of-information procedures to specify how they will try to escalate contact with members in case of emergencies (Comer et al., 2002; Kane & Sands, 1998). For all TM groups, providers should install toll-free phone lines so that participants in crisis will not be deterred by long-distance charges from calling the agency (Kane & Sands, 1998). For IM groups, e-mail messages and Web chat screens need to include standardized information about how to contact the sponsoring agency by phone. Group leaders of asynchronous IM groups should inform members how often and at what times they will check their e-mail. Agencies should also have policies specifying the kinds of follow-up support offered to members in distress who decide to drop out of the group (Meier, 2003).

Orientation to the Group

Organizers can use the informed-consent and assessment processes to help each member understand the entire process of group treatment (NASW, 1999; Sundel, Radin, & Churchill, 1985). All participants should receive information that describes (1) the goals of the group; (2) the procedures the group will use to achieve them; (3) how their participation in the group can help them achieve their personal goals; and (4) his or her own obligations to individual members, to the group leader, and to the group as a whole. For TM groups, orientation materials should also include information about how the mode of TM communication used for the group may affect their group experience, including risks to confidentiality and how members interact with each other.

Confidentiality Issues

In therapeutic group settings, members' privacy and confidentiality are always at risk to some degree, and members need to be informed of those risks (Gellman, 1999; Grohol, 2000). As a matter of principle, members should be advised that, if there is anything that they absolutely want kept secret, they should not divulge it to the group. Telephones and computer monitors focus the users' attention away from the surrounding environment, producing the illusion of privacy. As a result, some of the riskiest situations for TM group members are likely to happen in their local, social environments rather than their technological ones. For example, telephone group members may inadvertently allow calls to be screened or telephone conversations overheard (Rosenfeld, 1997). IM group members may use computers in places where passersby can read onscreen texts of e-mail messages from the group or carelessly leave printouts of message texts lying around where others can read them.

Some risks to confidentiality are specific to IMC. There is a slight possibility that Internet service employees might intercept messages as they are transmitted along the network. Employers have a legal right to read their employees' e-mail messages sent over the worksite's Internet service. E-mail messages can end up in the hands of unintended recipients because they were misaddressed or because members forward them without permission to people outside the group (Kane & Sands, 1998).

Regardless of the type of TM group, organizers must have procedures in place to insure privacy and to establish and enforce appropriate norms to minimize risk and to manage unauthorized disclosures that may occur. For example, group leaders who will be facilitating their groups from their homes or from sites away from the office should set up secure, second accounts. New regulations of the Health Insurance Portability and Accountability Act (HIPAA) represent the federal government's first efforts to protect the security, privacy, and confidentiality of consumer health information that is stored or exchanged electronically (New Mexico Health Policy Commission, 2003). It is not clear yet how these regulations will apply to the management of IM treatment group records that include the full transcripts of all member interactions.

In the interim, many new technologies are being developed in response to growing concerns over Internet privacy issues (Privacy.net, 2003). When planning a group, organizers need to discover what new technologies are available to protect members' privacy, such as encrypted e-mail accounts, and decide whether they can be implemented without making those same protections barriers to services (MSN.com, 2002).

Group Structure

In designing group interventions, size and duration must be considered together (Toseland & Rivas, 2001). Telephone and IM chat groups must be kept small (4–6 members) to insure that all members get sufficient "air time" to express their views during time-limited sessions. Researchers have not yet reached consensus on the optimal size for asynchronous IM groups. In theory, asynchronous IM groups can also be larger than synchronous ones because turn taking is not a problem, but how much bigger is still an empirical question. Early evidence suggests that brief therapeutic (e.g., 6–12 weeks) asynchronous groups should be similar in size to F2F treatment groups. Much larger groups may need to last much longer (e.g., 12 months) to allow members enough time to accumulate impressions of each other and contribute their thoughts (Lorig et al., 2002; Walther, 1993).

Group Composition

As with many other aspects of TM groups, we still know little about the characteristics of members best suited for each kind of TM group. Until we know more, TM therapeutic group members' sociodemographic characteristics, prior experiences, and types of problems must be matched to the purpose of the group, just as they are in F2F groups (Vinter, 1985). IM group members cannot see or hear each other, so they may take longer than members of F2F or phone groups to recognize their shared concerns. This suggests that IM groups may need to be more homogeneous than F2F groups, but it is still uncertain how to decide which characteristic(s) are key (Meier, 1999).

Intervention Modalities

TM communication appears to be appropriate for many different therapeutic modalities. Clinicians have had satisfactory experiences using psychodynamic approaches in IM (Colon, 1997) and phone groups (Springer & Stahmann, 1998; Wilson, 2000). Meier (2003) has shown that a brief, solution-focused, asynchronous IM group was feasible and satisfying to members (Meier, 2003). Most researchers have used TM support groups for their studies that are similar to brief, closed-membership, semi-structured, F2F groups. Thus far, research has shown these groups to be effective ways to offer emotional and informational support. Clinicians working with individual clients report that IM communication appears to be particularly well suited for cognitive-behavioral "coaching" and narrative therapies (Grohol, 1999), but the effectiveness of these intervention techniques in therapeutic group contexts has yet to be systematically evaluated.

Group Leader Roles

Social workers can feel reassured knowing that their training and practice wisdom concerning F2F groups are generally applicable to TM groups. However, organizers may need to adapt the ways that group leaders are trained in light of the differences between F2F and TM group communication. Here I suggest ways to modify group leader training and describe what group leaders in different kinds of TM groups need to do to form their groups and keep them going.

Training

In any group, the leader must feel comfortable and have the skills to help the group achieve its goals. In TM groups, the leader must not only have interpersonal leadership skills and be knowledgeable about group content but must also understand how to communicate effectively through the group's electronic medium (Schopler, Abell, & Galinsky, 1998). Leaders of phone groups need to be skilled in interpreting voice, tone, and pace. IM group leaders must have good keyboarding skills and the ability to express themselves in the informal writing styles appropriate for e-mail or on-line chat. To help leaders learn these skills, organizers can organize role plays of the type of TM group to be offered, using coworkers as members. IM group leaders can join public on-line self-help groups to learn more about IM group communication and about people whose concerns are similar to those in the groups they will be leading (Abell & Galinsky, 2002; Comer, Meier, & Galinsky, in press).

Early-Stage Tasks

Getting to Know the Members of the Group

The initial challenge for both group members and the leader is to develop coherent images of who else is in the group. Where appropriate, organizers can expedite this process by asking group members to submit brief, written self-descriptions prior to the start of the group. The group leader can compile and distribute these descriptions by mail (phone groups) or e-mail (IM groups) to all the members, so that they can to refer to them later to remind them about who is in the group (Meier, 2003). With digital cameras now widely available, members may also want to include pictures of themselves to illustrate their written descriptions.

"Starting" the Group

The group leader's tasks in beginning a group session will be different in synchronous and asynchronous TM groups. For phone and IM chat groups, the leader "arrives" 5–10 minutes before the scheduled start of the group session so that he or she can welcome members and reassure them that they have gotten connected to the "right place." Once that happens, the leader announces that the group is starting and summarizes any discussions that occurred before the last member "arrived." The procedures for starting the group are different in asynchronous IM groups. Here, the group leader announces that the group has officially begun by posting a welcoming first message, which is sent out to all members simultaneously. All the group's messages are stored on the host computer, so members never miss any of the group interactions.

Recognizing Who Is "Present"

TM group members may find it harder to experience themselves as part of a group than F2F group members do because of the absence of visual cues. Members and group leaders have to be more explicit in acknowledging each other's "presence." In all TM groups, the leader should prompt members to use each other's names when referring to other members' prior comments (Galinsky et al., 1993; Meier & Campbell, 2002). In asynchronous IM groups, members can help each other know that their messages will be read promptly by committing to checking their e-mail for messages from the group every day. Leaders should keep track of who contributes to the discussions and follow up to insure that all who do are acknowledged.

Promoting Member Participation in the Early Stages

As in any group, TM group leaders must promote participation by helping members learn to manage their interactions. Early on in the group, members should discuss how TM communication differs from F2F communication and the implications of those differences for how they will interact with each other. In addition to discussing the group's focal topics, members should also be encouraged to comment about group process and how TMC may be affecting it (Meier, 2000).

Synchronous TM groups (chat and telephone) are more challenging to facilitate than asynchronous groups because members have to learn turn-taking procedures. The group leader can help insure that everyone has an opportunity to contribute by asking members to start the discussion about the first topic in a round-robin format. In telephone groups, the leader can call on members in a specified order (e.g., by their first names). In chat groups, the sequence can be set using the on-screen list that displays the order in which they logged on to the chat room (Meier & Campbell, 2002).

In asynchronous IM groups, it is helpful if there are explicit norms about how many messages members are expected to post each week. For example, they can be asked to post at least two messages. These norms insure that, when members check their e-mail, there will be at least a few new messages to read. This will help members and the leader know who is "present" and will keep members engaged without making participation burdensome.

Middle-Stage Tasks

Sustaining Participation

To insure that some member concerns are not ignored, all group leaders must encourage "quiet" members to contribute and must moderate dominant members' participation. TM group leaders must be more active than F2F group leaders over the life of the group in managing member participation levels. In phone and IM chat groups, the leader should explicitly ask silent members for their comments in every session. In asynchronous IM groups, the group leader has much less control over member participation. A core group of members usually posts the majority of the messages, whereas other members "lurk," posting messages only occasionally. If a member's level of participation drops significantly, the leader should contact him or her privately by e-mail or phone to confirm whether he or she has simply lost interest or is overwhelmed by other life demands and does not have the time or energy to write. The leader can help sustain group cohesion by encouraging such members to inform the group themselves about what is going on or get their permission to let the other members know.

Conflict Resolution

As members get to know each other and how the group works, they are more likely to want to take more control of the group. In the normal course of events, they may begin to express dissatisfaction with the way the group is organized or the way the group leader is running it and demand changes in group structure and goals (Galinsky et al., 1993). Research on TM group interventions rarely reports on this phase of group development, however, so we know little about how best to facilitate it.

"Real time" conflicts in telephone and chat groups are likely to be expressed in ways similar to those in F2F groups, and the group leader can address their concerns immediately. In asynchronous groups, however, conflicts need to be handled differently but also as quickly as possible. The absence of visual cues reduces the level of social control and allows members to experience their feelings more intensely and to be less restrained in expressing them. Because responses are delayed, members' grievances have more time to fester. Similarly, members on the receiving end of provocative or hostile e-mail messages may feel the attack more intensely than they would with aggressive comments in F2F groups.

As in F2F groups, the leader should intervene by acknowledging the validity of members' differences of opinion. The leader can interpret such challenges to the group as evidence that members may be feeling safer with each other and that they are taking more responsibility for the group and feeling a greater sense of ownership. Members should also be encouraged to consider whether and how (1) IMC itself may have contributed to the development of the conflict and (2) they will have to invent new kinds of conflict resolution strategies that are better suited to the constraints of IM communication (Munro, 2002).

Sustaining Participation

Over time, TM group members learn what kind of support they provide each other, what kinds of problems they can solve, and how much conflict they can tolerate and resolve (Galinsky et al., 1993; Meier, 1999; Meier et al., 1995). By this time, it will be obvious who the active, core members are and which members are more passive. Member activity levels may shift in response to changes in discussion topics. If the discussion becomes too emotionally intense, some members may begin to participate less. In telephone groups, members who become uncomfortable will talk less. In IM groups, anxious members may decide to lurk, following the group's discussion but not contributing much.

With the group now largely able to maintain itself, the group leader can shift his or her efforts to keeping less active members engaged in the group. The group leader can contact inactive members privately to discover whether they are experiencing problems that prevent them from participating in the group. If needed, the leader can help them obtain assistance from their local providers.

Coping with the Limits of Group Support

As members gain trust in each other, they may reveal that they are having health or other life crises that are beyond the group's ability to remedy. In TM support groups in which members share a common problem, the group leader may have to help members cope with the fear that, some day, they too could face the same crises. In IM groups, members who are not in crisis also may need help coming to terms with the limits of the group's capacity to help and how geographic distance is a real barrier to offering instrumental support (Meier, 1999). Some members might suggest sending help or gifts via the World Wide Web. Organizers should anticipate this possibility and decide in advance whether to support or discourage this form of TM helping.

Late-Stage Tasks

A couple of weeks prior to the end date of the group, leaders should remind members that the group will be ending and help them cope with their feelings about the group's termination. It is particularly important to give asynchronous IM group members a longer lead time. The combination of lags in times at which members receive the message and not having scheduled, time-bounded group sessions may cause some to lose track of how much time has passed (Meier, 1999). As in F2F groups, leaders should encourage members to review their experience with the group and to let others know what they found helpful and their feelings about the group's ending.

Organizers should decide in advance whether it is therapeutically appropriate to encourage group members to stay in touch with each other after the group ends. If it is, they should provide members with information about the ways they can use TMC to do this. Members should consider whether to change TMC modes and, if so, how. For example, telephone groups whose members also have Internet access may want to begin to communicate by e-mail. Members of listserv groups may decide to gather periodically in a chat group, or vice versa. To protect members from undue social pressure, group leaders should contact each one privately to find out what he or she wants to do. Once members have made their decisions, group leaders should provide whatever information is needed so that those who want to stay connected can do so

PROSPECTS FOR THE FUTURE
OF TECHNOLOGY-MEDIATED GROUP WORK

Writing about these rapidly evolving technologies is a risky enterprise. Many of the technical details presented here may be obsolete by the time this book is published. No one knows when we will be presented with innovations that further transform our interactions with each other in ways that are inconceivable today. So readers are advised to view the information and conclusions presented here as tentative markings on our mental maps of TM communities.

With that caveat in mind, we can still take advantage of widespread accessibility of TMC and our growing comfort with it to invent new kinds of services. Wireless cell phones and Internet connectivity vastly increase the number of times and ways groups can communicate with each other, regardless of where individual members may be (Rheingold, 2002). Because most Internet users can now navigate seamlessly between e-mail and the World Wide Web, opportunities for IM multifunctional group interventions are expanding. At the same time, advances in text-to-speech, speech-to-text, and automatic translation software are also reducing barriers to group services for otherwise underserved populations, such as the hearing impaired (DeafSpot.net, 2002), people with disabilities that prevent them from using a keyboard or a mouse (ScanSoft.com, 2002), or people with visual impairments (Sensus Accessibility Consultants, 2003) or poor English skills (Systran Information and Translation Technologies, 2003). More research is needed to understand how to best use these resources with IM therapeutic groups. Finally, researchers and practitioners need to explore the possible advantages of combining TM and F2F group formats in situations in which members live near enough to meet periodically in person.

Our knowledge base of research and practice wisdom on TM group interventions is still in its infancy. It is hard for social work students and practitioners to get systematic training in the skills they need to be effective TM group leaders. Although on-line training programs in on-line individual counseling and coaching are beginning to appear on the Web, there are no accredited organizations offering professional training in TM groups.

If social workers are to take advantage of these new technologies on behalf of consumers and to advance the profession, they must become advocates for system-wide changes. They should demand further research on TM groups to develop and test the viability and effectiveness of new practice models (Meier & Comer, in press). Schools of social work need to add course content to their curricula to help students and practitioners learn how to adapt their expertise with F2F groups to TM groups. The Association for the Advancement of Social Work with Groups, and other professional associations that promote social group work, should go beyond merely sponsoring listservs for their members. They should actively encourage members to collaborate in systematically developing TM group interventions and standards of practice—or, at least, to be open to these new communication media as potential resources for service provision. Finally, practitioners must begin lobbying their licensing boards and insurance companies, demanding a reexamination of the growing body of research evidence that shows the promise of TM groups, and for policy changes and funding that will provide consumers greater access to these services.

NOTES

1. In this chapter, the abbreviation "TM" is used to refer to "technology-mediated," "TMC" for "technology-mediated communication," "IM" for "Internet-mediated," and "IMC" for "Internet-mediated communication."
2. SAHAR is the anglicized transliteration of the Hebrew acronym for "Support and Listening on the Net."

REFERENCES

Abell, M. L., & Galinsky, M. J. (2002). Introducing students to computer-based group work practice. *Journal of Social Work Education, 38*(1), 39–54.

American Psychological Association. (1997). *APA statement on services by telephone, teleconferencing and Internet: A statement by the Ethics Committee of the American Psychological Association.* Retrieved October 15, 2001, from: *http://www. apap.org/ethics/stmn01.html.*

Barak, A. (2001, November). *SAHAR: An Internet-based emotional support service for suicidal people.* Paper presented at the meeting on Psychology and the Internet: A European perspective, Farnborough, UK.

Barak, A., & Wander-Schwartz, M. (1999). *Empirical evaluation of a brief group therapy conducted in an Internet chat room.* Retrieved July 22, 2002, from: *http://www.brandeis.edu/pubs/jove/HTML/v5/cherapy3.htm.*

Blundo, R. G., Mele, C., Hairston, R., & Watson, J. (1999). The Internet and demystifying power differentials: A few women online and the housing authority. *Journal of Community Practice, 6*(2), 11–26.

Boberg, E. W., Gustafson, D. H., Hawkins, R. P., Chan, C., Bricker, E., Pingree, S., et al. (1995). Development, acceptance, and use patterns of a computer-based education and social support system for people living with AIDS/HIV infection. *Computers in Human Behavior, 11*, 289–311.

Brennan, P. F. (1998). Computer network home care demonstration: A randomized trial in persons living with AIDS. *Computers in Biology and Medicine, 28*, 489–508.

Brennan, P. F., & Fink, S. V. (1997). Health promotion, social support, and computer networks. In R. L. Street, W. R. Gold, & T. Manning (Eds.), *Health promotion and interactive technology: Theoretical applications and future directions* (pp. 157–169). Mahwah, NJ: Erlbaum.

Brennan, P. F., Moore, S. M., & Smyth, K. A. (1992). Alzheimer's disease caregivers' uses of a computer network. *Western Journal of Nursing Research, 14*(5), 662–673.

Brennan, P. F., & Ripich, S. (1994). Use of home-care computer network by persons with AIDS. *International Journal of Technology Assessment in Health Care, 10*(2), 258–272.

Brown, R., Pain, K., Berwald, C., Hirschi, P., Delehanty, R., & Miller, H. (1999). Distance education and caregiver support groups: Comparison of traditional and telephone groups. *Journal of Head Trauma Rehabilitation, 14*(3), 257–268.

Childress, C. (1998). *The risks and benefits of online therapeutic interventions.* Retrieved November 15, 2001, from: *http://www.ismho.org/issues/9801.htm.*

Clinical Social Work Federation. (2001). *CSWF position paper on Internet text-based therapy.* Retrieved October 12, 2001, from: *http://www.cswf.org/therapy.html.*

Coate, J. (1998). *Cyberspace innkeeping: Building online communities.* Retrieved July 8, 2002, from: *http://www.cervisa.com/innkeeping.html.*

Colon, Y. (1997). *Chattering through the fingertips: Doing group therapy online.* Retrieved July 8, 1997, from: *http://www.echonyc.com/~women/Issue17/public-colon.html.*

Comer, E., Meier, A., & Galinsky, M. J. (1999, October 21). *Studying innovations in group work practice: Applications of the Intervention Research Paradigm.* Paper presented at the American Association for the Advancement of Social Work with Groups, Denver, CO.

Comer, E., Meier, A., & Galinsky, M. J. (2002, February). *Teaching social workers how to develop and evaluate innovative group interventions: A training module for social work educators.* Paper presented at the Council on Social Work Education, 2002 Annual Program Meeting, Nashville, TN.

Comer, E., Meier, A., & Galinsky, M. J. (in press). Development of innovative group work practice using the Intervention Research Paradigm: Two cases. *Social Work*.

Deaf Spot.net. (2002). *Deaf Spot* [Home page]. Retrieved August 22, 2002, from: *http://www.deafspot.net*.

Evans, R. L., Fox, H. R., Pritzl, D. O., & Halar, E. M. (1984). Group treatment of physically disabled adults by telephone. *Social Work in Health Care*, 9(3), 77–84.

Evans, R. L., & Jaugreguy, B. M. (1982). Group therapy by phone: A cognitive behavioral program for visually impaired elderly. *Social Work in Health Care*, 7(2), 79–89.

Fenichel, M., Suler, J., Barak, A., Zelvin, E., Jones, G., Munro, K., et al. (2002). *Myths and realities of online clinical work: Observations on the phenomena of online behavior, experience and therapeutic relationships. A 3rd Year Report from ISMHO's Clinical Case Study Group*. Retrieved August 23, 2002, from: *http://www.rider.edu/users/suler/psycber/therapy.html*.

Finfgeld, D. L. (2000). Therapeutic groups online: The good, the bad and the unknown. *Issues in Mental Health Nursing*, 21, 241–255.

Fox, S., Rainie, L., Horrigan, J., Lenhart, A., Spooner, T., Lewis, O., & Carter, C. (2001). *Time online: Why some people use the Internet more than before and why some use it less*. Pew Internet and American Life Project. Retrieved November 1, 2001, from: *http://www.pewinternet.org/reports/toc.asp?Report=37*.

Galinsky, M., Rounds, K., Montague, A., & Butowsky, E. (1993). *Leading a telephone support group for persons with HIV Disease: A training manual for group leaders*. Chapel Hill: University of North Carolina, School of Social Work.

Galinsky, M. J., Schopler, J. H., & Abell, M. D. (1997). Connecting members through telephone and computer groups. *Health and Social Work*, 22(3), 181–188.

Gellman, R. (1999). The myth of patient confidentiality. *IMP Magazine*. Retrieved November 15, 2001, from: *http://www.cisp.org/imp/november_99/11_99gellman-insight.htm*.

Goodman, C. (1990). Evaluation of a model self-help telephone program: Impact on natural networks. *Social Work*, 35(6), 556–652.

Goodman, C., & Pynoos, J. (1988). Telephone networks connect caregiving families of Alzheimers's victims. *Gerontologist*, 28, 602–605.

Grinfeld, M. J. (1998). *Can telepsychiatry pay its own way?* Retrieved August 15, 2002, from: http://www.psychiatrictimes.com/p980851.html.

Grohol, J. M. (1999). *Best practices in e-therapy: Definition and scope of e-therapy*. Retrieved May 10, 2001, from: *http://psychcentral.com/best/best3.htm*.

Grohol, J. M. (2000, April 8). *Best practices in e-therapy: Confidentiality and privacy*. Retrieved November 9, 2000, from the International Society for Mental Health Online website: *http://www.ismho.org/issues/pp01.htm*.

Grumet, G. W. (1979). Telephone therapy: A review and case report. *American Journal of Orthopsychiatry*, 49, 574–584.

Gustafson, D. H., Hawkins, R., Boberg, E., Bricker, E., Pingree, S., & Chan, C. (1994). The use and impact of a computer-based support system for people living with AIDS and HIV infection. In J. G. Ozbolt (Ed.), *Proceedings of the 18th Annual Symposium on Computer Applications in Medical Care* (Vol. 18, pp. 604–608). Philadelphia: Hanley & Belfus.

Gustafson, D. H., Hawkins, R., Pingree, S., McTavish, F., Arora, N. K., Mendenhall, J., et al. (2001). Effect of computer support on younger women with breast cancer. *Journal of General Internal Medicine*, 16, 435–445.

Hampton, K., & Wellman, B. (2001). Long distance community in the network society: Contact and support beyond Netville. *American Behavioral Scientist*, 45(3), 477–496.

Heller, K., Thompson, M. G., Trueba, P. E., Hogg, J. R., & Vlachos-Weber, I. (1991). Peer support telephone dyads for elderly women: Was this the wrong intervention? *American Journal of Community Psychology*, 19(1), 53–74.

Hines, M. H. (1994). Using the telephone in family therapy. *Journal of Marital and Family Therapy*, 20(2), 175–184.

Houstra, T., & Mallon, B. (1999). Bridging the millenium: Technology in social work group treatment of spinal cord injured persons and their families. *SCI Psychosocial Process, 12*(3), 85, 88–91.

Humphreys, K., Winzelberg, A., & Klaw, E. (2000). Psychologists' ethical responsibilities in the Internet-based groups: Issues, strategies, and a call for dialogue. *Professional Psychology: Research and Practice, 31*(5), 493–496.

Jakobsen, K. R. (2002). Space-age medicine, stone-age government: How Medicare reimbursement of telemedicine services is depriving the elderly of quality medical treatment. *Specialty Law Digest: Health Care Law, 274,* 9–37.

Kane, B., & Sands, D. Z. (1998). *American Medical Informatics Association White Paper: Guidelines for the clinical use of electronic mail with patients.* Retrieved August 30, 2002, from: *http://www.amia.org/pubs/other/email_guidelines.html.*

Kaslyn, M. (1999). Telephone group work: Challenges for practice. *Social Work with Groups, 22*(1), 63–77.

Kiesler, S., & Sproull, L. (1986). Response effects in the electronic survey. *Public Opinion Quarterly, 50,* 402–413.

King, S., & Moreggi, D. (1998). Internet therapy and self-help groups: The pros and cons. In J. Gackenbach (Ed.), *Psychology and the Internet: Intrapersonal, interpersonal and transpersonal implications* (pp. 77–106). New York: Academic Press.

Kurtz, L. F. (1997). *Self-help and support groups: A handbook for practitioners.* Thousand Oaks, CA: Sage.

Lorig, K. R., Laurent, D. D., Deyo, R. A., Marnell, M. E., Minor, M. A., & Ritter, P. L. (2002). Can a back pain e-mail discussion group improve health status and lower health care costs? A randomized study. *Archives of Internal Medicine, 162*(7), 792–796.

Mark, J., Cornebise, J., & Wahl, E. (1997, April). *Community technology centers: Impact on individual participants and their communities.* Retrieved February 11, 2003, from: *http://www.ctcnet.org/eval.html.*

Marson, S. M. (1997). A selective history of Internet technology and social work. *Computers in Human Services, 14*(2), 35–49.

McCarty, D., & Clancy, C. (2002). Telehealth: Implications for social work practice. *Social Work, 47*(2), 153–161.

Meier, A. (1993). Addendum B: Focus on AIDS caregivers. In M. Galinsky & K. Rounds (Eds.), *Leading a telephone support group for persons with HIV disease: A training manual for group leaders* (pp. 1–56). Chapel Hill: University of North Carolina, School of Social Work.

Meier, A. (1997). Inventing new models of social support groups: A feasibility study of an online stress management support group for social workers. *Social Work with Groups, 20*(4), 35–53.

Meier, A. (1999). *A multi-method evaluation of a computer-mediated, stress management support group for social workers: Feasibility, process, and effectiveness.* Unpublished doctoral dissertation, University of North Carolina, Chapel Hill.

Meier, A. (2000). Offering social support via the Internet: A case study of an online support group for social workers. *Journal of Technology in Human Services, 17*(2/3), 237–266.

Meier, A. (2003). *Colon Cancer Caregivers' Online Support Group Project: Research and intervention feasibility and outcomes* (Final report). Chapel Hill: University of North Carolina, Lineberger Comprehensive Cancer Center.

Meier, A. (in press). In-person counseling and Internet self-help groups: Synthesizing new forms of social work practice. In P. Ephross & G. Greif (Eds.), *Group work with populations at risk.* New York: Oxford University Press.

Meier, A., & Campbell, M. K. (2002, August 11). *Internet-mediated "chat" focus groups: Feasibility and ethical issues for human services researchers.* Paper presented at the Technology Conference, Charleston, SC.

Meier, A., & Comer, E. (in press). Evidence-based group work practice. In P. Ephross & G. Greif (Eds.), *Group work with populations at risk.* New York: Oxford University Press.

Meier, A., Galinsky, M., & Rounds, K. (1995). Telephone support groups for caregivers of persons with AIDS. *Social Work with Groups, 18*(1), 99–108.

Menon, G. M. (2000). The 79-cent campaign: The use of on-line mailing lists for electronic advocacy. *Journal of Community Practice, 8*(3), 73–61.

MSN.com. (2002). *All about Hotmail: Frequently asked questions.* Retrieved August 29, 2002, from: *http://lc1.law13.hotmail.passport.com/cgi-bin/dasp/dasp/ua_info.asp?_lang=EN&pg=faq&id=2&fs=1&cb=_lang%3dEN&ct=1030642968#q10.*

Munro, K. (2002). *Conflict in cyberspace: How to resolve conflict online.* Retrieved August 23, 2002, from: *http://www.rider.edu/users/suler/psycyber/conflict.html.*

Nartz, M., & Schoech, D. (2000). Use of the Internet for community practice: A Delphi study. *Journal of Community Practice, 8*(1), 37–59.

National Association of Social Workers. (1999). *NASW code of ethics.* Retrieved July 19, 1999, from: *http://www.socialworkers.org/pubs/code/code.asp.*

National Board of Certified Counselors. (2002). *The practice of online counseling.* Retrieved September 25, 2002, from: *http://www.nbcc.org/ethics/webethics.htm.*

New Mexico Health Policy Commission. (2003). *The HIPAA awareness and preparedness program: What you need to do and how to do it.* Retrieved May 25, 2003, from: *http://hpc.state.nm.us/hipaaap/deskreference.pdf.*

Nua Internet Surveys. (2002). *How many online: US and Canada.* Retrieved November 1, 2002, from: *http://www.nua.com/surveys/how_many_online/n_america.html.*

Oxley, E. L. (1996). *Memo: Social work by Internet.* Unpublished manuscript.

Pinsoneault, T. B. (1996). Equivalency of computer-assisted and paper-and-pencil administered versions of the Minnesota Multiphasic Personality Inventory-2. *Computers in Human Behavior, 12*(2), 291–300.

Potts, S., & Verbiest, S. (1993). Appendix A: Focus on women and HIV disease. In M. Galinsky & K. Rounds (Eds.), *Leading a telephone support group for persons with HIV disease: A training manual for group leaders* (pp. 2–18). Chapel Hill: University of North Carolina, School of Social Work.

Privacy.net. (2003). *Privacy.net* [Home page]. Consumer.net. Retrieved May 22, 2003, from: *http://privacy.net/.*

Reamer, F. G. (1986). The use of modern technology in social work: Ethical dilemmas. *Social Work, 31*(6), 469–472.

Rheingold, H. (2002). *Smart mobs: The next social revolution.* Cambridge, MA: Perseus.

Roffman, R. A., Beadnell, B., Ryan, R. J., & Downey, L. (1995). Telephone group counseling in reducing AIDS risk in gay and bisexual males. *Journal of Gay and Lesbian Social Services, 2*(3/4), 145–157.

Roffman, R. A., Picciano, J. F., Ryan, R., Beadnell, B., Fisher, D., Lowney, L., & Kalishman, S. C. (1997). HIV-prevention group counseling delivered by telephone: An efficacy trial with gay and bisexual men. *AIDS and Behavior, 1*(2), 137–154.

Rosenfeld, M. (1997). *Counseling by telephone.* Thousand Oaks, CA: Sage.

Rothman, J., & Thomas, E. J. (1994). *Intervention research: Design and development for human service.* New York: Haworth Press.

Rounds, K. A., Galinsky, M. J., & Despard, M. R. (1995). Evaluation of telephone support groups for persons with HIV disease. *Research on Social Work Practice, 5*(4), 442–459.

Rounds, K. A., Galinsky, M. J., & Stevens, L. S. (1991). Linking people with AIDS in rural communities: The telephone group. *Social Work, 36*(1), 13–18.

Sarri, R. C., & Galinsky, M. J. (1985). A conceptual framework for group development. In M. Sundel, P. Glasser, R. Sarri, & R. Vinter (Eds.), *Individual change through small groups* (2nd ed., pp. 70–86). New York: Free Press.

ScanSoft.ComHome page. (2002). *ScanSoft: Productivity without boundaries.* Retrieved August 22, 2002, from: *http://www.scansoft.com/.*

Schopler, J. H., Abell, M. D., & Galinsky, M. J. (1998). Technology-based groups: A review and conceptual framework for practice. *Social Work, 43*(3), 254–267.

Schopler, J. H., Galinsky, M. J., & Abell, M. D. (1997). Creating community through telephone and computer groups: Theoretical and practice perspectives. *Social Work with Groups, 20*(4), 19–34.

Sensus Accessibility Consultants. (2003). *Sensus Internet browser.* Retrieved October 4, 2003, from: *http://www.sensus.dk/sib1ouk/htm.*

Smaglik, P., Hawkins, R. P., Pingree, S., Gustafson, D. H., Boberg, E., & Bricker, E. (1998). The quality of interactive computer use among HIV-infected individuals. *Journal of Health Communication, 3,* 53–68.

Smokowski, P. R., Galinsky, M. J., & Harlow, K. (2001). Using technologies in group work: Part 2: Technology-based groups. *Groupwork, 13*(1), 91–115.

Springer, A. K., & Stahmann, R. F. (1998). Parent perception of the value of telephone family therapy when adolescents are in residential treatment. *American Journal of Family Therapy, 26,* 169–176.

Stein, L., Rothman, B., & Nakanishi, M. (1993). The telephone group: Accessing group service to the homebound. *Social Work with Groups, 16*(1/2), 203–215.

Stewart, M. J., Hart, G., Mann, K., Jackson, S., Langille, L., & Reidy, M. (2001). Telephone support group intervention for persons with hemophilia and HIV/AIDS and family caregivers. *International Journal of Nursing Studies, 38*(2), 209–225.

Suler, J. (2001a). *Assessing a person's suitability for online psychotherapy.* Retrieved August 23, 2002, from: *http://truecenterpoint.com/ce/essentials1.html.*

Suler, J. (2001b). Assessing a person's suitability for online therapy: The ISMHO Clinical Case Study Group. *Cyberpsychology and Behavior, 4*(6), 675–679.

Sundel, M., & Glasser, P. (1985). Individual change through small groups [Preface]. In M. Sundel, P. Glasser, R. Sarri, & R. Vinter (Eds.), *Individual change through small groups* (2nd ed., pp. i–xv). New York: Free Press.

Sundel, M., Radin, N., & Churchill, S. R. (1985). Diagnosis in group work. In M. Sundel & P. Glasser & R. Sarri & R. Vinter (Eds.), *Individual change through small groups* (2nd ed., pp. 70–86). New York: Free Press.

Systran Information and Translation Technologies. (2003). *Systran Standard 4.0.* Retrieved April 23, 2003, from: *http://www.systransoft.com/Products/Standard.html.*

Telebridge. (2002). *Telebridge teleconferencing: Answers to frequently asked questions.* Retrieved April 15, 2002, from: *http://www.telebridge.com/faq.html.*

Toseland, R. W., & Rivas, R. F. (2001). *An introduction to group work practice* (4th ed.). Boston: Allyn & Bacon.

Tropp, D. (1987). Teleconferencing: Supportive group work by telephone. *Australian Social Work, 40*(4), 31–34.

Vinter, R. (1985). Essential components of social group work practice. In M. Sundel, P. Glasser, R. Sarri, & R. Vinter (Eds.), *Individual change through small groups* (2nd ed., pp. 11–34). New York: Free Press.

Walther, J. B. (1993). Impression development in computer-mediated interaction. *Western Journal of Communication, 57,* 381-398.

Weiner, L. S. (1998). Telephone support groups for HIV positive mothers whose children have died of AIDS. *Social Work, 43*(3), 279–285.

Weiner, L. S., Spencer, E. D., Davidson, R., & Fair, C. (1993). National telephone support groups: A new avenue toward psychosocial support for HIV-infected children and their families. *Social Work with Groups, 16*(3), 55–71.

White, M., & Dorman, S. M. (2001). Receiving social support online: Implications for health education. *Health Education Research, 16*(6), 693–707.

Wilson, D. S. (2000). Group therapy by telephone. In J. K. Aronson (Ed.), *Use of the telephone in psychotherapy* (pp. 265–276). Northvale, NJ: Aronson.

Winzelberg, A. (1997). The analysis of an electronic support group for individuals with eating disorders. *Computers in Human Behavior, 13*(3), 393–407.

Winzelberg, A. J., Classen, C., Alpers, G. W., Roberts, H., Koopman, C., Adams, R. E., et al. (2003). Evaluation of an Internet support group for women with primary breast cancer. *Cancer, 97*(5), 1164–1173.

Winzelberg, A. J., Taylor, C. B., Sharpe, T., Eldredge, K. L., Dev, P., & Constantinou, P. S. (1998). Effectiveness of an Internet-based program for reducing risk factors for eating disorders. *International Journal of Eating Disorders, 24*(4), 339–349.

Zabinski, M. F., Pung, M. A., Wilfley, D. E., Epstein, D. L., Winzelberg, A., Celio, A., & Taylor, C. B. (2001). Reducing risk factors for eating disorders: Targeting at-risk women with a computerized psychoeducational program. *International Journal of Eating Disorders, 29*(4), 401–408.

Zabinski, M. F., Wilfley, D. E., Pung, M. A., Winzelberg, A., Eldredge, K. L., & Taylor, C. B. (2001). An interactive, Internet-based intervention for women at risk for eating disorders: A pilot study. *International Journal of Eating Disorders, 29*(4), 129–137.

Author Index

Subject Index

517